S0-AAD-665

LYME DISEASE AND
RELATED DISORDERS

ANNALS OF THE NEW YORK ACADEMY OF SCIENCES
Volume 539

LYME DISEASE AND RELATED DISORDERS

Edited by Jorge L. Benach and Edward M. Bosler

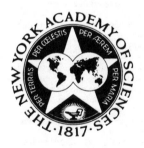

The New York Academy of Sciences
New York, New York
1988

Copyright © 1988 by The New York Academy of Sciences. All rights reserved. Under the provisions of the United States Copyright Act of 1976, individual readers of the Annals are permitted to make fair use of the material in them for teaching or research. Permission is granted to quote from the Annals provided that the customary acknowledgment is made of the source. Material in the Annals may be republished only by permission of The Academy. Address inquiries to the Executive Editor at The New York Academy of Sciences.

Copying fees: For each copy of an article made beyond the free copying permitted under Section 107 or 108 of the 1986 Copyright Act, a fee should be paid through the Copyright Clearance Center, Inc., 21 Congress Street, Salem, MA 01970. For articles more than 3 pages the copying fee is $1.75.

Cover (soft cover only): Borrelia burgdorferi *adhered to human endothelial cells. Photograph was taken with an AMRAY scanning electron microscope at a magnification of 10,000× by Andrew Szczepanski of the Department of Pathology, State University of New York at Stony Brook.*

Library of Congress Cataloging in Publication Data

Lyme disease and related disorders.

(Annals of the New York Academy of Sciences, ISSN 0077-8923; v. 539)
Result of the International Conference on Lyme Disease and Related Disorders, held by the New York Academy of Sciences and the State of New York Dept. of Health on Sept. 14–16, 1987 in New York, N.Y.
Includes bibliographies and index.
1. Lyme disease—Congresses. I. Benach, Jorge Luis, 1946–   . II. Bosler, Edward M. III. International Conference on Lyme Disease and Related Disorders (1987: New York, N.Y.) IV. New York Academy of Sciences. V. New York (State). Dept. of Health. VI. Series.
[DNLM: 1. Borrelia—congresses. 2. Lyme Disease—congresses. W1 AN626YL v.539 / WE 344 L9855 1987]
Q11.N5   vol. 539   500 s   88-25460
[RC155.5]   [616.9′2]
ISBN 0-89766-474-4
ISBN 0-89766-475-2 (pbk.)

SP
Printed in the United States of America
ISBN 0-89766-474-4 (cloth)
ISBN 0-89766-475-2 (paper)
ISSN 0077-8923

ANNALS OF THE NEW YORK ACADEMY OF SCIENCES

Volume 539
August 26, 1988

LYME DISEASE AND RELATED DISORDERS[a]

Editors and Conference Organizers
JORGE L. BENACH AND EDWARD M. BOSLER

CONTENTS

[a]This volume is the result of the International Conference on Lyme Disease and Related Disorders, which was held by the New York Academy of Sciences and the State of New York Department of Health on September 14–16, 1987, in New York, NY.

Part V. Treatment

Poster Session I: Basic Research Poster Papers

Poster Session II: Veterinary, Clinical, and Epidemiological Poster Papers

Financial Support

- THIS CONFERENCE WAS WHOLLY SUPPORTED BY THE STATE OF
  NEW YORK DEPARTMENT OF HEALTH.

The New York Academy of Sciences believes it has a responsibility to provide an open
forum for discussion of scientific questions. The positions taken by the participants in the
reported conferences are their own and not necessarily those of the Academy. The
Academy has no intent to influence legislation by providing such forums.

Preface

JORGE L. BENACH

State of New York Department of Health
Health Sciences Center
State University of New York
Stony Brook, New York 11794

This volume of the *Annals* contains reports by scientists from 17 countries in North America, Europe, and Asia. The exceptional scientific interest in a single disease demonstrated in this volume and in the conference of which it is the result reflects the increasing public health importance of Lyme disease.

Lyme disease has become a serious health threat in many areas of the world. Indeed, the increasing incidence of Lyme disease in New York State was the primary reason why the State of New York Department of Health conceived and entirely funded this conference for the purpose of disseminating the latest scientific information to health-care providers, researchers, and the public.

New clinical manifestations of this spirochetosis continue to be reported, creating additional problems in clinical diagnosis and in therapy. Because Lyme disease has protean manifestations and a tendency to mimic other common diseases, its clinical diagnosis is no simple task. We have also learned from the conference that laboratory diagnosis of Lyme disease is inconclusive in the early disease stages and that numerous questions about the significance of antibodies in the later or chronic stages remain to be resolved. I expect all will agree that Lyme disease is not a simple entity to diagnose either at the laboratory or clinical levels. Eventually, if it has not happened already, we will know most of the common clinical manifestations of Lyme disease and, with improved diagnostic tools, learn to recognize atypical presentations. We who are engaged in investigations on Lyme disease meet these research challenges with enthusiasm.

However, for health care practitioners to whom Lyme disease is just one more disease to be considered, these difficulties can lead to a delayed and possibly wrong diagnosis. Thus, in participating in a conference such as this, Lyme disease investigators have endeavored to simplify the information-seeking process by including the latest research results in one volume. The proceedings of this conference, along with those of the previous New Haven and Vienna meetings,[a] can serve as the basis for the initial and continuing education of the health-care practitioner regarding Lyme disease.

As Lyme disease gains in significance, investigators will be called upon with increasing frequency to provide scientific information to health-care professionals. The simplest and most efficient manner for dissemination of scientific medical information is through centralized literature searches. Unfortunately, searches on the topic of "Lyme disease" inevitably will overlook many important publications in which a different nomenclature has been used. In this conference alone, there were 11 names used for what is now obviously a single global disease. The nomenclature issue is not a real problem for those of us working on Lyme disease; we all know the history as well as

---

[a]Published in the *Yale Journal of Biology and Medicine* (**57**: 1–268, 1984) and the *Zentralblatt für Bakteriologie, Mikrobiologie und Hygiene, Series A* (**263**: 1–501, 1986), respectively.

the names used by investigators around the world. Bear in mind, however, that a physician confronted with a case of Lyme disease for the first time may not be aware of all of the names used for the same clinical entity. His sole concern is to obtain all the information relevant to a patient's needs. The health-care professional should not be impeded by a nomenclature problem, and we need to address this issue in a future conference. A serious attempt at resolving the nomenclature issue will demonstrate our resolve to eliminate unnecessary parochialism from our field of investigation.

In preparing this introduction, I had hoped to summarize the conference. This became an obvious difficulty after the first day and an absolute impossibility by the end of the conference. There were some 90 presentations ranging from basic genetic research to epidemiological studies from diverse areas of the world. Clearly, a summary of this volume might be just a shade smaller than the volume itself. Each presentation is thus left to speak for itself without any editorializing.

It is obvious that there has been an explosive growth of knowledge about this disease and its agent in the last 5 years. It would not be presumptuous to speculate that the number of presentations, as well as investigators, may double at a future conference.

We know today that Lyme disease is a chronic borreliosis with protean manifestations and a world-wide distribution. However, we still do not know how *Borrelia* can cause a chronic disease and interact with and injure nearly all organ systems, or why the disease is globally ubiquitous. We need to welcome additional investigators to these enticing challenges.

In closing, as Chairman of the Conference on Lyme Disease and Related Disorders, I would like to thank first and foremost the Commissioner of Health of the State of New York, Dr. David Axelrod, who understood the need for this conference and gave it his wholehearted support. The financial contributions of the Foundation for Microbiology and of Mr. Ron Steven are gratefully acknowledged.

Although putting together this conference was a pleasurable task involving colleagues, Academy and State Health Department professionals, and many friends and interested persons, there were times when we needed strong organizational skills. These were generously provided by Ms. April Golden of our staff. Dr. Dennis J. White, Director of the Arthropod-Borne Disease Unit of the New York State Department of Health, knows that without him this conference would not have occurred. It is important that he knows we know it too. Finally, I would like to thank the conference participants for bringing their impressive knowledge and professionalism.

Introduction

Borrelia burgdorferi Infection:
A Neurologist's Perspective

LOUIS REIK

Department of Neurology
University of Connecticut Health Center
Farmington, Connecticut 06032

The clinical investigations reported at this conference and elsewhere underscore the worldwide importance of *Borrelia burgdorferi* as a nervous system pathogen. We now know that *B. burgdorferi* infection affects the nervous system and its coverings in a high percentage of cases, causing a wide range of acute, chronic, and progressive central and peripheral nervous system abnormalities. We also know that these abnormalities can occur alone, either without any antecedent extraneural symptoms at all or else years after a symptomatic primary infection. The nervous system abnormalities caused by *B. burgdorferi* can thus mimic a variety of other neurologic conditions, and nervous system borreliosis must be a frequent diagnostic consideration for the neurologist in an endemic area.

We know less about the pathology and pathogenesis of these abnormalities. Meningitis probably does result directly from invasion of the cerebral spinal fluid (CSF) by *B. burgdorferi:* the spirochete has been cultured from CSF[1] and antibiotics shorten the course.[2] Similarly, at least some central nervous system (CNS) abnormalities may be caused directly through parenchymal invasion, as *B. burgdorferi* has been demonstrated histologically within brain tissue.[3] But clinical evidence suggests that some other CNS abnormalities are due to vasculopathy. The evidence includes the diffuse and multifocal pattern of neurologic abnormalities in some patients,[4] the occurrence of apparent transient ischemic attacks in some patients with encephalopathy,[5] the relatively high incidence of hemiparesis in some series,[6] computerized tomographic (CT) abnormalities in some cases suggesting cerebral infarction,[7,8] and, in one case, cerebral angiographic changes consistent with vasculitis.[7] Although obliterative endarteritis has been demonstrated histologically in synovium and myocardium, the presence of such changes in CNS vessels can only be inferred from the clinical evidence at present. The limited amount of pathologic material available has not shown clear-cut vasculitis. Moreover, other mechanisms may be operating within the CNS as well. The detection of abnormalities compatible with demyelination in CT and magnetic resonance (MR) images from patients with cerebral symptoms,[9,10] and the demonstration of cross-reaction of anti-*B. burgdorferi* antibodies with neuronal antigens,[11] both suggest that indirect immunopathological mechanisms may be involved.

B. burgdorferi infection probably damages the peripheral nervous system through more than one mechanism also. While spinal radiculitis and cranial neuritis could result from direct extension of inflammation from the meninges, the clinical patterns of mononeuritis simplex and multiplex and asymmetrical radiculoplexitis suggest a vasculitic cause. Indeed, sensory nerve biopsies from patients with meningopolyneuritis,[12] distal axonopathy of late Lyme disease,[13] and the neuropathy of acrodermatitis chronica atrophicans[14] have all shown axonal degeneration, loss of large myelinated fibers, and epineurial perivasculitis with occasional vessel wall infiltration and luminal thrombosis. The electrophysiologic findings in many cases are also compatible with a vasculitic cause.[15] Yet in other cases the electrophysiologic changes indicate demyelination,[15,16] and servere weakness in Lyme disease can resolve over weeks,[4,15] a time course more consistent with recovery from demyelination and conduction block than from Wallerian degeneration. Therefore, both segmental demyelination and axonal lesions apparently do occur in Lyme disease. Whether both are caused by the same vasculopathy or the demyelination is caused by other indirect immunopathological mechanisms is not clear.

Other questions about *Borrelia burgdorferi* of importance to the neurologist also remain. We know neither how soon after inoculation the spirochete reaches the human nervous system nor how often it does so. We also do not know why neurologic symptoms and signs of inflammation begin only later on in the course, and then only in certain individuals. It is now clear that *B. burgdorferi* can persist within the nervous system for years, causing progressive illness, and increasing evidence suggests also that the spirochete can remain latent there for years before producing clinical symptoms. The long-term risk for late neurologic disease, its possible forms, the events that cause the end of latency and the beginning of symptoms, and the best treatment regimens both to prevent and to eradicate late nervous system disease all remain to be defined.

Neither is it clear how best to diagnose nervous system borreliosis, particularly in late cases. Is a positive serologic test sufficient when serum antibodies can persist in significant titers for years after apparently successful treatment? The reports by Dr. Ackermann[17] and Dr. Stiernstedt[18] and their colleagues suggest that measurement of antiborrelial antibodies in the CSF may provide one clue. But what of the patient with CNS abnormalities, a positive serologic test, and a normal CSF? Is a reactive CSF the best measure of disease activity and predictor of antibiotic response, as in nervous system syphilis?[19]

Answers to these questions will depend ultimately on continued study of naturally occurring human infections and laboratory infections in experimental animals. Meanwhile the neurologist's best weapons against this disease are a high index of suspicion and the frequent use of serologic tests. Every neurologic patient with a positive serologic test should undergo lumbar puncture and determination of CSF antibody titer. Antibiotics should be prescribed if pleocytosis, elevated protein, or locally synthesized antiborrelial antibodies are present. Moreover, it seems prudent at present to prescribe the same antibiotic treatment for those patients with CNS abnormalities, a positive serum antibody test, and a normal CSF but no explanation for their symptoms other than nervous system borreliosis, especially if the deficits are progressive.

REFERENCES

1. STEERE, A. C., R. L. GRODZICKI, A. N. KORNBLATT, J. E. CRAFT, A. G. BARBOUR, W. BURGDORFER, G. P. SCHMID, E. JOHNSON & S. E. MALAWISTA. 1983. N. Engl. J. Med. **308:** 733–740.
2. STEERE, A. C., A. R. PACHNER & S. E. MALAWISTA. 1983. Ann. Intern. Med. **99:** 767–772.
3. MACDONALD, A. B. & J. M. MIRANDA. 1987. Hum. Pathol. **18:** 759–761.
4. REIK, L., A. C. STEERE, N. H. BARTENHAGEN, R. E. SHOPE & S. E. MALAWISTA. 1979. Medicine **58:** 281–294.
5. KOHLER, J., J. KASPER, U. KERN, U. THODEN & B. REHSE-KUPPER. 1986. Lancet **2:** 35.
6. STIERNSTEDT, G. 1985. Scand. J. Infect. Dis. Suppl. **45:** 1–70.
7. MIDGARD, R. & H. HAKON. 1987. Arch. Neurol. **44:** 781–783.

8. WEDER, B., P. WIEDERSHEIM, L. MATTER, A. STECK & F. OTTO. 1987. J. Neurol. **234:** 40–43.
9. REIK, L., L. SMITH, A. KHAN & W. NELSON. 1985. Neurology **32:** 1302–1305.
10. PACHNER, A. R. & A. C. STEERE. 1986. Neurology **36** (Suppl. 1): 286.
11. SIGAL, L. H. & A. H. TATUM. 1988. This volume.
12. VALLAT, J. M., J. HUGON, M. LUBEAU, M. J. LEBOUTET, M. DUMAS & R. DESPROGES-GOTTERON. 1987. Neurology **37:** 749–753.
13. HALPERIN, J. J., H. L. PASS, A. K. ANAND, B. J. LUFT, D. J. VOLKMAN & R. J. DATTWYLER. 1988. This volume.
14. KRISTOFERITSCH, W. 1988. This volume.
15. PACHNER, A. R. & A. C. STEERE. 1985. Neurology **35:** 47–53.
16. STERMAN, A. B., S. NELSON & P. BARCLAY. 1982. Neurology **32:** 1302–1305.
17. ACKERMANN, R., B. REHSE-KUEPPER, E. GOLLMER & R. SCHMIDT. 1988. This volume.
18. STIERNSTEDT, G., M. KARLSSON, B. SKOLDENBERG, B. SVENUNGSSON & R. GUSTAFSSON. 1988. This volume.
19. SIMON, R. P. 1985. Arch. Neurol. **42:** 606–613.

Early and Late Cutaneous Manifestations in *Ixodes*-borne Borreliosis (Erythema Migrans Borreliosis, Lyme Borreliosis)[a]

EVA ÅSBRINK AND ANDERS HOVMARK

Department of Dermatology
Karolinska Institute at Södersjukhuset
Stockholm, Sweden

COURSE AND CLASSIFICATION

The parallels between syphilis and *Ixodes*-borne borreliosis (erythema migrans borreliosis, Lyme borreliosis) are striking. Sir William Osler's description of syphilis as the great imitator of other diseases[1] is also true for the current borreliosis. Dermatologic as well as neurologic manifestations may present in a multiplicity of fashions. Both spirochetoses are infections with a potentially long-lasting course. Isolation of spirochetes from the skin of a patient with acrodermatitis chronica atrophicans with a disease duration of greater than 10 years shows the possibility of long-term survival of borreliae in humans.[2]

There are both historical and traditional reasons for the somewhat confusing nomenclature and the multiplicity of terms that are applied to this borreliosis and its different manifestations. In contrast to syphilis, where much of the course of the disease and its different stages (characterized by Philippe Ricord by 1838) was known long before the discovery of *Treponema pallidum* in 1905, the course of *Ixodes*-borne borreliosis was only fully realized and understood when the infecting agent, *Borrelia burgdorferi,* was revealed. In Europe different manifestations such as erythema migrans (EM), lymphadenosis benigna cutis (LABC), acrodermatitis chronica atrophicans (ACA), and the lymphocytic meningoradiculitis later named Bannwarth's syndrome have been recognized since the first decades of this century. These various clinical syndromes, which were at least partly defined long before the causative borreliae were discovered, had previously been described as separate entities. The arthritis was first recognized in the 1970s in the United States by Allen Steere as a new form of inflammatory arthritis, initially named Lyme arthritis, and the credit for delineating Lyme disease belongs to him.[3–5]

The differences in the current clinical descriptions of *Ixodes*-borne borreliosis may also appear somewhat confusing. Owing to the wide clinical spectrum, clinicians from many specialties encounter these patients. Different selections of patients may thus result in some dissimilarities in the clinical descriptions. Universal heterogeneity among the spirochetes involved may also explain some of the dissimilarities, however.

Syphilis is divided into early ("infectious") and late infection, the former comprising the primary and secondary stages. Syphilis of more than 2 years' duration, including latent syphilis of more than 2 years' duration, is classified as late infection.[6] In *Ixodes*-borne borreliosis somewhat varying classifications have hitherto been used.

---

[a]This work was supported by grants from the Edward Welander Foundation and from the Swedish Medical Research Council (grant no. 7935).

4

As ACA, which is generally accepted as being a late (tertiary) manifestation, may sometimes start less than 1 year after the primary skin manifestation EM,[7] a shorter time interval than 2 years is perhaps more adequate for a designation as late borreliosis. The time relations of early and late borrelial manifestations are not always definite, but clinical observations indicate that probably very few patients will still reveal early cutaneous lesions such as EM or Borrelia lymphocytoma (BL) after the first year of the infection, and that very few will develop late lesions such as ACA before that time.

Both overlapping between different stages and longer or shorter asymptomatic intervals (latent periods) may occur in both syphilis and borreliosis. Any or all of the various stages may develop in the individual patient and the infection may not become manifest until the second or third stage is reached. From the Oslo study of the natural course of untreated syphilis, it was found that 28% of the patients with early syphilis developed recognized late complications.[8] The corresponding figure in *Ixodes*-borne borreliosis may be lower but is still not known.

With the increasing knowledge about the clinical spectrum of this infection and about the course of the illness, efforts must be made to attain a well defined and unitary nomenclature and classification. In view of the many parallels with syphilis in clinical

TABLE 1. Course and Classification of *Ixodes*-borne Borreliosis[a]

EARLY	
Stage 1	*erythema migrans*
Stage 2	*multiple erythema migrans-like lesions*
	Borrelia lymphocytoma
	meningo-polyneuritis
	arthritis (acute/subacute)
	carditis
LATE	
Stage 3	*acrodermatitis chronica atrophicans*
	chronic joint/bone manifestations
	chronic neurologic manifestations

[a]Cutaneous manifestations are indicated by *italics*.

features and course, it would seem reasonable to use a similar classification. The classification used by the present authors is shown in TABLE 1.

EARLY CUTANEOUS MANIFESTATIONS

Erythema Migrans

Afzelius was the first to describe a case of erythema migrans following a tick bite.[9] Some years later Lipschütz[10] described another patient with long-standing erythema migrans and therefore changed the name to erythema chronicum migrans. As this skin lesion resolves spontaneously and sometimes after only a few weeks, the shorter designation, erythema migrans, proposed by Afzelius seems more appropriate.

EM can now be defined as an early erythematous skin lesion caused by *Ixodes*-borne borreliae. EM, like the primary chancer in syphilis, appears at the site of inoculation of spirochetes. The average incubation period is 1 to 3 weeks (range: 3 days to 16 weeks).[11-16]

A history of a tick bite at the site of the skin lesion is a helpful clue in making the correct diagnosis. However, in most studies fewer than half of the patients can recall having had a tick bite.[11–13,15,17]

This may be due partly to the fact that the nymphal ticks, which often transmit infection, are so small that they often escape notice or are not recognized as ticks. The question whether vectors other than *Ixodes* ticks may be important in transmitting these borreliae to humans is still not solved.

The classical EM lesion is an expanding erythema that fades in the center, leaving only the annular border erythematous. In some patients, however, a homogeneous erythema may persist. The size of the ring or the distance the erythema has migrated corresponds in many cases to the duration of the disease. Sometimes, however, the erythema may also remain stationary for a long time. Successful spirochetal cultivations from skin biopsies have proved that atypical variants such as vesicular, scaling, or purpuric-hemorrhagic lesions can occur.[18]

EM may appear almost anywhere on the skin, but is most commonly found on the lower extremity.[14,15,19] In children the face is a common site. The erythema may be so unobtrusive that it is neglected or escapes notice. Sometimes it is only clearly visible after the skin has been warmed up, for example in a hot bath. Localized swelling without erythema may also be encountered at the site of the tick bite and the spirochetal inoculation. Because of their sometimes asymptomatic nature or when located, for example, on the back, EM lesions may not be observed by the patient and go undiagnosed.

The EM lesion will heal spontaneously, often within weeks to months, but it may persist for up to a year.[12,19] Relapsing lesions may occur in untreated[19] or inadequately treated patients[12,20] and secondary and/or tertiary stage manifestations may sometimes follow. In patients who develop secondary stage manifestations, EM may sometimes still be present when these manifestations occur. However, the erythema often seems to be of shorter duration in patients who later develop meningitis[21] than in those who do not develop secondary manifestations.[19] Slight itching, burning, or dysesthesia at the site of the EM and regional lymphadenopathy are frequently but not always present.[12,14,17,19]

EM may occur with or without constitutional symptoms such as headache, fever, arthralgia-myalgia, or malaise.[12,13,15,17–19,22] These symptoms are usually mild and transitory but can be severe and long-lasting, and the changing and intermittent course with symptoms lasting for only hours at a given site is characteristic. Some patients appear mildly encephalopathic and complain of emotional changes, irritability, impairment of memory and concentration, and dizziness. Profound fatigue, sometimes persisting for many months, may occur and be disabling. Lumbar punctures performed on these patients are often normal (ref. 12 and own observations).

Constitutional symptoms may sometimes precede the EM or appear alone, and flu-like symptoms of an intermittent and changing nature appearing in the summer or autumn in persons exposed to an endemic area should give reason to suspect borreliosis. The convalescent phase appears to be longer in patients displaying more pronounced constitutional symptoms before treatment than in those with minor symptoms. Transient eruptions of macular or maculopapular exanthema, urticaria, malar rash, or periorbital edema in addition to the EM lesion may also develop,[12,14,18] but seem to be uncommon.

Diagnosis

Frequently the EM lesion and the medical history are classic enough for a presumptive diagnosis. The histopathologic findings are unspecific unless spirochetes can be demonstrated in the tissue with specific staining methods. Usually a sparse perivascular and sometimes interstitial lymphocytic infiltrate with plasma cells is found in biopsy specimens taken from the periphery of the skin lesion. A skin biopsy may be essential to rule out such differential diagnoses as erythema multiforme, erythematodes, tinea, or granuloma annulare and establish the correct diagnosis.

The present serologic tests with the use of ELISA and immunofluorescence methods have been found in most studies to be positive in only a minority of cases with uncomplicated EM.[11,23-26] Nonspecific laboratory tests do not provide much diagnostic help, but an elevated sedimentation rate, elevated serum IgM levels, circulating immune complexes, and abnormal liver function tests have been described.[12] In our experience such laboratory abnormalities are uncommon in uncomplicated EM.[19]

Multiple Erythema Migrans-like Lesions

The initial EM may be followed by similar but generally smaller and often nonmigrating lesions. More than ten lesions are uncommon, but may occur. Spirochetes have been isolated not only from primary but also from such secondary lesions.[12,18] The multiple secondary lesions are probably due to a hematogenous spread of spirochetes, analogous to the cutaneous eruptions in secondary syphilis. Thus, these secondary lesions ought to be classified as a stage 2 manifestation of borreliosis. In our experience the constitutional symptoms are often more severe and the laboratory abnormalities more frequent in these patients with multiple lesions than in those with a solitary EM. Multiple lesions have been reported in a higher frequency in the United States (25–48%[12,14]) than in Europe (8% or less[27,28]).

No acquisition of immunity seems to occur after EM infection, and thus reinfection may develop during subsequent summers.[19,25,29]

Borrelia Lymphocytoma

Lymphadenosis benigna cutis (LABC), which may appear in a solitary and a multiple form, was initially described as a radiosensible disease of unknown origin characterized by a dense lymphocytic infiltrate in the dermis and/or subcutis.[30] Many of the skin lesions that were previously diagnosed as LABC were probably of borrelial origin, but it is still an open question whether all these lesions are *Borrelia*-induced. Investigations regarding patients with LABC dispersa are still lacking. It is now often possible to distinguish clinically and serologically between *Borrelia*-induced lymphocytic skin infiltrates and infiltrates of other or unknown origin. The term Borrelia lymphocytoma therefore seems appropriate for naming the lymphocytic infiltrates of known borrelial etiology.[31,32]

Borrelia lymphocytoma (BL) can be defined as a localized dense dermal lymphoreticular proliferation caused by *Ixodes*-borne borreliae. Although BL may appear at the site of a tick bite, it sometimes also appears at a distance from the causative tick bite.[32] It may sometimes take as long as 6 to 10 months after the tick bite before a BL develops (FIG. 1, No. 1).[32,33]

BL may occur together with or be preceded by EM[32] and may sometimes also occur together with secondary stage manifestations such as meningitis, chorioiditis or acute arthritis,[32] or with tertiary manifestations such as ACA.[30,34] Clinically there is a tumor-like bluish-red swelling or nodule which, in the majority of cases, is accompanied by regional lymphadenopathy. Predilection sites are the ear lobes in children (FIG. 2) and the nipples-areola mammae in adults. To our knowledge, there is still only one spirochetal isolate from a BL lesion.[33] The duration of an untreated BL is usually many months.

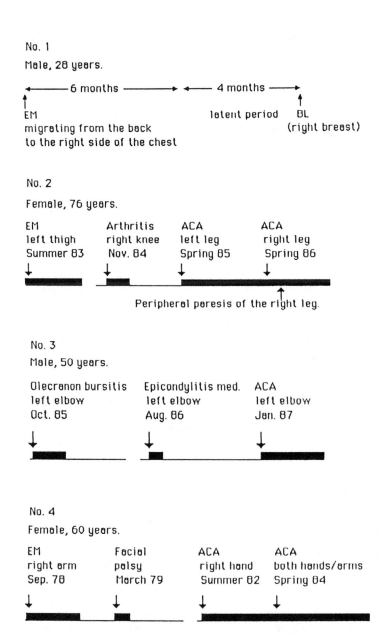

FIGURE 1. Sequence of different clinical events in one patient with Borrelia lymphocytoma (*BL*) and in three patients with acrodermatitis chronica atrophicans (*ACA*); *EM*, erythema migrans.

Diagnosis

The solitary lesions at the predilection sites are often typical enough to permit the diagnosis to be made. Failure to diagnose an infected child who for months has had a bluish-red, swollen ear lobe is usually due to unfamiliarity with this condition. Breast lesions in adults are sometimes initially misdiagnosed as malignancies.[32]

Histopathologically a dense dermal lymphocytic infiltrate with an admixture of plasma cells and occasionally eosinophils is found. The presence of reaction centers in the dermal infiltrate is a helpful diagnostic sign, but not an obligatory finding. Malignant lymphoma may sometimes be difficult to differentiate from BL both clinically and histopathologically.

The majority of patients with BL display elevated serum IgG titers to *Borrelia*.[31,32] Since BL may sometimes develop after an untreated EM and may occur far from the site of the tick bite and occasionally also may develop many months after the causative

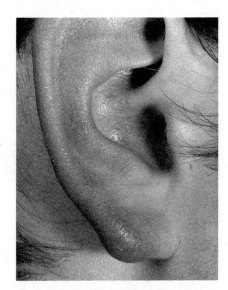

FIGURE 2. Ear lobe with Borrelia lymphocytoma of 6-month duration.

tick bite, and as BL and secondary stage manifestations such as meningitis and acute arthritis may appear simultaneously, we consider it reasonable and logical to classify BL as a secondary rather than a primary stage manifestation (TABLE 1).

LATE CUTANEOUS MANIFESTATIONS

Acrodermatitis Chronica Atrophicans

ACA is a late (tertiary) skin manifestation of *Ixodes*-borne borreliosis and starts with an inflammatory phase that may be followed by an atrophic phase. ACA has mainly been observed in the elderly, but may also occur in young persons. It is predominant in females. The onset is usually gradual and insidious and characterized by the appearance of a bluish-red discoloration and doughy swollen skin, which starts on one extremity, most commonly at an acral site such as the hand, foot, or olecranon area. However, red-violaceous patches on different sites of the extremities may also occur. Sometimes the erythema may be inconspicuous, and swelling of the soft tissue, sometimes resembling lymphedema or angioneurotic edema, may dominate the clinical picture. The erythema and swelling may initially also vary in intensity (wax and wane). ACA primarily involves one or more extremities, but occasionally extensive involvement of the trunk may occur.

A concomitant annular migrating erythema, as in EM, may sometimes appear in the proximity of cutaneous ACA lesions. Solitary or multiple fibrotic nodules near joints, particularly in the olecranon area, may develop in patients with ACA.

ACA does not resolve spontaneously like the early cutaneous lesions. The inflammatory phase may persist for many years (or decades), but gradually it becomes replaced by atrophy of the skin and sometimes also of underlying structures. However, cutaneous atrophy may be absent for a long time and is not an obligatory clinical or histologic sign for a diagnosis of ACA, which seems to be a not uncommon misunderstanding, probably because of the designation of this condition.

It is common for patients with ACA to have, besides the skin lesions, signs and symptoms of the infection in other organs such as the nervous system, the joints, and/or bones. Involuntary loss of weight may also occur.[35] Thirty to forty-five percent of the patients suffer from a polyneuropathy, which is often most pronounced in the limbs with cutaneous involvement.[35,36] It is mainly sensory, but peripheral nerve paralysis may occur (FIG. 1, No. 2). Fairly frequent complaints are paresthesia-hyperesthesia, weakness in the muscles, muscle cramps, and/or sensations of heaviness, mainly of the affected limb. In some patients pain in the limb with cutaneous involvement may dominate the clinical picture. Sometimes it is difficult to differentiate between pain caused by arthralgia and that caused by neuritis or periostitis. A not unusual characteristic feature, which may be used as a diagnostic sign, is pain, arising from impacts against bony prominences, such as the olecranon, malleolae, and knuckles, underlying ACA skin lesions.

In 1952 Gans and Landes reported on mental disturbances in a patient with ACA.[37] Profound fatigue[35] and personality changes may sometimes accompany ACA (own observations). There are also neurophysiological indications that central nervous system involvement may occur. In a recent study, nine out of 26 patients with ACA showed pathological auditory brainstem responses, which in eight of the nine cases were restored to normal or improved after intravenous antibiotic treatment.[38]

There have previously been conflicting data in the literature concerning joint and bone manifestations as part of the disease in patients with ACA. In one study joint and bone involvement underlying the cutaneous lesions were found radiographically in 16 out of 50 patients.[20] Subluxations/luxations of small joints in the hands or feet, arthritis of large joints, and/or periosteal thickening of bones were found. The latter is reminiscent of the so-called dactylitis syphilitica described in late benign syphilis. In an enlarged study of 86 patients with ACA, episodic attacks of joint effusions of a knee preceding or occurring simultaneously with the ACA were found in 17 patients.[39] Eighteen of the 86 patients exhibited subluxations or luxations of small joints, mainly of the toes.[39] Chronic joint and bone involvement underlying the cutaneous lesions was more often seen in patients with long-standing (years to decades) ACA than in those with a short duration of the disease. A swollen and/or painful foot or heel (FIG. 3), causing shoe problems, was a characteristic symptom and was exhibited by about one-third of the 86 patients.[41]

Periarticular manifestations such as bursitis in the knee or olecranon areas, epicondylitis, retro/subcalcaneal bursitis, and Achilles tendinitis on the same extremity as the cutaneous involvement have been found in patients following an untreated EM[39] and/or preceding ACA[20,39] (FIG. 1, No. 3).

The concordance in the site of the early and late cutaneous lesions and the changes in underlying or closely located articular-periarticular tissues or bones suggests that spirochetes may sometimes persist at or close to the initial site of the spirochetal inoculation.

Diagnosis

ACA may be the first indication of *Ixodes*-borne borrelial infection, but a careful medical history will reveal that many patients have histories consistent with preceding primary and/or secondary stage manifestations of borreliosis. A history of EM often on the same extremity on which ACA lesions had developed 6 months to 10 years later was found in 17 of our 95 patients (18%). In some of the patients the ACA had also been preceded by secondary neurologic manifestations (radiculitis, cranial neuritis)[20,35] and/or arthritis[20,39] (FIG. 1, Nos. 2, 4).

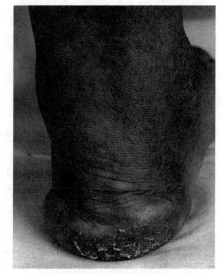

FIGURE 3. A swollen discolorated heel with acrodermatitis chronica atrophicans of more than 3-year duration.

ACA is often clinically overlooked or misinterpreted, and several visits to physicians without the illness being diagnosed is rather the rule than the exception for these patients.[35] Failure to diagnose an infected patient is often due to unfamiliarity with the disease, but sometimes also to an atypical clinical picture. ACA lesions on the legs are often misdiagnosed as circulatory insufficiency, such as venous insufficiency, eczema hypostaticum, disturbed arterial circulation, or they may be attributed to aging or cold injury. Fibrotic nodules may be mistaken for rheumatoid nodules, gouty tophi, or erythema nodosum. Juxtaarticular nodules may also be seen during the late stage of both syphilis and yaws. Joint involvement or pain may be the reason for seeking medical help, and in these cases the cutaneous ACA lesions may be neglected and the association missed.

ACA should not be diagnosed on clinical grounds alone, but verified by histopathologic examination and specific serologic tests. Acral cyanosis and atrophy of other origins have to be differentiated from ACA. The histopathological picture essential for the diagnosis of ACA is telangiectases in combination with a patchy and/or interstitial lymphocytic infiltrate, with plasma cells in the dermis and sometimes also in the subcutis. The epidermis may be thin and is often hyperkeratotic, and a liquefaction degeneration may be observed. Vacuoles, which probably represent lymph spaces, are sometimes found at different levels of the dermis.[7]

Elevated serum IgG titers to *Borrelia* have hitherto been found in all patients with ACA.[23,24,26,40,41] Characteristically the titers are often very high. After treatment the titers usually decrease, but in many patients seropositivity remains for years after treatment. Parallels may be drawn between ACA and late syphilis, where treponemal tests may remain elevated despite antibiotic therapy. The ACA patients with the highest serum titers to *Borrelia* have cross-reactive antibodies to treponemal antigens that are detectable in the FTA-ABS test but are nonreactive in TPHA and TPI tests.[24]

There are no characteristic unspecific laboratory findings, but hyperglobulinemia is frequent and an increased erythrocyte sedimentation rate may also occur.[35]

During the last 4 years 4.9 cases of ACA per 100,000 population were in average diagnosed each year in southern Stockholm. The incidence per 100,000 population for 1 year in the same area was at least 16.0 for EM and 1.7 for BL. There have hitherto been very few reports on patients with ACA and, to our knowledge, no reports on patients with BL in connection with Lyme disease in the United States. It is still an open question whether these dissimilarities in the clinical spectrum can be explained by slight spirochetal differences on either side of the Atlantic Ocean, or at least partly, by different levels of awareness and familiarity with these cutaneous borrelial manifestations.

Sclerotic and Atrophic Skin Lesions

Sclerotic skin lesions may develop in about 10% of patients with ACA[7,35,42] and also in patients with Borrelia lymphocytoma.[32] These lesions may be indistinguishable from localized scleroderma (morphea) and lichen sclerosus et atrophicus (LSA) both clinically and histopathologically. Thus, a *Borrelia* infection may cause sclerotic lesions that cannot be distinguished from localized scleroderma or LSA. *Borrelia*-induced sclerotic lesions may probably also develop in patients without other signs of borreliosis, but it is still controversial how often this happens.[43-45] In our experience, the majority of patients with localized scleroderma (morphea) or LSA do not display elevated serum titers of antibodies to *Borrelia*.[46] However, to evaluate the results of serologic studies in patients with sclerotic skin lesions, the history concerning antibiotic therapy must be known. It may be impossible to distinguish on clinical or histological grounds antibiotic-treated ACA patients with residual sclerotic skin lesions from patients merely with scleroderma. On the other hand, sclerotic lesions in patients with ACA may dominate the clinical picture and a diagnosis of localized scleroderma or lichen sclerosus et atrophicus may be given without the inflammatory ACA lesions being noticed.[7]

Elevated serum titers of antibodies to *Borrelia* have also been reported in solitary patients with atrophoderma,[47] eosinophilic fasciitis,[48] and anetoderma.[43] Atrophoderma and eosinophilic fasciitis are rare conditions that are often regarded as variants of scleroderma. Anetoderma is characterized by a macular atrophy sometimes preceded by erythema, and response of the early inflammatory stage to penicillin has been reported. Small, rounded, atrophic lesions consistent with anetoderma may also develop in patients with ACA.[49] The term "dermatitis atrophicans maculosa" has been used in connection with ACA to describe an uncommon disseminated form of macular atrophy.[49]

The case report of Buchwald in 1883 of "diffuser idiopathischer Hautatrophie" is considered to be the first report of ACA in its atrophic form.[50] This end stage of extremely advanced atrophy seems to be uncommon nowadays, probably because of the extensive use of antibiotics. Doses sufficient for other infections may perhaps modify the appearance and course of ACA. However, atrophy of the skin, resembling crumpled cigarette paper with clearly visible veins, is still seen. Often there is a clinical picture with both inflammatory and atrophic lesions in different regions in the same patient. Atrophic and sclerotic skin lesions may also occur in treponemal infections.

It is evident that borreliae may cause sclerotic skin lesions of varying types and also atrophy, including macular atrophy of the anetoderma type. It must be remembered, however, that the etiology of sclerotic skin lesions, as well as of anetoderma, is heterogeneous and that these conditions represent patterns of reaction rather than etiological entities.

CONCLUSIONS

Ixodes-borne borreliosis may vary considerably in its dermatologic manifestations. The early skin lesions generally heal with no residue, but late lesions may lead to atrophy, sclerosis, or ulceration of the skin and also to irreversible changes of underlying joints or bones and to concomitant neurologic manifestations.

As in syphilis, *Ixodes*-borne borreliosis may be divided into three stages, and EM, BL, and ACA can each be attributed to one of the stages and be regarded as the three dermatologic hallmarks of this borreliosis.

Besides these rather distinct skin lesions, more unspecific cutaneous signs, such as macular and urticarial rashes, and varying sclerotic and atrophic skin lesions may appear. The whole spectrum of dermatologic borrelial manifestations is probably still not known and remains to be settled in the future.

Secondary syphilis has been defined as the stage when generalized manifestations occur on the skin.[51] By analogy with syphilis, we therefore consider that multiple disseminated erythematous skin lesions should be regarded as belonging to the secondary stage and that the designation erythema migrans should be applied only to denote the primary erythema and not to disseminated secondary lesions.

As in syphilis, the difficulties in treatment seem to increase with the severity of the symptoms and the duration of the disease. We consider that a unitary clinical classification may be important as a basis in helping to understand the course and nature of this infection and in establishing the optimal treatment for different manifestations of *Ixodes*-borne borreliosis. Our proposal for classification of cutaneous borrelial manifestations is seen in TABLE 1.

ACKNOWLEDGMENTS

We thank Istvan Agocs, Södersjukhuset, for taking the photographs.

REFERENCES

1. BEAN, R. B. & W. B. BEAN. 1961. Sir William Osler: Aphorisms from His Bedside Teachings and Writings. Charles C Thomas. Springfield, IL.
2. ÅSBRINK, E. & A. HOVMARK. 1985. Successful cultivation of spirochetes from skin lesions of patients with erythema chronicum migrans Afzelius and acrodermatitis chronica atrophicans. Acta Pathol. Microbiol. Immunol. Sect. B 93: 161–163.

3. STEERE, A. C., S. E. MALAWISTA, D. R. SNYDMAN, R. E. SHOPE, W. A. ANDIMAN, M. R.
    ROSS & F. M. STEELE. 1977. Lyme arthritis: An epidemic of oligoarticular arthritis in
    children and adults in three Connecticut communities. Arthritis Rheum. **20:** 7–17.
4. STEERE, A. C., S. E. MALAWISTA, J. A. HARDIN, S. RUDDY, P. W. ASKENASE, W. A.
    ANDIMAN. 1977. Erythema chronicum migrans and Lyme arthritis. Ann. Intern. Med.
    86: 685–698.
5. STEERE, A. C., M. S. GRODZICKI, A. N. KORNBLATT, J. E. CRAFT, A. G. BARBOUR, W.
    BURGDORFER, G. P. SCHMID, E. JOHNSON & S. E. MALAWISTA. 1983. The spirochetal
    etiology of Lyme disease. N. Engl. J. Med. **308:** 733–739.
6. WORLD HEALTH ORGANIZATION. 1982. Treponemal Infections. Technical Report Series
    674. World Health Organization.
7. ÅSBRINK, E., E. BREHMER-ANDERSSON & A. HOVMARK. 1986. Acrodermatitis chronica
    atrophicans—a spirochetosis. Clinical and histopathological picture based on 32 patients.
    Am. J. Dermatopathol. **8:** 209–219.
8. GJESTLAND, T. 1955. The Oslo study of untreated syphilis. Acta Derm. Venereol.
    (Stockholm) Suppl. **35:** 1.
9. AFZELIUS, A. 1910. Verhandlungen der dermatologischen Gesellschaft zu Stockholm.
    Arch. Dermatol. Syph. **101:** 404.
10. LIPSCHÜTZ, B. 1914. Über eine seltene Erythemform (Erythema chronicum migrans).
    Arch. Dermatol. Syph. **118:** 349–356.
11. ÅSBRINK, E., B. HEDERSTEDT & A. HOVMARK. 1984. The spirochetal etiology of erythema
    chronicum migrans Afzelius. Acta Derm. Venereol. (Stockholm) **64:** 291–295.
12. STEERE, A. C., N. H. BARTENHAGEN, J. E. CRAFT, G. J. HUTCHINSON, J. H. NEWMAN,
    D. W. RAHN, L. H. SIGAL, P. N. SPIELER, K. S. STENN & S. E. MALAWISTA. 1983. The
    early clinical manifestations of Lyme disease. Ann. Intern. Med. **99:** 76–82.
13. BERGER, B. 1984. Erythema chronicum migrans of Lyme disease. Arch. Dermatol.
    120: 1017–1021.
14. WEBER, K., A. PUZNIK & T. BECKER. 1983. Erythema-migrans-Krankheit. Beitrag zur
    Klinik und Beziehung zur Lyme-Krankheit. Dtsch. Med. Wochenschr. **108:** 1182–1190.
15. STIERNSTEDT, G. 1985. Tick-borne Borrelia infection in Sweden. Scand. J. Infect. Dis.
    Suppl. **45:** 1–70.
16. KRISTOFERITSCHS, W., G. SPIEL & P. WESSELY. 1983. Zur Meningopolyneuritis (Garin-
    Bujadoux, Bannwarth). Nervenarzt **54:** 640–646.
17. WEBER, K. & U. NEUBERT. 1986. Clinical features of early erythema migrans disease and
    related disorders. Zbl. Bakt. Hyg. A **263:** 209–228.
18. ÅSBRINK, E., I. OLSSON & A. HOVMARK. 1986. Erythema chronicum migrans Afzelius in
    Sweden: A study on 231 patients. Zbl. Bakt. Mikrobiol. Hyg. A **263:** 229–236.
19. ÅSBRINK, E. & I. OLSSON. 1985. Clinical manifestations of erythema chronicum migrans
    Afzelius in 161 patients: A comparison with Lyme disease. Acta Derm. Venereol.
    (Stockholm) **65:** 43–52.
20. HOVMARK, A., E. ÅSBRINK & I. OLSSON. 1986. Joint and bone involvement in Swedish
    patients with *Ixodes ricinus*-borne *Borrelia* infection. Zbl. Bakt. Hyg. A **263:** 275–284.
21. HÖRSTRUP, P. & R. ACKERMANN. 1973. Durch Zecken übertragene Meningopolyneuritis
    (Garin-Bujadoux, Bannwarth). Fortschr. Neurol. Psychiatr. **41:** 583–606.
22. NEUBERT, U. 1984. Zur Ätiologie von Erythema-migrans-Krankheit und Lyme-Erkran-
    kung. Hautarzt **35:** 563–570.
23. STANEK, G., G. WEWALKA, V. GROH, R. NEUMANN & W. KRISTOFERITSCH. 1985.
    Differences between Lyme disease and European arthropod-borne Borrelia infections.
    Lancet **i:** 401.
24. ÅSBRINK, E., A. HOVMARK & B. HEDERSTEDT. 1985. Serologic studies of erythema
    chronicum migrans Afzelius and acrodermatitis chronica atrophicans with indirect
    immunofluorescence and enzyme-linked immunosorbent assays. Acta Derm. Venereol.
    (Stockholm) **65:** 509–514.
25. SHRESTHA, M., R. GRODZICKI & A. STEERE. 1985. Diagnosing early Lyme disease. Am. J.
    Med. **78:** 235–240.
26. WILSKE, B., G. SCHIERZ, V. PREAC-MURSIC, K. WEBER, H.-W. PFISTER & K. EINHÄUPL.
    1984. Serological diagnosis of erythema migrans disease and related disorders. Infection
    12: 331–337.

27. SONCK, C. E. 1965. Erythema chronicum migrans with multiple lesions. Acta Derm. Venereol. **45:** 34–36.
28. ÅSBRINK, E. 1985. Erythema chronicum migrans Afzelius and acrodermatitis chronica atrophicans. Early and late manifestations of Ixodes ricinus-borne Borrelia spirochetes. Acta Derm. Venereol. (Stockholm) Suppl. **118:** 1–63.
29. WEBER, K., G. SCHIERZ, B. WILSKE, U. NEUBERT, H. E. KRAMPITZ, A. G. BARBOUR & W. BURGDORFER. 1986. Reinfection in erythema migrans disease. Infection **1:** 32–35.
30. BÄFVERSTEDT, B. 1943. Über Lymphadenosis benigna cutis. Eine klinische und patologisch-anatomische Studie. P. A. Norstedt. Stockholm.
31. WEBER, K., G. SCHIERZ, B. WILSKE & V. PREAC-MURSIC. 1985. Das Lymphocytom—eine Borreliose? Z. Hautkr. **60:** 1585–1598.
32. ÅSBRINK, E., A. HOVMARK & I. OLSSON. 1988. Lymphadenosis benigna cutis solitaria— Borrelia lymphocytoma in Sweden. Zbl. Bakt. Hyg. In press.
33. HOVMARK, A., E. ÅSBRINK & I. OLSSON. 1986. The spirochetal etiology of lymphadenosis benigna cutis solitaria. Acta Derm. Venereol. (Stockholm) **66:** 479–484.
34. GOTTRON, H. 1938. Lymphadenosis cutis circumscripta im Bereich der Mamille bei gleichzeitiger Acrodermatitis chron. atrophicans der Extremitäten. Zbl. Hautkr. **59:** 633.
35. ÅSBRINK, E., A. HOVMARK & I. OLSSON. 1986. Clinical manifestations of acrodermatitis chronica atrophicans in 50 Swedish patients. Zbl. Bakt. Mikrobiol. Hyg. A. **263:** 253– 261.
36. HOPF, H. C. 1975. Peripheral neuropathy in acrodermatitis chronica atrophicans (Herxheimer). J. Neurol. Neurosurg. Psychiatry **38:** 452–458.
37. GANS, O. & E. LANDES. 1952. Akrodermatitis atrophicans arthropathica. Hautarzt **3:** 151–155.
38. SANDSTRÖM, M., G. BREDBERG, E. ÅSBRINK, A. HOVMARK & C. HOLMKVIST. Brainstem response audiometry in chronic Ixodes-borne borreliosis. Scand. Audiology. Submitted.
39. ÅSBRINK, E. 1987. Erythema migrans and acrodermatitic chronica atrophicans: Association with joint manifestations. Presented at Eurorheumatology: Eleventh European Congress of Rheumatology. Athens.
40. ÅSBRINK, E., A. HOVMARK & B. HEDERSTEDT. 1984. The spirochetal etiology of acrodermatitis chronica atrophicans Herxheimer. Acta Derm. Venereol. (Stockholm) **64:** 506– 512.
41. ACKERMANN, R., H. P. BOISTEN, J. KABATZKI, U. RUNNE, K. KRÜGER & W. P. HERRMANN. 1984. Serumantikörper gegen Ixodes-ricinus Spirochäte bei Acrodermatitis chronica atrophicans (Herxheimer). Dtsch. Med. Wochenschr. **109:** 6–10.
42. GOTTRON, H. A. 1938. Gleichzeitiges Vorhandensein von Acrodermatitis chronica atrophicans und circumscripter Sklerodermie. Zbl. Hautkr. **57:** 7.
43. RUFLI, T., S. LEHNER, A. AESCHLIEMANN, A. CHAMOT, F. GIGON & J.-P. JEANNERET. 1986. Zum erweiteren Spektrum zeckenübertragener Spirochätosen. Hautarzt **37:** 597– 602.
44. HANSEN, K., J. SERUP & S. HÖYBYE. 1987. Antibodies to *Borrelia burgdorferi* and localised scleroderma. Lancet **i:** 682.
45. ABERER, E., G. STANEK, M. ERTL & R. NEUMANN. 1987. Evidence for spirochetal origin of circumscribed scleroderma (morphea). Acta Derm. Venereol. (Stockholm) **67:** 225–231.
46. OLSSON, I., A. HOVMARK, E. ÅSBRINK & E. BREHMER-ANDERSSON. 1988. Sclerotic skin lesions as manifestations of *Ixodes*-borne borreliosis. This volume.
47. BÜCHNER, S. & TH. RUFLI. 1987. Atrophoderma Pasini-Pierini (abstract). Presented at Lyme borreliosis: Update Europe, Baden, Austria, June 2–4.
48. GRAHMANN, F., J. SCHMIDLI & C. MEIER. 1987. Shulman syndrome as precursor of acrodermatitis chronica atrophicans Herxheimer. A further manifestation of Lyme borreliosis (abstract). Presented at Lyme borreliosis: Update Europe. Baden, Austria, June 2–4.
49. HAUSER, W. 1958. Atrophien. Dermatologie und Venereologie, Bd II/2. H. A. Gottron & V. W. Schönfeld, Eds. Thieme. Stuttgart.
50. BUCHWALD, A. 1883. Ein Fall von diffuser idiopatischer Hautatrophie. Vjschr. Derm. **15:** 553–556.
51. ROOK, A., D. S. WILKINSON, F. J. G. EBLING, R. H. CHAMPION & J. L. BURTON, Eds. 1986. Textbook of Dermatology, Vol. 1. 4th edit. Blackwell. Oxford.

Chronic Neurologic Manifestations of Erythema Migrans Borreliosis

RUDOLF ACKERMANN,[a]

BRUNHILDE REHSE-KÜPPER,[b]

ECKHARD GOLLMER,[b]

AND ROGER SCHMIDT[b]

[a]Medizinisch-Diagnostisches Laboratorium
Hohenzollernring 14
5000 Cologne 1, Federal Republic of Germany

[b]Universitäts-Nervenklinik-Köln
Joseph-Stelzmann-Strasse 9
5000 Cologne 41, Federal Republic of Germany

European erythema migrans and North American Lyme borreliosis, like syphilis, affect the nervous system. *B. burgdorferi* as well as related European *Borrelia* strains tend to persist in this organ and induce chronic diseases, as does *T. pallidum*.

Nervous system involvement in the form of meningitis occurs in the second stage of syphilis. During the second stage of tick-borne borreliosis, analogously, we see meningopolyneuritis. In tertiary syphilis, the central nervous system is implicated by parenchymatous inflammation or vasculitis. Recent observations have shown that there exists a tertiary borreliosis which also involves the parenchyma of the central nervous system.[1-6]

This remarkable late neurologic manifestation of *Borrelia* infection shows a disseminated encephalomyelitis. Severe defects are frequent. Because of its nonspecific appearance it remained unknown to us in our sophisticated medical age for a long time. In contrast to syphilis it does not display distinct entities such as tabes dorsalis, general paresis, optic atrophy, or cerebrospinal vasculitis.

For the same reason it can be classified only by its symptomatology as mostly spinal or multiple-sclerosis-like and as mostly cerebral (TABLE 1). We probably still have much to learn about the clinical spectrum. Diagnosis can easily be missed if we do not look for intrathecally synthesized *Borrelia* antibodies. In order to prevent defects, however, early diagnosis and therapy are necessary.

Besides this progressive borrelia encephalomyelitis, we must consider further tertiary manifestations of the nervous system: sensorimotor polyneuritis associated with acrodermatitis chronica atrophicans is well known in Europe. How often the central nervous system is involved simultaneously is still unknown.

As a further tertiary manifestation, we recently observed a latent, mostly subclinical borrelial infection of the nervous system in patients who had had meningopolyneuritis many years earlier.[7]

We report here on 48 cases with tertiary neuroborreliosis, 44 with progressive borrelia encephalomyelitis and four with latent tertiary neuroborreliosis seen between 1985 and 1987 in the Federal Republic of Germany.

MATERIAL AND METHODS

The patients were seen in our clinic or in one of 18 other neurologic departments of the Federal Republic of Germany, which kindly provided us with clinical data.

TABLE 1. Tertiary Neuroborreliosis: Classification

I. Progressive encephalomyelitis
  A. Mostly spinal (MS-like)
  B. Mostly cerebral (multifocal encephalitis or psychosis)
II. Polyneuritis (ACA-associated)
III. Latent infection (subclinical)

Antibodies against *I. ricinus* borrelial strain N 34 were determined by a modified ELISA.[8,9] In order to demonstrate intrathecally synthesized *Borrelia* antibodies, we compared the antibody activity of CSF and serum per weight unit IgG. If a locally synthesized fraction is present the observed CSF value is higher and the serum-CSF difference reflects the intensity of the antibody production in the central nervous system. This method circumvents the calculation of ratios and also takes into consideration the barrier permeability.[10]

RESULTS

Progressive Borrelia Encephalomyelitis

Progressive borrelia encephalitis was diagnosed on the basis of neuropsychiatric findings, inflammatory alterations of the CSF, and in all cases intrathecally synthesized *Borrelia* antibodies. The average age of the 44 patients (24 male, 20 female) was 45.4 years. The youngest patient was 7, the oldest 79 years old. Most of the patients (57%) were in their fifth or sixth decennium (FIG. 1).

At the time diagnosis was made the illness had lasted seven months to 12 years, with a mean duration of 2.8 years (FIG. 2). In seven of the cases the duration was less than 1 year, but in none of the cases less than 7 months. When the infection took place could not be defined in most of the cases. Only five patients (with histories of 9 months

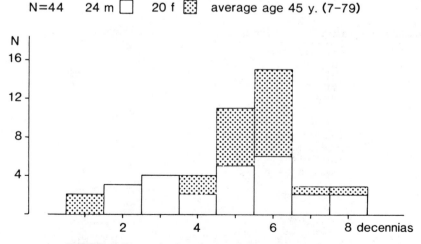

FIGURE 1. Progressive *Borrelia* encephalomyelitis: age duration.

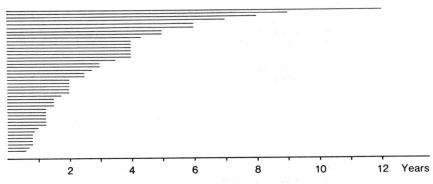

FIGURE 2. Progressive *Borrelia* encephalomyelitis: duration (*n* = 44).

and 1, 3, 4, or 5 years, respectively) reported symptoms at the beginning of their illness consistent with meningopolyneuritis Garin-Bujadoux-Bannwarth. None of the patients remembered an erythema chronicum migrans or other diseases typical for borreliosis.

The patients frequently complained of gait difficulties, ataxia, bladder dysfunction, visus disorders, hypacusis, or feeble memory and mental concentration. The most frequent wrong diagnoses were tuberculous meningoencephalitis, multiple sclerosis, and viral encephalitis.

Physical examination was normal, with the exception of two male patients 15 and 18 years old who had been sick since ages 5 and 8 years. They both showed retarded growth and sexual development. The older one also showed kyphosis of the spine.

Neurologic examination revealed signs of cranial nerves in 22 of the patients. Retrobulbar neuritis with visus impairment showed in four patients, engorged pupilla with visus deficiency in one patient. Most frequent were facial palsies, mostly unilateral, and impairment of hearing, mostly bilateral, in 12 patients each. Involvement of the n. oculomotorius with diplopia and palsies of the n. glossopharyngicus and n. hypoglossus were rare.

TABLE 2. Progressive *Borrelia* Encephalomyelitis: Clinical Signs (*n* = 44)

Cranial nerve palsies	
II	5
III	3
VII	12
VIII	12
IX	1
XII	1
Para- and tetraspastic pareses	29
Flaccid pareses	2
Sensibility disorders	9
Bladder dysfunction	11
Ataxia	17
Dysarthric speech	5
Seizures	3
Retarded growth	2
Retarded sexual development	2
Organic mental disorder	14

The most frequent neurologic signs were para- and tetraspastic pareses, which showed in two-thirds of the 44 patients (TABLE 2). Twelve of these 29 patients had only slight pareses, but 17 showed distinct or severe spastic pareses causing gait disturbancies and demanding crutches. Slight hemipareses, mostly transitory, were seen in four cases. In contrast to the motor signs, sensibility disorders were less frequent and mostly only slight. However, one patient showed a distinct sensorimotor transversal syndrome at TH XI with urinary bladder dysfunction. Ataxia (in one-third of the patients) was also a frequent sign, caused in part by spasticity or sensibility disorders. Additionally, however, four patients showed lateral nystagmus and six patients intention tremor. Bladder dysfunction, in some cases combined with bowel dysfunction, showed in 10 of the patients, dysarthric speech in five, and seizures in only three patients.

Organic mental alterations, combined often with neurologic signs, showed in 14 patients. Twelve of these cases had only slight difficulties with memory and mental concentration or showed slight alterations of their affectivity. Only two of the patients had severe mental disorders with dementia-like deficiencies, loss of orientation, and even altered consciousness.

Electroencephalogram was normal or showed only slow waves or slight dysrhythmias. Cranial computer tomogram displayed hypodense foci of different distribution in five of seven cases. Nuclear magnetic resonance showed foci in addition and was positive in all three cases.

TABLE 3. Progressive *Borrelia* Enchephalomyelitis: CSF Findings[a] ($n = 44$)

Cells (per mm³)	145 (1–566)[a]
Protein (mg/dl)	269 (32–1114)
Antibody titer (per μg IgG)	147 (8–1024)

[a]Expressed as median (range in parentheses).

Mononuclear pleocytosis and impaired blood-CSF barrier were predominant CSF findings (TABLE 3). Cells, mostly lymphocytes and plasma cells and rarely polynuclear cells, ranged from 1 to 566/mm³ with an average value of 145/mm³. Locally synthesized IgG, IgM, and IgA could frequently be demonstrated. Oligoclonal IgG bands could be demonstrated regularly. All 44 patients, including those with normal cell and protein content, showed positive *Borrelia* antibody titer in their CSF.

When antibodies were compared per weight unit IgG in CSF and serum, all patients showed higher *Borrelia* antibody titers in their CSF, indicating the presence of additional antibodies from local synthesis in the nervous system (FIG. 3). The antibody titer in serum per μg IgG ranged from 1 to 128 (mean value 20.8) and in CSF from 8 to 1025 (mean value 91.1). The antibody titer in CSF was one dilution step higher in four cases, two steps in 12 cases, three steps in 21 cases, and four and five steps in three cases each.

The clinical syndromes of the 44 patients are listed in TABLE 4.

After antibiotic therapy, the disorders disappeared only partially. Most of the patients with neuropsychiatric signs before treatment retained to a lesser degree sequelae such as spastic gait, hypacusis, and slight mental disorders.

However, one of the patients with severe mental disorder and dementia-like deficiencies recovered nearly completely and was able to work again as a psychologist. The second patient still has to stay in a psychiatric hospital 2 years after therapy because of his mental condition. In CSF, first cells and then protein become normal. Antibody titer declines more slowly and is often still positive after 1 year.

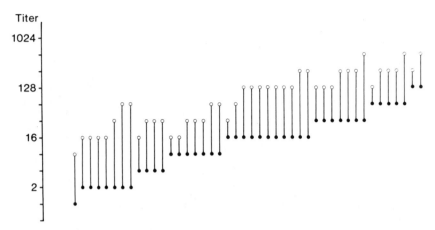

FIGURE 3. Progressive *Borrelia* encephalomyelitis: Antibody titer per microgram IgG in serum and CSF as determined by ELISA ($n = 44$).

Latent Neuroborreliosis

Four patients with latent *Borrelia* infection of the nervous system were detected during a follow-up examination or by chance. Three of them had gone through meningopolyneuritis Garin-Bujadoux-Bannwarth (3, 6 and 12 years earlier) without antibiotic therapy. The diseases had healed by themselves. One patient showed still slight facial palsy, another loss of Achilles reflexes. The fourth patient had complained of migrating pain for 6 years. He did not display any clinical signs. CSF of all four patients showed normal cell count, protein and IgG content, and in particular no intrathecally sythesized IgG as measured by laser nephrelometry. However, all four patients showed two- to fourfold higher *Borrelia* antibody titer per µg IgG in CSF than in serum (TABLE 5).

DISCUSSION

The recently discovered tertiary neuroborreliosis differs distinctly from the well-known meningopolyneuritis Garin-Bujadoux-Bannwarth of the second stage. The early clinically unique manifestation begins 4 to 10 weeks after the infection and heals generally within 4 to 5 months even without antibiotic treatment. Half of the patients remember a tick bite or an erythema. In contrast, borrelia encephalomyelitis begins later and does not heal by itself. The interval between the infection and the onset is difficult to determine because most of the patients do not remember former borreliosis

TABLE 4. Progressive *Borrelia* Encephalomyelitis: Clinical Syndromes ($n = 44$)

Meningitis	34
Myelitis	29
Cranial nerve palsies	22
Encephalitis	18
Mono- and polyneuritis	2

TABLE 5. Latent Neuroborreliosis

| Patient Age (y) | Sex | History | Clinical Symptoms | Serum Antibody | CSF | | *Borrelia* Antibody per μg IgG CSF/serum |
					Cells (per mm³)	Protein (mg/dl)	
59	F	MP[a] 3 y ago	none	750 U	1	42	1024/256[b]
59	M	MP 6 y ago	facial palsy	760 U	2	41	256/32
73	M	MP 12 y ago	Achilles refl. neg.	1600 U	1	53	256/128
71	M	since 6 y ago	migrating pain	145 U	0	51	32/4

[a]Meningopolyneuritis Garin-Bujadoux-Bannwarth.
[b]Reciprocal titer as determined by ELISA.

symptoms. However, five of our patients reported symptoms of a meningopolyneuritis 9 months to 5 years earlier. Obviously pathogenesis is identical with syphilis: infection of the nervous system during the early generalization can persist and evoke severe diseases many years later.

Multilocular symptomatology of progressive borrelia encephalomyelitis resembles many inflammatory, vascular, and neoplastic diseases of the central nervous system. Severe mental disorders can occur that resemble general pareses. More often clinical symptoms such as spinal motor signs, ataxia, bladder dysfunction, slight mental disorders, and in some cases opticus neuritis resemble those found in multiple sclerosis. Contradictory findings, however, are impaired blood-CSF barrier and higher pleocytosis, which are similar to those in tuberculous meningoencephalitis, mycosis, sarcoidosis, neoplastic meningiosis, and neurosyphilis. However, as in neurosyphilis, etiologic diagnosis can be made on the basis of specific CSF antibodies. But in order to prove the activity of the pathogen in the nervous system the presence of intrathecally synthesized antibodies must be demonstrated. Indeed, all our patients showed such autochthonous specific humoral reactions in their CSF, most with high titer.

The utility of CSF findings for diagnosis and evaluation of therapy is well-known from neurosyphilis. Nearly 40 years ago Dattner, a former coworker of Wagner von Jauregg in Vienna, and Thomas postulated activity signs of the CSF when they studied penicillin treatment of neurosyphilis in New York. Because of the similarity of the two spirochetoses, we believe that such indicators are equally important in neuroborreliosis. Half a year after specific therapy cell count should be back to normal. Also, after 1 year CSF protein should be falling or fixed at a low value. In neurosyphilis CSF antibodies persist even after sufficient treatment for several years. How long intrathecally synthesized *Borrelia* antibodies can persist has to be investigated.

Four of our patients showed *Borrelia* antibodies in their CSF as a single finding. Three of them had a borrelia meningopolyneuritis 3, 6, and 12 years ago. Though not treated with antibiotics, all four patients displayed no relevant clinical signs. They also showed no CSF activity, corresponding to the Dattner-Thomas concept. Cells, total protein, and IgG values were within normal range. Therefore one can interpret their CSF *Borrelia* antibody titers as a harmless residual finding. But intrathecally synthesized antibodies additionally present in all cases mean that the pathogen is still active in their nervous system and that the patients have a latent neuroborreliosis.

It cannot be predicted whether this latent infection finally will heal by itself, remain in a stable equilibrium, or relapse at any time. Therefore, those patients should be treated specifically and regularly reexamined.

Our observations demonstrate that intrathecally synthesized antibodies are the most sensitive diagnostic criterion. Using this sign the whole clinical spectrum of tertiary neuroborreliosis can be explored.

REFERENCES

1. KLENCK, W., R. HEITMANN & R. ACKERMANN. 1985. Rezidivierende Erythema-chronicum-migrans-Krankheit des Nervensystems: Querschnittsmyelitis als Rückfall einer Meningopolyneuritis Garin-Bujadoux-Bannwarth. Aktuel. Neurologie 1: 20–23.
2. ACKERMANN, R., E. GOLLMER & B. REHSE-KÜPPER. 1985. Progressive Borrelien-Enzephalomyelitis. Chronische Manifestation der Erythema-migrans-Krankheit am Nervensystem. Dtsch. Med. Wochenschr. 110(26): 1039–1042.
3. REIK, L., JR., L. SMITH, A. KHAN & W. NELSON. 1985. Demyelinating encephalopathy in Lyme disease. Neurology 32: 267–269.
4. ACKERMANN, R., B. REHSE-KÜPPER & E. GOLLMER. 1986. Progressive *Borrelia* encephalomyelitis. Zbl. Bakt. Hyg. A 263: 297–300.

5. PACHNER, A. R. & A. C. STEERE. 1986. CNS manifestations of third stage Lyme disease. Zbl. Bakt. Hyg. A **263:** 301–306.

6. WEDER, B., P. WIEDERSHEIM, L. MATTER, A. STECK & F. OTTO. 1987. Chronic progressive neurological involvement in *Borrelia burgdorferi* infection. J. Neurol. **234:** 40–43.

7. GOLLMER, E., R. SCHMIDT, J. KABATZKI, S. HARTUNG, B. REHSE-KÜPPER & R. ACKERMANN. *Borrelia* meningopolyneuritis Garin-Bujadoux-Bannwarth: Catamnesis of 25 cases. Zbl. Bakt. Hyg. In press.

8. CRAFT, J. E., R. L. GRODZICKI & A. C. STEERE. 1984. Antibody response in Lyme disease: Evaluation of diagnostic tests. J. Infect. Dis. **149(5):** 789–795.

9. REHSE-KÜPPER, B. & R. ACKERMANN. 1986. Demonstration of locally synthesized antibodies in cerebrospinal fluid. Zbl. Bakt. Hyg. A **263:** 407–411.

10. FELGENHAUER, K., H.-J. SCHÄDLICH, M. NEKIC & R. ACKERMANN. 1985. Cerebrospinal fluid virus antibodies: A diagnostic indicator for multiple sclerosis? J. Neurol Sci. **71:** 291–299.

Nervous System Abnormalities in Lyme Disease

JOHN J. HALPERIN,[a] HAROLD L. PASS,[b]
AZAD K. ANAND,[c] BENJAMIN J. LUFT,[d]
DAVID J. VOLKMAN,[d]
AND RAYMOND J. DATTWYLER[d,e]

Departments of [a]Neurology, [b]Psychiatry, [d]Internal Medicine,
and [e]Pathology
State University of New York
Stony Brook, New York 11794

[c]Long Island Diagnostic Imaging PC
Stony Brook, New York 11790

INTRODUCTION

Borrelia burgdorferi, the tick-borne spirochete that causes Lyme disease, has only recently been identified and characterized.[1-3] However, long before its etiologic role was defined, a number of the clinical syndromes it causes were well-known. In particular, it has long been recognized that neurologic abnormalities occur frequently in this infection[4-7]; there is now considerable evidence to suggest that this may be related to direct nervous system invasion.[8-10] The triad of aseptic meningitis, cranial neuritis, and painful radiculitis has been emphasized as the pathognomic form of nervous system involvement.[11] More recently, numerous reports have illustrated the rather protean manifestations of this disease, including myopathies,[12] neuropathies,[6,13-15] plexopathies,[7,11] focal encephalitis,[16-19] a multiple-sclerosis-like illness,[20-24] and psychiatric disorders.[21]

In evaluating patients with chronic Lyme borreliosis it rapidly became apparent to us that although the typical clinical triad occurred in some, far more patients had a variety of less dramatic symptoms, which despite their more subtle nature were quite disabling. Most patients with this chronic infection developed marked fatigue. Many developed difficulties with memory and intellectual function. Others developed intermittent limb paresthesias. In view of this broad range of symptoms, often with rather minimal findings on clinical examination, we began a series of detailed, systematic studies in an effort to identify and quantify the abnormalities underlying these patients' difficulties.

PATIENTS

During the 2-year period ending June 1, 1987, over 100 patients with definite late Lyme borreliosis were evaluated in the Lyme Disease Clinic at University Hospital, Stony Brook, NY. All patients were from areas highly endemic for Lyme disease[25] (primarily Suffolk County, NY, but also Westchester County, NY, and southern Connecticut). Standard criteria for a diagnosis of definite late Lyme disease were used: (1) either (or both) well-documented erythema chronicum migrans or evidence of immunologic reactivity to *B. burgdorferi,* determined either by specific ELISA[26] or an assay of cellular immune reactivity to the organism[27]; and (2) evidence of late, disseminated disease, *i.e.,* cardiac, rheumatologic or neurologic abnormalities. Only patients with disease of at least 4-weeks duration were included in these studies.

METHODS

In each case, other possible diagnoses were sought and excluded. All patients were examined by a neurologist (JJH). Those who described abnormalities of memory or cognition underwent one or more of the following procedures: (1) electroencephalo-gram (EEG); (2) lumbar puncture in which cerebrospinal fluid (CSF) was studied for cells, protein, glucose, anti-*B. burgdorferi* antibody titer, IgG index, oligoclonal bands, and myelin basic protein (MBP); (3) neuropsychological testing; (4) computerized tomographic (CT) scanning of the brain; (5) magnetic resonance imaging (MRI) of the brain. All patients—whether or not they had symptoms of peripheral nerve dysfunction—underwent nerve conduction studies. Two patients with clinically and neurophysiologically evident peripheral neuropathy underwent sural nerve biopsy. All patients were treated with appropriate antibiotics, and many were restudied at varying intervals after treatment.

Neurophysiologic Testing

Eighty-two patients underwent nerve conduction studies at least once, and 47 were restudied at least one additional time following treatment. Testing was performed using surface electrodes and either a Mystro® (TECA Corp., Pleasantville, NY) or 1500 (DISA Electronics, Franklin Lakes, NJ) electromyography apparatus. Skin temperature was maintained at or above 33°C for all studies. All patients underwent a standardized battery of tests[14,15] of (1) motor conductions (unilateral median, ulnar, peroneal and tibial nerves) including F responses[28,29]; (2) orthodromic sensory conduc-tions (unilateral median, ulnar, radial, and sural nerves); (3) H reflexes (both tibial nerves, recording from the soleus); and (4) blink reflexes.[30] Only one patient was unable to tolerate the entire set of tests, requiring that his study be abbreviated. Patients were considered to have a peripheral neuropathy if two or more different nerves were abnormal.

Pre- and posttreatment results were compared for each serially studied patient. Mean sensory conduction velocity (CV), sensory amplitude, motor CV, motor ampli-tude, motor terminal latency (TL), F response latency, H reflex latency, and blink reflex latencies were calculated for each patient, and the mean change of each of these values for each individual was calculated. These data were then analyzed for all 47 serially studied patients (whether or not the patient changed clinically or neurophysio-logically), and statistical comparisons were performed using Student's one-tailed *t* test for paired data.

Neuropsychological Testing

Seventeen patients underwent detailed neuropsychological testing, both before and after antibiotic treatment. A standardized battery of tests was used, consisting of (1) the California Verbal Learning Test (CVLT); (2) the Wechsler Memory Scale

(WMS); (3) the Information and Block Design subtests from the revised Wechsler Adult Intelligence Scale (WAIS-R); (4) the Symbol Digit Modalities Test; (5) Trailmaking Tests, parts A and B; (6) the booklet version of the Categories Test; (7) the Purdue Pegboard; and (8) a Beck Depression Inventory. Patients were studied prior to antibiotic treatment, and were restudied 5 to 28 weeks following treatment. Pre- and posttreatment scores were compared using a series of correlated t tests. Alternate test forms were used where necessary (WMS, CVLT) to minimize practice effects.

Magnetic Resonance Imaging

Ten patients with evidence of memory or intellectual dysfunction, but without focal abnormalities on neurologic examination, underwent MRI scanning of the brain using a GE scanner with a 1.5 Tesla field. T1- and T2-weighted axial images were obtained

TABLE 1. Neurophysiologic Abnormalities

	No. of Patients with Abnormality
Sensory conduction	
Conduction velocity (CV)	30
Amplitude	32
CV or amplitude	44
Motor conduction	
Terminal latency (TL)	29
Conduction velocity	4
Amplitude	13
TL, CV, or amplitude	34
F responses	34
H reflex	12
Blink reflexes	
V	2
VII	4
Carpal tunnel syndrome	21

using spin echo sequences, with repetition times (TR) of 2000 milliseconds. To obtain T1-weighted images, an echo delay time (TE) of 25 ms was used. To obtain T2-weighted images, the TE was increased to 80 milliseconds. All scans were acquired with multislice software and 10-mm slice thickness.

Sural Nerve Biopsy

Using standard techniques, portions of the biopsied sural nerve[15] were prepared for light and electron microscopy, teased fiber analysis, quantitation, and immunofluorescence. Immunofluorescent studies were performed to find evidence of deposition of IgG, IgA, IgM, C3, C4, fibrinogen, and properdin. In addition, sections were studied using a specific polyclonal rabbit antibody against *B. burgdorferi* (kindly provided by Dr. Jorge Benach).

TABLE 2. Neurophysiologic Studies: Mean Change ($n = 47$)

	Mean	SD	p Value
Sensory amplitude	+1.75 μV	3.20	<.0005
Sensory CV	+1.90 m/s	4.61	<.005
Motor amplitude	−0.09 mV	1.57	
Motor CV	+0.28 m/s	4.53	
Motor terminal latency	−0.17 ms	0.41	<.005
H reflex latency	−0.99 ms	4.72	
F response latency	−0.35 ms	2.03	
Blink reflex latencies	no change		

RESULTS

Neurophysiologic Testing

The average age of the patients studied was 40.5 years; the average duration of symptomatic Lyme disease was 30 months. Many had been previously treated unsuccessfully. Fifty-one described intermittent paresthesias of the limbs. Only four patients had histories of a Bell's palsy. Significant neurophysiologic abnormalities were observed in 60 patients; in 39, two or more nerves were abnormal. Sensory conductions were abnormal in 43 patients, motor conductions in 34, F responses in 34, and blink reflexes in 6 (TABLE 1). When patients were restudied following antibiotic treatment (TABLE 2), the only quantities that improved significantly (for the cohort as a whole) were sensory CV, sensory amplitude, and motor terminal latency (all of which may reflect the functioning of the distal axons).

No patient without a clear history of a Bell's palsy or facial numbness had subclinical abnormalities of the blink reflex. Twenty-one patients had neurophysiologic evidence of median nerve entrapment in the carpal tunnel (TABLE 1). Even excluding these patients, the presence of a neurophysiologically demonstrable neuropathy correlated very strongly ($p < 0.0005$, Student's one-tailed t-test) with the presence of intermittent limb paresthesias (TABLE 3). Similarly, the mean number of abnormal nerves was significantly greater in patients with paresthesias than in those without (TABLE 3); ($p < 0.0005$, chi-square).

The sural nerve biopsies demonstrated changes consistent with a mild axonal neuropathy. Several small perivascular collections of lymphocytes were found. Immu-

TABLE 3. Neurophysiologic Abnormalities

	n	Mean No. Abnormal Nerves	SD	Less than 2 Abnormal Nerves	2 or More Abnormal Nerves
Patients with paresthesias	51	2.55	1.89	18	33
Patients without parethesias	31	0.77	0.91	25	6
		$p < .0005$		$p < .0005$	
Abnormalities Due to Entrapment in the Carpal Tunnel Excluded					
Patients with paresthesias		2.31	1.85	22	29
Patients without paresthesias		0.68	0.82	26	5
		$p < 0.0005$		$p < 0.0005$	

nofluorescent staining failed to demonstrate evidence of *B. burgdorferi,* IgG, IgA, IgM, or C4.

Neuropsychological Testing

The average age of the patients studied was 39.2 years; the mean duration of symptomatic Lyme disease was 32.6 months. The group was quite well educated, with an average of 15.1 years of education. All patients had clinically apparent deficits of memory or cognition, but only four had any other deficits on neurologic examination (two with findings of peripheral neuropathy, one with a facial paresis, and one with a lumbosacral radiculopathy). In one patient, who was the most encephalopathic of the group, the EEG demonstrated mild generalized slowing and the CSF was abnormal (protein 114 mg%, normal glucose, 280 monocytes/mm^3). CT scan of the brain was normal. One other patient had a mildly abnormal EEG (but normal CSF and CT scan). One additional patient had a mild CSF pleocytosis (16 monocytes, normal protein and glucose). All other CSFs and EEGs were normal.

TABLE 4. Neuropsychological Measures

	Pretreatment Mean	Posttreatment Mean	
California Verbal Learning Test			
Immediate recall (trial 5)	10.25	13.06	$p < .001$
Free recall (2-minute delay)	9.00	11.76	$< .01$
Cued recall (2-minute delay)	10.00	12.47	$< .01$
Free recall (30-minute delay)	8.75	11.94	$< .01$
Cued recall (30-minute delay)	9.69	12.65	$< .01$
Recognition list	14.19	14.56	
Wechsler Memory Scale			
Logical memory (total score)	16.65	21.12	$p < .01$
Logical memory (30-minute delay)	11.44	16.06	$< .025$
Digits total	10.88	11.47	
Visual reproduction	9.53	12.24	$< .001$
Visual reproduction (30-minute delay)	8.44	10.24	$< .025$
Associate learning	20.12	22.82	$< .025$
Memory quotient	102.35	118.65	$< .01$
Attention/Concentration/Speed			
Symbol-Digit Modalities Test			
Written	48.71	55.35	$p < .001$
Oral	53.18	63.41	$< .001$
Trailmaking Test, part A	29.29	25.24	
Controlled oral word association	44.71	44.88	
Conceptual Ability			
Trailmaking Test, part B (s)	68.29	58.47	
Booklet Categories Test	52.85	33.20	$p < .01$
Psychomotor and Perceptual Motor			
Purdue Pegboard			
Dominant hand	13.81	14.93	$p < .025$
Nondominant hand	13.37	14.73	$< .01$
Simultaneous	11.69	12.47	
Block Design Subtest (WAIS-R, scaled)	11.00	12.37	$< .01$

TABLE 5. MRI Scans

	Age	Sex	Duration	Subjective Memory Deficit	Neuropsychological Testing Deficit	MRI
			Patients Describing Intellectual Difficulties Beyond Mild Memory Impairment			
1	49	F	15 y	+	severe	+
2	48	F	1 y	+	moderate	+
3	41	M	6 (?) mos.	+	moderate	+
4	32	F	8 mos.	+		+
5	31	M	7 mos.	+	moderate	−
			Patients with Minimal Subjective Intellectual Impairment			
6	42	M	4 y	+	mild-moderate	−
7	40	F	6 mos.	−		−
8	34	F	2 y	+/−		−
9	29	F	8 mos.	−		−
10	49	M	2 y	+/−		−

Serial neuropsychological testing demonstrated both initial deficiencies and significant improvement following treatment (TABLE 4). Memory testing was notable in that, despite the patients' high level of education, initial scores on the CVLT (trial 5) were definitely deficient. In contrast, initial scores on the WMS subtests, while probably abnormal for this group, would not ordinarily be classified as deficient. Following treatment, however, the results of both batteries improved significantly.

Results of the symbol-digit modalities test, which tests attention, concentration, and speed, were initially in the low normal range, but improved significantly with treatment. The trailmaking and controlled oral word association tests, which test more automatic aspects of the same functions, were normal prior to treatment, and changed little on retesting.

Performance on the Booklet Categories Test, a difficult test of conceptual ability, was definitely deficient prior to treatment, and improved significantly with treatment. Less improvement was seen on part B of the Trailmaking Test, which is a less complex test of similar functions.

Psychomotor and perceptual motor function, as tested by both the Block Design subtest of the WAIS-R and the Purdue Pegboard, improved significantly with treatment. In contrast, tests of orientation and over-learned intellectual abilities (WAIS-R information subtest, WMS information, mental control, and orientation subtests), which are typically resistant to deterioration in mild encephalopathies, were not significantly impaired initially and did not change significantly with treatment.

Finally, the Beck Depression Inventory did not demonstrate evidence of significant depression (usual cutoff, >15 indicating depression) before (7.63) or after treatment (4.42). Furthermore, most of the positive responses the patients did provide on the pretreatment questionnaire (to such questions as "Do you feel tired?", "Have you lost interest in other people or activities?") probably were a direct reflection of their feeling chronically ill.

MRI Scanning

The average age of the patients studied was 39.5 years (TABLE 5); the mean duration of symptomatic Lyme disease was 32.3 months. All had symptoms of memory difficulty. Patients 1 through 6 felt they had significant intellectual dysfunction. Formal neuropsychological testing was performed in patients 1, 2, 3, 5, and 6, and moderate dysfunction was demonstrated in all. Spinal fluid was normal in the two patients[1,4] in whom it was obtained. In neither were oligoclonal bands or myelin basic protein detected; IgG index was normal in both. None had any focal deficits on neurologic examination, nor any history suggestive of focal central nervous system (CNS) dysfunction in the past.

MRI scans on patients 5 through 10 were completely normal. In each of patients 1 through 4, the patients with the most significant intellectual deficits, punctate, hyperresonant areas were seen in the white matter of the cerebral hemispheres (FIGS. 1 and 2). These lesions were dense on both T1- and T2-weighted images. They were not associated with any mass effect. No other abnormalities were seen.

CONCLUSIONS

In these studies we have demonstrated that late Lyme borreliosis is often associated with significant, quantifiable nervous system abnormalities. Using neurophysiologic techniques, we have been able to document the presence of significant peripheral nerve abnormalities in 40–50% of our patients with late disease. Although the clinical neurologic examination was normal in many of these patients, most described symptoms of intermittent limb paresthesias. Only a few had radicular-type pain or

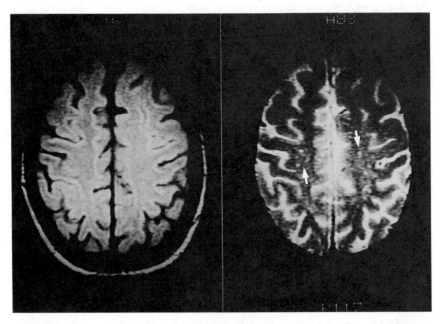

FIGURE 1. MRI scan of brain, axial plane, patient 2. Image on the left is a T1-weighted image, image on the right is T2-weighted. Numerous punctate hyper-resonant lesions (*arrows*) are evident in the cerebral white matter on the T2-weighted image; they are present but quite faint on the T1-weighted image.

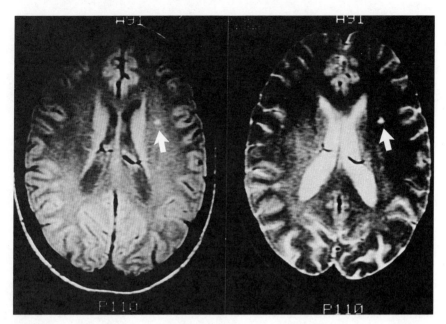

FIGURE 2. MRI scan of brain, axial plane, patient 4. Image on the left is a T1-weighted image, image on the right is T2-weighted. One large hyper-resonant lesion (*arrow*) is evident in the cerebral white matter in both images.

other symptoms as dramatic as those described in the literature. However, the type of electrophysiologic abnormality we have observed is somewhat similar to what has been described in other patients with radiculoneuritis in Lyme borreliosis.[6,13,31] Similarly, the findings on nerve biopsy are qualitatively similar to what has been described in earlier reports.[13] Our findings suggest to us that late Lyme borreliosis is frequently associated with peripheral nerve damage, and that previous reports have only described the most extreme examples of this phenomenon. By using very sensitive neurophysiologic tests in part of a prospective, broad survey of patients with late Lyme borreliosis, we have been able to demonstrate more subtle abnormalities in a much larger proportion of patients with late disease.

The pattern of abnormalities on biopsy and on electrophysiologic testing suggests that this neuropathy is primarily axonal in nature, and may affect the distal axons preferentially. Furthermore, these abnormalities appear to be readily reversible with appropriate antibiotic treatment. The observations that these abnormalities reverse rapidly, often before there has been an appreciable change in antibody titer, and that there appears to be no abnormal deposition of antibody or complement in damaged nerves, suggest to us that this neuropathy is related to the presence of the causative organism, rather than to the patient's immune response to it. However, this issue will require considerable further study.

Our observations of the central nervous system abnormalities closely parallel those we have made in the peripheral nervous system. We have noted that many patients with late Lyme disease describe specific difficulties with memory and intellectual function, often in association with incapacitating fatigue. Using extensive, standard-ized neuropsychological tests, we have been able to demonstrate that these patients (1) are not depressed; and (2) have readily identifiable, quantifiable, and reversible deficits of (a) immediate and delayed auditory-verbal and visual memory, (b) the ability to learn and retrieve new information, (c) sustained attention and concentration, (d) perceptual-motor tasks, and (e) problem-solving and conceptual flexibility. Patients' performance on these tests, and their improvement following successful treatment, correlated well with their subjective perceptions of their intellectual deficits. It is important to note that none of these patients had clinical evidence of focal CNS disease, and EEGs, examinations of the CSF, and most other laboratory investigations were generally normal.

Finally, in an effort to understand the pathogenesis of this central nervous system dysfunction, we have obtained MRI scans on 10 patients with this clinical syndrome. Four of the five most severely affected patients had clear abnormalities on MRI scans. These abnormalities had the MRI characteristics of edema or inflammation (bright on both T1- and T2-weighted images),[32] yet showed no evidence of local mass effect, as would be expected in focal infectious processes. The abnormalities most closely resemble those seen in multiple sclerosis (MS),[33] although the lesions we have demonstrated are generally smaller than those seen in that disorder. Furthermore, none of the patients with these abnormalities on MRI scan had clinical findings suggestive of MS. In addition, all four had normal visual and auditory evoked responses, tests which commonly are abnormal in multiple sclerosis. Finally, we examined the spinal fluid of the two patients with the most dramatic MRI abnormalities, and neither had any of the typical abnormalities seen in MS. From this we conclude that the CNS dysfunction we have observed in patients with late Lyme disease may reflect the presence of a mild inflammatory encephalomyelitis, and once again conclude that previously published observations of encephalitis and of a multiple-sclerosis-like illness in Lyme disease may well represent only the most severe, extreme cases of this more common phenomenon.

These parallel observations suggest to us that Lyme disease is frequently associated with both peripheral and central nervous system disease, that these disorders are associated with local inflammatory changes, and that the induced neurologic changes are often reversible. The detailed pathogenesis of these disorders remains completely unclear, but we feel that the application of these precise, quantitative methods in a systematic fashion will prove very helpful in further elucidating the mechanisms underlying these disorders.

REFERENCES

1. BURGDORFER, W., A. G. BARBOUR, S. F. HAYES, J. L. BENACH, E. GRUNWALDT & J. P. DAVIS. 1982. Lyme disease: A tick borne spirochetosis? Science **216:** 1317–1319.
2. BENACH, J. L., E. M. BOSLER, J. P. HANRAHAN, J. L. COLEMAN, G. S. HABICHT, T. F. BAST, D. J. CAMERON, J. L. ZIEGLER, A. G. BARBOUR, W. BURGDORFER, R. EDELMAN & R. A. KASLOW. 1983. Spirochetes isolated from the blood of two patients with Lyme disease. N. Engl. J. Med. **308:** 740–742.
3. STEERE, A. C., R. L. GRODZICKI, A. N. KORNBLATT, J. E. CRAFT, A. G. BARBOUR, W. BURGDORFER, G. P. SCHMID, E. JOHNSON & S. E. MALAWISTA. 1983. The spirochetal etiology of Lyme disease. N. Engl. J. Med. **308:** 733–740.
4. GARIN-BUJADOUX, C. 1922. Paralysie par les tiques. J. Med. Lyons **3:** 765–767.
5. BANNWARTH, A. 1941. Chronische lymphocytare Meningitis, entzundliche Polyneuritis und "Rheumatismus." Ein Beitrag zum Problem "Allergie und Nervensystem." Arch. Psychiat. Nervenkr. **113:** 284–376.
6. HOPF, H. C. 1975. Peripheral neuropathy in acrodermatitis chronica atrophicans. J. Neurol. Neurosurg. Psychiatry **38:** 452–458.

7. REIK, L., A. C. STEERE, N. H. BARTENHAGEN, R. E. SHOPE & S. E. MALAWISTA. 1979. Neurologic abnormalities of Lyme disease. Medicine (Baltimore) **58:** 281–294.
8. HENRIKSSON, A., H. LINK, M. CRUZ & G. STIERNSTEDT. 1986. Immunoglobulin abnormalities in CSF and blood over the course of lymphocytic meningoradiculitis. Ann. Neurol. **20:** 337–345.
9. WILSKE, B., G. SCHIERZ, V. PREAC-MURSIC, K. VON BUSCH, R. KUHBECK, H. W. PFISTER & K. EINHAUPL. 1986. Intrathecal production of specific antibodies against *Borrelia burgdorferi* in patients with lymphocytic meningoradiculitis. J. Infect. Dis. **153:** 304–314.
10. PREAC-MURSIC, V., B. WILSKE, G. SCHIERZ, H. W. PFISTER & K. EINHAUPL. 1984. Repeated isolation of spirochetes from the cerebrospinal fluid of a patient with meningoradiculitis Bannwarth. Eur. J. Clin. Microbiol. **3:** 564–565.
11. PACHNER, A. R. & A. C. STEERE. 1985. The triad of neurologic manifestations of Lyme disease: Meningitis, cranial neuritis, and radiculoneuritis. Neurology **35:** 47–53.
12. SCHMUTZHARD, E., J. WILLEIT & F. GERSTENBRAND. 1986. Meningopolyneuritis Bannwarth with focal nodular myositis. Klin. Wochenschr. **64:** 1204–1208.
13. VALLAT, J. M., J. HUGON, M. LUBEAU, M. J. LEBOUTET, M. DUMAS & DESPROGES-GOTTERON. 1987. Tick-bite meningoradiculoneuritis. Neurology **37:** 749–753.
14. HALPERIN, J. J. & R. J. DATTWYLER. 1987. Lyme neuropathy. Abstr. Am. Acad. Clin. Neurophysiol. **2:** 14.
15. HALPERIN, J. J., B. W. LITTLE, P. K. COYLE & R. J. DATTWYLER. 1987. Lyme disease—cause of a treatable peripheral neuropathy. Neurology. **37:** 1700–1706.
16. ACKERMAN, R., E. GOLLMER & K. REHSE. 1985. Progressive borrelia encephalomyelitis. Chronic manifestation of erythema chronicum migrans disease of the nervous system. Dtsch. Med. Wochenschr. **110:** 1039–1042.
17. BRODERICK, J. P., B. A. SANDOK & L. E. MERTZ. 1987. Focal encephalitis in a young woman 6 years after onset of Lyme disease: Tertiary Lyme disease? Mayo Clin. Proc. **62:** 313–316.
18. DIRINGER, M. N., J. J. HALPERIN & R. J. DATTWYLER. 1987. Lyme meningoencephalitis—report of a severe penicillin-resistant case. Arthritis Rheum. **30:** 705–708.
19. WOKKE, J. H. J., J. VAN GIJN, A. ELDERSON & G. STANEK. 1987. Chronic forms of *Borrelia burgdorferi* infection of the nervous system. Neurology **37:** 1031–1034.
20. HANSEN, K., C. RECHNITZER, N. S. PEDERSON, M. ARPI & O. JESSEN. 1987. Borrelia meningitis in Denmark. Zbl. Bakt. Hyg. A 348–350.
21. PACHNER, A. R. & A. C. STEERE. 1986. Neurologic involvement in the third stage of Lyme disease: CNS manifestations can mimic multiple sclerosis and psychiatric illness. Neurology **36** (Suppl. 1): 286.
22. PACHNER, A. R. & A. C. STEERE. 1986. CNS manifestations of third stage Lyme disease. Zbl. Bakt. Hyg. A **263:** 301–306.
23. REIK, L., L. SMITH, A. KHAN & W. NELSON. 1985. Demyelinating encephalopathy in Lyme disease. Neurology **35:** 267–269.
24. STIERNSTEDT, G., B. SKOLDENBERG, A. GARDE, *et al.* 1987. Clinical manifestations of *Borrelia* infection of the nervous system. Zbl. Bakt. Hyg. A **289–296.**
25. SCHMID, G. P., P. HORSLEY, A. C. STEERE, J. P. HANRAHAN, J. P. DAVIS, G. S. BOWEN, M. T. OSTERHOLM, J. S. WEISFELD, A. W. HIGHTOWER & C. V. BROOME. 1985. Surveillance of Lyme disease in the United States, 1982. J. Infect. Dis. **151:** 1144–1149.
26. RUSSELL, H., J. S. SAMPSON, G. P. SCHMID, H. W. WILKINSON & B. PLIKAYTIS. 1984. Enzyme linked immunosorbent assay and indirect immunofluorescence assay for Lyme disease. J. Infect. Dis. **149:** 465–470.
27. DATTWYLER, R. J., J. THOMAS, J. L. BENACH & M. G. GOLIGHTLY. 1986. Cellular immune responses in Lyme disease: The response to mitogens, live *Borrelia burgdorferi*, NK cell function and lymphocyte subsets. Zbl. Bakt. Hyg. A **263:** 151–159.
28. LACHMAN, T., B. T. SHAHANI & R. R. YOUNG. 1980. Late responses as aids to diagnosis in peripheral neuropathy. J. Neurol. Neurosurg. Psychiatry **43:** 156–162.
29. SHAHANI, B. T., F. POTTS & J. DOMINGUE. 1980. F response studies in peripheral neuropathies. Neurology **30:** 409–410.
30. SHAHANI, B. T. & R. R. YOUNG. 1983. The blink, H and tonic vibration reflexes. *In*

Electrodiagnosis of Neuromuscular Diseases. 3d edit. J. Goodgold & A. Eberstein, Eds.: 258–263. Williams & Wilkins. Baltimore, MD.

31. GRAF, M., W. KRISTOFERITSCH, U. BAUMHACKL & J. ZEITLHOFER. 1987. Electrophysiologic findings in meningopolyneuritis of Garin-Bujadoux-Bannwarth. Zbl. Bakt. Hyg. A 324–327.

32. BUONANNO, F. S., J. P. KISTLER, L. D. DeWITT, C. L. KRAMER & K. R. DAVIS. 1985. Nuclear magnetic resonance imaging of the brain. In Head and Spine Imaging. C. F. Gonzalez, C. B. Grossman & J. C. Masdeu, Eds.: 889–916. Wiley. New York.

33. EDWARDS, M. K., M. R. FARLOW & J. C. STEVENS. 1986. Multiple sclerosis: MRI and clinical correlation. Am. J. Roentgenology 147: 571–574.

Neuropathy Associated with Acrodermatitis Chronica Atrophicans

Clinical and Morphological Features

W. KRISTOFERITSCH,[a] E. SLUGA,[a,e] M. GRAF,[a]
H. PARTSCH,[b] R. NEUMANN,[c] G. STANEK,[d]
AND H. BUDKA[e]

[a]Department of Neurology
[b]Department of Dermatology
Wilhelminenspital der Stadt Wien
Vienna, Austria

[c]2d Department of Dermatology
[d]Hygiene Institute
[e]Neurological Institute
University of Vienna
Vienna, Austria

Neurological manifestations of Lyme borreliosis are varied but well-known in the second stage. Their usual pattern consists of painful peripheral nerve involvement such as meningopolyneuritis Garin-Bujadoux-Bannwarth (MPN-GBB), cranial nerve paresis, and meningitis.[15,17,23] Sometimes encephalitis and myelitis have been observed.[3] Apart from these well-described and self-limiting neurological disorders, several cases of chronic central nervous system (CNS) disease have been attributed to Lyme borreliosis.[1,21] In most cases this association was based principally on serological findings, although this may suffer from a strong bias, as up to 32% of apparently healthy individuals may show elevated *Borrelia* antibody titers.[11] As we were looking for well-defined cases of chronic Lyme borreliosis, we concentrated our neurological investigations on patients with acrodermatitis chronica atrophicans (ACA), which is a chronic skin disorder with established borrelial etiology. However, in these patients no CNS involvement was detected. Yet, we saw a significant number of patients with peripheral neuropathy, which we are going to discuss here.

PATIENTS AND METHODS

Over a period of 2 years, from 1985 to 1987, 65 patients from the Vienna region were looked at. In all the patients clinical diagnosis of ACA was confirmed serologically by ELISA testing as described previously.[22] Patients were all referred from two dermatology departments. Clinical and electroneurographical examinations were performed in each case. Sural nerve biopsies from four patients were investigated by light and electron microscopy.

Fifteen patients were found to have diseases or conditions other than ACA (diabetes mellitus, neoplastic disease, chronic alcoholism, radiotherapy) possibly causing peripheral neuropathy. They are excluded from the clinical part of our study.

Twenty-one of the 50 other patients received antibiotic treatment prior to their neurological examinations. The interval between the onset of treatment and the neurological examination was 8.4 ± 7.1 months. Nine of these treated patients with infiltrative stage of ACA at the beginning of therapy did not show any gross cutaneous alterations at the time of their neurological examination (TABLE 1). Skin lesions were found on one extremity in 32 patients, on two extremities in 12 patients, on three extremities in two, and on all four extremities in four patients. TABLE 1 provides biographical data and information on the stage of ACA in the 50 patients without other known cause for peripheral neuropathy.

Neurological Examinations

All patients were investigated by the same person. For the clinical diagnosis of neuropathy, hypesthesia and/or hyporeflexia or paresis had to be present. In patients older than 60 years isolated absence or diminution of ankle jerks or of pallesthesia without other signs or symptoms of peripheral nerve involvement were not considered to justify a diagnosis of peripheral neuropathy.[5]

Electroneurography (ENG)

In all patients motor nerve conduction velocities (NCV), compound action potentials (CAP), and distal latencies (DL) were measured usually in the peroneal or median nerve of at least one extremity involved by ACA. In 46 of the 50 patients sensory nerve conduction velocities were recorded with surface electrodes after antidromic stimulation of the median nerve or orthodromic stimulation of the sural nerve. Sensory nerve action potentials (SNAP) of the sural nerve were measured in 43 patients. The results were compared with those of a matching control group. An isolated decrease of CAP with more than 2.5 standard deviation, or a decrease of the NCV of less than 34 m/s with concomitant decrease of the CAP below 1 mV was considered suggestive of an axonal degeneration.[18] Slowing of NCV of more than 40% was indicative of a primary demyelination.

Morphology

Sural nerve samples of four patients were examined by light (paraffin and semithin sections) and electron microscopy. Direct immunofluorescence was carried out on

TABLE 1. Stage of ACA in 50 Patients

Patients	Without Therapy (n = 29)	With Therapy (n = 21)	Total (n = 50)
Age (y)	62.2 ± 16.4	59.2 ± 15.6	60.9 ± 16.0
Sex (M/F)	7/22	9/12	16/34
Infiltrative ACA (n)	21	2	23
Atrophic ACA (n)	8	10	18
Healed[a] ACA (n)	—	9	9
Months from therapy to neurological examination	—	8.4 ± 7.1	—

Plus-minus values are means ± 1 SD; n = number of patients.
[a]Healed = no visible skin alterations after therapy.

TABLE 2. Complaints in Patients Suffering from ACA-associated Neuropathy (Total in Sample = 24)

Complaint	No. of Patients	%
Pain	8	62
Paresthesias	6	46
Weakness	3	23
Muscle cramps	1	8
Restless legs	1	8
Total reporting complaints	13	54

frozen nerve sections using antisera specific for human IgG, IgA, IgM, and for the complement factor C3 and fibrinogen. Silver staining according to Dieterle[8] was performed in order to demonstrate borreliae. There were no reasons to admit a previous MPN-GBB in these four patients. Two patients, designated SM and LO on the figures, had mild diabetes mellitus in addition to ACA.

RESULTS

Twenty-four of the 50 patients without any evidence of neuropathy other than ACA showed clinical and/or electroneurographical signs of neuropathy.

Clinical Results

Thirteen of the 24 patients with signs of peripheral nerve involvement reported complaints indicative of polyneuropathy (TABLE 2). Pain was mentioned by five and paresthesia by three of the 26 other patients without any signs of neuropathy. Although pain was usually mild, four patients described it as severe, burning, and sharp. Three of the 24 patients with neuropathy suffered from migratory pain after tick bite or presumptive erythema chronicum migrans prior to the apparition of ACA and may therefore have suffered previously from MPN-GBB. The complaints began on the average 30 ± 40 months prior to our investigation. Diagnosis of neuropathy was established on clinical grounds in 19 patients. In six of them hypesthesia and hypalgesia were restricted to patchy areas usually within the region involved by ACA (FIG. 1). In three patients this hypesthetic zone seemed to be situated within the supply area of a cutaneous nerve. Analogously to similar cases of vasculitis, we considered this form of peripheral sensory nerve involvement as cutaneous neuritis.[19] In four patients these patchy hypesthetic areas were the only neurological abnormalities, whereas in the two others additional paresis or hyporeflexia was observed that could not be associated with the sensory loss. Neurological signs in these two patients and in five others, who showed a distally located asymmetrical neuropathy that did not correspond to the distribution of individual nerves but was more diffuse, were classified as asymmetric polyneuropathic. Eight other patients had signs of a distal symmetric polyneuropathy (TABLES 3 and 4). In the cases with polyneuropathy all sensory qualities were usually affected and the area of sensory deficit was frequently not restricted to the region affected by ACA.

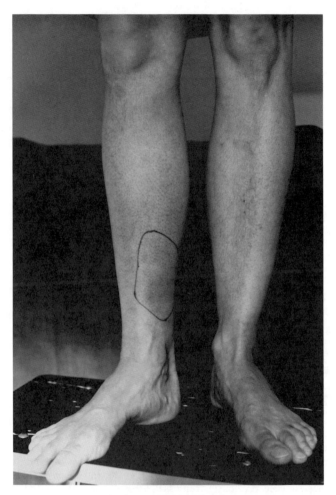

FIGURE 1. Cutaneous neuropathy in a patient with infiltrative ACA on the right lower extremity. Circled area indicates hypesthetic zone.

TABLE 3. Neurological Findings in 24 Patients with ACA-associated Neuropathy

Sensory Deficit	n	Paresis (n)	Reflex Disturbances (n)	Abnormal ENG[a] (n)
Patchy	6	1	1	1
Asymmetric	5	1	3	2
Symmetric	7	2	5	6
No deficit	6	—	1	6

n = Number of patients.
[a]ENG = electroneurography.

TABLE 4. Pattern of Peripheral Nerve Involvement in 24 Patients with ACA

Pattern of Neuropathy	n	%
Cutaneous	4	17
Distal asymmetric	7	29
Distal symmetric	8	33
Subclinical	5	21

n = Number of patients.

ENG Findings

Abnormal ENG results were found in 15 patients. In five of them, who showed no other clinical signs and symptoms of peripheral nerve involvement, subclinical neuropathy was detected (TABLE 4). In seven cases ENG alterations were compatible with axonal degeneration. No patient fulfilled the ENG criteria for primary demyelination as mentioned above.

Clinical and/or ENG signs of peripheral nerve involvement could be detected in five patients on extremities not overtly involved by ACA. Neuropathy could also be seen in cases with resolution of skin lesions after treatment. But extremities affected by ACA displayed the neurological deficit in a more severe way. On the other hand, neurological deficits were not necessarily present even in cases with long duration of ACA or profound skin involvement. The frequency of peripheral neuropathy was significantly lower ($\chi^2 = 5.366, p < 0.05$) in treated than in untreated patients (TABLE 5).

Morphological Results

Light microscopic examination of sural nerve specimens revealed consistently perivascular lymphoid cell infiltration of the median-sized and small epineurial vessels and of the epineurial soft tissue (FIG. 2). The infiltration was predominantly perivascular, but the vessel wall was also infiltrated, occasionally with obliteration of the lumen (FIG. 2). Necrosis, fibrosis, or polymorphonuclear infiltration of the vessel wall were not seen. Inflammatory infiltration of endoneurial vessels were not present. In clinically severely affected patients mononuclear cells could be sporadically detected in the endoneurium (FIG. 3b). In particular, semithin sections revealed disseminated loss of predominantly large myelinated fibers (FIG. 3). The amount of nerve fiber damage corresponded well with the intensity of epineurial vascular infiltration. In different fascicles nerve fiber degeneration was observed in varying

TABLE 5. Skin Alteration, Therapy, and ACA-associated Neuropathy in 24 Patients

Stage of ACA (n/N)		Without Therapy (n/N)	With Therapy (n/N)
Infiltrative	14/23	14/21	0/2
Atrophic	8/18	4/8	4/10
Healed	2/9	—	2/9
Total	24/50	18/29	6/21

n = Number of patients with ACA-associated neuropathy.
N = Total number of patients in sample.

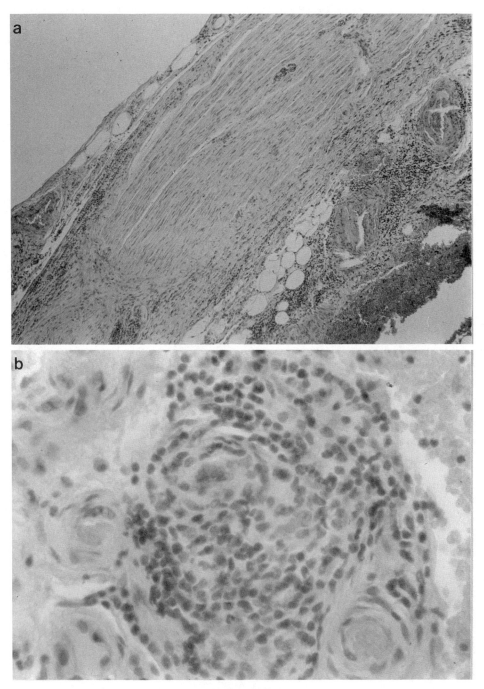

FIGURE 2. (a) Mononuclear cell infiltration of the epineurium with perivascular predominance (hematoxylin and eosin stain, paraffin section, magnification 60×; sural nerve of patient SM). (b) Infiltration of a small vessel with mononuclear cells obliterating its lumen (hematoxylin and eosin stain, paraffin section, magnification 630×; sural nerve of patient SM).

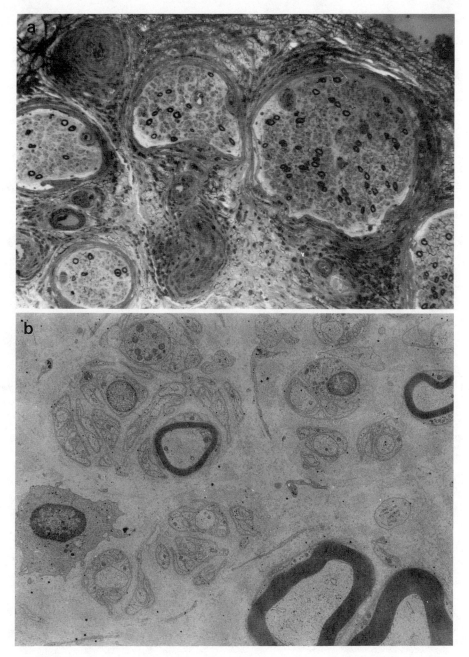

FIGURE 3. (a) Loss of myelinated fibers. Different fascicular involvement. Perivascular infiltration of the epineurial vessels (toluidine blue, semithin section, magnification 252×; sural nerve of patient SM). (b) Lymphocyte in the endoneurium of a sural nerve fascicle, myelinated and Remak fibers (electron microscopy, magnification 6000×; patient SM).

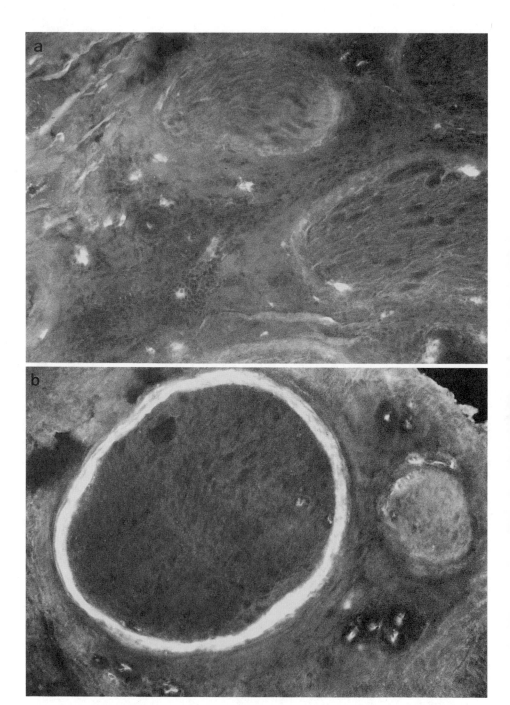

FIGURE 4. (a) IgM-positive mononuclear cells in epineurial and subperineurial distribution (magnification 252×, patient SM), and (b) IgM staining of the perineurium demonstrated by immunofluorescence (magnification 252×, patient LO).

distribution and intensity. No signs of primary segmental demyelination could be detected by electron microscopy. IgM- and IgA-, but not IgG-positive mononucleated cells, were found predominantly in the epineurium distributed perivascularly by direct immunofluorescence. Few were found under the perineurium (FIG. 4). One patient also showed IgA- and IgM-staining of the perineurium. Staining for C3 and fibrinogen was negative. No borrelial structures could be seen by silver staining or electron microscopy.

DISCUSSION

We could demonstrate in 62% of patients with untreated ACA and no other indications for neuropathy clinical and/or electroneurographical signs of peripheral nerve involvement. In 48% of a sample of ACA patients, including also treated cases, clinical signs of neuropathy could be detected. This frequency is similar to that described in the only two hitherto published systematic neurological studies on patients with ACA. H. C. Hopf[13,14] and M. Kaiser, in collaboration with H. C. Hopf,[16] found in 40% of a sample of treated and untreated patients with ACA clinical signs of predominantly sensory polyneuropathy. H. C. Hopf was convinced at the end of his detailed study "that a close association between ACA and peripheral neuropathy in cases with ACA exists."[13] Yet etiology and pathomechanism of this neurological disorder remained obscure and Hopf's postulate unfortunately did not induce further neurological studies. The recent discovery of *B. burgdorferi* as etiologic agent of multisystemic Lyme borreliosis,[4,6,24] which apart from joints also involves skin and nervous system, and its association with ACA[2] gave rise to this neurological reappraisal.

Peripheral nerve involvement occurs in patients with ACA as subclinical neuropathy, as sensory cutaneous neuropathy, which is identical with neuropathy of the "local type" observed by Hopf,[13] and as asymmetric and symmetric polyneuropathy. A similar pattern of different forms of neuropathy has been described in several infectious diseases,[20] but also more markedly in vasculitis.[19]

The neurological disorder in ACA is mild, but shows a chronic course. Neurological deficits are predominantly sensory and distally distributed. Distal location is also characteristic for the cutaneous lesions of ACA. All patients with peripheral nerve involvement had their major neurological deficits in regions affected with ACA. Thus, the local inflammatory process or the presence of antigen seems to be most important for the manifestation of neuropathy. Yet, there is need for another condition to be fulfilled in this process, since in several cases peripheral neurological deficit appeared even in extremities free from skin lesions, and conversely peripheral nerve involvement could not be seen in some cases with severe and long-standing ACA. These observations correlate distinctly with those by Hopf[13] and Kaiser.[16]

Neuropathological examinations of nerve biopsies in ACA, which have not been described previously, showed in all four investigated cases inflammatory mononuclear infiltration around small and medium-sized epineurial vessels. On several occasions the vessel wall was also infiltrated, but did not show destruction or fibrinoid degeneration, necessary for the diagnosis of classical necrotizing vasculitis.[10] The presence of perivascular infiltrates of inflammatory cells together with axonal degeneration and a decrease in the population of myelinated fibers have been accepted to be suggestive for vasculitic neuropathy.[26] Differential fascicular involvement and the relation between the intensity of vascular infiltration and the amount of nerve fiber loss strongly points to an ischemic origin of ACA-associated neuropathy. The two patients with additional mild diabetes mellitus also showed this relation, which suggests that their neuropathy was mainly not due to diabetes mellitus, but was related to ACA.

We were not able to detect borreliae in our specimens, nor did we find signs of immune complex vasculitis, so the cause for the epineurial inflammatory infiltrations remains unknown. We have also no sound explanation for the perineurial distribution of IgA and IgM.

There is a striking similarity of our nerve biopsy findings with those reported in patients with MPN-GBB,[7,9,12,25] the other borrelial disease affecting the peripheral nervous system. Perivascular infiltration of the epineurial vessels and axonal nerve fiber degeneration in ACA were almost identical with the findings in sural nerve biopsies in cases with MPN-GBB. Perivascular cuffing of endoneurial vessels and degenerating perineurial cells could additionally be detected in MPN-GBB,[9,12,25] indicating a more pronounced disorder. This may be expressed clinically by the more acute and severe course of MPN-GBB. The extent of morphological changes seems to be greater in neuropathy of MPN-GBB than in ACA-related neuropathy. If other recent investigations[7,9,12,25] are considered, our results demonstrate that a common pathologic mechanism underlies the peripheral nerve involvement in clinically different borrelial diseases.

REFERENCES

1. ACKERMANN, R., B. REHSE-KÜPPER & E. GOLLMER. 1986. Progressive *Borrelia* encephalomyelitis. Zbl. Bakt. Hyg. A **263**: 297–300.
2. ÅSBRINK, E., A. HOVMARK & B. HEDERSTEDT. 1984. The spirochetal etiology of acrodermatitis chronica atrophicans Herxheimer. Acta Derm. Venereol. (Stockholm) **64**: 505–512.
3. BAUMHACKL, U., W. KRISTOFERITSCH, E. SLUGA & G. STANEK. 1986. Neurological manifestation of *Borrelia burgdorferi*-infections: the enlarging clinical spectrum. Zbl. Bakt. Hyg. A **263**: 334–336.
4. BENACH, J. L., E. M. BOSLER, J. P. HANRAHAN, J. L. COLEMAN, G. S. HABICHT, T. F. BAST, D. J. CAMERON, J. L. ZIEGLER, A. G. BARBOUR, W. BURGDORFER, R. EDELMAN & A. R. KASLOW. 1983. Spirochete isolated from the blood of two patients with Lyme disease. N. Engl. J. Med. **308**: 740–742.
5. BRYNDUM, B. & J. MARQUARDSEN. 1964. The tendon reflexes in old age. Gerontol. Clin. **6**: 257–265.
6. BURGDORFER, W., A. G. BARBOUR, S. F. HAYES, J. L. BENACH, E. GRUNWALDT & J. P. DAVID. 1982. Lyme disease—tick-borne spirochetosis? Science **216**: 1317–1319.
7. CAMPONOVO, F. & C. MEIER. 1986. Neuropathy of vasculitic origin in a case of Garin-Bujadoux-Bannwarth syndrome with positive borrelia antibody response. J. Neurol. **233**: 69–72.
8. DURAY, P. H., A. KUSNITZ & J. RYAN. 1985. Demonstration of the Lyme disease spirochete *Borrelia burgdorferi* by a modification of the Dieterle stain. Lab. Med. **16**: 685–687.
9. ENGELHARDT, A., F. GROHMANN & B. NEUDÖRFER. 1988. Vasculitic neuropathy in a case of Bannwarth's syndrome. Zbl. Bakt. Hyg. In press.
10. FAUCI, A. S., B. F. HAYNES & P. KATZ. 1978. The spectrum of vasculitis: Clinical, pathologic, immunologic, and therapeutic considerations. Ann. Intern. Med. **89**: 660–676.
11. GERN, L., E. FROSSARD, A. WALTER & A. AESCHLIMANN. 1988. Presence of antibodies against *Borrelia burgdorferi* in a human population of the Swiss plateau. Zbl. Bakt. Hyg. In press.
12. GREHL, H. & C. MEIER. 1988. Pathogenesis of neurological complications in Lyme borreliosis. Nerve biopsy findings and observations in tissue culture. Zbl. Bakt. Hyg. In press.

13. HOPF, H. C. 1966. Acrodermatitis chronica atrophicans (Herxheimer) und Nervensystem. Monographien aus dem Gesamtgebiet der Neurologie und Psychiatrie **114:** 1–130.
14. HOPF, H. C. 1975. Peripheral neuropathy in acrodermatitis chronica atrophicans (Herxheimer). J. Neurol. Neurosurg. Psychiatry **28:** 452–458.
15. HÖRSTRUP, P. & R. ACKERMANN. 1973. Durch Zecken übertragene Meningopolyneuritis (Garin-Bujadoux, Bannwarth). Fortschr. Neurol. Psychiatr. **41:** 583–606.
16. KAISER, M. 1972. Neurologische Komplikationen bei Acrodermatitis chronica atrophicans und ihre Beeinflussung durch die Penicillintherapie. M.D. Thesis, Universität Göttingen, Göttingen.
17. KRISTOFERITSCH, W., G. SPIEL & P. WESSELY. 1983. Zur Meningopolyneuritis (Garin-Bujadoux, Bannwarth): Klinik und Laborbefunde. Nervenarzt **54:** 640–646.
18. MAMOLI, B. & G. BRUNNER. 1984. Elektrophysiologische Untersuchungen bei Neuropathien. Wien. Klin. Wochenschr. **96** (Suppl. 147): 9–14.
19. MOORE, P. M. & A. S. FAUCI. 1981. Neurologic manifestations of systemic vasculitis. Am. J. Med. **71:** 517–524.
20. NEUDÖRFER, B., J. M. SCHRÖDER & D. CLAUS. 1987. Polyneuritiden und Polyneuropathien. Edition Medizin, VCH. Weinheim.
21. PACHNER, A. R., & A. C. STEERE. 1986. CNS manifestations of third stage Lyme disease. Zbl. Bakt. Hyg. A **263:** 301–306.
22. STANEK, G., A. HIRSCHL & W. KRISTOFERITSCH. 1986. IFA and ELISA in the serological diagnosis of Lyme borreliosis. Mitt. Österr. Ges. Trop. Parasitol. **8:** 1–6.
23. STEERE, A. C., N. H. BARTENHAGEN, J. E. CRAFT, G. J. HUTCHINSON, J. H. NEWMAN, A. R. PACHNER, D. W. RAHN, L. H. SIGAL, P. N. SPIELER, E. TAYLOR & S. E. MALAWISTA. 1986. Clinical manifestations of Lyme disease. Zbl. Bakt. Hyg. A **263:** 201–205.
24. STEERE, A. C., R. C. GRODZICKY, A. N. KORNBLATT, J. E. CRAFT, A. G. BARBOUR, W. BURGDORFER, G. P. SCHMID, E. JOHNSON & S. E. MALAWISTA. 1983. The spirochetal etiology of Lyme disease. N. Engl. J. Med. **308:** 733–739.
25. VALLAT, J. M., J. HUGON, M. LUBEAU, M. J. LEBOUTET, M. DUMAS & R. DESPROGES-GATTERON. 1987. Tick-bite meningoradiculoneuritis: Clinical, electrophysiologic, and histologic findings in 10 cases. Neurology **37:** 749–753.
26. WEES, S. J., I. N. SUNWOO & S. J. OH. 1981. Sural nerve biopsy in systemic necrotizing vasculitis. Am. J. Med. **71:** 525–532.

Clinical Manifestations and Diagnosis
of Neuroborreliosis

GÖRAN STIERNSTEDT,[a] ROLF GUSTAFSSON,[b]
MATS KARLSSON,[a] BO SVENUNGSSON,[b]
BIRGIT SKÖLDENBERG[a]

[a]Department of Infectious Diseases
Danderyd Hospital
S-182 88 Danderyd, Sweden

[b]Department of Infectious Diseases
Roslagstull Hospital, Box 5901
S-114 89 Stockholm, Sweden

In Sweden, the first case of erythema chronicum migrans (ECM) was described in 1909 by Afzelius.[1] By 1930 Hellerström had reported that ECM might be complicated by subsequent meningitis.[2] Hellerström was also the first to use penicillin for the treatment of neuroborreliosis when he successfully treated a patient with ECM and associated meningitis in 1950.[3] From these observations one might conclude that neuroborreliosis has existed in Sweden for more than 50 years. However, it was not until Steere in 1975 described Lyme disease in the Unites States[4] and Burgdorfer in 1982 isolated the etiologic agent[5] that ECM with or without meningitis received real interest in Sweden. Serological assays have been available in Sweden since 1984 and the number of serologically verified cases of Lyme borreliosis has steadily increased (TABLE 1).[6] The total number of cases of Lyme borreliosis has increased threefold from 1984 to 1986 (TABLE 1). The majority of serologically verified cases of Lyme borreliosis suffer from neuroborreliosis, but one must remember that cases of ECM, the most common manifestation of Lyme borreliosis, are seldom serologically verified. More than 200 cases of neuroborreliosis were diagnosed in 1986.[6] *Borrelia is today the most common bacterial pathogen of the nervous system in Sweden.*

Lyme borreliosis is usually divided into three distinct stages (TABLE 2), often with symptom-free intervals between the stages. These stages might overlap and they might also occur alone. In stage 1, ECM might be accompanied by symptoms imitating meningitis, but CSF is in most cases normal and consequently neuroborreliosis should not be regarded as a stage 1 manifestation. Most patients with neuroborreliosis are usually classified as stage 2. In this stage most patients have meningitis and/or predominantly symptoms from the peripheral nervous system. Stage 3 of neuroborreliosis is less frequent and in this stage symptoms from the central nervous system usually appear. However, on clinical grounds it is difficult to distinguish if patients with neuroborreliosis belong to stage 2 or 3, as patients with neurological manifestations of Lyme borreliosis often lack a symptom-free interval between stage 2 and 3. Furthermore, there is today no definition derived from disease duration that could be used to classify a patient as stage 2 or 3.

CLINICAL MANIFESTATIONS OF NEUROBORRELIOSIS

In a previous study on clinical manifestations of neuroborreliosis in Sweden, we described 46 patients treated at two different departments of infectious diseases in

TABLE 1. Serologically Verified Cases of Lyme Borreliosis and Neuroborreliosis in Sweden 1984–86

	1984	1985	1986
Lyme borreliosis, total	112	256	374
Neuroborreliosis	72	167	208

Stockholm during a 9-year period from 1975 to 1983.[7] In the present study, data will be presented of 75 other patients with neuroborreliosis treated at the same clinics during a 3-year period from 1984 to 1986. These 75 patients fulfilled at least one of the following inclusion criteria:

1. Pleocytosis in cerebrospinal fluid (CSF) and positive *Borrelia* serology in serum and/or CSF.
2. Neurological signs and positive serology in serum and/or CSF.
3. Neurological signs following ECM within 3 months.

Groups 2 and 3 were included in order to search for patients without pleocytosis in CSF and also for patients who might be serologically negative.

Demographic data of the 75 patients in comparison with corresponding data of the 46 patients in the previous study[7] are shown in TABLE 3. Most patients with neuroborreliosis were women, but there was a slight tendency towards a more even sex distribution in the present study in comparison with the previous study. Ages of patients have varied between 4 and 82 years. However, no conclusions regarding the age distribution could be drawn, since children with neuroborreliosis in Sweden often are treated at pediatric departments and therefore not included in the studies. Data from all serologically verified cases of Lyme borreliosis in Sweden show that the incidence is highest among children between 5 and 15 years of age, and among adults over 50 years of age. Boys dominate among children whereas women predominate among adults.

Clinical manifestations are presented in TABLE 4. Symptoms such as fatigue, headache, migrating myalgias, and low-grade fever are important and common but rather unspecific. Among symptoms found in the peripheral nervous system, facial palsy and radicular pain are the most common. The present and other studies have shown that *Borrelia* might cause different kinds of peripheral paresis.[8] *Borrelia* may also affect most cranial nerves. It is important to stress that occasionally involvement of cranial nerves may have serious consequences for the individual patient. Impaired hearing has appeared when the auditory nerve is affected. Another serious manifestation reported is blindness.[9] In 1987 we saw one patient with bilateral atrophy of the opticus nerve caused by *Borrelia*. The patient became almost completely blind.

TABLE 2. Clinical Stages of Lyme Borreliosis

Stage 1	Erythema chronicum migrans (ECM)
	Lymphadenosis benigna cutis (LABC)
Stage 2	Carditis
	Neurological disease
	Arthritis
Stage 3	Chronic neurological disease
	Chronic arthritis
	Acrodermatitis chronica atrophicans Herxheimer (ACA)

TABLE 3. Some Demographic Data of Swedish Patients with Neuroborreliosis.

	Series II 1984–86	Series I[a] 1975–83
No. of patients	75	46
Male : female ratio	0.74	0.64
Age (median)	48	50
Age (range)	6–77	4–82

[a]From Stiernstedt et al.[7]

Central nervous system manifestations that appear to be most common are paraparesis and ataxia. Several reports of dementia and personality changes occurring in neuroborreliosis patients have been published.[8,10] One patient in the present study had loss of hearing, disorientation and change of personality.

Another way of showing the broad clinical spectrum of neuroborreliosis is by examples of how the symptoms and signs listed were interpreted by the patients and physicians before the diagnosis of neuroborreliosis was set. In our experience, patients with neuroborreliosis might appear within all medical disciplines. Radicular pain may

TABLE 4. Symptoms and Signs in 75 + 46 Swedish Patients with Neuroborreliosis

	% of Patients	
	Series II 1984–86 ($n = 75$)	Series I[a] 1975–83 ($n = 46$)
General or Meningeal Symptoms		
Fatigue	72	65
Headache	64	54
Fever		
≥ 37.5	49	50
≥ 38.5	20	15
Weight loss	40	59
Malaise	29	46
Vomiting	19	26
Neck stiffness	28	17
Peripheral Nerve Symptoms		
Facial nerve	35	37
Abducens nerve	4	9
Oculomotor nerve	0	2
Auditory nerve	1	4
Trigeminal nerve	1	4
Glossopharyngeal nerve	1	0
Vestibular nerve	1	0
Other peripheral paralysis	5	9
Dysesthesia	13	24
Radicular pain	55	65
CNS Symptoms		
Hemiparesis	0	7
Paraparesis	4	4
Ataxia	4	2
Dementia	1	0

[a]From Stiernstedt et al.[7]

be interpreted as abdominal pain, and when accompanied by vomiting diagnosed as gastric ulcer. In several of our patients gastroscopy has been performed. One Swedish patient was colecystectomized because of right-sided radicular pain interpreted as gall bladder disease. Other patients have been diagnosed as renal calculus and subjected to investigations of their urinary tract. Orthopedic surgeons are also likely to have contact with neuroborreliosis patients. The combination of lumbar pain and radiating pain in one leg imitates a herniated disk, and several of our patients have been investigated with CT scan and/or myeolgraphy. Cervical pain is common among patients with neuroborreliosis, and several patients have been diagnosed as having cervical rhizopathy.

The ophthalmologists must be aware that *Borrelia* might cause eye muscle paresis and, as mentioned above, unilateral or bilateral blindness. For the otolaryngologists neuroborreliosis is also a reality. According to Swedish investigations, *Borrelia* is the etiology of 15–25% of Bell's palsy cases in Sweden.[11,12] Vestibular neuritis, impaired hearing, and possibly deafness might also be caused by *Borrelia*.

To specialists in internal medicine neuroborreliosis might imitate stroke, but we also know of patients with neuroborreliosis who have been hospitalized with suspected myocardial infarction because of severe thoracal radicular pain. Extreme fatigue, anorexia, and loss of weight has resulted in endocrine investigations. Myalgias and athralgias might indicate rheumatological disease to the physician.

To the neurologist neuroborreliosis might appear as a multiple-sclerosis-like disease. Neuroborreliosis might also imitate brain tumor. Furthermore, the syndrome of pseudotumor cerebri, *i.e.,* papilloedema and high intracranial pressure with normal CSF, may have *Borrelia* as one of several possible etiologies.[13] One child with this syndrome has been recognized in Sweden (study unpublished).

Neuroborreliosis might imitate cancer. Symptoms such as loss of weight and pain appear malignant. Furthermore we have also found that mononuclear cells found in CSF might appear atypical and malignant. Two patients in Sweden have been misdiagnosed as having meningeal lymphoma. One of them also received radiation treatment of the head, which she survived.

To specialists in infectious diseases, neuroborreliosis might appear as subacute meningitis and has most probably often been misdiagnosed as viral meningitis. One striking finding is how mild the meningitis might appear. Several patients have only slight headache and very mild discomfort, and they might look completely healthy and show no neck stiffness. Although high fever is unusual in patients with *Borrelia* meningitis, it may in a few patients be a dominating symptom. Patients with neuroborreliosis have been hospitalized for fever of unknown origin, and weeks have passed before a lumbar puncture has been performed and the diagnosis settled.

Different psychiatric symptoms may be associated with neuroborreliosis. Mental depression and personality changes might lead to psychiatric hospitalization. Other patients have been suspected of suffering from anorexia nervosa. One of our patients was hospitalized at an alcoholism ward for tremor, bilateral leg paresis, and change of personality. *Borrelia* has also been reported to cause dementia.[8,10]

DIAGNOSIS OF NEUROBORRELIOSIS

Neuroborreliosis is a great disease imitator, as can be seen from the overview given above. On the other hand, none of the symptoms discussed are specific to *Borrelia,* and consequently diagnostic tests are of utmost importance. However, not only specific serological tests but also more nonspecific clinical clues such as tick bite and ECM are

TABLE 5. Preceding Markers in 75 + 46 Swedish Patients with Neuroborreliosis

	% of Patients	
	Series II 1984–85 ($n = 75$)	Series I[a] 1975–83 ($n = 46$)
Tick bite	56	28
ECM	43	35
None	33	—

[a]From Stiernstedt et al.[7]

important. Neuroborreliosis is also in most instances associated with CSF abnormalities, which could be diagnostically useful in combination with the symptoms and signs of the individual patient.

Clinical Markers for Neuroborreliosis

Important clinical markers for neuroborreliosis are tick bite and ECM. ECM is of course the most important one and should be regarded as a specific marker for neuroborreliosis. The number of patients remembering preceding tick bite and/or erythema migrans has increased significantly in the present study in comparison with our previous study (TABLE 5). This finding is probably explained by the increased knowledge of the markers among both patients and physicians. Still, however, 33% of our patients with neuroborreliosis lacked both preceding ECM and tick bite.

In a Swedish study of neuroborreliosis in children five of nine patients studied had unilateral facial palsy.[14] All five of these patients had had preceding ECM localized to the face at the same side on which the paresis later developed. In the present study of 75 patients, 26 suffered from facial palsy, 10 of whom reported of a preceding ECM. In five of these 10 patients the preceding skin lesion was situated in the face, and in all five patients it was localized to the same side as the subsequent facial palsy. Forty-two of 75 patients in the present study had radicular pain. In 12 of these 42 patients the radicular pain was strictly localized to one extremity during the whole course of the neuroborreliosis. Ten of these 12 patients had had a preceding ECM, and in eight of these 10 patients the skin lesion was situated at the same side as the subsequent radiculoneuritis. We think that these findings support neural spread as one mechanism by which the spirochete reaches the central nervous system.

TABLE 6. Cerebrospinal Fluid Parameters in 75 Swedish Patients with Neuroborreliosis

Spinal leukocytes ($\times 10^6/l$) $\geq 5 \times 10^6/l$ Mean: $215 \times 10^6/l$ Range: $0–1400 \times 10^6/l$	70/75 patients (93%)
Spinal protein (g/l) >0.5 g/l Mean: 1.3 g/l Range: 0.3–6.2 g/l	56/68 patients (82%)
CSF/blood glucose ratio <0.5	10/68 patients (15%)

Cerebrospinal Fluid Abnormalities

Pleocytosis in CSF is in many patients with neuroborreliosis a very important clue to the diagnosis. The combination of certain neurological signs, such as radicular pain and/or facial palsy, in combination with pleocytosis is often strong evidence that the patient's actual disease has a borrelial etiology. In the present study the cell count in CSF varied between 0 and $1400 \times 10^6/1$ CSF, with a mean cell count of $215 \times 10^6/1$ CSF (TABLE 6). Five of 75 patients had a normal cell count. One of these patients had an elevated CSF protein of 0.8 g/l and consequently the CSF was normal for all parameters in 4 of 75 patients. Percentage of mononuclear cells was more than 90% in 53 of 70 (76%) of the patients. Only two out of 70 (3%) patients had less than 50% mononuclear cells (TABLE 6).

Spinal protein was normal (≤ 0.5 g/l) in 12 out of 68 (18%) patients (data missing from seven patients). Another seven patients had a protein content of CSF that was only slightly elevated (0.6–0.7 g/l). The mean protein content was 1.3 g/l CSF (TABLE 6), which is a significant decrease in comparison with the previous study (2.4 g/l CSF). The explanation of this decrease is the shorter mean disease duration in the present study. High CSF protein content is mainly seen in patients with a long duration of the disease. Another parameter, the CSF:blood glucose ratio, is also influenced by the

TABLE 7. Result of *Borrelia* CSF and Serum Serology in 75 Swedish Patients with Neuroborreliosis

	Patients Serologically Positive in:			
	Serum + CSF	Serum Only	CSF Only	Negative Serum + CSF
No. of patients (%)	36 (48)	12 (16)	18 (24)	9 (12)
Median disease duration, weeks	6	3	3	1
Range, weeks	0.5–90	0–8	1–6	0–3
No. of patients with preceding ECM (%)	13 (36)	7 (58)	6 (33)	7 (78)

duration of disease. Consequently, a much lower percentage of the patients in the present study, 10 of 68 (15%), had a ratio of <0.5 as compared with 40% in the previous study.[7]

In previous reports,[7,15] we have stressed the typical pattern of intrathecal immunoglobulin production with raised IgG index and oligoclonal bands in electrophoresis or isoelectric focusing of CSF. However, we have found that today many patients lack these indications of intrathecal IgG production, again because of disease duration. A disease duration of 4–5 weeks is neccessary before the IgG index rises and oligoclonal bands in CSF appear.

Serological Diagnosis of Neuroborreliosis

Antibodies to *Borrelia* were measured by an ELISA assay using sonicated whole cell antigen.[16] Antibody titers were determined in both CSF and serum in all 75 patients studied. Twelve out of 75 (48%) patients were positive in both CSF and serum serology (TABLE 7). Eighteen out of 75 (24%) were positive only in CSF serology and 12 out of 75 (16%) were positive only in serum serology. Nine out of 75 (12%) were negative in all serological assays. The total sensitivity of the CSF assay was 72% and the total sensitivity of the serum assay was 64%. The median disease duration differed between patients in these different groups. The nine patients who were negative in all serological assays had a median disease duration of only 1 week and none of the patients in this group had a disease duration of more than 3 weeks. Both patients positive only in serum serology and patients positive only in CSF serology had a median disease duration of 3 weeks. The longest median disease duration (6 weeks) showed patients positive both in CSF and serum serology.

Most probably, the matter of positivity in serum or CSF or both depend on the duration of immune stimulation in serum and CSF, respectively. If the primary immune response takes place in serum, the serum response will appear before the CSF response. If the antibody response in serum is inadequate when the spirochete is localized to the skin, the primary immune response in patients with neuroborreliosis will appear intrathecally. If, however, the disease duration and duration of immune stimulation is long enough, the patients will become positive in both serum and CSF. Further support for this theory was the tendency towards a higher percentage of patients with preceding ECM, 58%, among patients who were only positive in serum serology as compared with approximately 35% among patients who were positive in only CSF serology or who were positive in both serum and CSF serology (TABLE 7). It seems likely that the chance of having a primary serum antibody response is higher in patients with preceding ECM than without. This finding might also partly explain previous differences reported for American and European patients with neuroborreliosis. Positive serum titers have been found in nearly 100% of American neuroborreliosis patients. To my knowledge nearly all patients in the American studies have had ECM before neurological infection developed. In European studies, most patients lacked preceding ECM.

The whole-cell antigen used so far in most ELISA assays might also explain reported differences in sensitivity of serum and CSF antibody estimation. When using such an antigen, the level of nonspecific antibody titers in serum is high. It seems likely that the background is lower in CSF, which probably contains fewer cross-reacting substances. Dr. Hansen and collaborators in Denmark have recently presented data that pointed in this direction.[19] When they used the whole-cell antigen, CSF serology was much more sensitive than serum serology. This difference in sensitivity was almost completely eliminated when they used a preparation of flagella antigen. This antigen also resulted in a significantly lower background in serum. We achieved corresponding results when using Western blot technique. Patients with a short disease duration who were negative in serum serology had in many cases *Borrelia*-specific antibodies when examined with Western blot.[20] These specific antibodies were often directed towards the 42 kDa protein, which is identical with the flagella antigen.

Although the serum serology might become more sensitive if a purer antigen is used, the importance of performing CSF serology in cases of neuroborreliosis should be stressed. One problem with the serum assay is that many patients have specific *Borrelia* antibodies due to earlier clinical or subclinical infection. Such infections are far from uncommon, especially as *Borrelia* has turned out to be much more common than earlier believed. Several studies have shown that subclinical infections exist.[21,22] This means that although a purer antigen is used, we still have patients with elevated titers not due to unspecific background but instead due to earlier infection. In such cases, the IgM-assay is of course of special importance to settle if the elevated titer is due to an old infection or is a result of the patient's actual disease. However, one problem with *Borrelia* is that the IgM response might also be rather long-lasting. We also know that the IgM assay is more problematic than the IgG assay, with a greater interassay variation. Consequently, we might also have positive IgM titers due to previous infection. The chance that positive CSF titers are due to previous infection is logically much less. Therefore, positive CSF titers are much more specific than slightly or moderately elevated serum titers.

In order to achieve a great degree of specificity in the CSF assay, the leakage of antibodies over the CSF-blood barrier must be taken into consideration, especially in patients who are seropositive and who have a highly damaged barrier. Estimation of the barrier damage may be performed by comparing the CSF : serum titer ratio with the corresponding albumin ratio[16] or with the corresponding ratio of antibody titers towards a control antigen, e.g., measles.

Demonstration of intrathecally produced specific antibodies points toward a direct connection with the patients' ongoing neurological disease. However, one must be aware that there may be one exception to this rule. According to preliminary results, patients with neuroborreliosis may have signs of intrathecal synthesis of *Borrelia* antibodies for months and even years after adequate treatment. Therefore, in a few cases, CSF antibodies might also be due to previous infection, but most probably such an infection is symptomatic and could be recognized in the patient's disease history.

The relation between serum and CSF antibody titer is complex. Serum and CSF should be regarded as two different compartments of antibody synthesis with a certain degree of transportation between the two compartments. The antibody level in these two compartments will depend on the degree of barrier damage, the duration of immune stimulation in the two compartments, and previous exposure to *Borrelia*.

There is one further disadvantage with the present whole-cell antigen. We have examined the same serum and CSF samples in ELISA using different *Borrelia* strains as antigen and also different batches of the same antigen. Although such tests are difficult to standardize, our results indicated considerable variations between different strains and also between different batches of the same strain. The explanation of these results are probably that the composition of different antigenic proteins varies between strains and batches. A better standardization with the same amount of protein in different batches is desirable.

Other Methods of Diagnosing Neuroborreliosis

Cultivation of spirochetes from the CSF is one further possibility for diagnosing neuroborreliosis. However, the chance of success seems small and the reports in the literature of such isolations are sparse. We have succeeded so far in only four out of approximately 50 attempts in patients with *Borrelia* infection of the nervous system verified by serology. Furthermore, it usually takes weeks before detection of spirochetes in the culture is possible, a great disadvantage, and cultivation of spirochetes from CSF will most probably remain a method reserved for scientific work.

To demonstrate specific *Borrelia* antigen in CSF would be the ideal method to dignose neuroborreliosis, since it would be a rapid method. We have tried but not succeeded so far. Unfortunately, there is a great possibility that the antigen concentrations in CSF are too small to allow detection. The difficulties in cultivating spirochetes from CSF may support this theory.

SUMMARY

Lyme borreliosis has in a few years turned out to be a health problem not only in the United States, but also in many European countries. When it affects the nervous system, Lyme borreliosis acts as the great disease imitator. Because of this characteristic it is often difficult to diagnose on clinical grounds. Patients with neuroborreliosis might appear within all medical disciplines. Clinical markers, such as preceding tick bite and/or ECM, are important clues to the diagnosis. Mononuclear pleocytosis and elevated CSF protein are present in most patients with neuroborreliosis. Final evidence for the diagnosis is the demonstration of specific antibodies in serum and/or CSF. Measurement of antibody titers should be carried out in both serum and CSF, since these methods are complementary when trying to obtain a serological diagnosis of neuroborreliosis.

REFERENCES

1. AFZELIUS, A. 1910. Verhandlungen der Dermatologischen Gesellschaft zu Stockholm. Arch. Dermatol. Syph. **101:** 404.
2. HELLERSTRÖM, S. 1930. Erythema chronicum migrans Afzelii. Acta Derm. Venereol. **11:** 315–321.
3. HELLERSTRÖM S. 1951. Erythema chronicum migrans Afzelius with meningitis. Acta Derm. Venereol. **31:** 227–234.
4. STEERE, A. C., S. E. MALAWISTA, J. A. HARDIN, S. RUDDY, P. W. ASKENASE & W. A. ANDIMAN. 1977. Erythema chronicum migrans and Lyme arthritis. The enlarging clinical spectrum. Ann. Intern. Med. **86:** 685–698.
5. BURGDORFER, W., A. G. BARBOUR, S. F. HAYES, J. L. BENACH, E. GRUNWALDT & J. P. DAVIS. 1982. Lyme disease—a tick-borne spirochetosis? Science **216:** 1316–1319.
6. LANNER, M., B. HEDERSTEDT, E. ÅSBRINK, A. HOVMARK & G. STIERNSTEDT. 1987. Serodiagnosis of Borrelia infection during 1986 in Sweden. Presented at Lyme Borreliosis: Update Europe, Baden, Austria.
7. STIERNSTEDT, G., B. SKÖLDENBERG, A. GÄRDE, G. KOLMODIN, H. JÖRBECK, B. SVENUNGSSON & A. CARLSTRÖM. 1986. Clinical manifestations of Borrelia infections of the nervous system. Zbl. Bakt. Hyg. A **263:** 289–296.
8. PACHNER, A. R. & A. C. STEERE. 1985. The triad of neurologic manifestation of Lyme disease: meningitis, cranial neuritis, and radiculoneuritis. Neurology **35:** 47.
9. STEERE, A. C. et al. 1985. Unilateral blindness caused by infection with the Lyme disease spirochete, Borrelia burgdorferi. Ann. Intern. Med. **103:** 382–384.
10. REIK, L., W. BURGDORFER & J. O. DONALDSON. 1986. Neurologic abnormalities in Lyme disease without erythema chronicum migrans. Am. J. Med. **81:** 73.
11. JONSSON, L., G. STIERNSTEDT & L. THOMANDER. 1987. Tick-borne Borrelia infection in patients with Bell's palsy. Arch. Otolaryngol. Head Neck Surg. **113:** 303–306.
12. ASBRINK, E., I. OLSSON, A. HOVMARK, et al. 1985. Tick-borne spirochetes as a cause of facial palsy. Clin. Otolaryngol. **10:** 279–284.
13. RAUCHER, H. S., D. M. KAUFMAN, J. GOLDFARB, R. I. JACOBSON, B. ROSEMAN & R. R. WOLFF. 1985. Pseudotumor cerebri and Lyme disease: A new association. J. Pediatr. **107:** 931–933.
14. JÖRBECK, H. J. A., P. M. GUSTAFSSON, H. C. F. LIND & G. T. STIERNSTEDT. 1987. Tick-borne Borrelia-meningitis in children. An outbreak in the Kalmar area during the summer of 1984. Acta Paediatr. Scand. **76:** 228–233.
15. STIERNSTEDT, G. 1985. Tick-borne Borrelia infection in Sweden. Scand. J. Infect. Dis. Suppl. **45:** 1–70.
16. STIERNSTEDT, G. T., M. GRANSTRÖM, B. HEDERSTEDT & B. SKÖLDENBERG. 1985. Diagnosis of spirochetal meningitis by enzyme-linked immunosorbent assay and indirect immunofluorescence assay in serum and cerebrospinal fluid. J. Clin. Microbiol. **21(5):** 819–825.
17. CRAFT, J. E., R. L. GRODZICKI & A. C. STEERE. 1984. Antibody response in Lyme disease: Evaluation of diagnostic tests. J. Infect Dis. **149:** 789–795.
18. RUSSELL, H., J. S. SAMPSON, G. P. SCHMID, H. W. WILKINSON & B. PLIKAYTIS. 1984.

Enzyme-linked immunosorbent assay and indirect immunofluorescence assay for Lyme disease. J. Infect. Dis. **149:** 465–470.

19. HANSEN, K. *et al.* 1987. Improved serodiagnosis of lymphocytic meningoradiculitis (Bannwarth's syndrome) by an ELISA for IgG and IgM antibodies in serum and CSF against the *Borrelia burgdorferi* flagellum (abstract no. 40). International Conference on Lyme Disease and Related Disorders, New York, Sept. 14-16.

20. KARLSSON, M. *et al.* 1988. Western blot analysis of serum and cerebrospinal fluid antibodies to *Borrelia* strains in patients with *Borrelia* meningitis. This volume.

21. HANRAHAN, J. P., J. L. BENACH, J. L. COLEMAN, E. M. BOSLER, D. L. MORSE, D. J. CAMERON, R. EDELMAN & R. A. KASLOW. 1984. Incidence and cumulative frequency of endemic Lyme disease in a community. J. Infect. Dis. **150:** 489–496.

22. STEERE, A. C., E. TAYLOR, M. L. WILSON, J. F. LEVINE & A. SPIELMAN. 1986. Longitudinal assessment of the clinical and epidemiological features of Lyme disease in a defined population. J. Infect. Dis. **154:** 295–300.

Borrelia burgdorferi in the Nervous System: The New "Great Imitator"

ANDREW R. PACHNER

Department of Neurology
Georgetown University School of Medicine
Washington, D.C. 20007

Lyme disease, first described in 1977,[1] is becoming an increasingly severe public health problem. Neurological manifestations have always been a prominent feature of the illness; Bannwarth's syndrome,[2] also called syndrome of Garin-Bujadoux,[3] a lymphocytic meningoradiculitis now known to be caused by *B. burgdorferi*, has been a relatively common illness for decades in Europe. A subacute meningitis, frequently accompanied by radiculoneuritis or cranial neuritis, is the most common presentation of Lyme disease in Europe, and has been the subject of numerous publications on both sides of the Atlantic.[4-7] What has become clear over the last few years is that the clinical presentation of Lyme disease in the nervous system is not limited to this meningoradiculoneuritis[8-12] and that a number of clinical syndromes associated with CNS damage occur, especially in the later stages of the disease.

LYME MENINGORADICULONEURITIS

The meningoradiculoneuritis of Lyme disease generally is relatively easy to diagnose because of frequent association with ECM or a tick bite weeks to months earlier, its occurrence in the summer or early fall, and the lymphocytic pleocytosis in the CSF clearing quickly with penicillin, along with the majority of the symptoms. Radicular pain is seen more frequently in Europe than in the Unites States, but in all other respects Lyme meningitis is indistinguishable from the Bannwarth-Garin-Bujadoux syndrome. Sometimes the peripheral involvement at this stage of the disease, which can take the form of pain and/or weakness determined by the distribution of roots ("radiculitis") or peripheral nerves ("plexitis" or "neuritis"), can mimic the Guillain-Barré syndrome or a cervical disk, but in general the diagnosis can be made easily by neurologists in endemic areas. The occasional culturing of *B. burgdorferi* from cerebrospinal fluid of patients with Lyme meningitis indicates that it is probably due to direct invasion by the organism. Occasionally, patients have lingering symptoms of malaise and/or fatigue, but we have not seen any patients develop recurrent meningitis, arthritis, or later CNS involvement after adequate intravenous penicillin therapy for 10–14 days of 20 million units per day in divided doses. This form of involvement of the nervous system occurs within the second stage of the disease, weeks to a few months after the initial infection; the ECM and flu-like illness occur within a few days to a week or two after infection.[13] Occasionally CNS involvement (long-tract signs, significant encephalitis, posterior fossa involvement) can be seen in the second stage (case report no. 1, see APPENDIX), but this is unusual.

CNS INVOLVEMENT IN LYME DISEASE

There is ample evidence that

1. Chronic, parenchymal CNS involvement, manifesting months to years after initial infection, can occur if Lyme disease is not adequately treated in its early stages.
2. This form of the disease can be very difficult to diagnose definitively.
3. CNS involvement in *B. burgdorferi* infection can mimic other diseases.
4. This "tertiary" form does not respond to intravenous penicillin as well as does the second stage meningitis.

In the last 2 years (1985–87) my outpatient experience in Connecticut with neruological manifestations of Lyme disease has been predominantly with CNS involvement as opposed to second-stage disease. This is because both ECM and Lyme meningitis, previously felt to be arcane problems needing referral to the medical center, now are treated routinely by community physicians in endemic areas of Connecticut. Of 58 patients primarily referred for diagnosis or treatment of Lyme disease, 13 had no evidence for Lyme disease, and their neurologial symptoms either resolved spontaneously or developed into other disease processes (lumbosacral disk, depression, neuropathy of unknown cause, etc.). Ten patients had Lyme meningitis and were treated successfully with i.v. penicillin. Nine patients (all female) were in a borderline group, because of absence of definite positive serology or absence of a clear relationship of Lyme disease to their neurological picture.

The diagnosis of CNS Lyme disease in 26 patients was made on the basis of the presence of CNS abnormalities without another documented cause, a positive serology for *B. burgdorferi*, and residence in an area endemic for Lyme disease; supporting data included past or present symptoms or signs of Lyme disease in other organ systems and resolution of CNS abnormalities with penicillin therapy. Patients with all five of these criteria were considered to have definite CNS Lyme disease. We have not found selective concentration of anti-*B. burgdorferi* antibody in the CSF to be helpful diagnostically, even in patients with Lyme meningitis. CSF or blood cultures have not proved to be helpful because of very low yield. In one of our patients a brain biopsy obtained because of the possibility of herpes encephalitis revealed spirochetes, but this is obviously not a diagnostic procedure that can be commonly used. Seventeen of the 26 patients with CNS Lyme disease did not have all five criteria, sometimes because they refused treatment or other manifestations of Lyme disease were not present.

Seventeen males and nine females had third-stage CNS manifestations. Fifteen were from Connecticut, six from Westchester County or Long Island in New York, three from endemic areas of New Jersey, and two from Massachusetts (Boston and Nantucket). The most common presentation (13 pts.) was diffuse, chronic brain involvement leading to behavioral changes (case report 2), memory difficulty, or subacute encephalitis (case report 3). Nine of these patients were 18 or younger at the time of their first symptoms. Treatment with i.v. PCN was generally successful in five, unclear in another three, and clearly unsuccessful in two. Successful therapy in one patient with dementia was documented with serial neuropsychological testing.

Six patients had relapsing-remitting episodes of focal CNS disease, sometimes mimicking multiple sclerosis (MS). In fact, one of these patients, case report 4, had been diagnosed as having MS by the chairman of a major medical center in the Northeast; he responded completely to i.v. PCN, with a 2-year F/U period. In another patient, the possibility exists that Lyme disease and MS coexist, since antibiotic therapy did not prevent two subsequent episodes of demyelination (case report 5); alternatively, "MS"-like Lyme disease in the brain may not universally respond to i.v. penicillin (case report 6).

Four patients had chronic, incapacitating fatigue as their major chronic complaint. Their neurological examination was normal. In some of these, fatigue was not constant, and often weeks would go by without symptoms. The patient would then be disabled with enervating fatigue for a few weeks, after which normal strength would return. One patient had only seizures (without prior Lyme meningitis), and two patients had had Lyme meningitis with neuritis that had gone unrecognized and presented with severe progressive radiculoneuritis.

Treatment with 2 weeks of i.v. PCN (20 million units per day) was clearly successful in 12 patients, clearly unsuccessful in seven patients, of unclear outcome in four patients, and not tried in three patients.

Experience at Other Medical Centers

Although it was initially questioned whether Lyme disease caused CNS abnormalities, investigators in both America and Europe have recently reported several patients with CNS abnormalities usually associated with more typical stage 2 neurologic manifestations of Lyme disease, and in some cases, these abnormalities were progressive and led to permanent neurologic deficit. Ackermann and his colleagues in West Germany reported eight patients (one in detail) with CNS involvement, most commonly spastic parapareses.[12] This infection, which they called progressive borrelial encephalomyelitis, lasted for 1 to 8 years, and sometimes left permanent deficits, including dementia. In one series from Sweden, seven patients with stage 2 neurologic involvement also had CNS symptoms, including hemiparesis, spastic paraparesis, or ataxia.[7] In Denmark, three of 18 reported patients had severe CNS lesions—transverse myelitis and spastic paraparesis, focal encephalitis with hemiparesis, and dementia with gait disturbances.[14] Several similar cases have been noted in Hungary and Yugoslavia.[15,16] In the United States, Reik et al. reported two patients with encephalitis, seizures, dementia, or myelitis due to Lyme disease.[10,17]

SUMMARY

There are many obvious similarities between Lyme disease and syphilis. The major ones are their spirochetal etiology, the ability of the spirochetes to stay alive in human tissue for years, occurrence of clinical manifestations in stages, early disease in the skin and later disease in the brain, and susceptibility to antibiotic treatment. Thus, one can assume that many of the same lessons learned from the centuries of experience with syphilis will apply to Lyme disease. One of these lessons that should be constantly borne in mind is that spirochetal disease of the brain can mimic many other neurological diseases. Thus, the "effective clinician"[18] must take special care to consider Lyme disease primarily because of the excellent response to antibiotics early in its course in relationship to some of the diseases it mimics.

Lyme meningitis, occurring in the "second stage" of the disease, usually is fairly easily recognized because it occurs in the summer or early fall, often is associated with ECM or a recent history of it, and has a characteristic clinical picture of lymphocytic meningoradiculoneuritis. Many patients with Lyme meningitis or ECM have very mild symptoms, and it is likely that a large percentage of patients go undiagnosed and untreated. The frequency of progression of these patients to third-stage disease is unknown but may be quite high. This can be inferred from a similar situation in the other major late manifestation of Lyme disease: Lyme arthritis. A large number of patients present with joint involvement as their only manifestation of Lyme disease. Similarly, patients may present with symptoms of third-stage Lyme disease affecting the CNS, but they may not be recognized because of the lack of earlier stages usually associated with the disease.

Thus, serology has become a very important tool for identifying patients exposed to *B. burgdorferi*. At the present time, serologic tests are the key to diagnosis of Lyme disease in its later stages, since, as in neurosyphilis, cultures and tests for antigen have not proven useful.[19] Lyme arthritis and acrodermatitis atrophicans (ACA) both are associated with quite high antibody titers to the organism, while the test is understandably unreliable for identification of patients with ECM. Antibody titers in Lyme meningoradiculoneuritis are generally positive but often are not as high as those in ACA or arthritis. The antibody response in serum in CNS Lyme disease seems to be related to the presence of other manifestations; patients who have had both arthritis and CNS disease have quite high titers, while those with only CNS disease sometimes do not. For instance, our patient with brain-biopsy documented infection, who also had *B. burgdorferi*-reactive lymphocytes in his CSF, had a relatively low titer of serum antibody (1 : 400 with normal being less than 1 : 200).[20] Unfortunately, there is a great deal of variability in the performance of anti-*B. burgdorferi* antibody titers[21]; what is considered normal in one lab is considered positive in another, and vice versa. Interpretation may thus be difficult, and if a strong suspicion exists for the presence of Lyme disease and antibody response is negative at one laboratory, it would be advisable to confirm the titers at another lab.

CNS infection usually is associated with an inflammatory response, and, in our patients with Lyme meningoradiculoneuritis, a lymphocytic pleocytosis was found in all.[27] However, in CNS involvement in Lyme disease, pleocytosis may not be present. A comparable situation exists in HIV-3 infection: in chronic infection of the brain, a CSF pleocytosis is uncommon, the protein concentration is normal, and there is no significant selective concentration of anti-HIV antibody in the CSF. In six of our patients who best fulfilled diagnostic criteria for CNS Lyme disease,[9] a pleocytosis was absent in two, and none had selective concentration of anti-*B. burgdorferi* antibody.

The lack of response of some of these patients to antibiotics, the lack of correlation of clinical manifestations with signs of infection, and the difficulty in finding organisms in affected tissues raises the possibility that some manifestations are parainfectious, rather than infectious. Supporting this hypothesis are the findings of (i) antibody in the serum of patients with Lyme meningoradiculoneuritis cross-reacting with peripheral nerve antigens,[22] and (ii) T-cell clones from the CSF of Lyme patients reacting with myelin basic protein.[23] Thus, it is possible that the underlying pathogenesis of nervous system involvement may differ between patients, or even for different manifestations within the same patient. This may have direct application to treatment: patient AD (case report no. 6), who had progressive disease unresponsive to intravenous antibiotics, had a prolonged disease-free interval after cyclophosphamide treatment.

Recommendations

Diagnosis

The index of suspicion for the *B. burgdorferi* infection as the causative agent of neurological syndromes in endemic areas must be very high. Our patients with Lyme neurological involvement all had positive antibody titers, and positive serology was used as a diagnostic criterion; in chronic infections of the brain, antibody in the serum is not always detectable,[24] and it is conceivable that some patients have *B. burgdorferi* in the brain, but do not have positive serologies. However, until more studies are performed and antibody-negative patients identified, serology (from a trustworthy laboratory) remains the best way of identifying patients with CNS Lyme disease, especially those without other manifestations of the disease. Thus, it is my feeling that every patient entering a hospital in an area endemic for Lyme disease for a neurological evaluation should be tested for the presence of anti-*B. burgdorferi* antibody; this test could then replace the VDRL, which in many hospitals is still routinely done on admission.

Treatment

Patients who fulfill diagnostic criteria for CNS involvement in Lyme disease should be treated with parenteral antibiotics. Our choice is penicillin G, 20 million U intravenously per day in six divided doses, for a 70 kilogram man.[28] Others have treated late manifestations refractory to penicillin with ceftriaxone, 2 g b.i.d. i.v. or i.m., and have reported excellent responses[25]; others[26] have not found ceftriaxone successful in treatment of patients with arthritis who have not responded to penicillin. Arguments can be mustered for either side on the issue of optimal treatment; the most important consideration is that the patient be diagnosed and treated aggressively.

REFERENCES

1. STEERE, A. C., S. E. MALAWISTA, D. R. SNYDMAN, *et al.* 1977. Lyme arthritis: An epidemic of oligoarticular arthritis in children and adults in three Connecticut communities. Arthritis Rheum. **20:** 7–17.
2. BANNWARTH, A. 1941. Chronische lymphozytare Meningitis, entzundliche polyneuritis und rheumatismus. Arch. Psychiatr. Nervenkr. **113:** 284–376.
3. GARIN, C. & C. BUJADOUX. 1922. Paralysie par les tiques. J. Med. Lyon. **71:** 765–777.
4. PACHNER, A. R. & A. C. STEERE. 1985. The triad of neurological manifestations of Lyme disease: Meningitis, cranial neuritis, and radiculoneuritis. Neurology **35:** 47–53.
5. PACHNER, A. R. 1986. Spirochetal diseases of the nervous system. Neurologic Clinics **4:** 207–222.
6. SCHMUTZHARD, E., G. STANEK & P. POHL. 1985. Polyneuritis cranialis associated with *B. burgdorferi.* J. Neurol. Neurosurg. Psychiatr. **48:** 1182–1184.
7. STIERNSTEDT, G., B. SKOLDENBERG, A. GARDE, G. KOLMODIN, H. JORBECK, B. SVENUNGS-SON & A. CARLSTROM. 1986. Clinical manifestations of *Borrelia* infections of the nervous system. Zbl. Bakt. Hyg. A. **263:** 289–296.
8. PACHNER, A. R. & A. C. STEERE. 1986. Neurological manifestations of third stage Lyme disease. Zbl. Bakt. Hyg. A. **263:** 301.
9. PACHNER, A. R. & A. C. STEERE. Central nervous system manifestations of Lyme disease. In press.
10. REIK, L., L. SMITH, A. KHAN, *et al.* 1985. Demyelinating encephalopathy in Lyme disease. Neurology **35:** 267–269.
11. PFISTER, H., K. M. EINHAUPL, B. WILSKE & V. PREAC-MURSIC. 1986. Bannwarth's syndrome and the enlarged neurological spectrum of arthropod-borne borreliosis. Zbl. Bakt. Hyg. A. **263:** 343–347.
12. ACKERMANN, R., E. GOLLMER, B. REHSE-KUPPER. 1985. Progressive Borrelien-Enzephalo-myelitis. Chronische Manifestation der Erythema-chronicum-migrans Krankheit am Nervensystem. Dtsch. Med. Wochenschr. **110:** 1039–1042.

13. STEERE, A. C., N. H. BARTENHAGEN, J. E. CRAFT, G. J. HUTCHINSON, J. H. NEWMAN, A. R. PACHNER, D. W. RAHN, L. H. SIGAL, E. TAYLOR & S. E. MALAWISTA. 1986. Clinical manifestations of Lyme disease. Zbl. Bakt. Hyg. A **263:** 201–205.
14. HANSEN, K., C. RECHNITZER, N. PEDERSEN, M. APRI & O. JESSEN. 1986. Borrelia meningitis in Denmark. Zbl. Bakt. Hyg. A **263:** 348–350.
15. LAKOS, A., L. TELEGDY, G. KALI, G. PRINZ, E. BAN & J. BUDAI. 1986. Lyme disease imitating multiple sclerosis (Abstract). Presented at the Ninth International Congress on Infectious and Parasitic Diseases, Munich.
16. STRIE, F., L. VIDMAR, R. RAKAR, M. GAJSEK & G. KOLAR. 1986. Lyme borreliosis in Slovenia (Abstract). Presented at the Ninth International Congress on Infectious and Parasitic Disease, Munich.
17. REIK, L., W. BURGDORFER & J. DONDALDSON. 1986. Neurologic abnormalities in Lyme disease without erythema chronicum migrans. Am. J. Med. **81:** 73–78.
18. TUMULTY, P. A. 1973. The Effective Clinician. Saunders. Philadelphia, PA.
19. TRAMONT, E. C. 1987. Syphilis in the AIDS era. N. Engl. J. Med. **316:** 1600–1601.
20. CRAFT, J. E., R. L. GRODZICKI & A. C. STEERE. 1984. Antibody response in Lyme disease: Evaluation of diagnostic tests. J. Infect. Dis. **149:** 789–795.
21. HEDBERG, C. W., M. T. OSTERHOLM, K. L. MACDONALD & K. W. WHITE. 1987. An interlaboratory study of antibody to *Borrelia burgdorferi.* J. Infect. Dis. **155:** 1325–1327.
22. SIGAL, L. 1988. IgM in the sera of patients with Lyme neurologic disease bind to cross-reacting neuronal and *Borrelia burgdorferi* antigens. This volume.
23. MARTIN, R. 1988. *Borrelia burgdorferi* as a trigger for autoimmune T-cell reactions within the central nervous system. This volume.
24. RAGNI, M. V. *et al.* 1987. Isolation of human immunodeficiency virus and detection of HIV DNA sequences in the brain of an ELISA antibody-negative child with acquired immune deficiency syndrome and progressive encephalopathy. J. Pediatr. **110:** 892–894.
25. DATTWYLER, R. J., J. J. HALPERIN, H. PASS & B. J. LUFT. 1987. Ceftriaxone as effective therapy in refractory Lyme disease. J. Infect. Dis. **155:** 1322–1325.
26. STEERE, A. C. 1987. Personal communication.
27. PACHNER, A. R., A. C. STEERE, L. H. SIGAL & C. J. JOHNSON. 1985. Antigen-specific proliferation of CSF lymphocytes in Lyme disease. Neurology **35:** 1642–1644.
28. STEERE, A. C., A. R. PACHNER & S. MALAWISTA. 1983. Successful treatment of the neurological abnormalities of Lyme disease with high-dose intravenous penicillin. Ann. Intern. Med. **99:** 767–772.

OTHER PERTINENT REFERENCES

BRODERICK, J. P., B. A. SANDOK & L. E. MERTZ. 1987. Focal encephalitis in a young woman 6 years after the onset of Lyme disease: Tertiary Lyme disease? Mayo Clin. Proc. **62:** 313–316.
BURGDORFER, W., A. G. BARBOUR, S. F. HAYES, *et al.* 1982. Lyme disease—a tick-borne spirochetosis? Science **216:** 1317–1319.
CLARK, J. R., R. D. CARLSON, C. T. SASAKI, A. R. PACHNER & A. C. STEERE. Facial paralysis in Lyme disease. The Laryngoscope **95:** 1341-1345.
MACDONALD, A. B. 1986. Borrelia in the brains of patients dying with dementia (letter to the editor). J. Am. Med. Assoc. **256:** 2195.
REIK, L., A. C. STEERE & N. H. BARTENHAGEN, *et al.* 1979. Neurologic abnormalities of Lyme disease. Medicine **58:** 281–294.
STEERE, A. C., W. P. BATSFORD & M. WEINBURG, *et al.* 1980. Lyme carditis: Cardiac abnormalities of Lyme disease. Ann. Int. Med. **93:** 8–16.
STEERE, A. C., R. L. GRODZICKI, A. N. KORNBLATT, *et al.* The spirochetal etiology of Lyme disease. N. Engl. J. Med. **308:** 733–740.
STIERNSTED, G., B. SKOLDENBERG, B. VANDVIK, B. HEDERSTEDT, A. GARDE, H. KOLMODIN, H. JORBECK & B. SVENUNGSSON. 1984. Chronic meningitis and Lyme disease in Sweden. Yale J. Biol. Med. **57:** 491–497.

APPENDIX: CASE REPORTS

1. CNS Involvement in Second-Stage Lyme Disease

A 55-year-old woman developed headache, neck pain, and low-grade fever in June, 1984. After 3 weeks, she noted bilateral facial weakness and marked difficulty walking. On admission to the hospital, she had bilateral peripheral facial palsy, was unable to stand with her feet together, and had poor heel-to-shin coordination and a broad-based ataxic gait. Motor and sensory testing were normal, as were deep tendon reflexes. Lumbar puncture revealed a marked spinal fluid pleocytosis with elevated protein, and MRI scan showed multiple areas of increased density periventricularly consistent with the plagues of demyelination. Routine blood tests were normal, but the IgG antibody titer to *B. burgdorferi* was elevated. She was treated with intravenous penicillin G, 20 million U a day for 10 days, and during the following month had complete resolution of her symptoms.

2. Behavioral Changes

Between 1982 and 1984, a 12-year-old boy had four attacks of swelling of the right knee; the diagnosis of Lyme arthritis was confirmed serologically. After the last attack, he was treated with doxycycline, 100 mg twice a day for 30 days. Two months later, the patient became withdrawn and depressed. He no longer interacted with his friends, spent most of this time alone, and would no longer do his school work. He ate very little and began to exercise compulsively. His weight dropped 14 kg. On admission to a psychiatric hospital, he was grossly depressed and uncommunicative. He was diagnosed as having anorexia nervosa.

Because of the history of Lyme disease, he was transferred to Yale-New Haven Hospital. Serum and CSF antibody titers to *B. burgdorferi* were elevated, but neurologic evaluation was normal. He was treated with intravenous penicillin, 20 million U a day for 14 days, and within several weeks he began to eat more, gain weight, and communicate. During the following several months, his behavior returned to normal, he went back to school, and has remained asymptomatic for the past 2 years.

3. Subacute Encephalitis

A previously normal 21-year-old man developed progressive confusion, agitation, and disorientation in November 1985. One month later, on admission to the hospital, his mental status was grossly impaired with disorientation, inappropriate laughter, and violent outbursts. There were no focal findings. Lumbar puncture revealed a lymphocytic pleocytosis and the electroencephalogram showed diffuse slowing with minimal right-sided predominance, but CT and brain scans, angiogram, CSF cytologies, and bacterial and fungal cultures were normal. Routine blood tests, including the erythrocyte sedimentation rate, were normal, and serologic tests for cryptococcal antigens and for viruses, including human immunodeficiency virus, were negative. However, the antibody titer to *B. burgdorferi* was elevated in serum and CSF. CSF and peripheral blood mononuclear cells were exposed to *B. burgdorferi* antigen *in vitro*; cells from both sites showed significant proliferation, and those in CSF were 2 to 5 times more active.

Although the patient lacked clear focal findings, he underwent a right temporal lobe brain biopsy because of the possibility of herpes encephalitis. The biopsy specimen showed focal areas of microgliosis without inflammatory infiltrate, but intranuclear viral inclusions were not present. In addition, appropriate stains for toxoplasmosis, acid-fast organisms, other bacteria, and fungal-yeast forms were negative; and culture of the specimen in modified Kelly's medium was negative. However, spirochetes, morphologically compatible with *B. burgdorferi,* were seen extracellularly in 5 of 36 Dieterle-stained tissue sections. He was treated with penicillin, 20 million units a day intravenously for 14 days. During therapy he became less agitated, and during the following 3 months his behavior and mental status returned to normal and he resumed his premorbid employment.

4. "Multiple Sclerosis"

During the summer of 1983, a 37-year-old man from central New Jersey developed low-grade fever, malaise, migratory myalgias and arthralgias, sore throat, followed within several weeks by macular, erythematous lesions on the trunk and legs lasting for one week. These symptoms were followed by increasing pain in the neck, back, and legs, profound fatigue, and a 35-kg weight loss. By October he began to have weakness in the right leg, then in the left, and then in both upper arms. On examination, a neurologist documented mild deltoid and marked hip flexor weakness bilaterally, pathologically brisk reflexes, and a left Babinski sign. During the following month, he had difficulty obtaining and maintaining an erection and two brief episodes of left facial palsy. Cerebrospinal fluid showed a lymphocytic pleocytosis with elevated responses and CT scan of the head, with and without contrast, were normal. A diagnosis of multiple sclerosis was made.

During the following months his weakness improved, but he experienced migratory joint pain in the left wrist, shoulder, and ankle. In May 1984, the knees became swollen for several months and the IgG antibody titer to *B. burgdorferi* was elevated. He was treated with intravenous penicillin G, 20 million U per day for two weeks. Within several weeks, his fatigue, weakness, and joint pain began to improve, and after several months he felt normal but still had mild residual hip flexor weakness.

5. "Multiple Sclerosis"

In July 1976, a six-year-old girl developed a "flu-like" illness followed 2 weeks later by knee swelling. During the next 5 years she had many short attacks of headache and stiff neck or of arthritis or arthralgia, primarily in the knees. In October 1982, she again experienced headache followed two days later by progressive numbness and paresthesias from the toes to the buttocks. On examination, mental status, cranial nerves, and motor and sensory testing were normal. However, she had decreased sensation below L4, mild weakness in foot dorsiflexion and plantar flexion, hyperreflexia without clonus in the legs compared to the arms, and an equivocal Babinski sign. Cerebrospinal fluid showed a lymphocytic pleocytosis with five oligoclonal bands, but tests for myelin basic protein were negative, and myelography was normal. The sedimentation rate was 24 mm/h, and the serum and CSF antibody titers to *B. burgdorferi* were elevated. The patient was treated with intravenous penicillin G, 10 million U a day for 10 days. Within several weeks, all of her neurologic symptoms resolved.

Five months later, in April 1983, she developed vertigo with nystagmus and ataxia associated with a CSF pleocytosis. This episode, which was treated with Antivert, resolved within several weeks. Ten months later, in February 1984, she experienced a blind spot surrounded by bright lights in the right eye for several days. She again had a CSF pleocytosis, but visual evoked responses were normal. She has been well during the subsequent 3 years.

6. "Brain Stem Glioma"

In late August of 1982, a 61-year-old man, who had returned from his summer vacation on Nantucket Island to his home in Illinois, developed the sudden onset of double vision, and then numbness on the left side of his tongue, weakness of his face, and progressive numbness of the fingers of the right and left hands. Neurologic examination in an Illinois hospital during the winter of 1982 showed facial weakness, decreased convergence bilaterally with double vision on left lateral gaze, bilateral peripheral facial weakness, decreased strength of the triceps, wrist and finger flexors on the left, and diminished triceps and brachioradialis reflexes on the left. Lumbar puncture, brain stem evoked responses, CT and MRI scans, and myelography were normal. An intramedullary brain stem tumor was suspected. He was treated with high-dose prednisone. In 1983, despite this therapy, he experienced increasing facial numbness, progressive loss of sensation in his hands and arms, and developed disabling fatigue.

During the spring of 1984 he noticed difficulty with urination, and cystometrogram revealed a neurogenic bladder. In addition, he developed swelling of his right knee and left olecranon bursitis for approximately 2 months. *B. burgdorferi* serology was strongly positive. In July, on admission to Yale-New Haven Hospital, cerebrospinal fluid was normal except for three oligoclonal bands, and an MRI scan demonstrated multiple areas of increased density in periventricular regions consistent with the plaques of demyelination. He was treated with intravenous penicillin G, 20 million U a day for 10 days. Afterwards he felt less fatigued, and the prednisone dose was reduced. However, despite repeated courses of high-dose penicillin accompanied by probenecid, his neurologic deficit has worsened and MRI scan has shown pontine, in addition to periventricular, plaques.

Clinical Pathologic Correlations of Lyme Disease by Stage

PAUL H. DURAY

Department of Pathology
Fox Chase Cancer Center
Philadelphia, Pennsylvania 19111

ALLEN C. STEERE

Department of Internal Medicine
Division of Rheumatology
Tufts University School of Medicine
Boston, Massachusetts 02111

INTRODUCTION

It is now known that erythema migrans disease (as described by Afzelius and Herxheimer[1]), acrodermatitis chronica atrophicans,[2] lymphocytoma of Bafverstedt,[3] meningopolyneuritis (Garin-Bujadoux-Bannwarth syndrome),[4,5] and Lyme disease (as described by Steere in North America)[6,7] are all one and the same disease caused by *B. burgdorferi*.[8] All of these disorders are histopathologically characterized by variable infiltrates of perivascular lymphocytes and plasma cells, and vascular damage and fibrin deposits in the synovia of arthritis patients.[9]

Primarily cutaneous and neural in involvement, the disease has come to be understood as a multisystemic infectious syndrome involving the cardiovascular system, central and peripheral nervous system, and reticuloendothelial and gastrointestinal systems.[10,11] Involvement of these and specialized systems produces clinical symptoms that can correlate with varying degrees of tissue damage caused by a complex interplay of cells of the immune system and humoral factors such as interleukin-1 (IL-1), circulating immune complexes, prostaglandins, collagenases, and possibly compounds derived from arachidonic acid.[12,13]

Experience in both hemispheres now points to ever-expanding clinical and pathologic lesions that heretofore have been referred to by a variety of seemingly unrelated terms. Many of these involve the skin in chronic phases. Increasing evidence points to the continuing presence of spirochetes in these lesions. This paper summarizes these alterations as seen histopathologically.

MATERIALS AND METHODS

Tissues of human patients infected with *B. burgdorferi* have been obtained by consultations and contributions from clinicians and pathologists from both hemispheres. Tissues largely have been submitted previously formalin fixed and embedded in paraffin from postmortem examinations, surgical biopsies, dermatologic punch biopsies, synovectomies obtained both from arthroscopy as well as open joint surgery, and endocardial biopsies by trans-venous catheterization. Tissue samples have been submitted from acute stage illness, chronic and convalescent stages, and from patients in quiescent periods of the disease. In some instances the material was confined to glass

65

slides and/or photomicrographs. Whenever available, paraffin blocks were recut for histochemical studies utilizing reticulin stains, Mallory trichrome stains, Giemsa stains for mast cells, Putt's fibrin stain for fibrin products and fibrinogen, Verhoeff Van Gieson stain for elastin, alcian blue stains at pH 1.8 and 2.4 for stromal mucopolysaccharides, modified Dieterle stain for spirochetes, and routine hematoxylin and eosin stains. Avidin-biotin immunohistochemistry utilizing monoclonal antibodies H5332, H3TS, and H9724 obtained from Dr. Alan Barbour and hyperimmune human polyclonal antibody obtained from Dr. Allen C. Steere was used to identify spirochetes in formalin-fixed tissue sections. Chromagen substrates used in the immunohistochemical analyses consisted of diaminobenzidine and alkaline phosphatases, chromagen I and III.

Tissue samples have been examined from the states of California, Minnesota, Wisconsin, Texas, Michigan, Pennsylvania, New Jersey, New York, Maryland, North Carolina, and Massachusetts. Countries in the Western Hemisphere include the Netherlands, Sweden, France, West Germany, Italy, and Austria.

Notes on Histogenesis

The spirochete disseminates by the vascular system following a variable period of time in the skin upon tick inoculation.[14] Humoral and cellular immune responses play a major role in all clinical pathologic stages as well as a number of enzymes, including collagenase and derivatives of the arachidonic acid pathway, namely prostaglandin, and biologic response modifiers such as IL-1. Circulating immune complexes and elevated IgM, IgA, and later IgG, become elevated in the circulation[15] as well as some deposition of IgG in the synovia of the joints. Lymphocytes—both B-cell and T-cell (helper and suppressor)—proliferate at one time or another in most of the organ systems that will be discussed subsequently, and are accompanied by varying numbers of macrophages, dendritic immune cells, and tissue mast cells. The plasma cell and its precursors are a mainstay inflammatory responder in most if not indeed all visceral and organ system sites of involvement. Visceral damage and alteration are caused by an interplay of these humoral and cellular elements, presumably in response to the continuing presence of spirochetal antigen(s),[14] either from viable and proliferating spirochetes or from degenerating forms. Although T cells seem to be a major responder in the central nervous system and elsewhere, B cells which differentiate into plasma cells comprise a major response in the deep dermis, fascia, soft tissues, myocardium, dermis, and synovium. Not only are plasma cells plentiful in the spleen, lymph nodes and bone marrow, they are also represented by large and somewhat atypical-appearing precursor B cells as well. Mild-to-moderate vasculopathies in the form of mild vasculitis and hypercellular vascular occlusion are often seen in multiple sites, and appear to be temporally related. These vascular alterations are not fully explained, but may reflect secondary damage by immune cells and possibly immune complexes. Tissue necrosis in any site appears lacking with one minor exception: lymphadenitis in stage I. Multinucleated giant cells, granulomas, gummas, and fibrin microthrombi of vessels appear not to be found in human Lyme disease thus far.

CLINICAL PATHOLOGIC CORRELATION BY STAGE

Stage I

The tick bite site in the skin yields an ulceropapule consisting of partially denuded and peripherally hyperplastic epithelium, overlaying an inflammatory infiltrate in the dermis of lymphocytes, plasma cells, macrophages, and mast cells, acutely and followed by plasma cells later on (TABLE 1). In some circumstances discrete, somewhat unusual appearing, hemorrhagic nodules are seen in the deep dermis below the inflammatory infiltrate. At this stage spirochetes are hard to see but are nevertheless present. Erythema chronicum migrans, the hallmark of stage I involvement, is reflected histologically by mild-to-moderate perivascular infiltrates of mostly lymphocytes and minor components of plasma cells and mast cells. Vasculitis is not seen at this stage, and there is no vascular proliferation. Spirochetes at this stage are seen randomly near the epidermis but appear preferentially in the reticular dermal collagen. We have also seen them in lymphstasis in the subcutaneous soft tissues. Spirochetes stain poorly with the specific monoclonal antibodies in the skin but stain readily with polyclonal human immune serum followed by an avidin-biotin immunohistochemical procedure. Collagen is intact in ECM in the first stage, and the infiltrate is confined to the immediate perivascular regions. The epidermis appears normal. In Europe mainly, and rarely in the U.S., cutaneous lymphoid hyperplasia may be seen in the earlobes or the nipple skin.[16] This consists of benign but remarkably hyperplastic and crowded lymphocytic follicles with discrete germinal centers in the dermis, yielding an

TABLE 1. Stage I

Tick papule
Erythema chronicum migrans
Secondary lesions
Lymphocytoma cutis (lymphadenosis benigna cutis)
Ear lobe
Nipple/areolae
Conjunctivitis; uveitis; pharyngitis
Interstitial pneumonitis
Myalgia-arthralgia
Early meningitis (meningismus)
Encephalopathy
Lymphadenopathy
Splenomegaly
Hepatitis
Orchitis
Hematuria; proteinuria

appearance of tonsillar tissue. Numerous names have been given to this stage, including pseudolymphoma, lymphoid hyperplasia, follicular hyperplasia, lymphocytoma cutis, Spiegler-Fendt lymphoid hyperplasia, and lymphadenosis benigna cutis of Baverstedt. Secondary lesions of ECM occur as the spirochete disseminates to other regions of the skin, and the perivascular infiltrate is the same in the secondary deposits. In later biopsies of ECM, mast cells become more numerous near the lymphoid cells.

Soon after the onset of ECM, the organism disseminates hematogenously, with what appears to be random dispersal throughout the body. The immune response involves virtually all of the organs and structures of the reticuloendothelial system including the bone marrow, and clinical pain and discomfort seems to correlate with hyperplasia of lymph nodes and spleen and bone marrow. Diffuse visceral involvement in this acute stage mimics infectious mononucleosis or disseminated viral syndromes. These include conjuctivitis, pharyngitis, pneumonitis with dry cough and mild pleuritic pain, hepato-splenic tenderness, lymph node swelling of the neck and groin, and orchitis. There is lymphoid hyperplasia of the lymph nodes and spleen consisting of prominent germinal centers and numerous perifollicular lymphocytes, with proliferation of plasma cell precursors and mature plasma cells. The plasma cell precursors are

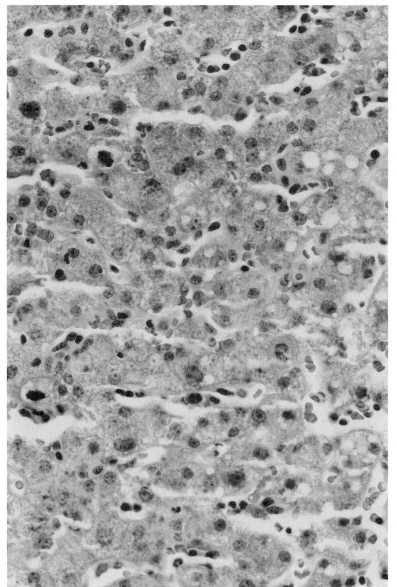

FIGURE 1. Photomicrograph of stage I Lyme hepatitis from an elderly woman. Liver cells are swollen with microvesicles of fat with numerous sinusoidal leukocytes. Near the top are two liver cells in mitosis. Hematoxylin and eosin stain; magnification 500×.

large, appear tumor-like, and can resemble Reed-Sternberg cells. Others look like typical immunoblasts (FIG. 1). In one example, cervical lymph nodes show cell degeneration with karyorrhexis and nuclear debris of lymphoid elements. This patient had repeated high fevers and marked discomfort of neck nodes. Large atypical immunoblasts can also be seen in the spleen and bone marrow. The red pulp of the spleen is congested, not unlike that seen in infectious mononucleosis. Spirochetes can be demonstrated in the lymph nodes, spleen and bone marrow and liver. There is a transient hepatitis reflected by elevated liver cell enzymes such as SGOT, SGPT, and GGT. The liver can vary from a mild lymphocytic portal triaditis all the way to liver cell derangement that simulates acute viral hepatitis. The cells at this stage appear swollen with clear cytoplasm and microvesicles of fat (FIG. 2). Numerous leukocytes are seen in the sinusoids, and there is Kupffer cell hyperplasia. Plasma cells are present and randomly distributed throughout the sinusoids and portal tracts. One hepatitis case from Wisconsin showed a remarkable number of mitoses of liver cells, itself a very

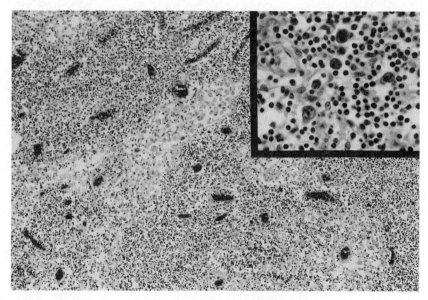

FIGURE 2. Peripheral lymph node from stage I Lyme disease patient with lymphadenopathy. An increase in macrophages is seen in the lymphatic spaces. High power shows the presence of moderately atypical-appearing immunoblasts and precursor B cells (inset).

unusual finding in non-neoplastic conditions of the liver. In stage I the lungs are involved by a hypercellular interstitial pneumonitis with irregular alveolar spaces (FIG. 3). The interstitial infiltrate is nonspecific and does not appear to resemble the interstitial lymphocytic pneumonitis of classic influenza. Cells are mixed with macrophages and tissue histiocytes in addition to lymphocytes. The alveolar spaces are irregular in shape.

Stage II

Stage II (TABLE 2) begins weeks to several months following the initial infection and is largely characterized by the involvement of the cardiovascular and central

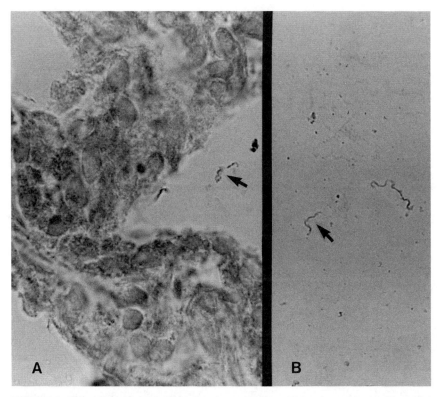

FIGURE 3. Photomicrograph of a stage I patient with interstitial pneumonitis. (**A**) Interstitial thickening by inflammatory cells. *Arrows* show spirochetes labeled with H5332 monoclonal antibody, specific for *Borrelia burgdorferi*. (**B**) Positive control from a culture of spirochetes. Avidin-biotin immunohistochemical technique; magnification 900×.

TABLE 2. Stage II

Lymphocytoma cutis (LABC)
Iritis, panophthalmitis
Meningitis-pleocytosis
Encephalitis-like
Perivascular cuffs, vasculopathic
Mild spongioform changes
Focal microgliosis
No apparent abnormality
Cranial neuritis (bilateral Bell's Palsy)
Radiculoneuritis
Myelitis
Myocarditis
Endocarditis
Endomyocarditis, vasculitis
Fibrinous pericarditis
Myositis, perivascular cuffs
Fasciitis (Schulman-like)

nervous system. By this time the acute reactive phase with diffuse involvement of the reticuloendothelial system and elevated serum IgM levels have subsided. Cardiovascular system involvement is manifested by one or more forms of cardiac arrhythmia. Patients may have either an incomplete (first or second degree) AV block or a complete AV block. Some patients appear not to be aware of their arrhythmias during this stage. Fortunately most of these forms are benign and transient. Nevertheless severe forms do occur and can be manifested by slow idioventricular rhythms. We previously recorded a terminal case of Lyme myocarditis in a middle-aged man with refractory arrhythmia.[17] We examined several sections of the myocardium from this case, but had no opportunity to dissect the cardiac conduction system. Nevertheless a transmural inflammatory infiltrate involved all three layers of the myocardium including the endocardium. The infiltrate consisted of lymphocytes, plasma cells, and

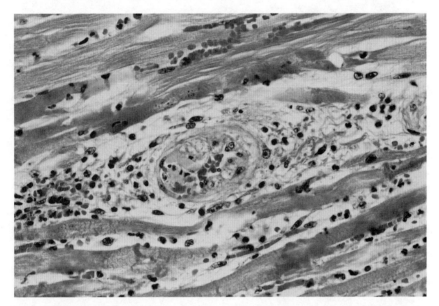

FIGURE 4. Lyme myocarditis with perivascular lymphocytes and plasma cells and vascular damage with disruption of the endothelium and debris in the lumen.

macrophages. Scattered branches of intramyocardial veins showed sparse lymphocytes in the tunica media. Lymphocytes and scattered macrophages were also present in the tunica adventitia and the immediate perivascular stroma. The stroma showed laminations suggesting early obliterative vasculopathy. Necrotizing vasculitis was not present, but rare vessels showed luminal amorphic debris and vasculopathy (FIG. 4). The lymphocytes and plasma cells diffusely infiltrated the interstitium of the myocardium in all sections examined. The endocardium showed a band-like infiltrate of lymphocytes and plasma cells of more or less uniform thickness. In another case of myocarditis from a middle-aged woman in Pennsylvania, early traces of myocardial fiber degeneration were present along with neutrophils in addition to lymphocytes and plasma cells. This patient survived the myocarditis phase following intravenous penicillin therapy. Fibrinous pericarditis occurred in another case, wherein symptoms of pericardial

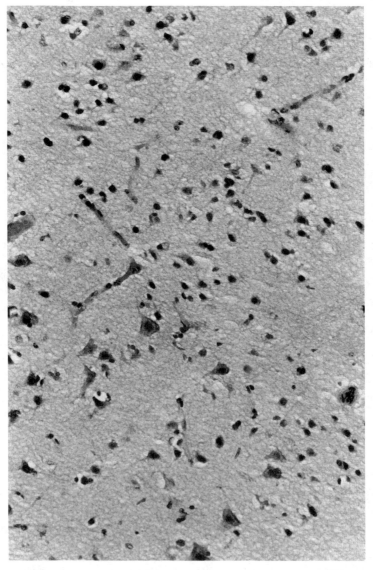

FIGURE 5. Stage II Lyme cerebritis demonstrated by an increase in microglial cells and round cells. Hematoxylin and eosin; magnification 250×.

constriction were clinically evident. That patient also survived. Spirochetes can be demonstrated in multiple sections of the myocardium, but they were absent in the fibrinous pericarditis samples. This characteristic band-like infiltrate of the endocardium can be demonstrated even in limited biopsies taken of the right ventricle by trans-venous catheter.

Clinical signs and symptoms of meningoencephalitis are fully developed in stage II. Patients have headache, photophobia, and signs of meningismus. This stage is paralleled by CSF pleocytosis. In terminal cases seen thus far, band-like infiltrates of lymphocytes and plasma cells are seen in the leptomeningeal layers. Some cases have shown mild spongioform changes of the cerebral cortex, and others have shown an increase in oligodendrocytes, which at times are situated in cuffs around small vessels. Microgliosis of a focal nature was seen in one young male in coma who responded to intravenous penicillin therapy (FIG. 5). Spirochetes were demonstrated in that case. Patients have either severe encephalopathy including stupor and coma, or varied forms of psychoneurosis including depression. Many of these are also found in stage III disease. These encephalopathic stages may be entirely absent, and patients present with various combinations of cranial neuritis.[30] Bilateral Bell's palsy is a prominent feature in some stage II patients, and almost constitutes a firm clinical sign that a given patient in an endemic area with bilateral Bell's palsy has Lyme disease until proven otherwise. Also the clinical triad of cranial neuritis, meningitis, and radiculoneuritis also constitutes Lyme disease in an endemic area unless proven otherwise.[18] Aggregates and groups of lymphocytes are found infiltrating the autonomic ganglia directly as well as the afferent and efferent rootlets. Plasma cells are not so prominent as are the lymphocytes in this stage. We have not seen spirochetes in the ganglia, but the assumption is that they are directly present.

We have had recent experience with a lesion that is not uncommonly seen in late stage II in Europe, and that consists of a lesion manifested clinically by extreme pain in one or more proximal muscle groups such as the musculature of the thigh or forearm. This pain is not that of the stage I myalgia but is one of pain at rest as well as in motion. Clinically there is swelling and tenderness of involved muscle groups. This lesion appears to be independent of peripheral neuropathy or central nervous system involvement, although they may coexist. Biopsy shows perivascular infiltrates of lymphocytes and plasma cells of vessels within the muscle itself. The myocardial fibers show minimal swelling but no sarcoplasmic degeneration or direct myopathy such as peripheralization of nuclei. In one case we demonstrated spirochetes in the interstitium and overlying muscle fibers. These perivascular lymphoid infiltrates within muscle are virtually identical to those found in polymyositis and dermatomyositis. The duration of Lyme myositis is not known, but it probably can persist for variably long periods.

Stage III

Stage III (TABLE 3) is the chronic phase of Lyme disease, usually beginning months after initial onset, and lasting into many years. Stage III is characterized by involvement of the joints (intermittent oligoarthritis), peripheral nervous system, skin and subcutaneous soft tissue. The arthritis is one of an intermittent nature with periods of activity alternating with quiescence. Knee, wrist, and shoulder are more common, with the knee joint being the most characteristically involved.[19] Clinically there is swelling and pain of the involved joint, and unlike rheumatoid arthritis rarely will more than three joints be involved. It is now well known that Lyme arthritis is reflected by varying degrees of hypertrophic, proliferative synovitis, consisting of aggregates of lymphocytes in the subsynovium, with admixtures of plasma cells, macrophages, and numerous mast cells. Neutrophils are found in the synovial fluid, and with only minor exception are not usually seen in the synovium in Lyme arthritis. They probably are present in acute stages of the arthritis but give way within a short period of time to lymphocytes and plasma cells. Well-defined germinal centers are usually not seen in the synovia as they were in lesion of the skin called lymphadenosis benigna cutis. Synovial cells are hyperplastic, often more than four cells thick, and accompany the villous hypertrophy. Vessels are prominent and may actually be angiomatoid in appearance. Deposits of fibrin and fibrinogen are found not only on the surfaces of some villi, but also within the stroma of villi, and sometimes compose 50% or more of the total tissue volume as obtained by synovial curetting specimens. Putt's fibrin stain yields a rose-to-pink color against a background of blue collagen, confirming that fibrinogen and fibrin are present in this material. Despite this deposition, fibrin microthrombi are not seen within the vessels (FIG. 6). Not every case of Lyme arthritis shows this fibrin deposition, but it is prominent in some patients and exceeds the amount seen as a rule in rheumatoid arthritis or Reiter's disease.[9] This material is not seen in every example, and is not a requirement for Lyme synovitis.

TABLE 3. Stage III

Arthritis-synovitis vasculitis
Lymphoplasmacellular hyperplasia
Fibrinaceous deposits
Occlusive vessels
Myositis, fasciitis
Peripheral neuropathies: motor, sensory
EPI and endoneural vasculitis
Wallerian degeneration
Demyelination
Acrodermatitis chronica atrophicans, occluded vessels
Lymphocytoma cutis?
Linear scleroderma, morphea, fasciitis, vasculopathy
Ulnar fibrous nodules, occluded vessels
Lichen sclerosus

The small vessels in some cases have obliteration as a result of a hypercellularity of the inner lining of the vessels (FIG. 6). In some cases this produces the appearance of "onion skinning" of the type classically seen in the vasculopathy of vessels of the spleen in lupus erythematosus. This is also not seen in every case of Lyme arthritis, but when coexisting with prominent deposits of fibrin suggests the presence of Lyme arthritis, if the patient is in an endemic area.[9] Spirochetes are very sparse and are demonstrated in histologic sections only with great difficulty and in only a minority of cases (FIG. 6). A large number of cases show prominent hemosiderin deposits, especially in the deeper subsynovial regions. It is possible that exacerbations and flairs of the arthritis are heralded by stromal hemorrhages, leading to the hemosiderin and fibrin and fibrinogen depositions.

The peripheral nervous system can be involved in stage III, manifested mainly by peripheral neuropathies. There is overlap from stage II neural involvement. Most neuropathies in stage III appear to be cranial.[21,22] These neuropathies are sensorimotor, and involve the infiltration of predominantly lymphocytes and a few plasma cells along the perineurium. Fewer lymphocytes can infiltrate the internal segment of the nerves, where they can be clustered around small vessels. The vessels and the perineural

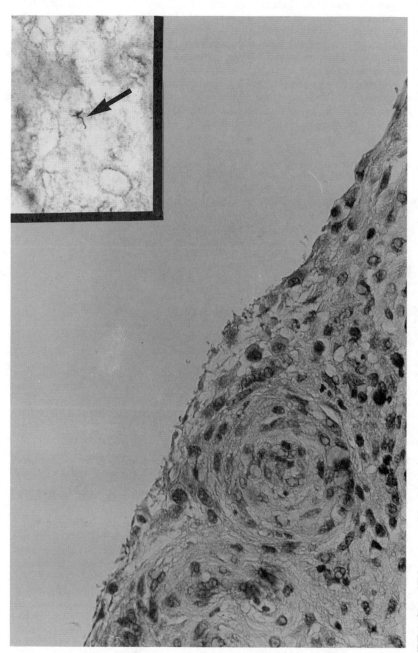

FIGURE 6. Stage III Lyme synovitis with hypercellular occluded vessel with perivascular plasma cells and lymphocytes. A synovial spirochete is seen by silver stain in the inset (magnification 1000×).

regions as well as within the nerve proper show a vasculopathy in the form of variable occlusion and lymphocytes. These changes also can be found in stage II involvement. In chronic and severe forms, there may be nerve fiber loss, demyelination, and changes not unlike that of Wallerian degeneration. Amyloid deposits are not seen.

The skin and subcutaneous tissues are involved in chronic, stage III Lyme disease, and seemingly more common in European patients. The hallmark is acrodermatitis chronicum atrophicans, a peculiar, often bilaterally symmetrical, reddish discoloration of the acral skin such as the feet, ankles, hands, and wrists, often with scaling and hyperkeratosis.[23] At times, a peripheral neuropathy accompanies this dermal change. The joints may also be involved at the same time.[24] The histology is characteristic in that there can be loss of rete ridges subjacent to which is a dermis infiltrated by

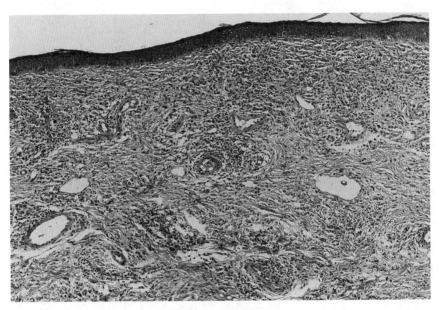

FIGURE 7. Photomicrograph of acrodermatitis chronicum atrophicans. There is loss of rete ridges followed by dilatation of the dermal vessels and a persistent infiltrate of lymphocytes and plasma cells.

lymphocytes, plasma cells, macrophages, scattered mast cells, and prominent blood vessels (FIG. 7). The vasculature shows a dilation which appears to be characteristic of ACA. The infiltrate can extend into the subcutaneous fat where a panniculitis becomes prominent. Scattered blood vessels in the involved dermis can show occlusion like that seen in the synovia and peripheral nerves. The blood vessels of the subcutaneous fat show increasing numbers of plasma cells and more severe damage than those in the upper dermis. Spirochetes can be demonstrated in sections of ACA and can also be cultured from ACA. It is becoming clear that lesions resembling morphea (linear scleroderma) can be found in stage III Lyme disease. Histologically they resemble scleroderma strongly, with a thickened dermis by excess collagen which extends below the eccrine sweat glands and into the fibrous septae that support the pannus. Perivascular lymphocytes and plasma cells are also present in these cases. Another sclerodermoid manifestation of stage III Lyme disease is related to linear scleroderma and has the clinical and histologic appearance of eosinophilic fasciitis. Here there are more perivascular plasma cells, especially in the deeper dermis, and there is an underlying lymphocytic and plasmacytic fasciitis. Perhaps fewer eosinophils than are found in classic eosinophilic fasciitis are present in this form, but they can be found. Two cases of lichen sclerosus (et atrophicus) have now been seen in chronic Lyme disease patients by us and by others.[23] Both had the upper papillary dermal homogenization of the collagen with an edematous appearance as seen in classic LSEA, and also had the band-like mid-dermal lymphocytic infiltration. Again in both of these cases, the deeper dermal vessels showed occlusive changes.

Recent experience in Europe shows that some patients with evidence of exposure to *B. burgdorferi* have skin lesions that histologically are identical to granuloma annulare.[25,26] Granuloma annulare may indeed be another chronic cutaneous manifestation of stage III Lyme disease, but we have had no experience with this in North American cases so far.

Another European lesion, not uncommon in West Germany, is the condition referred to as ulnar fibrous nodules.[27] These peculiar thickenings found over the outer aspect of the forearms near the elbow joints consist of homogenized nodular collagen deposits which contain thickened and occluded blood vessels, with perivascular infiltrates of macrophages and plasma cells. We have seen spirochetes by silver staining in our examination of these nodules, supporting the premise that the spirochete survives for long periods of time in skin and soft tissue structures.

LYME DISEASE IN MATERNAL INFECTIONS

It is clear that *B. burgdorferi* can be transmitted in the blood of infected pregnant women across the placenta into the fetus. This has now been documented with resultant congenital infections[28] and fetal demise.[29] Spirochetes can be recovered or seen in the infant's tissues including the brain, spleen and kidney. The chorionic villi of the placenta show an increase in Hofbauer cells as in luetic placentitis. Inflammatory changes of fetal or neonatal changes are not as pronounced as in the adult, but cardiac abnormalities, including intracardiac septal defects, have been seen.[28,29] It is not known why inflammatory cells are so sparse from maternal transmission, but it is possible that an immature immune system plays a role.

SUMMARY

Lyme disease is capable of producing a wide variety of clinical pathologic conditions and lesions having in common histologic features of collagen-vascular disease. The plasma cell is an omnipotent inflammatory responder in most tissues involved by Lyme disease, ranging from relatively acute to lesions that have gone on for years. Vascular thickening also seems to be prominent, and in the dermis is accompanied by scleroderma-like collagen expansion. The disease in some ways resembles the responses seen in lupus erythematosus such as mild cerebritis with lymphocytes and plasma cells in the leptomeninges. Lymphoplasmacytic panniculitis of Lyme disease resembles lupus profundus, both in the infiltrate and the plasma cell-blood vessel relationship. The onion skin thickened vessels of the synovia resemble the vessels of lupus spleens, while the scleradermoid thickening of the dermis and various skin lesions of stage III Lyme disease suggest a collagen-vascular disorder. Finally, the perivascular lymphoid infiltrate in clinical myositis does not differ from that seen in polymyositis or dermatomyositis. All of these histologic derangements suggest immunologic damage in response to persistence of the spirochete, however few in number.

REFERENCES

1. AFZELIUS, A. 1910. Verhandlungen der dermatologischen Gesellschaft zu Stockholm. Arch. Dermatol. Syph. (Berlin) **101:** 405–406.
2. FRITZ, A. & B. LANGERHOLM. 1983. Acrodermatitis chronica atrophicans, erythema chronicum migrans and lymphadenosis benigna cutis—spirochetal diseases? Acta Derm. Venereol. (Stockholm) **63:** 432–436.
3. BAFVERSTEDT, B. 1950. Lymphadenosis benigna cutis (LABC): Its nature, course and prognosis. Acta Derm. Venereol. (Stockholm) **40:** 10–18.
4. GARIN, C. & C. BUJADOUX. 1922. Paralysie par les tiques. J. Med. Lyon **71:** 765–767.
5. BANNWARTH, A. 1941. Chronische lymphocytare Meningitis, entzundliche Polyneuritis and "Rheumatismus." Arch. Psychiatr. Nervenkr. **113:** 284–376.
6. STEERE, A. C., S. E. MALAWISTA, D. R. SNYDMAN, *et al.* 1977. Lyme arthritis: An epidemic of oligoarticular arthritis in children and adults in three Connecticut communities. Arthritis Rheum. **20:** 7–17.
7. STEERE, A. C., S. E. MALAWISTA, J. A. HARDIN, S. RUDDY, P. W. ASKENASE & W. A. ANDIMAN. 1977. Erythema chronicum migrans and Lyme arthritis: The enlarging clinical spectrum. Ann. Intern. Med. **86:** 685–698.
8. BURGDORFER, W., A. G. BARBOUR, S. F. HAYES, J. L. BENACH, E. GRUNWALDT & J. P. DAVID. 1982. Lyme disease—a tick-borne spirochetosis? Science **216:** 1317–1319.
9. JOHNSTON, Y. E., P. H. DURAY, A. C. STEERE, *et al.* 1985. Lyme arthritis: Spirochetes found in synovial microangiopathic lesions. Am. J. Pathol. **118:** 26–34.
10. STEERE, A. C., S. E. MALAWISTA, N. H. BARTENHAGEN, *et al.* 1984. The clinical spectrum and treatment of Lyme disease. Yale J. Biol. Med. **57:** 3–14.
11. DURAY, P. H. 1987. The surgical pathology of human Lyme disease. An enlarging picture. Am. J. Surg. Pathol. **11** (Suppl. 1): 47–60.
12. STEERE, A. C., C. E. BRINKERHOFF, D. J. MILLER, H. DRINKER, E. D. HARRIS JR. & S. E. MALAWISTA. 1980. Elevated levels of collagenase and prostaglandin E2 from synovium associated with erosion of cartilage and bone in a patient with chronic Lyme arthritis. Arthritis Rheum. **238:** 591–599.
13. HABICHT, G. S., G. BECK & J. L. BENACH. 1987. Lyme disease. Sci. Am. **257:** 78–83.
14. STEERE, A. C., R. L. GRODZICKI, A. N. KORNBLATT, *et al.* 1983. The spirochetal etiology of Lyme disease. N. Engl. J. Med. **308:** 733–740.
15. HARDIN, J. A., A. C. STEERE & S. E. MALAWISTA. 1984. The pathogenesis of arthritis in Lyme disease: Humoral immune responses and the role of intraarticular immune complexes. Yale J. Biol. Med. **57:** 139–143.
16. ÅSBRINK, E., A. HOVMARK & I. OLSSON. 1987. Lymphadenosis benigna cutis in Sweden. Presented at Lyme Borreliosis: Update Europe, Baden, Austria. June 2–4, 1987.
17. MARCUS, L. C., A. C. STEERE, P. H. DURAY, A. E. ANDERSON & E. B. MAHONEY. 1985. Fatal pancarditis in a patient with co-existing Lyme disease and babesiosis. Ann. Intern. Med. **103:** 374–376.
18. PACHNER, A. R. & A. C. STEERE. 1985. The triad of neurologic abnormalities of Lyme disease: Meningitis, cranial neuritis, and radiculoneuritis. Neurology **35:** 47–53.
19. STEERE, A. C., A. GIBOFSKY, M. E. PATARROYO, R. J. WINCHESTER, J. A. HARDIN & S. E. MALAWISTA. 1979. Chronic Lyme arthritis: Clinical and immunogenetic differentiation from rheumatoid arthritis. Ann. Intern. Med. **90:** 286–291.
20. HERZER, P. & B. WILSKE. 1986. Lyme arthritis in Germany. Zbl. Bakt. Hyg. A **263:** 268–274.
21. PACHNER, A. R. & A. C. STEERE. 1986. CNS manifestations of third stage Lyme disease. Zbl. Bakt. Hyg. A **263:** 301–306.

22. BAUMWACKL, U., W. KRISTOFERITSCH, E. SLUGA & G. STANEK. 1986. Neurological manifestations of *Borrelia burgdorferi* infections: The enlarging clinical spectrum. Zbl. Bakt. Hyg. A **263:** 334–336.
23. ÅSBRINK, E., E. BREHMER-ANDERSSON & A. HOVMARK. 1986. Acrodermatitis chronica atrophicans—A spirochetosis: Clinical and histopathological picture based on 32 patients. Course and relationship to erythema migrans Afzelius. Am. J. Dermpathol. **8:** 209–219.
24. HOVMARK, A., E. ÅSBRINK & I. OLSSON. 1986. Joint and bone involvement in Swedish patients with *Ixodes* ricinus-borne borrelia infection. Zbl. Bakt. Hyg. A **263:** 275–288.
25. ABERER, E., R. NEUMANN, H. KLODGE & G. STANEK. 1987. Antibodies against *Borrelia burgdorferi:* Serological screening of dermatological patients. Presented at Lyme Borreliosis: Update Europe, Baden, Austria, June 2–4, 1987.
26. KUSKE, B., J. SCHMIDLI, T. HURZIKA, M. CUENI & T. RUFLI. 1987. Antibodies against *Borrelia burgdorferi* in patients with granuloma annulare. Presented at Lyme Borreliosis: Update Europe, Baden, Austria, June 2–4, 1987.
27. WEBER, K., G. SCHIERZ, B. WILSKE & V. PREAC-MURSIC. 1984. European erythema migrans diseases and related disorders. Yale J. Biol. Med. **57:** 15–21.
28. SCHLESINGER, P. A., P. H. DURAY, B. A. BURKE, A. C. STEERE & M. T. STILLMAN. 1985. Maternal fetal transmission of the Lyme disease spirochete, *Borrelia burgdorferi*. Ann. Intern. Med. **103:** 67–68.
29. MACDONALD, A. 1986. Human fetal borreliosis, toxemia of pregnancy, and fetal death. Zbl. Bakt. Hyg. A **263:** 189–200.
30. REIK, L., A. C. STEERE, N. H. BARTENHAGEN, R. E. SHOPEY & S. E. MALAWISTA. 1979. Neurologic abnormalities of Lyme disease. Medicine **58:** 281–294.

The Role of Interleukin-1 in the
Pathogenesis of Lyme Disease[a]

GAIL S. HABICHT,[b] GREGORY BECK,[b]
AND JORGE L. BENACH[b,c]

[b]*Department of Pathology*
[c]*New York State Department of Health*
State University of New York
Stony Brook, New York 11794

INTRODUCTION

Interleukin-1 (IL-1) is a family of cytokines produced by monocytes, macrophages, and a variety of related and nonrelated cells. It is a major immunoregulatory protein and is also the molecular orchestrator of nonspecific host defense mechanisms against infectious, inflammatory, and immunologic insults. When a host is faced with an endogenous or exogenous challenge a dramatic series of changes occurs, most of which are directed at eliminating the stimulus. These changes are part of the acute phase response that takes place within a few hours of challenge. Others may evolve over longer periods and suggest persistent disease or chronic infection. The acute phase response is systemic and includes fever, increased synthesis of hepatic acute phase proteins, decreased plasma iron and zinc, leukocytosis, fatigue, and decreased appetite. The acute phase response is mediated by IL-1.[1]

Lyme disease, first recognized as a focal outbreak of arthritis in Old Lyme, CT,[2] is caused by the bite of an *Ixodes* tick infected with the spirochete *Borrelia burgdorferi*. Primary Lyme disease consists of a skin lesion, erythema chronicum migrans (ECM), which may be followed by secondary manifestations involving the cardiovascular and the central and peripheral nervous systems.[3] Tertiary Lyme disease is characterized by recurrent pain and swelling of the large joints. Sixty percent of Lyme disease patients experience joint symptoms that develop months to years following the tick bite.[4] In many cases, arthritis is the only clinical manifestation of the disease.[2] Arthritis involves the large joints and is histologically similar to rheumatoid arthritis.[5]

Although the manifestations of Lyme disease are widespread and may be severe, it has been relatively difficult to demonstrate the presence of the spirochete in affected tissues. Silver staining has occasionally shown spirochetes in skin lesions,[6] especially the leading edge of erythema chronicum migrans, the myocardium[7] and synoviae[8] from Lyme disease patients. Spirochetes have been cultured only infrequently from blood[3,6] and synovial fluids.[9] That *Borrelia burgdorferi* are rarely identified in Lyme disease patients has led us to search for both spirochete and host-derived factors with the capacity to amplify the pathogenicity of the organism.

We have previously shown the Lyme disease spirochete to be a potent inducer of IL-1 production by cultured human and murine mononuclear phagocytes.[10] In addition, we have reported that *B. burgdorferi* possess a lipopolysaccharide (LPS) that

[a]This work was supported by grant no. AR36028 from the National Institutes of Health.

has powerful biological activities.[11] Lipopolysaccharides are known to induce IL-1 synthesis and release by a variety of cells.[1] In this paper we examine the role of spirochete-derived products and interleukin-1 in the development of arthritis in Lyme disease.

MATERIALS AND METHODS

Cell Culture

The human histiocytic tumor cell line U937 and the murine macrophage cell line P388D1 were grown in RPMI 1640 containing 10% heat-inactivated FCS, penicillin (100 U/ml), and streptomycin (100 μg/ml). Human IL-1 was produced by stimulating U937 cells with *B. burgdorferi* as described in detail.[10]

The Shelter Island isolate of the Lyme disease spirochete was grown and passaged as described previously.[11] Before use, spirochetes were washed in RPMI 1640 three times by resuspension after centrifugation at 9000 $\times$g at 4°C for 20 min. The spirochetes were then resuspended in RPMI 1640 at a concentration of 1×10^8/ml.

Cells from Lyme disease or routine autopsy synovial fluids were obtained by centrifugation at 3000 $\times$g at 4°C for 10 min. The cells were washed in saline, and resuspended in 5 ml of RPMI 1640 containing 10% heat-inactivated FCS, penicillin (100 U/ml), and streptomycin (100 μg/ml). The cells were then seeded into T 25 tissue culture flasks and after an overnight incubation at 37°C in 5% CO_2 in air, the nonadherent cells were removed and fresh medium added. Cells were examined and the medium was replaced every 4 days. After 25 days, the cells had reached confluency and all cells were removed by the addition of trypsin/EDTA (0.5% trypsin and 0.02% disodium salt of EDTA) for 20 min at 37°C. The medium was changed at this time to MEM containing 20% heat-inactivated FCS and the cells placed into T 75 tissue culture flasks. After an additional 21 days, differential trypsinization was done to separate populations of cells based on their adherence to plastic in the presence of trypsin.[12] Trypsin/EDTA was added to monolayers for 5 min at 37°C. Medium was then added and the cells released by the trypsin/EDTA treatment were removed and seeded into new flasks. The original flasks received new medium and were returned to the incubator.

IL-1 Assay: Thymocyte Proliferation Assay

Samples were assayed for lymphocyte activation factor (LAF) activity[1] as a measure of IL-1 activity with thymocytes from 4- to 8-week-old BALB/c mice, as previously described.[10] Neutralization of IL-1 activity by anti-IL-1 antibodies was performed using an IgG fraction of rabbit anti-human IL-1 antibody kindly provided by Dr. Robert C. Newton of DuPont (Glenolden, PA). The antibody was produced by injection of purified α and β human monocyte-derived IL-1 into rabbits. This antibody (1 : 320 dilution) is capable of approximately 50% inhibition of 1 U of human IL-1 when assayed in the thymocyte proliferation assay.[13,14] It also inhibited the activity of IL-1 in a fibroblast proliferation assay and in a chondrocyte stimulation assay but had no effect on IL-2 assays. IL-1–containing samples were incubated for 30 min at room temperature with and without antibody before addition of thymocytes. For all assays, significance of differences was assessed by Student's *t*-test.

Preparation of Spirochete Lipopolysaccharide (LPS) and Peptidoglycan

LPS was isolated from *B. burgdorferi* by the petroleum-ether:chloroform:liquid-phenol extraction procedure as previously described.[11] Peptidoglycan was isolated as described by Beck and Habicht (this volume).

Release of IL-1 Activity by Stimulated, Cultured Synovial Fluid Cells

Synovial fluid cells from the T 75 flasks were removed from confluent cultures by trypsinization, washed, and grown to confluency in 24-well tissue culture dishes. At this time, the medium was removed, the plates were washed, and 1 ml of MEM containing either spirochetes (5×10^6) or spirochetal LPS (0 to 10 μg/ml) was added. Control cultures of spirochetes or spirochetal LPS in the absence of cells were also established. The plates were incubated for 24 hours. The supernatants were harvested and centrifuged at 9000 $\times$g for 10 min at 4°C and stored at -20°C until assayed for IL-1 activity as described above.

Patient Selection

Synovial fluids from eight patients with Lyme arthritis of long duration were obtained by sterile arthrocentesis of swollen joints only in cases where removal of fluid was therapeutically essential. Synovial fluids collected from five autopsy specimens served as controls.

IL-1 in Synovial Fluids

Joint fluids of Lyme disease patients were centrifuged to remove cells, diluted 1:2 in RPMI 1640, and sterilized by millipore filtration (0.22 μm, Millipore, Bedford, MA). Some of the fluid was assayed for IL-1 as described above. The remainder of the fluid was treated with type II hyaluronidase (10 μg/ml final concentration) for 60 min at 37°C.[15] The fluid was then centrifuged (5000 $\times$g), dialyzed (6000–8000 dalton cutoff) against PBS, and applied to a Sephadex G-50 column (Pharmacia, Piscataway, NJ). Fractions were collected (3 ml) and run in the thymocyte assay as described above.

RESULTS AND DISCUSSION

Synovial fluids from Lyme disease patients and autopsy controls were tested for their capacity to stimulate murine thymocyte proliferation in the presence of a submitogenic concentration of concanavalin A (0.4 μg/ml). This assay for lymphocyte activating factor (LAF) activity defines the biological activity of IL-1. While most Lyme disease specimens had significant IL-1 activity as measured at a 1:128 dilution (stimulation indices ranged from 4 to 10) only an occasional normal fluid showed such activity and then at a lower dilution (1 : 16). G-50 column chromatography of Lyme disease synovial fluids revealed that joint fluid IL-1 eluted in the 15,000–20,000 dalton range, a molecular weight consistent with that of IL-1 secreted by monocytes.[1] Like monocyte-derived IL-1 synovial fluid, IL-1 showed molecular weight heterogeneity.

Similar findings have been made with IL-1 activity in synovial fluids from rheumatoid arthritis patients.[16-18]

When the major peak of IL-1 activity from synovial fluid G-50 chromatography was concentrated and incubated with anti-human monocyte-derived IL-1 antibodies, the LAF activity was partially neutralized (39.3%; $p < 0.001$). Monocyte-derived IL-1 was neutralized under the same conditions by 39.5% ($p < 0.001$). Thus, synovial fluid IL-1 has the same size and immunologic profiles as monocyte IL-1.

Lyme disease synovial fluids were characterized by the presence of large numbers of polymorphonuclear cells and smaller numbers of mononuclear cells. The latter have been shown to have heightened reactivity to *B. burgdorferi* antigens.[19] In order to characterize further mononuclear cells in synovial fluids, cells were isolated and differentiated into two populations based on their sensitivity to differential trypsinization. The first population was fibroblast-like in appearance with large nuclei and abundant cytoplasm with numerous processes (type 1 cells). The second population was more epithelial-like (type 2 cells). Both cell types were found in both normal and Lyme disease synovial fluids. These cell types were examined for their ability to

TABLE 1. Stimulation of Cultured Synovial Fluid Cells

Cell Type	Stimulus	IL-1 Activity (^{3}H-Thymidine Uptake) (ΔMean dpm + SEM)	% Neutralization by Anti-IL-1
Normal synovial cells, type 1	5×10^6 spirochetes	6769 ± 1036^b	42.5 ± 18.8^a
	2.5 μg/ml LPS	5026 ± 1059^a	nd
Normal synovial cells, type 2	5×10^6 spirochetes	3374 ± 604^a	59.4 ± 4.6^a
	2.5 μg/ml LPS	5943 ± 1364^a	nd
Lyme synovial cells, type 2	5×10^6 spirochetes	$14,583 \pm 2475^a$	51.6 ± 8.5^a
	2.5 μg/ml LPS	5708 ± 595^b	nd

$^a p < 0.01$ compared to unstimulated cells or to no anti-IL-1.
$^b p < 0.001$ compared to unstimulated cells or to no anti-IL-1.
nd = Not determined.

produce IL-1 activity between the third and twelfth cell passages. The addition of 5×10^6 *B. burgdorferi* cells per ml to both cell populations resulted in enhanced release of IL-1 activity into the supernatant (TABLE 1). Spirochete-induced synovial fluid cell IL-1 activity was also partially neutralized by anti-human monocyte IL-1.

Since very few viable spirochetes have ever been identified in synovial fluids from Lyme disease patients, it is important to ask whether spirochete products also stimulate IL-1 production. LPS is shed from spirochetes *in vitro*[11] and is also a potent inducer of monocyte IL-1 production. To test its effect on IL-1 production, *B. burgdorferi* LPS was incubated with both type 1 and type 2 synovial fluid cells at concentrations ranging from 0.6–10 μg/ml. All concentrations tested induced small amounts of IL-1 activity (TABLE 1). In addition, we have shown that peptidoglycan from *B. burgdorferi* can induce murine macrophages to produce IL-1 (Beck and Habicht, this volume). It will be of interest to extend these studies to synovial cells, since peptidoglycans have been implicated in the pathogenesis of arthritides associated with gram positive bacterial infections.[20]

Several cell types in or near the joint capsule have been shown to be capable of secreting IL-1, including resident macrophages[1] and synoviocytes.[21] It has been postulated that local production of IL-1 in strategically located, specialized cells may participate in the pathogenesis of several inflammatory diseases, especially the destructive bone and joint diseases.[22,23] In Lyme disease the arthritic lesion involves pannus formation and erosion of bone and cartilage.[24] IL-1 stimulates pannus formation.[22] In a closed space like that of the joint, IL-1 may have destructive actions occurring in the absence of a systemic response, such that the hallmarks of ongoing infection such as fever or increased erythrocyte sedimentation rate may be sporadic or absent. Arthritis frequently occurs in Lyme disease patients in the absence of systemic changes.

IL-1 has several biological activities that affect cells in or near the synovium and may be involved in the pathogenesis of Lyme arthritis. These include the production of prostaglandin E_2 (PGE_2), which induces pain, and the release of proteolytic enzymes or their zymogens. Chondrocytes are stimulated to proliferate and to release PGE_2, latent collagenase, and plasminogen activator by IL-1.[24-26] Fibroblasts also produce PGE_2 and latent collagenase when stimulated by IL-1.[27,28] Synovial cells release PGE_2 in response to purified and recombinant IL-1.[28,29] Mononuclear-cell-conditioned medium containing IL-1 activity enhances the release of synovial cell plasminogen activator and neutral proteoglycanase activity. Plasmin, resulting from the presence of plasminogen activator, activates various mediators of inflammation and enzymes capable of inducing joint destruction including collagenase and neutral proteoglycanase. The activities of osteoblasts and osteoclasts are also affected by IL-1. Studies with porcine cells suggest that IL-1 acts on osteoblasts, causing them to produce a factor that acts at short range to activate osteoclasts to initiate bone resorption.[30] In other studies IL-1 seems to activate osteoclasts directly.[31] Osteoblasts also proliferate in the presence of IL-1.[32]

That IL-1 may play a role in the pathogenesis of Lyme arthritis is supported by the present observation of IL-1 activity in synovial fluids from Lyme disease patients. Steere *et al.* have reported elevated levels of collagenase and PGE_2 production by synovial tissue from a patient with chronic Lyme arthritis.[33]

Many factors suggest that IL-1 is centrally involved in the pathogenesis of Lyme disease and especially of Lyme arthritis. The Lyme disease spirochete and at least two of its cellular components are powerful inducers of IL-1 formation *in vitro*. Several cell types capable of releasing IL-1 as well as cells responsive to IL-1 are found in or near the joint. Local production of and response to IL-1 may produce cryptic disease characterized by local tissue destruction such as that found in Lyme disease.

REFERENCES

1. DINARELLO, C. A. 1984. Interleukin-1. Rev. Infect. Dis. **6:** 51–95.
2. STEERE, A. C., S. E. MALAWISTA, J. A. HARDIN, S. RUDDY, P. W. ASKENASE & W. A. ANDIMAN. 1977. Erythema chronicum migrans and Lyme arthritis. The enlarging clinical spectrum. Ann. Intern. Med. **86:** 685–698.
3. BENACH, J. L., E. M. BOSLER, J. P. HANRAHAN, J. L. COLEMAN, G. S. HABICHT, T. F. BAST, D. J. CAMERON, J. L. ZIEGLER, A. G. BARBOUR, W. BURGDORFER, R. E. EDELMAN & R. A. KASLOW. 1983. Spirochetes isolated from the blood of two patients with Lyme disease. N. Engl. J. Med. **308:** 740–742.
4. STEERE, A. C., S. E. MALAWISTA, N. H. BARTENHAGEN, P. N. SPIELER, J. H. NEWMAN, D. W. RAHN, G. J. HUTCHINSON, J. GREEN, D. R. SNYDMAN & E. TAYLOR. 1984. The clinical spectrum and treatment of Lyme disease. Yale J. Biol. Med. **57:** 453–461.
5. STEERE, A. C., A. GIBOFSKY, M. E. PATARROYO, R. J. WINCHESTER, J. A. HARDIN & S. E.

MALAWISTA. 1979. Chronic Lyme arthritis. Clinical and immunogenetic differentiation from rheumatoid arthritis. Ann. Intern. Med **90:** 896–901.

6. STEERE, A. C., R. L. GRODZICKI, A. N. KORNBLATT, J. E. CRAFT, A. G. BARBOUR, W. BURGDORFER, G. P. SCHMID, E. JOHNSON & S. E. MALAWISTA. 1983. The spirochetal etiology of Lyme disease. N. Engl. J. Med. **308:** 733–740.

7. MARCUS, L. C., A. C. STEERE, P. H. DURAY, A. E. ANDERSON & E. B. MAHONEY. 1985. Fatal pancarditis in a patient with coexistent Lyme disease and babesiosis. Demonstration of spirochetes in the myocardium. Ann. Intern. Med. **103:** 374–376.

8. JOHNSTON, Y. E., P. H. DURAY, A. C. STEERE, M. KASHGARIAN, J. BUZA, S. E. MALAWISTA & P. W. ASKENASE. 1985. Lyme arthritis. Spirochetes found in synovial microangiopathic lesions. Am. J. Pathol. **118:** 26–34.

9. SNYDMAN, D. R., D. P. SCHENKIEN, V. P. BERARDI, C. C. LASTAVICA & K. M. PARISER. 1986. *Borrelia burgdorferi* in joint fluids in chronic Lyme disease. Ann. Intern. Med. **104:** 798–800.

10. HABICHT, G. S., G. BECK, J. L. BENACH, J. L. COLEMAN & K. D. LEICHTLING. 1985. Lyme disease spirochetes induce human and murine interleukin-1 production. J. Immunol. **134:** 3147–3154.

11. BECK, G., G. S. HABICHT, J. L. BENACH & J. L. COLEMAN. 1985. Chemical and biological characterization of a lipopolysaccharide extracted from the Lyme disease spirochete (*Borrelia burgdorferi*). J. Infect. Dis. **152:** 108–117.

12. FRESHNEY, R. I. 1983. Culture of Animal Cells. Alan R. Liss, New York. pp. 129–143.

13. BECK, G. & G. S. HABICHT. 1986. Isolation and characterization of a primitive interleukin-1-like protein from an invertebrate, *Asterias forbesi*. Proc. Natl. Acad. Sci. USA **83:** 7429–7433.

14. KELLEY, M. M., M. E. ROSEMILLER, A. J. DAULERIO & R. C. NEWTON. 1984. Development of an antibody specific for human interleukin-1. Lymphokine Res. **3:** 251.

15. STASTNY, P., M. ROSENTHAL, M. ANDRIES & M. ZIFF. 1975. Lymphokines in the rheumatoid joint. Arthritis Rheum. **18:** 237–243.

16. WOOD, D. D., E. J. IHRIE, C. A. DINARELLO & P. L. COHEN. 1983. Isolation of an interleukin-1-like factor from human joint effusions. Arthritis Rheum. **26:** 975–983.

17. FONTANA, A., H. HENGARTNER, E. WEBER, K. FEHR, P. J. GROB & G. COHEN. 1982. Interleukin-1 activity in the synovial fluid of patients with rheumatoid arthritis. Rheumatol. Int. **2:** 49–53.

18. NOURI, A. M. E., G. S. PANAYI & S. M. GOODMAN. 1984. Cytokines and the chronic inflammation of rheumatic disease. I. The presence of interleukin-1 in synovial fluids. Clin. Exp. Immunol. **55:** 295–302.

19. SIGAL, L. H., A. C. STEERE, D. H. FREEMAN & J. M. DWYER. 1986. Proliferative responses of mononuclear cells in Lyme disease. Reactivity to *Borrelia burgdorferi* antigens is greater in joint fluid than in blood. Arthritis Rheum. **29:** 761–769.

20. SCHWAB, J. H. 1981. Acute and chronic inflammation induced by bacterial cell wall structures. *In* Arthritis: Models and Mechanisms. H. Deicker & L. S. Schultz, Eds. Springer-Verlag. New York.

21. WOOD, D. D., E. J. IHRIE & D. HAMERMAN. 1985. Release of interleukin-1 from human synovial tissue *in vitro*. Arthritis Rheum. **28:** 853–862.

22. DINARELLO, C. A. 1985. An update on interleukin 1: From molecular biology to clinical relevance. J. Clin. Immunol. **5:** 287–297.

23. BECK, G., G. S. HABICHT, J. L. BENACH & F. MILLER. 1986. Interleukin 1: A common endogenous mediator of inflammation and the local Shwartzman reaction. J. Immunol. **136:** 3025–3031.

24. KRAKAUER, T., J. J. OPPENHEIM & H. E. JASIN. 1985. Human interleukin-1 mediates cartilage matrix degradation. Cell. Immunol. **91:** 92–99.

25. RIFAS, L., V. SHEN, K. MITCHELL & W. A. PECK. 1984. Macrophage-derived growth factor for osteoblast-like cells and chondrocytes. Proc. Natl. Acad. Sci. U.S.A. **81:** 4558–4562.

26. GOWEN, M., D. D. WOOD, E. J. EHRIE, J. E. MEATS & R. G. G. RUSSELL. 1985. Stimulation by human interleukin-1 of cartilage breakdown and production of collagenase and proteoglycanases by human chondrocytes but not by human osteoblasts *in vitro*. Biochim. Biophys. Acta **797:** 186–193.

27. SCHMIDT, J. A., S. B. MIZEL, D. COHEN & I. GREEN. 1982. Interleukin-1, a potential regulator of fibroblast proliferation. J. Immunol. **128:** 2177–2182.
28. MIZEL, S. B., J.-M. DAYER, S. M. KRANE & S. E. MERGENHAGEN. 1981. Stimulation of rheumatoid synovial cell collagenase and prostaglandin production by partially purified lymphocyte activating factor (interleukin-1). Proc. Natl. Acad. Sci. U.S.A. **78:** 2474–2477.
29. DAYER, J.-M., B. DE ROCHEMONTIEUX, B. BURRUS, S. DEMCZUK & C. A. DINARELLO. 1986. Human recombinant interleukin-1 stimulates collagenase and prostaglandin E_2 production by human synovial cells. J. Clin. Invest. **77:** 645–648.
30. THOMPSON, B. M., J. SAKLATVALA & T. J. CHAMBERS. 1986. Osteoblasts mediate interleukin-1 stimulation of bone resorption by rat osteoclasts. J. Exp. Med. **164:** 104–112.
31. STASHENKO, P., F. E. DEWHIRST, W. J. PEROS, R. L. KEND & J. M. AGO. 1987. Synergistic interactions between interleukin-1, tumor necrosis factor, and lymphotoxin in bone resorption. J. Immunol. **138:** 1464–1468.
32. GOWEN, M., D. D. WOOD & R. G. G. RUSSELL. 1985. Stimulation of the proliferation of human bone cells *in vitro* by human monocyte products with interleukin-1 activity. J. Clin. Invest. **75:** 1223–1229.
33. STEERE, A. C., C. E. BRINKERHOFF, D. J. MILLER, H. DRINKER, E. D. HARRIS, JR. & S. E. MALAWISTA. 1980. Elevated levels of collagenase and prostaglandin E2 from synovium associated with erosion of cartilage and bone in a patient with chronic Lyme arthritis. Arthritis Rheum. **238:** 591–599.

Pathogenesis of Lyme Arthritis

Implications for Rheumatic Disease[a]

ALLEN C. STEERE

Division of Rheumatology/Immunology
New England Medical Center
Tufts University School of Medicine
Boston, Massachusetts 02111

The chronic inflammatory arthritides include rheumatoid arthritis, juvenile arthritis, Reiter's syndrome, reactive arthritis, ankylosing spondylitis, arthritis associated with inflammatory bowel disease, psoriatic arthritis, and Lyme arthritis. The causes of most of these diseases remain unknown. Reiter's syndrome and reactive arthritis are thought to be triggered by various enteric or sexually transmitted pathogens. However, in the United States, where *Yersinia enterocolita* infection is rare, the specific agent responsible for these diseases is often unclear in a given case. Since 1982, the etiologic agent of Lyme arthritis, *Borrelia burgdorferi,* has been known with certainty.[1]

Several mechanisms have been hypothesized to explain rheumatoid arthritis. First, an unidentified microorganism, perhaps a virus, may be present in synovial tissue, which results in an immune response directed against the organism. Alternately, there may be molecular mimicry between components of a microorganism elsewhere, perhaps in bowel flora, and components of synovium; or perhaps nondegradable bacterial peptidoglycan is deposited in synovium where it elicits a chronic immune response. However, rheumatoid arthritis has more commonly been thought to be due to genetically determined autoimmune phenomena, such as complexes of IgG and IgM rheumatoid factor or immunity to collagen type II.

Because the cause of Lyme arthritis is now known with certainty, it provides an important opportunity to determine the pathogenesis of one form of chronic inflammatory arthritis. The following review details our studies of the last several years, completed or in progress, that bear upon this issue.

NATURAL HISTORY OF LYME ARTHRITIS

During the late 1970s, before the role of antibiotic therapy in Lyme disease was known, we enrolled patients in a prospective study to determine the natural history of Lyme arthritis. Through a surveillance system of community-based physicians, we attempted to find all patients with erythema chronicum migrans in the Lyme, Connecticut area. Fifty-five of these patients, who did not receive antibiotic therapy for erythema migrans, were followed longitudinally for a mean duration of 6 years. We believe that these patients provide the best information available on the natural history of Lyme arthritis.

Eleven of the 55 patients (20%) had no subsequent manifestations of Lyme disease.[2] From 1 day to 8 weeks after disease onset, 10 of the patients (18%) began to experience brief episodes of periarticular or musculoskeletal pain for as long as 6 years,

[a]This work was supported by grant no. AR-20358 from the National Institutes of Health.

but they never developed objective joint abnormalities. From 4 days to 2 years after disease onset, 28 of the patients (51%) experienced one episode or began to have intermittent attacks of frank arthritis, primarily in large joints; a few had polyarticular involvement. The total number of these patients who continued to have recurrences decreased by 10–20% each year. The remaining six patients (11%) developed chronic synovitis later in the illness; two of them (4%) had erosions, and one (2%) had permanent joint disability.

We believe that this experience makes several important points about pathogenesis. First, it shows that the majority of patients exposed to *B. burgdorferi* in the United States develop joint symptoms. However, these symptoms range from arthralgias, to intermittent attacks of arthritis, to chronic erosive disease. We favor the hypothesis that Lyme arthritis and arthralgias result from hematogenous spread of spirochetes to multiple joints early in the illness. Some patients experience vague, somewhat evanescent, migratory joint pain from this event while others develop frank arthritis, most commonly in knees. In the rat model of Lyme arthritis, it has been shown that the spirochete spreads hematogenously to many joints early in the illness and that clinically apparent arthritis develops only in the tibiotarsal joints weeks later.[3]

HOST FACTORS

The wide spectrum of joint involvement suggests that host factors play a major role in determining the severity and duration of Lyme arthritis. In our initial study of 10 patients with chronic Lyme arthritis, seven had the B cell alloantigen DR2 and four were positive for DR4.[4] Thus, in this preliminary assessment, there appeared to be an increased frequency of DR2 in patients with chronic Lyme arthritis. In collaboration with Dr. Robert Winchester at the Hospital for Joint Diseases, we have now typed 125 patients with different manifestations of Lyme disease, including erythema migrans alone, neurologic involvement, or arthritis. None of these groups had an increased frequency of a D locus antigen. However, when the 76 patients with arthritis were segregated according to duration of disease, 14 of 22 patients with chronic Lyme arthritis (64%) had DR4 compared with 12 of 54 patients with intermittent arthritis (22%, $p < .0001$) or with 31% of individuals in a normal population ($p < .005$). Since the frequency of DR4 is also increased in patients with rheumatoid arthritis, it is possible that similar mechanisms predispose to chronicity in these two diseases.

THE SYNOVIAL LESION

In past studies of sections stained with hematoxylin and eosin, the synovial lesions of Lyme arthritis have been noted to be similar to those of other chronic inflammatory arthritides, including rheumatoid arthritis.[5] In markedly inflamed synovium with lymphoid follicles, the lesion may have features of a peripheral lymph node, the primary site where T cell-dependent immune responses are mounted against foreign antigens. Thus, chronically inflamed synovium is sometimes called an ectopic lymphoid organ.

In order to extend these observations, we examined the synovial lesions of Lyme disease using monoclonal antibodies to *B. burgdorferi* and to lymphoid surface cell markers, and compared these lesions with those from rheumatoid synovium and tonsillar lymphoid tissue.[6] The synovial lesions of Lyme disease and rheumatoid arthritis were nearly identical and often consisted of the elements in normal organized lymphoid tissues. In both diseases, T cells, predominantly of the helper-inducer subset, were distributed diffusely in subsynovial lining areas, often with nodular aggregates of tightly intermixed T and B cells. IgD-bearing B cells were scattered within the aggregates, and a few follicular dendritic cells and activated germinal center B cells were sometimes present. Outside the aggregates, many plasma cells, high endothelial venules, scattered macrophages, and a few dendritic macrophages were found. HLA-DR and DQ expression was intense throughout the lesions. Thus, the lesion is typical of a chronic hypersensitivity immune response to foreign antigen.

In Lyme arthritis, we have attempted to find evidence of agent/antigen in the tissue using culture and immunohistologic techniques.[6] To date, of 18 synovial specimens cultured in modified Kelly's medium, none have been positive. For immunohistologic studies, we produced monoclonal antibodies against B. burgdorferi spirochetes, and by immunoperoxidase techniques stained the tissues with antibodies to the 31-kDa outer membrane polypeptide of the spirochete and the 41-kDa flagellar antigen. In six of 12 patients with Lyme arthritis but in none of the 12 with rheumatoid arthritis, a few spirochetes and globular antigen deposits were seen in and around blood vessels in areas of lymphocytic infiltration. Although background staining was minimal, it was still very difficult to find spirochetes or spirochetal antigen in the tissue, and many high-power fields of many sections had to be examined to find them.

The scarcity of organisms in the synovial lesion of Lyme arthritis is reminiscent of the lesions of tertiary syphilis or tuberculoid leprosy. In these diseases, it is very difficult to find organisms in the lesion, but the small number present are able to persist and trigger a florid chronic lymphoplasmacellular immune response. In Lyme arthritis, the antigenic stimulus for chronic synovial inflammation would appear to be a small number of spirochetes.

CELLULAR IMMUNITY

After the Lyme disease spirochete was discovered in 1982, it became possible to measure the specific immune response to these antigens. In 27 patients with early Lyme disease tested in 1983, the mean response of peripheral blood mononuclear cells to Lyme spirochetal Borrelia burgdorferi antigens (723 cpm) was similar to that of control subjects.[7] During convalescence, 2 to 3 weeks later, the patients' mean response was significantly higher (2075 cpm, $p < 0.008$). Compared with those with early disease, the peripheral blood mononuclear cells of 22 patients with Lyme arthritis reacted even more to B. burgdorferi (2923 cpm, $p < 0.0004$), and by far the greatest response was in concomitantly obtained synovial fluid mononuclear cells (15,238 cpm, $p < 0.001$). The peripheral blood mononuclear cells of patients with early Lyme disease reacted slightly less to phytohemagglutin and pokeweed mitogen than those of normal control subjects, but patients with arthritis had greater than normal mitogen responses. In contrast, mitogen reactivity among synovial fluid cells was markedly decreased and correlated inversely with the response to antigen. Thus, in patients with Lyme disease, the antigen-specific responses of mononuclear cells increase as the disease progresses and in those with arthritis, the greatest reactivity to antigen is found in cells in the inflamed joint. Such cells, rather than a direct effect of the organism, may play a key role in the resultant synovial pathology.

In both the rheumatoid arthritis and in Lyme disease, the ratio of T helper to T suppressor cells in joint fluid may be increased, the response to mitogens is less in joint fluid than in peripheral blood, and the background counts are greater in synovial fluid. However, in rheumatoid arthritis patients in our studies, neither peripheral blood nor joint fluid cells responded to B. burgdorferi antigens. This experience with Lyme disease makes us wonder whether rheumatoid lymphocytes might respond to antigens that are currently unknown.

HUMORAL IMMUNITY

In an effort to better understand the pathogenesis of the arthritis, we used immunoblotting to define the sequence in which IgM and IgG antibodies appeared to each of the protein antigens of *B. burgdorferi,* and compared the antibody responses in serum and joint fluid.[8] In 12 patients with early disease alone, both the IgM and IgG responses were restricted primarily to the 41-kDa flagellar antigen of the spirochete. This limited response disappeared within several months. In contrast, among six patients with prolonged illness, the IgM response to the 41-kDa protein sometimes persisted for months to years, and late in the illness during arthritis, a new IgM response sometimes developed to a 34-kDa component of the organism. The IgG response in these patients appeared in a characteristic sequential pattern over months to years to as many as 11 spirochetal antigens.

Although synovium is not a selective barrier like the blood-brain barrier, we hypothesized that additional antigens may be bound by antibodies produced locally in the joint, and therefore may be concentrated or present only in joint fluid. Among the nine patients tested, however, there were no qualitative differences in the paired joint fluid and serum responses. In addition, our analysis of serial sera in patients with different clinical manifestations did not reveal an association between arthritis and a particular polypeptide. Rather, progression of the disease was associated with gradual expansion of the immune response, regardless of the particular clinical manifestations. Although we did not implicate a particular spirochetal antigen as important in the pathogenesis of the arthritis, the appearance of a new IgM response and the expansion of the IgG response late in the disease, and the lack of such responses in the patients with erythema migrans alone, supports the view that *B. burgdorferi* remains alive throughout the illness.

It has been postulated that immune complexes, which include rheumatoid factor, may be important in the pathogenesis of rheumatoid arthritis. In our initial studies, using the C1q binding assay, abnormal C1q binding was uniformly present in the synovial fluid of affected joints, and always to a greater extent than in the circulation.[9] More recently, we have looked for evidence of spirochetal antigens in immune complexes but, to date, have been unable to find them. Thus, although immune complexes appear to be present in the joint fluid of patients with Lyme arthritis, their derivation and phlogistic potential remain unclear.

Lyme arthritis differs from rheumatoid arthritis with respect to the presence of rheumatoid factor. In a recent study, using a sensitive ELISA, 7 of 25 patients with Lyme arthritis had a positive test for IgM rheumatoid factor, but only one of the samples was positive by the more insensitive latex agglutination method.[10] In addition, we have been unable to find rheumatoid factor activity in cryoprecipitable complexes.[11] Although the precise role of rheumatoid factor in Lyme disease is unknown, it is probably similar to that of a number of chronic infections, and different from that in rheumatoid arthritis.

TREATMENT

In our initial studies, we tested parenteral penicillin regimens for treating Lyme arthritis.[12] In a double-blind placebo-controlled trial carried out from 1980 to 1982, 20 patients with established Lyme arthritis were assigned treatment with 2.4 million U of intramuscular benzathine penicillin weekly for 3 weeks (total 7.2 million U) and 20 patients received saline. Seven of the 20 penicillin-treated patients (35%) had complete resolution of arthritis soon after the injections and have remained well during a mean follow-up period of 5 years. In contrast, all 20 patients given placebo had one or more attacks of arthritis afterwards ($p < 0.02$). Because high-dose intravenous penicillin achieves peak blood drug levels more than 100 times as high as those attained by other routes of administration, we next did an observational study of one regimen—high-dose intravenous penicillin, 20 million U per day for 10 days—for the treatment of established Lyme arthritis.[12] Of 20 patients treated in this way in 1983, nine (45%) had complete resolution of arthritis and have remained well since. We concluded that established Lyme arthritis can often be treated successfully with parenteral penicillin. However, in contrast to our experience in treating neurologic disease with high-dose penicillin, which was uniformly effective,[13] neither of the regimens that we tested for arthritis appeared to be optimal.

We are currently testing prolonged oral antibiotic regimens and other parenteral ones for established Lyme arthritis. Such patients who have not previously received antibiotic therapy are being randomized to receive oral regimens of doxycycline or amoxicillin and benemid. Patients who did not respond to oral regimens were originally given high-dose intravenous penicillin for 2 or 3 weeks. For the past 10 months, such patients have been treated with intravenous ceftriaxone. To date, we have entered a total of 40 patients into one of these four treatment groups, and they have been followed for mean durations of 7 to 19 months since treatment. Although more patients and longer periods of follow-up are still needed before conclusions can be drawn, a few generalizations can be made. First, with each antibiotic regimen, joint effusions generally changed little during the course of antibiotics and in patients who responded, the effusions gradually decreased over a period of several months. Although patients given parenteral antibiotics had had arthritis for significantly longer than those receiving oral regimens, only about 50–70% of patients in each of the four treatment groups had resolution of arthritis within months. Another 10–30% of patients in each group, after resolution of the arthritis as above, had one or two short recurrent attacks of minor joint swelling, but did not require additional antibiotic therapy. The remaining approximately 10–20% of patients in each group had undiminished arthritis for 6 months or longer after treatment, which was usually terminated by arthroscopic synovectomy. Thus, in preliminary observations, none of the differences among groups were statistically significant.

The usual response of established Lyme arthritis to antibiotic therapy also provides evidence that spirochetes are still alive when arthritis is present. However, the slowness of this response and the difficulty in finding spirochetal antigens in synovium suggests that immune-mediated phenomena or small numbers of live attenuated spirochetes may propagate the synovial lesion for at least several months after treatment is given.

IMPLICATIONS FOR RHEUMATIC DISEASE

In summary, in the chronic inflammatory arthritides, it has been hypothesized that infectious agents may trigger, in genetically susceptible persons, an immune response that leads to chronicity. The current work on Lyme arthritis provides evidence in each of these areas. In Lyme arthritis, a few *B. burgdorferi* appear to survive in synovium, but it is very difficult to find them or parts of them in the tissue. At least part of the resultant immune response seems to be directed against the organism, and this response may account for much of the synovial pathology. However, infection and autoimmunity are not mutually exclusive, and this work does not rule out the possibilities that molecular mimicry, nondegradable bacterial fragments, or autoimmunity may play a role in some aspects of the pathogenesis of the synovial lesion. As in rheumatoid arthritis, chronicity of the arthritis may be greater in patients with the DR4 alloantigen. This experience lends greater credibility to the possibility that an infectious agent may be present in rheumatoid synovium.

REFERENCES

1. STEERE, A. C., R. L. GRODZICKI, A. N. KORNBLATT, J. E. CRAFT, A. G. BARBOUR, W. BURGDORFER, G. P. SCHMID, E. JOHNSON & S. E. MALAWISTA. 1983. The spirochetal etiology of Lyme disease. N. Engl. J. Med. **308:** 733–740.
2. STEERE, A. C., R. T. SCHOEN & E. TAYLOR. 1987. The clinical evolution of Lyme arthritis. Ann. Intern. Med. **107:** 725–731.
3. BARTHOLD, S. W., K. D. MOODY, G. A. TERWILLIGER, P. H. DURAY, R. O. JACOBY & A. C. STEERE. 1988. Experimental Lyme arthritis in rats infected with *Borrelia burgdorferi*. J. Infect. Dis. **157:** 842–846.
4. STEERE, A. C., A. GIBOFSKY, M. E. PATARROYO, R. J. WINCHESTER, J. A. HARDIN & S. E. MALAWISTA. 1979. Chronic Lyme arthritis: Clinical and immunogenetic differentiation from rheumatoid arthritis. Ann. Intern. Med. **90:** 896–901.
5. JOHNSTON, Y. E., P. H. DURAY, A. C. STEERE, M. KASHGARIAN, J. BUZA, S. E. MALAWISTA & P. W. ASKENASE. 1985. Lyme arthritis: Spirochetes found in synovial microangiopathic lesions. Am. J. Pathol. **118:** 26–34.
6. STEERE, A. C., P. H. DURAY & E. C. BUTCHER. 1988. Spirochetal antigens and lymphoid cell surface markers in Lyme synovitis: Comparison with rheumatoid synovium and tonsillar lymphoid tissue. Arthritis Rheum. **31:** 487–495.
7. SIGAL, L. H., A. C. STEERE, D. H. FREEMAN & J. M. DWYER. 1986. Proliferative responses of mononuclear cells in Lyme disease: Reactivity to *Borrelia burgdorferi* antigens is greater in joint fluid than in blood. Arthritis Rheum. **29:** 761–769.
8. CRAFT, J. E., D. K. FISCHER, G. T. SHIMAMOTO & A. C. STEERE. 1986. Antigens of *Borrelia burgdorferi* recognized during Lyme disease: Appearance of a new IgM response and expansion of the IgG response late in the illness. J. Clin. Invest. **78:** 934–939.
9. HARDIN, J. A., A. C. STEERE & S. E. MALAWISTA. 1979. Immune complexes and the evolution of Lyme arthritis: Dissemination and localization of abnormal C1q binding activity. N. Engl. J. Med. **301:** 1358–1363.
10. KUJALA, G. A., A. C. STEERE & J. S. DAVIS IV. 1987. IgM rheumatoid factor in Lyme disease: Correlation with disease activity, total serum IgM, and IgM antibody to *Borrelia burgdorferi*. J. Rheum. **14:** 772–776.
11. STEERE, A. C., J. A. HARDIN, S. RUDDY, J. G. MUMMAW & S. E. MALAWISTA. 1979. Lyme arthritis: Correlation of serum and cryoglobulin IgM with activity and serum IgG with remission. Arthritis Rheum. **22:** 471–483.
12. STEERE, A. C., J. GREEN, R. T. SCHOEN, E. TAYLOR, G. J. HUTCHINSON, D. W. RAHN & S. E. MALAWISTA. 1985. Successful parenteral penicillin therapy of established Lyme arthritis. N. Engl. J. Med. **312:** 869–874.
13. STEERE, A. C., A. PACHNER & S. E. MALAWISTA. 1983. Neurologic abnormalities of Lyme disease: Successful treatment with high-dose intravenous penicillin. Ann. Intern. Med. **99:** 767–772.

Specific Immune Responses in Lyme Borreliosis

Characterization of T Cell and B Cell Responses to *Borrelia burgdorferi*

RAYMOND J. DATTWYLER, DAVID J. VOLKMAN,
JOHN J. HALPERIN, BENJAMIN J. LUFT,
JOANNE THOMAS, AND MARC G. GOLIGHTLY

*State University of New York
at Stony Brook
School of Medicine
Stony Brook, New York 11794*

Lyme borreliosis, *Borrelia burgdorferi* infection, is a chronic progressive infection involving multiple organ systems including the skin, the central and peripheral nervous systems, the heart, liver, and kidney, and the musculoskeletal system.[1-3] As in other chronic infectious diseases, host responses to this infecting microorganism play a major role in shaping the clinical expression of this persistent spirochetosis. Untreated patients develop an antibody response to a limited number of antigens early in the course of infection. The humoral response gradually evolves to include a broader range of spirochetal antigens only later as the disease progresses.[4,5] A vigorous specific T cell response to *B. burgdorferi* is detectable early in the course of the infection, often preceding the development of a measurable humoral response.[6] The role that these immune responses play in the expression of the various clinical manifestations of this illness remains to be delineated. However, since spirochetes have been demonstrated in patients with high specific antibody levels against *B. burgdorferi*,[7,8] it is clear that the development of immunity to this organism does not effectively eradicate it from the host.

As with any infection, the immune response plays a pivotal role in the containment of the invading microorganism. In any chronic infection, the microbe must evolve strategies to avoid eradication by the host. Such strategies include suppression of the host's defenses; evasion of host defenses through antigenic mimicry or antigenic variation; or invasion of immunologically privileged sites.[9] The precise host-parasite relationship in *B. burgdorferi* infection remains largely undefined, but a clear understanding of this relationship will be critical for the development of optimal treatment regimens and for any attempts to promote the immunologic control of this infectious disease.

Erythema chronicum migrans (ECM) has classically been the best marker of Lyme borreliosis.[10] However, with the discovery of the causative organism, demonstration of an antibody response to *B. burgdorferi* has become a requirement for the diagnosis of late infection.[11,12] As in syphilis, prompt antibiotic treatment aborts the development of a sustained humoral response.[5,13] It has been felt that the failure of patients to mount a measurable specific antibody response after treatment of early Lyme borreliosis indicates the successful elimination of the organism.[14] However, persistent symptoms including arthralgias, tingling in the arms or legs, chronic fatigue, and other neurologic complaints are not uncommon in patients treated with oral

93

antibiotic regimens.[14,15] The presence of these symptoms has been attributed by some to a post-Lyme disease syndrome and not to the possibility of continued infection.

We have previously shown that Lyme borreliosis is associated with both the development of strong specific T cell response to whole *B. burgdorferi* and alteration of normal immune function.[6] In this study we further delineate human T and B cell responses in Lyme borreliosis and present a model that addresses interactions of T cells and B cells in developing anti-*B. burgdorferi* reactivity.

METHODS

Human Subjects

All subjects involved in this study were from Suffolk County, New York, an area highly endemic for Lyme borreliosis. For the purpose of this study, the subjects were grouped as follows:

- Early Lyme borreliosis: ECM with no significant antibody titer to *B. burgdorferi* as measured by a specific ELISA.
- Late Lyme borreliosis: Patients with signs and symptoms of active late Lyme borreliosis (cardiac, neurologic, and/or joint involvement) and a history of ECM.
- Normal controls: Normal healthy adults with no history of Lyme borreliosis or any rheumatic or immune disorder.

ELISA

The ELISA was performed as previously described,[16] with minor modifications. Briefly, 96-well microtiter plates were coated with a sonicate of *B. burgdorferi* (5 μg/ml) for 18 hours in 0.05 M sodium carbonate (pH 9.6), then washed in blocking buffer containing bovine serum albumin. Patient sera, positive, and negative controls were diluted 1 : 500. Aliquots of 100 μl of sera were added to duplicate wells, incubated, and then washed. Phosphatase substrate was added and after stopping the reaction the plates were read on an ELISA reader.

Immunofluorescent Assay

Indirect immunofluorescence assays (IFA) for the detection of both IgM and IgM antibodies against *B. burgdorferi* were performed by standard techniques. Briefly, slides coated with *B. burgdorferi* (Diagnostic Technology, Hauppauge, NY) were incubated with serial dilutions of patient sera for 60 minutes at room temperature, and washed three times in PBS. The slides were then incubated for 30 minutes with fluorescence-labeled anti-IgG or anti-IgM and washed and examined under a fluorescent microscope.

SDS-PAGE and Immunoblotting

Qualitative antibody analyses were performed as previously described[17] with slight modifications. Briefly, *B. burgdorferi* strain B31 was grown in BSK II media[18] and washed three times in phosphate-buffered saline (PBS). Spirochetes were resuspended in 2 ml of PBS containing 10 mM ethylene diamine tetracetic acid and 1 mM paramethylsulfonyl fluoride and sonicated in an Ultratip Labsonic System (Lab-Line Instruments, Melrose Park, IL) for 5 minutes. The protein concentration was measured by the Bradford procedure.[19] The mixture was made 2.5% in SDS and 2.5% in 2-mercaptoethanol, heated at 100°C for 3 min, and adjusted to 0.4–0.6 mg/ml of protein. SDS-PAGE was performed using a Might Small II apparatus (Hoeffer, San Francisco, CA) at 60 V for 2 hours. Blots were left overnight at 4°C in Tris buffer (50 mM Tris, 150 mM NaCl) containing 1% bovine serum albumin. Blots were next incubated with serum diluted 1 : 100 with Tris buffer for 2 h at 37°C and washed for 10 min with Tris buffer containing 0.5% Tween-20 and then for 10 min in Tris buffer alone. Bound Ig was detected with goat anti-human IgG and IgM conjugated to alkaline phosphatase (Sigma, St. Louis, MO). After a 2-h incubation at 37°C with a 1 : 5000 dilution of the conjugates, the blots were again washed in a two-step procedure and then incubated with BICIP-Substrate System (KPL, Gaithersburg, MD) for 20 minutes. The reaction was stopped by rinsing the blots in distilled water.

Preparation of B. burgdorferi *sonicates*

Organisms were pelleted by centrifugation at 10,000 g for 20 mins at 4°C, washed four times in cold 0.01 M PBS, and sonicated in an Ultratip Labsonic System for 5 minutes. Supernates were prepared by centrifugation of the sonicate at 4°C for 30 min at 10,000 g.

Lymphocyte Proliferative Assays

Lymphocyte proliferative assays were performed as previously described.[6] Briefly, mononuclear cells were isolated by Ficoll-Hypaque density gradient centrifugation (Pharmacia) and washed three times. They were adjusted to a final concentration of 1×10^6 cells per ml in RPMI 1640 containing 10% human AB serum, 0.5% penicillin/streptomycin, and 2% L-glutamine. Cells (1×10^5 per well) were pipetted into a 96-well microtiter plate (Costar) and stimulated (in triplicate) with whole *B. burgdorferi* at a concentration of 1×10^6 organisms per well. For the limiting dilution experiments centrifuged or uncentrifuged sonicates were added where appropriate in place of the whole organism. Control wells received media only. Cell cultures were incubated in a humidified atmosphere of 5% CO_2 at 38°C. One μCi well of ^{3}H-thymidine (S.a, 6.7 Ci/mmol) (NEN, Boston, MA) was added 18 hours prior to harvest. After 5 days the cultures were harvested by an automated cell harvester onto filter disks and counted in a liquid scintillation counting system. Counts were expressed as disintegrations per minute (dpm). The triplicates were averaged and a Stimulation Index (SI) was calculated for each patient:

$$SI = \frac{dpm \ (stimulated)}{dpm \ (unstimulated)} .$$

Limiting Dilution Analysis

Limited dilution analysis to determine the precursor frequency of antigen-specific T cells was modified from previously described methods.[21,22] Peripheral blood mononuclear cells (PBMC) were cultured at varying densities in 96-well, U-bottomed microtiter plates (Linbro, Flow Laboratories, McLean, VA) containing 10^4 irradiated (2400 rad) autologous PBMC. PBMC densities from 1×10^3 to 30×10^3 per well were analyzed. Twenty-four replicate wells at each cell density were cultured; 18 wells contained *Borrelia* antigen (either 10^5 whole *Borrelia* or 80 μg/ml of soluble antigen); six of the wells contained only medium. Cells were cultured for 6 days, and pulsed with 1 μCi of ^{3}H-thymidine 18 h prior to harvest. Wells were scored as containing at least one *Borrelia*-specific T cell if their thymidine incorporation (dpm) was greater than three standard deviations above the mean dpm of the six wells without antigen. The precursor frequency was obtained by plotting the logarithm of the percent negative wells against the average number of cells per well and extrapolating to the cell number at which 37% of the wells will score negative (the number at which there will be an average of one *Borrelia*-specific T cell per well).[22]

RESULTS

TABLE 1 compares the T cell blastogenic response to whole *B. burgdorferi* with response to the supernates from centrifuged *B. burgdorferi* sonicates at equivalent protein concentrations. Whole *B. burgdorferi* proved to be the best stimulator of specific T cell proliferation by a substantial margin. The superiority of whole *B. burgdorferi* was confirmed by limiting dilution analysis of the precursor frequency of antigen-specific T cells (FIG. 1). In the donor studied, the frequency of cells responding to whole *B. burgdorferi* was 1 per 5300 mononuclear cells, or approximately 1 per 3700 T cells. Using uncentrifuged *B. burgdorferi* sonicates as the stimulating antigen produced only a slight decrease in the calculated frequency of responding T cells (data not shown). Thus, there is little or no loss of antigenicity after simple sonication. In marked contrast, the precursor frequency when supernates from centrifuged *B. burgdorferi* sonicates were used as the stimulating antigen was less than 1 per 200,000 mononuclear cells, approximately one-fortieth the number of specific T cells capable of responding to the whole organism.

When the peripheral blood mononuclear cells from five patients with classic antibody-positive late Lyme borreliosis were cultured with whole *B. burgdorferi* there was a strong proliferative response. The mean dpm were 21,690 and the mean SI was 20.6. Five patients with virtually identical clinical histories, but with no significant

TABLE 1. Proliferative Responses to Soluble and Whole *B. burgdorferi* Antigens

Stimulus	Proliferation[a] dpm (± SEM)
Medium alone	163 (14)
PHA (2 μg/ml)	44,701 (2912)
B. burgdorferi supernatants	
8 μg/ml	5911 (1382)
80 μg/ml	14,789 (1652)
800 μg/ml	8660 (2222)
Whole *B. burgdorferi*	
2×10^4	75,552 (16,123)
2×10^5	87,205 (6282)
2×10^6	90,716 (4162)

[a]Proliferation measured by ^{3}H-thymidine incorporation

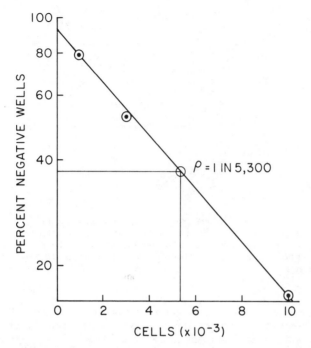

FIGURE 1. Limiting dilution analysis of precursor frequency for whole *B. burgdorferi* specific T cells. PBMC were as described in METHODS. The concentration at which 37% of the wells were negative represents an average frequency of one antigen-specific T cell per well.

humoral response to *B. burgdorferi* as measured by a specific ELISA, had T cell responses very similar to the sero-positive patients. Their mean response to *B. burgdorferi* was 20,861 dpm.

The sequential development of antibody responses to an expanding range of *B. burgdorferi* antigens as infection proceeds is illustrated in FIGURE 2. Immunoblots show specific IgG against *B. burgdorferi* detected in the serum of patients diagnosed with Lyme borreliosis at various times after ECM. Lane A is a normal control; lanes B through F are five individual patients with increasing duration of untreated *B. burgdorferi* infection. All patients were treated immediately after diagnosis with appropriate antibiotics. Subsequent IgG immunoblots demonstrated that once antispirochetal antibiotics are given, the expansion of the humoral response to additional *B. burgdorferi* antigens ceases.

DISCUSSION

The limiting dilution analysis data presented here reveal that in established *B. burgdorferi* infection, the frequency of T cells capable of responding to the whole organism is relatively high (approximately 1 in 3700 T cells). This frequency is comparable to the reported precursor frequency of other potent T-cell-dependent antigens, suggesting that *B. burgdorferi* has a large number of antigenic sites and/or

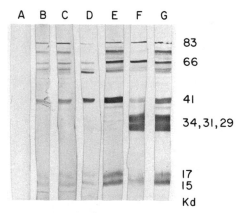

FIGURE 2. Immunoblots of individual patients illustrating the sequential development of the antibody response to *B. burgdorferi*. Lane A, normal control; lanes B–G, individual patients with increasing duration of untreated infection. These blots were probed with a 1 : 200 dilution of sera, and affinity-purified anti-human IgG alkaline phosphatase conjugates were used to detect specific bound IgG.

that infection produces a sizable expansion of reactive T cell clones. Despite there being little difference in the observed protein bands on SDS-PAGE analysis between supernatants and uncentrifuged sonicates, a marked loss of T cell antigenicity occurs when the sonicated organism is centrifuged (only approximately 1 in 140,000 T cells responding). Thus, particulate-associated antigens lost with high-speed centrifugation are highly effective stimuli of specific blastogenic responses. Since several major *Borrelia* proteins are membrane associated, removal of these particulate antigens may well alter the ability of phagocytes to present these antigens. The marked differences in the antigenicity between both whole *B. burgdorferi* and sonicates as compared to supernates from centrifuged sonicates explain the disparity between the vigorous T cell responses reported in this study and in our previous report (18,000 to 20,000 counts)[6] and the substantially lower responses reported by others (2000 to 2700 counts).[24-26] Therefore, one must be cautious in interpreting proliferative responses when centrifuged sonicates are used as the source of *B. burgdorferi* antigens. This puts into doubt any conclusions drawn from previous experiments on the cellular immune response in Lyme borreliosis in which centrifuged sonicates were used as the source of *B. burgdorferi* antigens. Studies are currently under way in our laboratory to identify T cell immunodominant antigens present in sonicate pellets produced by high-speed centrifugation.

In a previous study we demonstrated that in patients with ECM, the specific T-cell response to *B. burgdorferi* can develop prior to the development of a measurable humoral response.[6] The finding of a specific T cell response in the absence of a measurable humoral response in patients with early infection was not unexpected, since T cell help is required for the production of a mature humoral response to most antigens. The present study suggests that a disassociation of T and B cell immunity can also occur in patients with late Lyme borreliosis. There is ample precedent in human infectious diseases for the disassociation of specific T and B cell immunity. Mycobacterial, fungal, helminthic, and protazoan infections can at times be associated with specific T cell anergy to the infecting organism, while at the same time there is a high level of specific B cell activity.[26-28] The finding that patients with late Lyme borreliosis can have specific T cell activity against *B. burgdorferi* in the absence of a significant antibody response detectable by ELISA is the converse of these other situations. Although an ELISA assay failed to detect significant levels of specific antibody, these patients were not totally devoid of antibodies reacting to spirochetel antigens. Using a Western blot assay, a faint band of IgG antibody activity against the 41-kDa band was detectable in all five patients. In addition, two of these patients also had a faint IgM band against the 41-kDa antigen. However, antibody activity against the 41-kDa band is not specific for *B. burgdorferi* infection since the 41-kDa flagellar-associated antigen contains epitopes shared by treponemes and by other borreliae. Approximately half of our normal controls had similar faint bands. The finding of this incidence of reactivity against the 41-kDa antigen in normal controls is higher than that reported by other groups. We have no precise explanation for this difference. One possibility is that our assay is more sensitive. Another is the fact that our controls were all from a highly endemic area and many have had previous tick bites.

The mechanisms producing this disassociation of T and B cell responses remain to be precisely delineated. However, antibiotic therapy may play a role, since all five patients were treated with antimicrobials early in the course of their infection. Perhaps this treatment removed most of the organism at an early stage of the immune response. Early treatment has previously been noted to interrupt the development of an antibody response in patients treated at the ECM stage.[5] A similar abrogation of the antibody responses after early treatment occurs in syphilis.[13]

We propose a model of the specific immune response that may explain the observed phenomena (FIG. 3). Current theories maintain that antigens are presented by Ia-positive phagocytic cells, such as macrophages and dendritic cells to immature antigen specific T cells, triggering clonal expansion and maturation of these antigen-specific clones. In antigen-specific systems, mature T cells can only cooperate with cells in the immune system expressing both the appropriate Ia and the specific antigen,

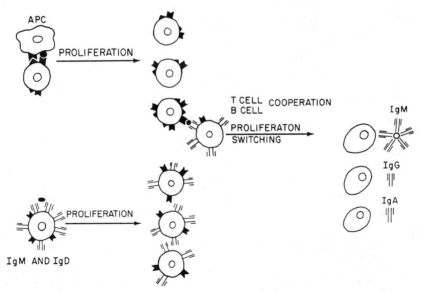

FIGURE 3. A model of T and B cell interaction in the development of the immune response to *B. burgdorferi*.

since the T cell receptor recognizes both Ia and antigen.[29] The lack of either will cause a failure of recognition. Thus, this model predicts that antigen initially triggers parallel clonal expansion of both T and B cells. Antigen-specific B cells, after this initial relatively T cell independent proliferation, must then present antigen to receive the requisite T cell help necessary for further maturation. Failing to do this, these committed but immature B cells never mature and may be lost. In the case of *B. burgdorferi* infection, early treatment with the resultant removal of antigen limits effective antigen-specific T and B cell interaction, blunting the development of a measurable antibody response. This effect may not be limited to early disease. It has been recognized that during the course of infection untreated patients sequentially develop antibody responses to additional antigens.[4,5] The progression of this sequential development appears to be arrested by antibiotic treatment as well.

This model postulates that removal of antigen at any point in the course of infection causes the failure of antigen-specific helper T cells to recognize specific B cells, aborting the development of a mature antibody response. However, this model apparently does not account for continued disease activity in the absence of a maturing antibody response. Late disease is felt to be secondary to persistent infection, thus antigen has to be present in the host. A possible explanation for this inconsistency is that although oral antibiotics can effectively eradicate the bulk of *B. burgdorferi*, the organism may invade immunologically privileged sites like the central nervous system where it can escape both effective treatment and the immune system. Since neither oral tetracycline nor low-dose penicillin enters the central nervous system in concentrations high enough to reach the reported mean inhibitory concentrations for the majority of *B. burgdorferi*, spirochetes reaching this immunologically privileged site may remain viable despite these treatments.[28]

On a more practical level, this study demonstrates that measurement of the specific T cell response to *B. burgdorferi* may document exposure to this spirochete. In addition to possibly forming the basis for the diagnosis of Lyme borreliosis, this may provide important information with regard to the pathophysiology of this infectious disease. It has been postulated in the past that the humoral immune response plays the key role in the pathophysiology of the later stages of this illness. Investigators have reported that elevated IgM levels, cryoglobulins, and circulating immune complexes are associated with active Lyme borreliosis and have proposed that immune complexes are responsible for the inflammatory arthritis of this disease.[30,31] In the absence of a significant maturing humoral response these mechanisms are unlikely to account for the observed symptoms and signs of Lyme borreliosis.

REFERENCES

1. HELLERSTROM, S. 1951. Erythema chronicum migrans Afzelius with meningitis. Acta Derm. Venereol. **31:** 227.
2. BURGDORFER, W., A. G. BARBOUR, C. F. HAYES, J. L. BENACH, E. GRUNWALDT & J. P. DAVIS. 1982. Lyme disease—a tick-borne spirochetosis? Science **216:** 1317.
3. MALAWISTA, S. E. & A. C. STEERE. 1986. Lyme disease: Infectious in origin, rheumatic in expression. Adv. Intern. Med. **31:** 147.
4. CRAFT, J. E., D. K. FISCHER, G. T. SHIMAMOTO & A. C. STEERE. 1986. Antigens of *Borrelia burgdorferi* recognized during Lyme disease. J. Clin. Invest. **78:** 934.
5. STIERNSTEDT, G., G. ERICKSSON, W. ENFORS, H. JORBECK, B. SVENUNGSSON, B. SKOLDEN-BERG & M. GRANSTROM, 1986. Erythema chronicum migrans in Sweden: Clinical manifestations and antibodies to *Ixodes ricinus* spirochete measured by indirect immunofluorescence and enzyme-linked immunosorbent assay. Scand. Infect. Dis. **18:** 217.

6. DATTWYLER, R. J., J. THOMAS, J. L. BENACH & M. G. GOLIGHTLY. 1986. Cellular immune responses in Lyme disease. Zbl. Bkt. Hyg. A **263**: 151.
7. WOLKE, J. H. J., J. VAN GIJIN, A. ELDERSON & G. STARREK. 1987. Chronic forms of *B. burgdorferi* infection of the nervous system. Neurology **37**: 1031.
8. LASTAVICA, C. C., D. R. SNYDMAN, D. P. SCHENKEIN, V. P. BERARDI & K. M. PARISER. 1986. Demonstration of *Borrelia burgdorferi* in a patient with chronic Lyme arthritis. Zbl. Bkt. Hyg. A **263**: 288.
9. BLOOM, B. R. 1979. Games parasites play: How parasites evade immune surveillance. Nature **279**: 21.
10. STEERE, A. C., S. E. MALAWISTA, J. A. HARDIN, S. RUDDY, P. W. ASKENASE & W. A. ANDIMAN. 1977. Erythema chronicum migrans and Lyme arthritis. Ann. Intern. Med. **86**: 685.
11. BENACH, J. L., E. M. BOSLER, J. P. HANRAHAN, J. L. COLEMAN, G. S. HABICHT, T. F. BAST, D. J. CAMERON, J. L. ZIEGLER, A. G. BARBOUR, W. BURGDORFER, R. EDELMAN & R. A. KASLOW. 1983. Spirochetes isolated from the blood of two patients with Lyme disease. N. Engl. J. Med. **308**: 740–742.
12. STEERE, A. C., R. L. GRODZICKI, A. N. KORNBLATT, J. E. CRAFT, A. G. BARBOUR, W. BURGDORFER, G. B. SCHMID, E. JOHNSON & S. E. MALAWISTA. 1983. The spirochetal etiology of Lyme disease. N. Engl. J. Med. **308**: 733–740.
13. FITZGERALD, T. J. 1981. Pathogenesis and immunology of *Treponema pallidum*. Ann. Rev. Microbiol. **34**: 29.
14. STEERE, A. C., G. J. HUTCHINSON, D. W. RAHN, L. H. SIGAL, J. E. CRAFT, E. T. DE SANNA & S. E. MALAWISTA. 1983. Treatment of the early manifestations of Lyme disease. Ann. Intern. Med. **99**: 22.
15. HALPERIN, J. J., P. K. COYLE & R. J. DATTWYLER. 1986. Lyme disease. A spirochete-associated, treatable polyneuropathy. Clin. Res. **34**: 519A.
16. CRAFT, J. E., R. J. GRODZICKI & A. C. STEERE. 1984. Antibody response in Lyme disease: Evaluation of diagnostic tests. J. Infect. Dis. **149**: 789.
17. TOWBIN, J., R. STAEHELIN & J. GORDON. 1979. Electrophoretic transfer of proteins from polyacrylamide gels to nitrocellulose sheets: Procedure and some applications. Proc. Natl. Acad. Sci. U.S.A. **76**: 4350.
18. BARBOUR, A. G. 1984. Isolation and cultivation of Lyme disease spirochetes. Yale J. Biol. Med. **57**: 521.
19. BRADFORD, M. M. 1976. A rapid and sensitive method for the quantitation of microgram quantities or protein utilizing the principle of protein-dye binding. Anal. Biochem. **72**: 248.
20. VOLKMAN, D. J., L. A. MATIS & A. S. FAUCI. 1984. Development and characterization of interleukin-2-independent antigen-specific human T cell clones that produce multiple lymphokines. Cell. Immunol. **88**: 323.
21. NUTMAN, T. B., E. A. OTTESEN, A. S. FAUCI & D. J. VOLKMAN. 1984. Parasite antigen-specific human T cell lines and clones: Major histocompatibility complex restriction and B cell helper function. J. Clin. Invest. **73**: 1754.
22. LEFKOVITS, I. & H. WALDMANN. 1979. Limiting Dilution Analysis of Cell in the Immune System. Cambridge Univ. Press. Cambridge. p. 262.
23. SIGAL, L. H., C. M. MOFFAT, A. C. STEERE & J. M. DWYER. 1984. Cellular immune findings in Lyme disease. Yale J. Biol. Med. **57**: 595.
24. MOFFAT, C. M., L. H. SIGAL, A. C. STEERE, D. H. FREEMAN & J. M. DWYER. 1984. Cellular immune findings in Lyme disease: Correlation with serum IgM and disease activity. Am. J. Med. **625**:
25. SIGAL, L. H., A. C. STEERE, D. H. FREEMAN & J. M. DWYER. 1986. Proliferative responses of mononuclear cells in Lyme disease. Arthritis Rheum. **29**: 261.
26. DATTWYLER, R. J., J. THOMAS & L. C. HURST. Antigen-specific T cell anergy in progressive mycobacterium marinum infection in man. Ann. Intern. Med. In press.
27. STIERNSTEDT, G., B. SKOLDENBERG, D. A. GARDE, G. KOLMODIN, H. JORBACK, B. SVENUNGSSON & B. CARLSTROM. 1985. Clinical manifestations of borrelia infection of the nervous system. Zbl. Bkt. Hyg. A **263**: 289.

28. DATTWYLER, R. J. & J. J. HALPERIN. 1987. Failure of tetracycline therapy in early Lyme disease. Arthritis Rheum. **30:** 448.
29. BENACERRAF, B. 1981. Role of MHC gene products in immune regulation. Science **212:** 1229.
30. HARDIN, J. A., A. C. STEERE & S. E. MALAWISTA. 1981. Immune complexes and the evolution of Lyme arthritis: Dissemination and localization of abnormal C1q binding activity. N. Engl. J. Med. **301:** 1358.
31. STEERE, A. C., J. A. HARDIN, S. RUDDY, J. G. MUMMAU & S. E. MALAWISTA. 1979. Lyme arthritis: Correlation of serum and cryoglobulin IgM with activity and serum IgG with remission. Arthritis Rheum. **22:** 471.

Modulation of Natural Killer Cell Activity by *Borrelia burgdorferi*[a]

MARC GOLIGHTLY, JOSEPHINE THOMAS,
DAVID VOLKMAN, AND RAYMOND DATTWYLER

Department of Pathology and the Department of Medicine
State University of New York at Stony Brook
Stony Brook, New York 11794

INTRODUCTION

Natural killer (NK) cells are a heterogenous subpopulation of peripheral blood lymphocytes (PBL) that have the ability to kill various tumors and tumor cell lines in the absence of prior sensitization. These cells have generated considerable interest and have been implicated in natural resistance to tumors,[1-5] resistance to viral infection,[5-7] transplantation rejection,[5,8] and immunoregulation of both T and B cells.[9-11] Recently, there has been evidence that NK cells or large granular lymphocytes (LGLs) are also involved in host resistance against bacterial infections. This has been demonstrated by the bactericidal activity of NK-like cells against certain bacteria such as *Shigella* and *Salmonella*.[12-14] In addition to these interactions, there are several reports that demonstrate bacterial activation and/or recruitment of NK and NK-like cells presumably through the production or action of interferon, interleukin-2, and/or lipopolysaccharide (LPS).[12,16-18] Under certain conditions this augmentation may be inhibited by LPS,[17] which attests to the complex nature of the microorganism-host interactions. Furthermore, the NK cell killing of infected host cells[15] or local inflammation secondary to the killing of extracellular microorganisms may be responsible for the tissue destruction seen in various bacterial infections.

The humoral and cellular responses in Lyme borreliosis have recently been under active investigation. While the humoral antibody response to *Borrelia burgdorferi* is well characterized, the cellular immune response is not well defined. However, it is known that a strong specific T cell response to *B. burgdorferi* occurs early in the course of the disease. This response may even precede the development of a measurable antibody response in some cases.[19] Once established, this response is long lasting.

In this report, the cellular immune response to *B. burgdorferi* is further investigated. Specifically, the modulation of NK cells and NK cell activity by *B. burgdorferi* both *in vivo* and *in vitro* is characterized and discussed.

MATERIALS AND METHODS

Cell Preparations

Normal human peripheral mononuclear cells (PBMs) were obtained from healthy volunteers or from patients with Lyme disease by separation on Ficoll-Hypaque density gradients as previously described.[20]

[a]This work was supported in part by NIH grant no. CA39345–02 and by a Catacosinos Research Award.

Immunofluorescent Assays and Cell Sorting

For immunofluorescent phenotyping a microlabeling procedure was developed due to the constraints on cell numbers. This procedure is basically the same as the standard published labeling techniques,[21] with the exception that only $5-10 \times 10^4$ cells were labeled with appropriately reduced amounts of antibody. In addition, the labeling was done in conical tubes rather than the round bottom tubes standardly used. The monoclonal antibodies used were CD3 (Leu-4, T cells), CD4 (T4, helper-inducer cells), CD8 (T8, cytotoxic-suppressor cells), Leu-7 (NK cells), CD16 (Leu-11, cytotoxic NK cells), and NKH-1 (also NK cells). Leu series antibodies were from Becton-Dickinson, Mountainview, CA. T4, T8, and NKH-1 were from Coulter, Hialeah, FL.

Cytotoxic Assay

^{51}Cr *Release Assay.* Cytotoxic activity was determined in a chromium release microcytotoxicity assay as described in detail elsewhere.[23] Briefly, chromium-labeled target cells were added at 5×10^3 per well in V-bottom 96-well tissue culture plates. Effector cells were then added at various effector to target cell ratios in a total volume of 0.2 ml of RPMI 10% Ab. Each ratio was performed in triplicate. Total release was determined by substitution of 100 μl of 1% Triton X-100 for effectors. The plates were then centrifuged. After incubation at 37°C for 1–2 hours, they were centrifuged again and 100 μl collected from each well and counted in a gamma counter. The percent cytotoxicity was calculated according to the following formula:

$$\text{percent cytotoxicity} = \frac{\text{experimental release} - \text{spontaneous release}}{\text{total release} - \text{spontaneous release}} \times 100.$$

Statistical Analyses. Results are expressed as the mean ± SE % cytotoxicity from triplicate wells. Significance was established using single classification analysis of variance for two groups (equivalent to the Student's t-test for the difference between two means).

Targets. The suspension tumor cell line used as targets was the K562 human erythromyeloid cell line. The cells were maintained in RPMI 10% FCS. The cells were mycoplasma free as determined periodically by the Hoescht fluorescent staining method.[23]

IL-2 Lymphocyte Cultures. IL-2 cultures were set up as previously described[24] with modifications. Briefly, 20 BRMP U/ml of TCGF (interleukin-2, Cellular Products, Buffalo, NY) was incubated with the responding cells (usually plastic depleted and nylon fiber column passed) at a concentration of 1×10^6/ml in RPMI 10% for 3 days or more depending on the experiment.

RESULTS

NK Activity and Phenotypic Analysis in Lyme Borreliosis

PBL from patients with various stages and treatment of Lyme borreliosis were examined for NK functional activity against K562 tumor targets. These results were compared to normal controls drawn and processed on the same day. FIGURE 1 demonstrates that there was a marked and highly significant inhibition ($p < 0.0005$) of *in vivo* endogeneous NK activity in two patient populations: (1) patients in the early stages of Lyme disease (ECM stage) and before treatment, and (2) patients exhibiting chronic active stages of the disease. There was no significant inhibition of NK activity in three other patient populations: (1) patients in the early stages of Lyme disease (ECM stage) after treatment; (2) chronic inactive patients; and (3) seronegative chronic Lyme disease patients before treatment. The seronegative patients were diagnosed with Lyme disease based on the clinical symptoms and a positive mitogenic responsiveness of PBL to *B. burgdorferi*.

The phenotypic analysis of PBL from patients with early Lyme disease and chronic Lyme disease demonstrates that there were no significant changes in the absolute numbers of T cells (CD3) and T cell subsets (CD4 and CD8, FIG. 2). However, FIGURE 3 demonstrates that there was a significant ($p < 0.0001$) increase in the absolute

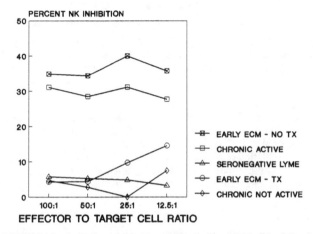

FIGURE 1. NK inhibition by *B. burgdorferi in vivo*. Patients exhibiting the following stages and treatment of Lyme borreliosis were tested by NK activity against K562 tumor targets and compared to normal healthy controls: (1) early ECM, no treatment ($n = 7$, $p < 0.0005$); (2) chronic active Lyme ($n = 11$, $p < 0.0005$); (3) seronegative Lyme ($n = 5$, not significant); (4) early ECM after treatment ($n = 5$, not significant); (5) chronic lyme, not active ($n = 4$, not significant).

number of circulating CD16$^+$ NK cells in the Lyme disease patients over the controls. It is interesting to note that while these patients exhibit an approximately fourfold *increase* in absolute numbers of CD16 NK cells, the NK activity is *decreased* by 30–40% without being normalized for the increase in absolute numbers. There was no significant change in the absolute number of Leu-7 and NKH-1 positive cells. In addition to the absolute numbers, these differences and similarities were also reflected in the percentage of fluorescent positive cells (data not shown).

Effect of B. burgdorferi *Culture on Normal PBL*

PBL from normal healthy donors were cultured for 7 days with and without *B. burgdorferi* in BSKII media or in RPMI-1640 with 10% FCS. On days 3, 5, and 7 the NK activity was examined. FIGURE 4 demonstrates that when lymphocytes are

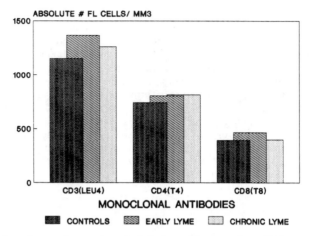

FIGURE 2. Lymphocyte phenotypic analysis in Lyme disease patients. PBL were examined in early Lyme, chronic Lyme, and normal healthy controls for expression of T cell antigens (CD3, CD4, and CD8). No significant differences were detected when compared to controls.

cultured in the presence of growing *B. burgdorferi* (in BSKII media) there is a marked inhibition ($p < .0005$) of NK activity on days 3, 5, and 7 when compared to lymphocytes cultured in BSKII media in the absence of spirochetes. This effect is not due to a selective depletion of or toxicity to endogeneous NK since viability studies and monoclonal antibody studies demonstrate no significant changes after culture with the organism (FIG. 5). The inhibition is directly attributable to the organism or its

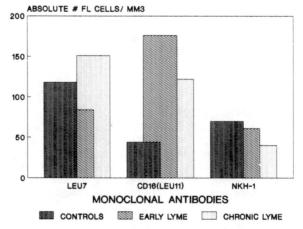

FIGURE 3. Lymphocyte phenotypic analysis in Lyme patients. PBL were examined in early Lyme, chronic Lyme, and normal healthy controls for expression of NK cell antigens (Leu-7, CD16, NKH-1). Early Lyme and chronic Lyme increased over control for CD16 ($p < 0.0001$ for both).

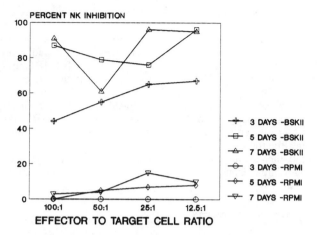

FIGURE 4. *B. burgdorferi* inhibition of NK *in vitro*. PBL from normal healthy donors were cultured for up to 7 days with spirochetes. On days 3, 5, and 7 NK activity was assessed and compared to those PBL cultured in the same media without spirochetes. In all cultures viability was >95%; $p < 0.0005$ for spirochete-PBL cultures in BSKII media.

products, since supernatants from the organism cultures also inhibit endogeneous NK without prior exposure (data not shown).

PBL cultured in the presence of *B. burgdorferi* in RPMI-1640 media exhibited no inhibition when compared to lymphocytes cultured in RPMI-1640 in the absence of spirochetes. Whether this lack of inhibition is related to inhibited spirochetal growth or metabolism is not known and is currently under investigation.

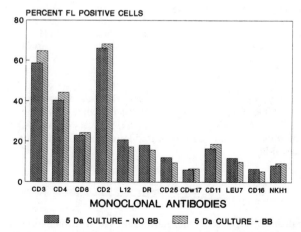

FIGURE 5. Lymphocyte phenotypic analysis of normal PBL after culture with *B. burgdorferi* in BSKII media. Cultures were grown for 5 days, then the PBL recovered and subjected to phenotypic analysis with monoclonal antibodies.

Effect of Interleukin-2 on PBL Cultured with **B. burgdorferi**

PBL from normal healthy donors were cultured for 5 days with and without spirochetes (in BSKII media). The PBLs were then washed and resuspended in RPMI-1640 10% FCS or RPMI-1640 10% FCS with 20 BRMP units/ml TCGF (IL-2) for an additional 3 days. The cytotoxic activity was then determined against K562 targets. Viability was greater than 98% (by trypan blue exclusion). FIGURE 6 demonstrates a representative experiment. PBL incubated with spirochetes for 5 days were unable to spontaneously recover NK activity when switched to RPMI-1640 in the absence of proliferating spirochetes (the majority of spirochetes are removed by the slow-speed centrifugations during the washes). However, PBL cultured with spirochetes for 5 days, then incubated with interleukin-2, recovered the cytotoxic activity to levels indistinguishable from IL-2-exposed PBL that were not cultured with *B*.

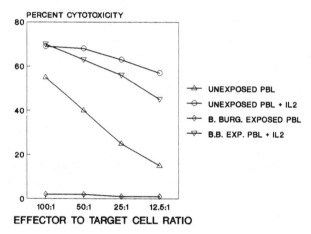

FIGURE 6. Recovery with IL-2 of NK-like activity from PBL cultured with *B. burgdorferi*. Normal healthy PBL were cultured with or without *B. burgdorferi* in BSKII media for 5 days. The cultures were then washed and cultured an additional three days with IL-2. NK activity was then determined; $p < 0.0001$ for *B. burgdorferi* exposed without IL-2 compared to *B. burgdorferi* exposed with IL-2.

burgdorferi. The cytotoxicity exhibited by both IL-2-stimulated populations was significantly ($p < 0.0001$) augmented over that of the control PBL never exposed to spirochetes or IL-2. Whether this is due to an actual recovery of the inhibited NK cells or due to the induction of lymphokine-activated killer (LAK) cells is under investigation and is discussed below.

DISCUSSION

It has been demonstrated that abnormalities in NK function and numbers exist in distinct populations of patients with Lyme borreliosis. Patients with chronic active disease and untreated patients in the early stages of the disease were found to exhibit a highly significant fourfold increase in the peripheral blood of the absolute number of NK cells expressing the CD16 (Leu-11) phenotype. The majority of these CD16[+] cells must also be Leu-7, based on the absolute numbers found. This increase may be the result of lymphokines (*i.e.*, IL-2, interferon) produced or actual bacterial antigens that have been reported to recruit previously inactive pre-NK cells into the cytotoxic NK pool.[17,18,25] However, this does not explain the significantly decreased NK cytotoxic ability of these patients' PBL. It is possible that this inhibition of NK activity is the result of a recruitment of inactive NK cells expressing CD16. However, this is unlikely since it has been reported that the majority of CD16[+], Leu-7[-] cells have cytotoxic activity.[26] Alternatively, the decrease in NK activity may be due to a direct effect of the *B. burgdorferi* organism or its products on the NK cell. It has been reported that LPS isolated from *Salmonella* has the ability to inhibit the bacterial augmentation of activated killers while leaving endogenous NK activity intact.[17] Thus, if a similar mechanism is occurring, it must also inhibit endogenous NK. It is also possible that *B. burgdorferi* produces a toxin that is responsible for the inhibition. An adenylate cyclase toxin can be extracted from *Bordetella* that will increase cAMP levels when added to NK cells, resulting in an inhibition of NK activity without killing the NK effector cells.[27]

It is interesting to note that the treated early Lyme and seronegative Lyme patients exhibit normal NK activity. This suggests that proliferating organisms and/or active interaction between *B. burgdorferi* and the immune system is required for inhibition of cytotoxic NK activity. These conditions may not occur in these patients, since treated early Lyme disease patients undergo a limited immune response due to the early eradication of the organism and the seronegative patients most likely have an aborted immune response due to the spirochetes being eliminated from the periphery and localized in immunologically privileged sites.[28]

The inhibition demonstrated *in vivo* was also observed *in vitro*. PBL cultured in the presence of proliferating organisms exhibited a marked diminution of NK activity, while PBL cultured in the presence of nonactively proliferating organisms did not demonstrate this decrease. This suggests that the inhibition may require active spirochetal metabolism. However, the requirement of a critical spirochete number cannot be ruled out since the inhibition occurs after the organisms have proliferated. Preliminary results suggest that the inhibition seen both *in vivo* and *in vitro* is due to an aberration in the lytic recycling ability of the NK cells and not in the actual recognition or lytic events associated with killing.

The *in vitro* inhibition of NK could be abrogated by additional culturing in the presence of interleukin-2. This may be due to actual recovery of the inhibited NK, recruitment of pre-NK cells into the cytotoxic NK pool, or the induction of lymphokine activated killer (LAK) cells. Preliminary evidence suggests that the majority of this "recovery" is due to LAK cells. However, contribution by the other mechanisms cannot be ruled out and is currently under investigation.

In summary, *B. burgdorferi* can induce a severe inhibition both *in vivo* and *in vitro* in NK cell cytotoxic capabilities. This is in contrast to other bacteria that are known to activate NK cells. While the inhibition appears to be directly related to spirochetal proliferation or concentration, the exact mechanism is unclear and is under active investigation. Interleukin-2 stimulation abrogates this inhibitory effect, possibly via the induction of LAK cells, which may be involved secondarily to the inhibited endogenous NK. More studies will be needed to elucidate these interactions and their full significance to the host-microorganism interaction.

REFERENCES

1. Pross, H. & M. Baines. 1976. Spontaneous human lymphocyte-mediated cytotoxicity against tumor target cells. Int. J. Cancer **13:** 593.

2. HALLER, O., M. HANSSON, R. KIESSLING & H. WIGZELL. 1977. Role of nonconventional natural killer cells in resistance against syngeneic tumor cells *in vivo*. Nature **270:** 609.
3. TAKASUGI, M., A. RAMSEYER & J. TAKASUGI. 1977. Decline of natural nonselective cell-mediated cytotoxicity in patients with tumor progression. Cancer Res. **37:** 413.
4. HANNA, N. & R. BURTON. 1981. Definitive evidence that natural killer (NK) cells inhibit experimental tumor metastasis *in vivo*. J. Immunol. **127:** 1754.
5. HERBERMAN, R. & J. ORTALDO. 1981. Natural killer cells: Their role in defenses against disease. Science **214:** 24–30.
6. LOPEZ, C., P. FITZGERLAD & T. SCHINDLER. 1985. Mechanisms of Cytotoxicity by NK Cells. R. Herberman & D. Callewaert, Eds.: 125. Academic. Orlando, FL.
7. LOPEZ, C. *et al.* 1983. Correlation between low natural killing of fibroblasts infected with herpes simplex virus type 1 and susceptibility to herpesvirus infections. J. Infect. Dis. **146:** 1030–1035.
8. NEMLANDER, A., E. SAKSELA & P. HAYRY. 1983. Are "natural killer" cells involved in allograft rejection? Eur. J. Immunol. **13:** 348–350.
9. TILDEN, A., T. ABO & C. BALCH. 1983. Suppressor cell function of human granular lymphocytes identified by the HNK-1 (Leu-7) monoclonal antibody. J. Immunol. **130:** 1171.
10. BRIEVA, J., S. TARGAN & R. STEVENS. 1984. NK and T cell subsets regulate antibody production by human *in vivo* antigen-induced lymphoblastoid B cells. J. Immunol. **132:** 611–615.
11. ROBLES, C. & S. POLLACK. 1986. Regulation of secondary *in vitro* antibody response by endogenous NK cells. J. Immunol. **137:** 2418.
12. TARKKANEN, J., E. SAKSELA & L. LANIER. 1986. Bacterial activation of human natural killer cells. J. Immunol. **137:** 2428–2433.
13. NENCIONI, L. *et al.* 1983. Natural and antibody-dependent cell mediated activity against *Salmonella typhimurium* by peripheral and intestinal lymphoid cells in mice. J. Immunol. **130:** 903.
14. MORGAN, D. *et al.* 1984. Cytotoxicity of human peripheral blood and colostral leukocytes against *Shigella* species. Infect. Immun. **46:** 25.
15. KLIMPEL, G., D. NIESEL & K. KLIMPEL. 1986. Natural cytotoxic effector cell activity against *Shigella flexneri*-infected HeLa cells. J. Immunol. **136:** 1081–1086.
16. NORMIER, G. *et al.* 1985. NK-cell stimulating properties of a membrane proteoglycane from non-capsulated *Klebsiella pneumoniae* biotype a. Acta Pathol. Microbiol. Scand. **93:** 233–243.
17. TARKKANEN, J. *et al.* 1986. Bacterial induction of human activated lymphocyte killing and its inhibition by lipopolysaccharide (LPS). J. Immunol. **136:** 2662–2668.
18. NAKANE, A. & T. MINAGAWA. 1985. Sequential production of alpha and beta interferons and gamma interferon in the circulation of *Listeria monocytogenes*-infected mice after stimulation with bacterial lipopolysaccharide. Microbiol. Immunol. **29:** 659–669.
19. DATTWYLER, R., J. THOMAS, J. BENACH & M. GOLIGHTLY. 1986. Cellular immune response in Lyme disease. Zbl. Bakt. Hyg. A **263:** 151–159.
20. BOYUM, A. 1968. Separation of leukocytes from blood and bone marrow. Scand. J. Clin. Lab. Invest. **21:** 77.
21. GOLIGHTLY, M. G., C. P. BRANDT, B. F. HAYNES & H. S. KOREN. 1982. Characterization of large granular lymphocytes before and after stimulation with interferon. *In* NK Cells and Other Natural Effectors. Ronald Herberman, Ed.: 79 Academic Press. New York.
22. SEELEY, J. & S. GOLUB. 1979. Studies on cytotoxicity generated in human mixed lymphocyte cultures. J. Immunol. **120:** 1414–1422.
23. CHEN, T. 1977. Microscopic demonstration of mycoplasma contamination in cell cultures and cell culture media. Exp. Cell Res. **104:** 255.
24. TILDEN, A., K. ITOH & C. BALCH. 1987. Human lymphokine-activated killer (LAK) cells. J. Immunol. **138:** 1068–1073.
25. BLANCHARD, D. *et al.* 1986. Interferon-induction by lipopolysaccharide. J. Immunol. **136:** 963–970.
26. LANIER, L. & M. LOKEN. 1984. Human lymphocyte subpopulations identified by using three-color immunofluorescence and flow cytometry analysis. J. Immunol. **132:** 151–156.

27. HEWLETT, E. *et al.* 1984. *Bordetella* extracytoplasmic adenylate cyclase: Actions as a bacterial toxin. Dev. Biol. Standard **21.**

28. DATTWYLER, R., J. THOMAS, D. VOLKMAN, M. GOLIGHTLY *et al.* 1988. Specific immune responses in Lyme borreliosis: Characterization of T cell and B cell responses to *Borrelia burgdorferi*. This volume.

Introduction

Lyme Disease: Antigens of *Borrelia burgdorferi* and Immune Responses to Them

GAIL S. HABICHT

Department of Pathology
State University of New York
Stony Brook, New York 11794

Although there has been rapid progress in our understanding of the epidemiology and etiology of Lyme disease since its description in the United States little more than a decade ago, many facets of this disease remain a mystery. People, cows, horses, and dogs may become ill when infected with *Borrelia burgdorferi* while the "natural" hosts, including wild mice and deer, remain unaffected despite the presence of readily demonstrable spirochetemias. In addition, most laboratory animals are resistant to disease induced by *B. burgdorferi*. Lyme disease patients are recognized clinically by the presence of the pathognomic rash, erythema chronicum migrans (ECM), and in the laboratory by the presence of antibodies specific for the spirochete—in fact, the higher the antibody titer, the more likely it is that a patient has an ongoing infection with *B. burgdorferi*. Why are these antibodies not protective? Why are they not destroying the spirochete? What are the implications of these observations for the development of vaccines against Lyme disease? The answers to these questions are no doubt complicated.

When the Lyme disease spirochete was discovered in the midgut of *Ixodes dammini* ticks collected from Shelter Island, New York, the conclusion that this was the etiologic agent of Lyme disease was substantiated by the demonstration of antibodies specific for the organism in the sera of patients but not of normal controls.[1] Indirect immunofluorescence revealed antibodies homogeneously reactive with the outer surface of the spirochete. SDS-PAGE of whole spirochete extracts showed numerous protein bands that were potential antigens. Bands at 34,000 (34 kDa), 41 kDa, and 60 kDa were prominent.[2] The 34-kDa and 41-kDa polypeptides were immunogenic in patients as demonstrated by Western blots. Sera from patients with early Lyme disease showed reactivity with the 41-kDa band while the late antibody response was specific for 31/34-kDa polypeptides.[3] Monoclonal antibodies have been used to identify the 41-kDa band as the spirochetal flagellin[4] and Benach *et al.*[5] have demonstrated that it consists of a family of several proteins.[5] Two outer surface spirochetal proteins have been designated OspA (31 kDa) and OspB (34 kDa).[6] OspA has a single, basic isoelectric point.[5]

The roles of the major outer surface proteins in spirochetal physiology are not well understood. Barbour[7] has shown that OspA and OspB are transcribed as a single messenger RNA. They are not found in the chromosomal DNA but rather in a supercoiled, circular, plasmid DNA. Plasmids are unstable in spirochetes cultured over long periods, which may account for the variable expression of OspA and OspB in different isolates of *B. burgdorferi*. Genes controlling lipopolysaccharide (LPS) expression have been found on plasmids in other bacteria[8] and the instability of plasmid DNA may explain why some laboratories have been able to detect LPS in *B. burgdorferi*[9] while others have not.[10]

Antigenic variability has been sought in isolates of spirochetes from ticks, patients, and animal carriers from various parts of Europe and the United States. American isolates show greater homogeneity than European isolates. Wilske *et al.*[11] demonstrated that European isolates were homogeneous with respect to the 41-kDa and 60-kDa polypeptides but showed molecular weight and antigenic heterogeneity of the OspA, OspB and pC proteins[11]; pC is another surface protein variably expressed on *B. burgdorferi*. Isolates from cerebrospinal fluid were more heterogeneous than those from the skin of ECM or of acrodermatitis atrophicans patients.

B. burgdorferi induces lymphocyte transformation as measured by ^{3}H-thymidine uptake in peripheral blood mononuclear cells[12] and joint fluid cells[13] from Lyme disease patients. Benach *et al.*[5] showed that both flagellin and OspA stimulated murine and human lymphocytes to proliferate, although responsiveness was not necessarily correlated with the presence of humoral immunity to the spirochete. Whether lymphocyte transformation in response to spirochetal antigens is related to disease resistance or to the presence of an ongoing infection remains to be determined.

Although either ECM or the presence of *B. burgdorferi* specific antibodies in a patient is diagnostic for Lyme disease, the expression of ECM is variable and there is a need for a diagnostic test that can detect early Lyme disease. Magnarelli[14] has examined over 4000 sera submitted for Lyme disease serology in Connecticut in a search for a laboratory correlate of early disease. Whole cells and cell sonicates were equally effective antigens in ELISA assays. Patients with early Lyme disease produce IgM antibodies specific for the 41-kDa flagellin,[3] whereas those with established disease produce predominantly IgG1 and IgG3 antibodies, as detected by ELISA.[15] A definitive serological test that would either confirm the clinical diagnosis of ECM or detect Lyme disease when patients present with nonspecific complaints is not yet available. Current efforts are being directed at detecting *B. burgdorferi* antigens in the urine of patients and infected animals.[16] Should this prove sensitive and feasible it would provide a noninvasive method for screening large numbers of individuals such as those with increased occupational risk for Lyme disease.

Because no complete laboratory animal model of Lyme disease is yet known, it has been difficult to study either vaccine development or pathogenesis. Experiments reported by Johnson *et al.*[16] show that the hamster experiences a transient spirochetemia and prolonged infection of other organs following injection of *B. burgdorferi*.[16] However, the animals are not noticeably sick. *B. burgdorferi* specific rabbit antibodies passively transferred to the hamster afforded protection if they were given before but not after bacterial challenge. In this respect the animal model is true to the human disease in that high titer antibodies coexist with ongoing infection. These observations suggest that the spirochete is sequestered in an immunologically privileged site and that it exerts its pathogenesis through components that escape immunological elimination.

REFERENCES

1. BURGDORFER, W. 1984. Discovery of the Lyme disease spirochete and its relation to tick vectors. Yale J. Biol. Med. **57:** 515–520.
2. BARBOUR, A. G., W. BURGDORFER, E. GRUNWALDT & A. C. STEERE. 1983. Antibodies of patients with Lyme disease to components of the *Ixodes dammini* spirochete. J. Clin. Invest. **72:** 504–515.
3. COLEMAN, J. L. & J. L. BENACH. 1987. Isolation of antigenic components from the Lyme disease spirochete: Their role in early diagnosis. J. Infect. Dis. **155:** 756–765.
4. BARBOUR, A. G., S. F. HAYES, R. A. HEILAND, M. E. SCHRUMPF & S. L. TESSIER. 1986. A *Borrelia*-specific monoclonal antibody binds to a flagellar epitope. Infect. Immun. **52:** 549–554.

5. BENACH, J. L., J. L. COLEMAN, J. C. GARCIA-MONCO & P. C. DEPONTE. 1988. Biological activity of *Borrelia burgdorferi* antigens. This volume.

6. BARBOUR, A. G., S. L. TESSIER & S. F. HAYES. 1984. Variation in a major surface protein of Lyme disease spirochetes. Infect. Immun. **45:** 94–100.

7. BARBOUR, A. G. & C. F. GARON. 1988. The genes encoding major surface proteins of *Borrelia burgdorferi* are located on a plasmid. This volume.

8. RILEY, L. W., L. N. JUNIO, L. B. LIBAEK & G. K. SCHOOLNIK. 1987. Plasmid-encoded expression of lipopolysaccharide O-antigenic polysaccharide in enteropathogenic *Escherichia coli*. Infect. Immun. **55:** 2052–2056.

9. BECK, G., G. S. HABICHT, J. L. COLEMAN & J. L. BENACH. 1985. Chemical and biological characterization of a lipopolysacharide extracted from the Lyme disease spirochete (*Borrelia burgdorferi*). J. Infect. Dis. **152:** 108–117.

10. TAKAYAMA, K., R. J. ROTHENBERG & A. G. BARBOUR. 1987. Absence of lipopolysaccharide in the Lyme disease spirochete, *Borrelia burgdorferi*. Infect. Immun. **55:** 2311–2313.

11. WILSKE, B., V. P. MURSIC, G. SCHIERZ, R. KÜHBECK, A. G. BARBOUR & M. KRAMER. 1988. Antigenic variability of *Borrelia burgdorferi*. This volume.

12. DATTWYLER, R. J., J. A. THOMAS, J. L. BENACH & M. G. GOLIGHTLY. 1986. Cellular immune response in Lyme disease: The response to mitogens, live *Borrelia burgdorferi*, NK cell function and lymphocyte subsets. Zbl. Bakt. Hyg. A **263:** 151–159.

13. SIGAL, L. H., A. C. STEERE, D. H. FREEMAN & J. M. DWYER. 1986. Proliferative responses of mononuclear cells in Lyme disease. Reactivity to *Borrelia burgdorferi* antigens is greater in joint fluid than in blood. Arthritis Rheum. **29:** 761–769.

14. MAGNARELLI, L. A. 1988. Serologic diagnosis of Lyme disease. This volume.

15. HECHEMY, K. E., H. L. HARRIS, M. J. DUERR, J. L. BENACH & C. B. REIMER. 1988. Immunoglobulin G (IgG) subclasses specific to *Borrelia burgdorferi* in patients with Lyme disease. This volume.

16. JOHNSON, R. C., C. KODNER, M. RUSSELL & P. H. DURAY. 1988. Experimental infection of the hamster with *Borrelia burgdorferi*. This volume.

Biological Activity of *Borrelia burgdorferi* Antigens[a]

JORGE L. BENACH,[b] JAMES L. COLEMAN,[b]
JUAN CARLOS GARCIA-MONCO,[c]
AND PAUL C. DEPONTE[b]

[b]New York State Department of Health
Health Sciences Center
State University of New York at Stony Brook
Stony Brook, New York 11794

[c]Hospital Nacional Marques de Valdecilla
Santander, Spain

INTRODUCTION

Outer surface protein A (OSP-A) and the flagellin bands of *Borrelia burgdorferi* are prominent in SDS-PAGE of whole spirochetes[1,2] and account for at least one-third of the total protein of this organism as measured by densitometry.[2] In the human patient, IgM and then IgG antibodies are produced initially to antigenic components of the periplasmic flagella (endoflagella) while antibodies to OSP-A (which is exposed on the outer surface) do not appear until later in the disease. Considering the anatomical abundance and exterior position of OSP-A, it would have been logical to assume that antibody recognition would have been reversed in the patient. In these experiments, we sought to measure the B- and T-cell repsonse to OSP-A and to flagellins in inbred Balb/c mice, which are refractory to *B. burgdorferi,* and in Syrian hamsters, which can harbor spirochetes for a long time with minimal evidence of disease and/or pathology.[3]

In addition to immunogenesis, bacterial antigens can have other roles in the disease process. In an inflammatory condition such as is Lyme disease, prominent antigens could induce significant migration of granulocytes, thereby contributing to the pathogenesis of the disorder.

B. burgdorferi is not easily isolated from human body fluids.[4] In laboratory animals and in reservoirs, successful isolations are mostly associated with tissues.[3,5] We have provided evidence that *B. burgdorferi* adhere strongly to cells of the tick midgut,[6] and other studies have shown that this organism binds to lymphocytes.[7] Adherence to cells is considered a first and important step in the pathogenesis of bacterial disease. In this study, we have attempted to explore the role of OSP-A and flagellins in cytoadherence.

Using eluted OSP-A and flagellins from SDS-polyacrylamide gels, we report here on the results of experiments designed to understand the role of these antigens in immunity, chemotaxigenesis, and cytoadherence.

[a]This work was partially funded by grant no. AI-23167 from the National Institutes of Health.

115

MATERIALS AND METHODS

Organisms and Animals

Borrelia burgdorferi B31 strain was used throughout all of the experiments in serum-free medium.[8] Balb/c mice and Syrian hamsters (outbred) were used for the studies on the development of antibodies to components of *B. burgdorferi* and as splenocyte donors for the studies on the cellular immune response.

Development of Antibody Response in Mice and Hamsters

Ten mice and ten hamsters were given a single intraperitoneal injection of 10^8 washed, live *B. burgdorferi* in RPMI-1640 supplemented with 10% heat-inactivated normal homologous serum. Animals were bled at weekly intervals and the sera was used for immunoblots and ELISA using *B. burgdorferi* as antigen- and class-specific anti-mouse conjugates: anti-mouse IgM (μ-chain specific) and anti-mouse and hamster IgG (γ-chain specific) conjugated with horseradish peroxidase (Hyclone Laboratories, Logan, UT). 4-Chloro-1-naphthol was used as enzyme substrate.

SDS-PAGE and Western Blots and Elution of Proteins

Spirochetal proteins (~ 10 μg) were separated by electrophoresis on 10% acrylamide slab gels using a Laemmli buffer system under reducing conditions.[9] Transfer of separated proteins to nitrocellulose was done by standard methods[10] on a Transblot® (BioRad, Richmond, CA). Molecular weight standards (Bethesda Research Laboratories, Gaithersburg, MD) were loaded on the outside lane of all gels. The elution procedures for OSP-A (~ 31 kDa) and for flagellins (~ 41 kDa) have been described.[2] Because the elution yields are small, several fractions from different elution runs were pooled. Only fractions that yielded single bands on silver stained gels were used in these experiments.[11]

Measurement of Antigen-Specific Cellular Immune Responses

Splenocytes from normal and previously infected mice (5 weeks after receiving 10^8 *B. burgdorferi*) were washed three times in RPMI-1640, counted and resuspended in culture medium (RPMI-1640 supplemented with 10% fetal calf serum, 100 U of penicillin G per ml and 100 μg of streptomycin per ml) and dispensed into sterile, flat-bottomed microtiter plates at 3×10^5 cells per well. Antigen-specific responses were measured by adding eluted OSP-A and flagellins at 0.01, 01, 1, and 2 μg/ml. Whole, washed spirochetes resuspended in RPMI-1640 were added at ratios of one cell to one spirochete, and then 10 : 1 and 100 : 1. Concanavalin A at 10 μg/ml was added to assess splenocyte function. Controls consisted of cells in culture medium. Human blood (from normal donors, nonreactive to *B. burgdorferi* by ELISA, and from Lyme disease patients with previously known reactivity to flagellins alone and to both flagellins and OSP-A) was collected in heparinized vacuum tubes, diluted 1 : 2 in RPMI-1640, layered in Ficoll-Paque® gradients (Pharmacia Fine Chemicals, Piscataway, NJ), and centrifuged for 45 minutes at 400 g. The resulting mononuclear bands were collected, washed twice, and the pellet resuspended in culture medium to deliver 3×10^5 cells per microtiter plate well. Antigens, spirochetes, concanavalin A, and controls were treated as described for the mouse cultures except that serum from a type AB blood donor was substituted for the fetal calf serum. All culture plates were incubated at 37°C in a 5% CO_2 atmosphere for 72 hours, and pulsed with 1 μCi of ^{3}H-thymidine 24 hours before harvest onto glass fiber filter paper with a multiple sample automatic harvester. Filter paper disks were placed in 3 ml of scintillation fluid (Betaflour, National Diagnostics, Sommerville, NJ) and ^{3}H-thymidine incorporation was measured as disintegrations per minute (dpm). Stimulation indices were calculated as the mean (four wells for each antigen, spirochete and mitogen concentration) of the treated cultures divided by the mean dpm of control cultures containing serum alone.

Chemotaxis Assay

This assay followed the modifications of the Boyden Chamber Method for measuring chemotaxis of polymorphonuclear cells (PMN).[12] Normal volunteers served as donors for the dextran (T-500, Pharmacia) sedimented PMNs from heparinized blood. PMN were suspended at a concentration of 2×10^6 cells/ml of Hanks balanced salt solution supplemented with 0.01-M HEPES, 2% bovine albumin, and 100 units of penicillin G and 100 μg of streptomycin. Three hundred μl of the PMN suspension was dispensed into the upper chamber of the chemotaxis unit (Boyden Chamber). The lower chamber also contained 300 μl of the various concentrations of the chemotactic agents (10^{-7}, 10^{-6}, 10^{-5} M OSP-A and flagellins) in the same medium. The separating membrane between the chambers was a 3.0-μ pore nitrocellulose disk (Millipore, Bedford, MA). Controls consisted of (1) a solution of formyl methionine, leucine and phenylalanine (FMLP, Sigma) prepared as a stock solution of 10^{-3} M in dimethyl sulfoxide (DMSO) and diluted further in medium to a concentration of 10^{-7} M; (2) medium alone; and (3) medium supplemented with DMSO as in the FLMP solution. The chambers were incubated for 90 minutes at 37°C. At the end of the incubation, the membranes were stained with hematoxylin and eosin and the leading front of the migrating cells were enumerated by light microscopy. Each concentration of OSP-A, mean flagellins and controls was done in triplicate. Results are expressed as mean percentages of the numbers of PMN migrating toward the FMLP solution.

Adhesion Assays

HEp-2 epithelial cells (ATCC no. CCL 23) were grown in Eagle's Minimum Essential Medium supplemented with 10% fetal calf serum and antibiotics at 37°C and 5% CO_2. These cells could also be grown in spirochete growth medium supplemented with 15% fetal calf serum under the same conditions. The ability to grow HEp-2 cells in spirochete medium allowed for incubation of both cells and spirochetes in an environment suitable for both. Cells were grown in 12-mm (diameter) sterile coverslips. Various concentrations of spirochetes were delivered in 50 μl of medium to cover the surface of the coverslip and incubated at 33°C for 1 hour. Adhesion of spirochetes to cells was measured by counting a predetermined number of cells with bound spirochetes in a darkfield microscope after rinsing the coverslip in PBS for 10 seconds each. Inhibition assays were performed by incubating spirochetes for 1 hour at 33°C with the following: 2 μg/ml of a murine IgM monoclonal antibody 11G1 (to an antigenic determinant in OSP-A),[13] supernatant fluid from the murine hybridomas producing monoclonal antibodies H5332 and H9724,[14,15] 2 μg/ml of two irrelevant murine monoclonal antibodies;[16,17] heat-killed spirochete preparations were made by

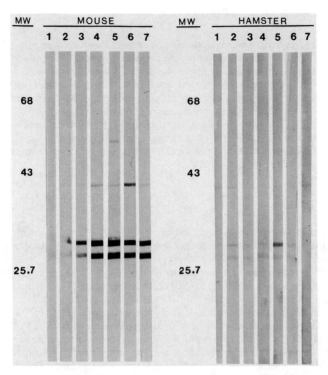

FIGURE 1. Sequential immunoblot analysis of the binding of mouse and hamster serum to spirochetal proteins. Mice and hamsters were inoculated with 10^8 *B. burgdorferi* and blots were made weekly for 7 weeks after inoculation. $M_r \times 10^3$ standards are shown.

TABLE 1. Uptake of ^{3}H-Thymidine by Splenocytes from Normal and Infected Mice Stimulated by Whole Spirochetes and Eluted Antigens

Antigen	Stimulation Index[d] Normal Mouse	Stimulation Index Infected Mouse
Con A[a]	125 ± 9	79 ± 7
B. burgdorferi,[b] 1 : 1	45 ± 5	87 ± 7
B. burgdorferi, 10 : 1	13 ± 3	82 ± 7
B. burgdorferi, 100 : 1	0.9 ± 0.2	0.5 ± 0.2
OSP-A[c] 0.01	9 ± 3	6 ± 2
OSP-A 0.1	50 ± 5	29 ± 4
OSP-A 1	53 ± 5	34 ± 4
OSP-A 2	37 ± 9	32 ± 4
Flagellin[c] 0.01	2 ± 0.8	3 ± 0.8
Flagellin 0.1	8 ± 3	13 ± 4
Flagellin 1	31 ± 7	19 ± 4
Flagellin 2	2 ± 0.6	5 ± 0.2

[a]Con A at 10 μg/ml.
[b]Ratio of spirochetes to cells.
[c]μg/ml.
[d]Stimulation index = mean dpm of quadruplicate cultures/mean dpm of control cultures containing serum alone.

Mean dpm ± SE of normal mouse control = 530 ± 34; mean dpm ± SE of infected mouse control = 1177 ± 68.

incubating at 56°C for 1 hour. For some experiments, the cells were incubated for 24 hours at 37°C with various concentrations (10, 20, 40 μg/ml) of tunicamycin and neuraminidase (sialidase, Sigma) before incubation with spirochetes.

RESULTS

Development of Antibody Response in Mice and Hamsters

A sequential series of immunoblots were done on mice and hamsters experimentally inoculated with 10^8 *B. burgdorferi*. In both species, a faint IgG response to OSP-A, OSP-B, and flagellins was noted in immunoblots but not in ELISA as early as

TABLE 2. Uptake of ^{3}H-Thymidine by Peripheral Mononuclear Cells from Control and Patients with Lyme Disease Stimulated by Whole Spirochetes and Eluted Antigen[a]

Antigen	Stimulation Index[d] Normal Human	Stimulation Index Lyme Disease Patient
Con A[a]	52 ± 6	32 ± 5
B. burgdorferi,[b] 1 : 1	2 ± 0.1	11 ± 2
B. burgdorferi, 10 : 1	3 ± 0.1	13 ± 2
B. burgdorferi, 100 : 1	0.3 ± 0.1	0.5 ± 0.2
OSP-A[c] 0.01	1 ± 0.1	2 ± 0.4
OSP-A 0.1	1 ± 0.3	5 ± 1
OSP-A 1	2 ± 0.3	7 ± 2
OSP-A 2	1 ± 0.1	10 ± 2
Flagellin[c] 0.01	3 ± 0.1	5 ± 1
Flagellin 0.1	3 ± 0.3	15 ± 2
Flagellin 1	3 ± 0.2	18 ± 3
Flagellin 2	4 ± 0.2	15 ± 1

[a]Con A at 10 μg/ml.
[b]Ratio of spirochetes to cells.
[c]μg/ml.
[d]Stimulation index = mean dpm of quadruplicate cultures/mean dpm of control cultures containing serum alone.
Mean dpm ± SE of normal mouse control = 1320 ± 52; mean dpm ± SE of Lyme disease patient control = 1998 ± 75.

1 week after infection (FIG. 1). The IgM response in mice was identical to that of the IgG. (IgM response was not measured in hamsters.) ELISA values were highest in week 5 for both species of animals.

Antigen-Specific Cellular Immune Responses in Mice and Patients

Results obtained from the stimulation of normal and infected splenocytes with whole *B. burgdorferi* and various concentrations of eluted OSP-A and flagellins are listed in TABLE 1. Normal mice appear to recognize whole *B. burgdorferi* at ratios of 1 and 10 spirochetes per splenocyte. An obviously cytotoxic effect was noted in cultures with 100 organisms per splenocyte. Cell proliferation was also noted with eluted

OSP-A and flagellins as antigens. Splenocytes from previously infected mice responded strongly to *B. burgdorferi* and to OSP-A but significantly less to flagellin. Uptake of ^{3}H-thymidine by peripheral mononuclear cells from normal controls stimulated by *B. burgdorferi*, OSP-A, and flagellins was negligible (TABLE 2). The patients selected for this assay were of two types: two patients had only IgG reactivity to flagellins by previous immunoblots, and two patients had multiple band reactivity by previous immunoblots including flagellins and OSP-A. Although the latter patients showed slightly more ^{3}H-thymidine uptake in cultures stimulated with OSP-A, in both types of patient most of the stimulation was due to the flagellins. As in the mouse cultures, spirochetes at a ratio of 100 : 1 cell were cytotoxic. Uptake of ^{3}H-thymidine in infected mouse and patient cultures stimulated by Con A was reduced compared to that of controls.

Chemotaxis Assays

The ability of various concentrations of OSP-A and flagellins to stimulate PMN chemotaxis was measured in modified Boyden Chamber assays (TABLE 3). The

TABLE 3. Chemotaxis of Human Neutrophils in a Modified Boyden Chamber Assay by Spirochetal Antigens[a]

Chemotactic Agent	Mean Percent ± SD
10^{-7}-M FMLP	100
10^{-7}-M OSP-A	21 ± 2
10^{-6}-M OSP-A	38 ± 3
10^{-5}-M OSP-A	50 ± 3
10^{-7}-M flagellin	39 ± 2
10^{-6}-M flagellin	62 ± 7
10^{-5}-M flagellin	78 ± 7
DMSO control	4 ± 0.8
Medium control	2 ± 0.8

[a]Results are given as mean percentages ± SD of triplicate experiments and expressed as fractions of the numbers obtained with a 10^{-7}-M solution or FMLP (100%).

concentrations of spirochetal antigens were chosen as molar equivalents of FMLP, a known chemotactic agent, so that comparisons could be made. Flagellins were approximately twice as effective as OSP-A in stimulating the migration of PMN and both stimulated migration in significantly higher numbers than the controls ($p < 0.01$). Neither spirochetal antigen was as effective as 10^{-7}-M FMLP (TABLE 3).

Adhesion Assays

HEp-2 cells grown in spirochete medium supplemented with 15% FCS and antibiotics were incubated with spirochetes in medium. These bacteria avidly bound to the cells (FIG. 2). Incubation of approximately 10 spirochetes per HEp-2 resulted in the binding of multiple organisms to all cells in the nearly confluent monolayer. Partial binding inhibition was obtained by preincubating the spirochetes with monoclonal antibodies directed to antigenic determinants in OSP-A and flagellins (TABLE 4). Preincubation of cells with 10, 20 and 40 µg/ml of tunicamycin and neuraminidase

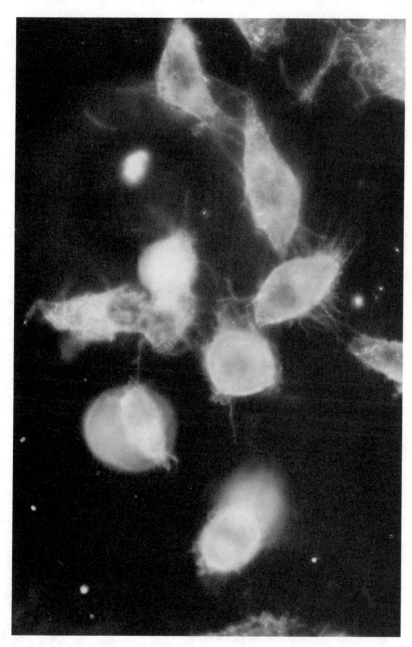

FIGURE 2. HEp-2 cells with adhered *B. burgdorferi* (40×, Kodak T-Max, 400 ASA, in dark field).

resulted also in partial inhibition. Heat-killed spirochetes did not bind HEp-2 cells. Irrelevant murine monoclonal antibodies did not inhibit the binding of bacteria to the cells.

DISCUSSION

Mice and hamsters develop a strong antibody response to both OSP-A and flagellins shortly after intraperitoneal inoculation of organisms. The OSP-A response in these animals is in contrast to the known pattern of antibody production in man. The cellular response of previously infected mice to whole spirochetes was quite pronounced, but so was the response of normal mice. Uptake of ^{3}H-thymidine by normal mouse splenocytes upon stimulation with OSP-A and flagellins was less than that noted for whole spirochetes. In all cases, whole spirochetes at ratios of 1 : 1 and

TABLE 4. Inhibition of Adherence of *B. burgdorferi* to HEp-2 Cells[a]

	Inhibition %
Spirochetes (treatment):	
Heat killed	100
mAb 11G1 (2 μg/ml)	45 ± 14
mAb 5332	40 ± 12
mAb 9724	27 ± 8
mAb anti-PMN-FcR	0
mAb antipancreatic carcinoma	0
Cells (treatment):	
Tunicamycin	
10 μg/ml	10 ± 3
20 μg/ml	14 ± 5
40 μg/ml	21 ± 9
Neuraminidase	
10 μg/ml	8 ± 2
20 μg/ml	22 ± 9
40 μg/ml	43 ± 14

[a]Mean percentage inhibition ± SD of three experiments.

10 : 1 were stimulatory to both normal and infected mice and always greater than to OSP-A and flagellins when cultured separately. Additional antigens from or factors released by spirochetes are needed for the full spectrum of the cellular response. The results obtained from mononuclear cell cultures of normal mice suggest a previous encounter with antigenically similar bacteria, yet immunoblots made from mice before infection failed to show reactivity to spirochetal antigens. The response to OSP-A in splenocyte cultures was greater than that seen in the cultures with flagellins. Peripheral mononuclear cell cultures of normal volunteers and of patients showed a pattern more consistent with the B-cell response. Cultures from normal volunteers showed negligible stimulation by spirochetes, OSP-A, and/or flagellins. The patient's response was greatest to the flagellins in both patients with antibodies to flagellins only as well as in patients with antibodies to OSP-A.

The role of OSP-A in human immunogenesis is obviously still not clear. There is now substantial evidence that, unlike in laboratory animals, antibody production of OSP-A in Lyme disease patients does not appear in all patients and almost always in patients with disease of long duration. A number of hypotheses could explain this phenomenon. Antigenic shifts in the phenotypic expression of this protein could delay recognition by the immune system. The classic examples of this phenomenon in relapsing fever *Borrelia* enhances the possibility that such a mechanism may exist.[18] Many human isolates would have to be studied, however, before the existence of such a mechanism can be proved. Modulation of the protein by the spirochete resulting in more or less shedding and formation could delay a response, particularly if posttranslation modifications of the protein were to take place. That the flagellins constitute the first recognized antigens suggests that the outer envelope bearing the OSP-A must be degraded or shed to expose the endoflagella.

The lower response of OSP-A in the patients may also indicate that this antigen is poorly immunogenic to man and may explain the delayed production of antibodies to this abudant protein. Endogenous human proteins could conceivably have sequences shared by or similar to OSP-A. Future investigations of possible cross-reactivity with endogenous proteins resulting in autoimmunity should consider OSP-A as a prime candidate. The denatured condition of eluted OSP-A and flagellins may account for the results in these assays. Eluted OSP-A and flagellins, however, conserve antigenic determinants to murine monoclonal antibodies and to both mouse and patient sera. Route of inoculation could influence the pattern of antibody formation. In these experiments mice and hamsters were inoculated intraperitoneally, whereas the normal route of inoculation in man is intradermal. Intradermally inoculated hamsters and mice, however, show a significantly delayed but identical pattern of antibody production, suggesting that this might not be the case (unpublished data). In both infected mice and patients there is reduced mitogenesis by Con A as compared to controls, suggesting a period of decreased mononuclear cell function. High ratios of spirochetes to cells are cytotoxic to both mice and patient cells.

Neither OSP-A nor flagellins in molar equivalents to a known and potent chemotactic agent such as FMLP is capable of eliciting a strong migration of PMN by itself. Earlier studies, however, have shown that whole spirochetes can induce extensive PMN migration *in vivo* at the sites of intradermal injection of these organisms.[19] Again, more spirochetal components are apparently needed for the full expression of inflammation in Lyme disease.

The affinity of spirochetes for cell surfaces is well-known; extensive literature exists on the interactions of *Treponema pallidum* with various cell types. There is increasing evidence that *B. burgdorferi* can adhere to cell surfaces in both the vertebrates and invertebrate hosts.[6,20,21] In these preliminary cytoadherence studies, OSP-A seems to have an important role in the interaction with the cells; to a lesser extent so do the flagellins. At this time, we have only succeeded in partially inhibiting adherence by treatment of spirochetes with monoclonal antibodies. The one conclusion that can be drawn is that the interaction of spirochetes with cell surfaces is complex, possibly involving more than one surface protein. Binding sites on the cell appear to be carbohydrates on surface glycoproteins and/or glycolipids.

The flagellins of *B. burgdorferi* elicit a strong but not protective antibody response in man. The abundant OSP-A appears to be poorly immunogenic to man but otherwise important in cytoadherence. Both may be involved, in addition to other components, in chemotaxigenesis with resulting inflammation. In particular, OSP-A, which is strongly immunogenic to experimentally infected laboratory animals but not to man, could be an antigen involved in cross-reactivity with endogenous proteins and thus promote late disease pathogenesis.

SUMMARY

OSP-A (~31 kDa) and flagellins (~41 kDa) are prominent antigens of *Borrelia burgdorferi*. Both OSP-A and flagellins are immunogenic in patients and in experimentally infected mice and hamsters, but the kinetics of antibody formation to each vary considerably between the species. The role of eluted OSP-A and flagellins in the cellular immune response, chemotaxigenesis, and cytoadherence was measured. Eluted OSP-A and flagellins stimulated the proliferation of normal and infected mouse splenocytes but only the peripheral mononuclear cells of patients. Both OSP-A and flagellins induced human neutrophil chemotaxis, but at significantly reduced levels as compared to other known chemotactic peptides. Live *B. burgdorferi* adhere to HEp-2 cells in culture. OSP-A and the flagellins are involved in adherence; monoclonal antibodies to determinants in these proteins partially inhibited adherence. Cytoadherence was also partially inhibited by treatment of the cells with tunicamycin and sialidase.

ACKNOWLEDGMENTS

Dr. Alan Barbour of the University of Texas at San Antonio provided monoclonal antibodies H5332 and H9724, Dr. Howard B. Fleit and Dr. Frederick Miller of SUNY at Stony Brook provided monoclonal antibodies AR2–20 and 3G8, respectively. The help given by Gregory Beck is gratefully acknowledged.

REFERENCES

1. BARBOUR A. G., W. BURGDORFER, E. GRUNWALDT & A. C.. STEERE. 1983. Antibodies of patients with Lyme disease to components of the *Ixodes dammini* spirochete. J. Clin. Invest. **72:** 504–515.
2. COLEMAN, J. L. & J. L. BENACH. 1987. Isolation of antigenic components from the Lyme disease spirochete: Their role in early diagnosis. J. Infect. Dis. **155:** 756–765.
3. JOHNSON, R. C., N. MAREK & C. KODNER. 1984. Infection of Syrian hamsters with Lyme disease spirochetes. J. Clin. Microbiol. **20:** 1099–1104.
4. BENACH, J. L., E. M. BOSLER, J. P. HANRAHAN, J. L. COLEMAN, G. S. HABICHT, T. F. BAST, D. J. CAMERON, J. L. ZIEGLER, A. G. BARBOUR, W. BURGDORFER, R. EDELMAN & R. A. KASLOW. 1983. Spirochetes isolated from the blood of two patients with Lyme disease. N. Engl. J. Med. **308:** 740–742.
5. ANDERSON, J. F., R. C. JOHNSON, L. A. MAGNARELLI & F. W. HYDE. 1986. Culturing *Borrelia burgdorferi* from spleen and kidney tissues of wild caught white-footed mice, *Peromyscus leucopus*. Zbl. Bakt. Hyg. A **263:** 34–39.
6. BENACH, J. L., J. L. COLEMAN, R. A. SKINNER & E. M. BOSLER. 1987. Adult *Ixodes dammini* on rabbits: A hypothesis of the development and transmission of *Borrelia burgdorferi*. J. Infect. Dis. **155:** 1300–1306.
7. FUMAROLA, D., M. COSTANZA CEDOLA, G. GUANTI, A. MATSUURA, T. UEDE & E. JIRILLO. 1986. Adherence of Lyme disease spirochetes to rat lymphocytes. Zbl. Bakt. Hyg. A **263:** 146–150.
8. BENACH, J. L., H. B. FLEIT, G. S. HABICHT, J. L. COLEMAN, E. M. BOSLER & B. P. LANE. 1984. Interaction of phagocytes with the Lyme disease spirochete: Role of the Fc receptor. J. Infect. Dis. **150:** 497–507.
9. LAEMMLI, V. K. & M. FAVRE. 1973. Maturation of the head of bacteriophage T4. I. DNA packaging events. J. Mol. Biol. **80:** 575–599.
10. TOWBIN, H., T. STAEHELIN & J. GORDON. 1979. Electrophoretic transfer of proteins from

polyacrylamide gels to nitrocellulose sheets: Procedures and some applications. Proc. Natl. Acad. Sci. U.S.A. **76:** 4350–4354.

11. TSAI, C. M. & C. E. FRASCH. 1982. A sensitive silver stain for detecting lipopolysaccharides in polyacrylamide gels. Anal. Biochem. **119:** 115–121.

12. CATES, K. L., C. E. RAY & P. G. QUIE. 1978. Modified Boyden chamber method of measuring polymorphonuclear leukocyte chemotaxis. *In* Leukocyte Chemotaxis. J. I. Gallin & P. G. Quie, Eds. Raven Press. New York.

13. BENACH, J. L., J. L. COLEMAN & M. G. GOLIGHTLY. 1988. A murine IgM monoclonal antibody binds to antigenic determinant in OSP-A, an immunodominant basic protein of the Lyme disease spirochete. J. Immunol. **140:** 265–272.

14. BARBOUR, A. G., S. L. TESSIER & W. J. TODD. 1983. Lyme disease spirochetes and ixodid tick spirochetes share a common surface antigenic determinant defined by a monoclonal antibody. Infect. Immun. **41:** 795–804.

15. BARBOUR, A. G., S. F. HAYES, R. A. HEILAND, M. E. SCHRUMPF & S. L. TESSIER. 1986. A *Borrelia* genus specific monoclonal antibody binds to a flagellar epitope. Infect. Immun. **59:** 549–554.

16. FLEIT, H. B., S. D. WRIGHT & J. C. UNKELESS. 1982. Human neutrophil Fc receptor distribution and structure. Proc. Natl. Acad. Sci. U.S.A. **79:** 3275–3279.

17. CHIN, J., R. ZUNA & F. MILLER. 1987. Reactivity of monoclonal anti-human pancreatic carcinoma antibodies AR2–20 and AR1–28 with tumors of nonpancreatic origin. Am. J. Pathol. **126:** 183–193.

18. BARBOUR, A. G., O. BARRERA & R. JUDD. 1983. Structural analysis of the variable major proteins of *Borrelia hermsii*. J. Exp. Med. **158:** 2127–2146.

19. HABICHT, G. S., G. BECK, J. L. BENACH & J. L. COLEMAN. 1986. *Borrelia burgdorferi* lipopolysaccharide and its role in the pathogenesis of Lyme disease. Zbl. Bakt. Hyg. A **263:** 137–141.

20. FITZGERALD, T. J., R. C. JOHNSON, J. M. MILLER & J. A. SYKES. 1977. Characterization of the attachment of *Treponema pallidum* (Nichols strain) to cultured mammalian cells and the potential relationship of attachment to pathogenicity. Infect. Immun. **18:** 476–480.

21. BASEMAN, J. B. & E. C. HAYES. 1980. Molecular characterization of receptor binding proteins and immunogens of virulent *Treponema pallidum*. J. Exp. Med. **151:** 573–580.

Antigenic Variability of *Borrelia burgdorferi*

BETTINA WILSKE,[a] VERA PREAC-MURSIC,[a]
GÜNTHER SCHIERZ,[a] RENATE KÜHBECK,[a]
ALAN G. BARBOUR,[b] AND MICHAEL KRAMER[c]

[a]*Max von Pettenkofer Institute*
University of Munich
D-8000 Munich, Federal Republic of Germany

[b]*Departments of Microbiology and Medicine*
University of Texas Health Science Center
San Antonio, Texas 78284

[c]*Dermatological Clinic*
University of Heidelberg
Heidelberg, Federal Republic of Germany

INTRODUCTION

Lyme borreliosis (LB), a multisystem disorder caused by the spirochete *Borrelia burgdorferi,* is a worldwide tick-borne disease. In the Federal Republic of Germany LB appears to be the predominant tick-borne human infection,[2] and *B. burgdorferi* can be demonstrated in a high percentage (up to 33%)[3] of the main vector *Ixodes ricinus.* Immunochemical analysis of North American strains revealed two abundant surface proteins, OspA and OspB.[4,5] OspA of North American strains are recognized by a monoclonal antibody (MAB) H5332 raised against strain B31, the American-type strain. In contrast, OspB are more heterogeneous, as shown by OspB-specific MAB.[5] Western blot analysis of European strains with MAB H5332 suggested heterogeneity of OspA, as strong, weak and negative reactions were observed.[6] Subsequent analysis with MAB and polyclonal antibodies (PAB) has clearly shown that European strains are heterogeneous with respect to their OspA.[7,8] In European strains another major protein of an approximate molecular weight of 20 kilodaltons (kDa), designated "pC" by us, may be present.[7,8] In contrast to OspA and OspB, pC is an important immunogen in the human disease.[8] Previously a preliminary serotyping system based on the reactivity of the *Borrelia* OspA with two MAB, H5332 and H3TS, was proposed by one of us: serogroup I (reactive to both MAB), serogroup II (only H5332 reactive), and serogroup III (nonreactive to both MAB).[9]

In the present study proteins of *B. burgdorferi,* relapsing fever borreliae (RFB), and treponemes are characterized by monoclonal and polyclonal antibodies using the Western blot technique. Our aims were (1) to examine *B. burgdorferi* isolates for common antigenic components and to differentiate them from RFB and treponemes; and (2) to characterize the variable proteins of *B. burgdorferi* in more detail.

MATERIAL AND METHODS

Strains

Treponemes. Treponema phagedenis and *T. pallidum* were obtained from Behringwerke AG (Marburg, FRG). *T. phagedenis* was cultured in thioglycolate broth as

126

previously described.[10] *T. pallidum* was provided as lyophilized purified whole cell preparation.

Relapsing Fever Borreliae. *Borrelia hermsii* was a strain from the Rocky Mountain Laboratory, Hamilton, MT. *B. turicatae* and *B. parkeri* were provided by Russell C. Johnson, University of Minnesota, Minneapolis, and *B. duttoni* by Heinz E. Krampitz, Tropeninstitut, München, FRG.

TABLE 1. *B. burgdorferi:* Source of Isolates and Characterization of Outer Membrane Protein OspA with MAB H5332 (Western Blot)

Isolate[a] (ref.)	Geographic Location	Isolated from	Reactivity of OspA with H5332
B31 (1)	US	*I. damini*	+
B. pac (19)	US	*I. pacificus*	+
Min. m. (19)	US	mouse	+
272 (19)	US	skin, EM	+
297 (19)	US	CSF	+
W12[b]	Austria	CSF	−
PBr (20)	FRG	CSF	+
PFei[c]	FRG	CSF	−
PKle[c]	FRG	CSF	+
PSpe[c]	FRG	CSF	+
PBi (20)	FRG	CSF	−
PKa (20)	FRG	CSF	+
ACAI (19)	Sweden	skin, ACA	+
PWe[c]	FRG	skin, ACA	+
PSto[c]	FRG	skin, ACA	+
PGau[c]	FRG	skin, ACA	+
PTr (20)	FRG	skin, ACA	+
PRui (20)	FRG	skin, ACA	+[e]
PKe (20)	FRG	skin, EM	+
PRi[c]	FRG	skin, EM	+
PJu[c]	FRG	skin, EM	+
PLe (20)	FRG	skin/EM	+
PKo (20)	FRG	skin/EM	+
IRS (19)	Switzerland	*I. ricinus*	+
FI (19)	Sweden	*I. ricinus*	−[f]
TN (8)	FRG	*I. ricinus*	+
T25 (8)	FRG	*I. ricinus*	−
T245[c]	FRG	*I. ricinus*	+
T21 (8)	FRG	*I. ricinus*	+
T24 (8)	FRG	*I. ricinus*	+
T17 (8)	FRG	*I. ricinus*	+
T26 (8)	FRG	*I. ricinus*	+
B45[d]	Berlin	*I. ricinus*	+
T39/40 (19)	US	*I. dammini*	+

[a]Reference 19 contains the original references of isolates from Sweden, Switzerland, and the US.
[b]Source: Gerold Stanek, Hygiene Institute Vienna, Austria.
[c]Source: Vera Preac-Mursic, Pettenkofer Institute, Munich, FRG.
[d]Source: Arno Schönberg, Robert von Ostertag Institute, West Berlin.
[e]Only a trace of an OspA in SDS-PAGE (FIG. 1); OspA with MAB H5332 detectable, but weak.
[f]No major OspA detected by SDS-PAGE.

Borrelia burgdorferi *Isolates*. For source of *B. burgdorferi* isolates, see TABLE 1. Six isolates from North America and 28 isolates from Europe were examined.

Borrelia Antibodies

Monoclonal Antibodies. The following monoclonal antibodies (see TABLE 2) were used in this study: H9724, reactive with *Borrelia* axial filament (41 kDa protein)[11]; H5332 and H3TS, reactive with the OspA of *B. burgdorferi* strain B31[7]; LA23, reactive with 41 kDa protein of strain B31; and LA5 and LA2, reactive with OspA of B31 (M. Kramer *et al.*, submitted).

Polyclonal Antibodies. The polyclonal antibodies used in this study and data of the immunization procedures are listed in TABLE 3.

Antibodies against Whole Borreliae. Sera 1 and 2 were delivered by rabbits immunized intravenously at 1-week (serum 1) and 2-week (serum 2) intervals, with approximately 10^8 borreliae washed 4–5 times in PBS with 0.005 $MgCl_2$ per injection. Immune sera 3–7 were produced in Balb/c mice immunized intraperitoneally with whole borreliae containing 200 μg protein (determined by the Bradford method[12]) per injection. The first injection was performed with complete Freund's adjuvant, the second 1 week later without adjuvant. Immune sera 8–12 were raised in rabbits

TABLE 2. Reactivity of *Borrelia* Proteins with Monoclonal Antibodies (MAB) as Tested by Western Blot

Borrelia Strain (Serotype)[a]	MAB for 40–41 kDa		MBA for OspA			
	H9724	LA23	H5332	H3TS	LA5	LA2
B31 (1)	+	+	+	+	+	+
PKa (1)	+	+	+	+	+	+
ACAI (2)[b]	+	+	+	−	−	−
PKo (2)	+	+	+	−	−	−
PSpe (2)	+	+	+	−	−	−
PBr (3)	+	+	+	−	+	−
PBi (4)	+	+	−	−	−	−
W12 (5)	+	+	−	−	−	−
TN (6)[c]	+	+	+	−	−	−
T25 (7)[d]	+	+	−	−	−	−
B. hermsii	+	−	−	nd[e]	nd	nd
B. duttoni	+	−	−	nd	nd	nd
B. turicatae	+	+	−	nd	nd	nd
B. parkeri	+	+	−	nd	nd	nd
T. pallidum	−	−	nd	nd	nd	nd
T. phagedenis	−	−	nd	nd	nd	nd

[a]*B. burgdorferi* serotype, see TABLE 4.
[b]All serotype 2 strains are negative in the Western blot with MAB LA5.
[c]TN is different from serotype 2 by negative reaction with PAB OspB/PKo.
[d]T25 is different from serotype 4 and 5 by very strong reactivity with PAB OspA/25 compared to only weak reaction of types 4 (PBi, FIG. 8) and 5 (data not shown).
[e]Not done.

TABLE 3. Polyclonal Antibodies against *B. burgdorferi*

No. and Identification	Antigen	Immunized Animals	No. of Immunizations (Application)
1. anti-PKA	PKa, whole cells	rabbits	10 (i.v.)
2. anti-PKo	PKo, whole cells	rabbits	4 (i.v.)
3. anti-T25	T25, whole cells	mice	2 (i.p.)
4. anti-TN	TN, whole cells	mice	2 (i.p.)
5. anti-PKo	PKo, whole cells	mice	2 (i.p.)
6. anti-PBr	PBr, whole cells	mice	2 (i.p.)
7. anti-B31	B31, whole cells	mice	2 (i.p.)
8. anti-PKa	PKa, whole cells	rabbits	2 (i.v.)
9. anti-PSpe	PSpe, whole cells	rabbits	2 (i.v.)
10. anti-PBr	PBr, whole cells	rabbits	2 (i.v.)
11. anti-PBi	PBi, whole cells	rabbits	2 (i.v.)
12. anti-W12	W12, whole cells	rabbits	2 (i.v.)
13. PAB OspA, PKo	OspA, PKo[a]	rabbits	2 (i.c.)
14. PAB OspA, PBr	OspA, PBr[a]	rabbits	3 (i.c.)
15. PAB OspA, T25	OspA, T25[a]	rabbits	3 (i.c.)
16. PAB OspB, PKo	OspB, PKo[a]	rabbits	3 (i.c.)
17. PAB OspB, PKa	OspB, PKa[a]	rabbits	2 (i.c.)
18. PAB pC, PKo	pC, PKo[a]	rabbits	3 (i.c.)

[a]Electroeluted protein from SDS-PAGE.

immunized intravenously with two injections on day 0 and day 8 with *Borrelia* cell suspensions containing 250 μg protein per dose.

Antibodies against Isolated Proteins. Whole borreliae (800–900 μg protein per gel) were subjected to SDS-PAGE (see below). Protein bands were isolated from the gel by electroelution with the Biotrap apparatus (Schleicher and Schüll, Dassel, FRG). The isolated proteins were tested for purity and antigenicity by Western blot with antisera against whole borreliae (see RESULTS). Rabbits were immunized once a week intracutaneously with the isolated proteins (first injection: 200 μl eluate and 200 μl complete Freund's adjuvant; further injections: 200 μl eluate and 200 μl incomplete Freund's adjuvant). By this method protein-specific antibodies (PAB) were prepared against the following proteins: OspA of strains PKo, PBr and T25; OspB of strains PKo and B31; and pC of strain PKo.

SDS-PAGE and Western Blot

SDS-PAGE and Western blot techniques used by us have been described in detail.[13] Briefly, for SDS-PAGE whole cell lysates of the spirochetes (30 μg protein per lane) were submitted to 15% SDS-PAGE and stained with Coomassie brilliant blue. For Western blot only 15 μg protein per lane were subjected to SDS-PAGE and spirochetal proteins were transferred to nitrocellulose paper in a transblot cell. The proteins were reacted with mouse or rabbit antibodies and immunocomplexes were detected by horseradish peroxidase (HRPO) conjugates: HRPO–anti-mouse immunoglobulin (1:750) or HRPO–anti-rabbit immunoglobulin (1:200) (Dakopatts, Copenhagen, Denmark).

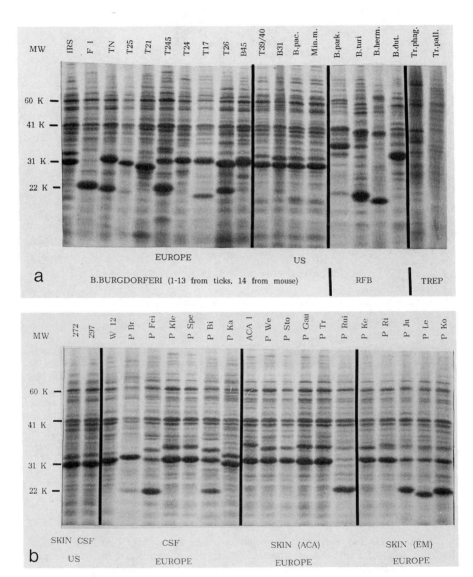

FIGURE 1. SDS-PAGE (15% gel) of spirochete proteins (whole cell lysate containing 30 μg protein per lane), Coomassie blue stain. Molecular weights (MW) of proteins are given in kilodaltons. (a) *B. burgdorferi* (tick isolates *n* = 13, mouse isolate); relapsing fever borreliae (RFB, *n* = 4); treponemes (TREP, *n* = 2). (b) *B. burgdorferi* (human isolates, *n* = 20).

RESULTS

Comparison of B. burgdorferi *Strains with RFB and Treponemes*

SDS-PAGE

FIGURE 1 shows the SDS-PAGE patterns of the spirochetes examined in this study. At first sight the patterns seem very heterogeneous, but if analyzed carefully some typical aspects of the different groups of spirochetes can be elaborated. First, in contrast to treponemes, borreliae (*B. burgdorferi* and RFB) have abundant major protein components.[14] As a rule, all *B. burgdorferi* strains tested have two protein components with constant molecular weights (MW) of 41 kDa and 60 kDa and they

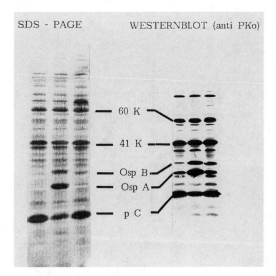

FIGURE 2. Phenotypic variations of three subcultures of one *B. burgdorferi* isolate. *Left:* SDS-PAGE of three subcultures of strain PKo. *Right:* Western blot of the same three subcultures reacted with rabbit immune serum against strain PKo (anti-PKo 1 : 500). OspA and OspB proteins are reactive in the Western blot even if not detected in SDS-PAGE.

have one, two, or three of the above-mentioned abundant major proteins of low MW: OspA (31–32 kDa), OspB (33–36 kDa), and pC (21–22 kDa). These proteins vary slightly in molecular size and occur combined or alone. All combinations except OspB alone or OspB/pC were observed among the 34 *B. burgdorferi* isolates. The MW of the proteins do not differ among subcultures of one isolate, but as shown in FIGURE 2, quantitative differences of the amount of OspA, OspB, or pC among subcultures of one strain may be observed. Heterogeneous patterns of low MW proteins are especially predominant in European isolates. A surprising finding was that the OspA of the European CSF and tick isolates have variable molecular weights, whereas the European skin isolates have OspA with identical MW of 32 kDa. The six North American isolates show very similar SDS-PAGE patterns: they have no major pC and the OspA have identical MW of 31 kDa. Unlike *B. burgdorferi,* the RFB tested have

40-kDa–range proteins of slightly different molecular size. Major OspA proteins are not observed, but traces of proteins in the 31-32–kDa range are present. Each individual RFB (analyzed here) shows one abundant major protein: *B. hermsii* and *B. turicatae* in the range of the pC of Bb, *B. parkeri* and *B. duttoni* in a MW range above the OspB of *B. burgdorferi*.

Immunological Analysis

For detection of common antigenic components, a spirochete panel of four *B. burgdorferi*, four RFB and two treponemes were subjected to Western blot analysis with an immune serum against *B. burgdorferi* (FIG. 3). This serum (anti-PKa, no. 1)—obtained after ten intravenous injections of whole borreliae—has a broad antibody

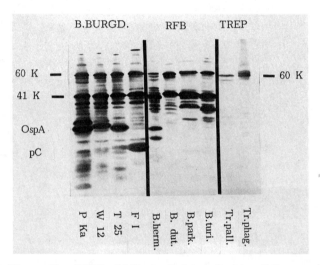

FIGURE 3. Western blot of SDS-solubilized cells from spirochetes (15 μg protein per lane) reacted with a rabbit immune serum against *B. burgdorferi* (strain PKa). The serum recognizes major proteins with variable molecular weights in the 30-kilodalton range (OspA) or in the 20-kilodalton range (pC) of four *B. burgdorferi* isolates and an OspA-like protein of *B. hermsii*.

spectrum against *B. burgdorferi* proteins. In all strains, including treponemes, a 60-kDa–range protein is recognized by this serum. In borreliae (RFB and *B. burgdorferi*) a 40-kDa–range protein was detected but no corresponding protein was detected in the treponemes. The anti-*B. burgdorferi* serum also detected an OspA-like protein in *B. hermsii*.

Western blot with MAB 9724 and MAB LA 23 revealed positive reactions with the 41-kDa proteins of all *B. burgdorferi* tested (TABLE 2, FIG. 5). In contrast, treponemes were nonreactive with both monoclonal antibodies. RFB differed in their patterns with the two MAB: while H9724 was reactive with the four RFB strains, LA 23 was only reactive with *B. turicatae* and *B. parkeri*. Spirochetes were further tested with antibodies against electroeluted OspA and pC proteins (see FIG. 4). Western blot analysis with both antisera (PAB OspA/PKo and PAB pC/PKo, FIG. 5) show strong

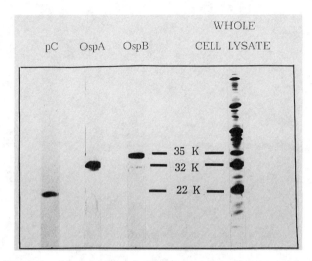

FIGURE 4. Electroeluted proteins of strain PKo. Preparations of major proteins OspA, OspB, and pC were tested for purity and antigenic reactivity with rabbit immune serum against strain PKo (diluted 1 : 500) by Western blot. Molecular weights of proteins are given in kilodaltons.

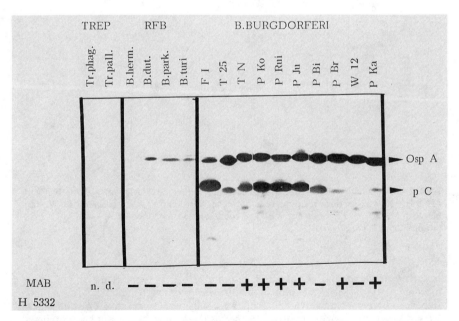

FIGURE 5. Reactivity of borreliae and treponemes with rabbit antibodies against the OspA (PAB OspA/PKo) and the pC (PAB pC/PKo) of *B. burgdorferi* strain PKo. PAB OspA/PKo and PAB pC/PKo were tested with a mixture of the two antibodies in a final dilution of 1 : 2000. Bottom: Reactivity of borreliae with MAB H5332.

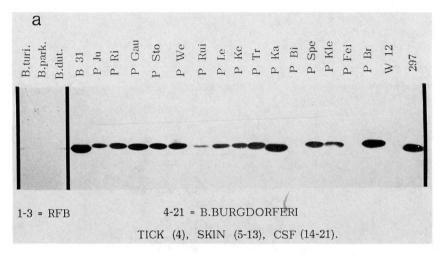

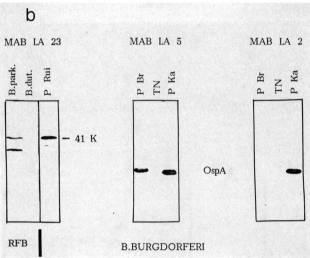

FIGURE 6. Reactivity of borreliae with monoclonal antibodies (MAB). **(a)** Western blot with MAB H5332 (strains: three relapsing fever borreliae (RFB) and 18 *B. burgdorferi*). **(b)** Western blot with MAB LA 23 (strains: two RFB and one *B. burgdorferi*), MAB LA 5, and MAB LA 2 (strains: three *B. burgdorferi*).

reactivity of OspA and pC of all *B. burgdorferi*—if present as major proteins—meaning that at least one protein per isolate is strongly reactive. In contrast, treponemes were nonreactive and RFB were only weakly reactive (*B. duttoni, B. parkeri, B. turicatae*) or negative (*B. hermsii*). A monoclonal antibody of broad reactivity with *B. burgdorferi* is H5332.[4] This OspA-specific antibody is positive with most of the strains tested (TABLE 3, FIG. 6). RFB and treponemes are negative. Nonreactivity of *B. burgdorferi* was observed under two conditions: either the strain has no major OspA (FI) or the OspA is present but nonreactive (three human isolates and one tick isolate).

Immunological Analysis for Detection of Differences between B. burgdorferi *Isolates*

A panel of five *B. burgdorferi* isolates was tested with the corresponding mouse antisera by Western blot (FIG. 7). Sera from shortly immunized mice are predominantly reactive with 41 kDa OspA, OspB, and pC. The strongest reactivity in Western blot was obtained with the homologous serum, indicating antigenic heterogeneity of the three major variable proteins (OspA, OspB, and pC). OspA from H5322-nonreactive strains react with OspA-specific polyclonal antibodies (anti-OspA/PKo, see above) or anti-OspA/T25 raised against the OspA of a H5332 negative strain (FIG. 8). The blot shows a very strong reaction with the homologous OspA (of T25) compared to weak reactions with the heterologous strains. Similar results were obtained with another protein-specific antibody (anti-OspA/PBr).

For a more systematic approach to antigenic analysis we concentrated our efforts on serotyping the isolates from patients. Twenty human isolates were available: two from the United States and 18 from Europe. Twelve strains were isolated from human skin, six from erythema migrans (EM) and six from acrodermatitis chronica atrophicans (ACA). Eight strains were isolated from human CSF. The antigenic characteristics of the proteins of these strains are summarized in TABLE 4. The human isolates were divided into five serotypes according to antigenic characteristics (mainly at OspA and OspB proteins). Serotype 1 (corresponding to serogroup I of Barbour) is characterized by positive reactions with MAB H5332 and MAB H3TS. Serotype 1 is further characterized by positive reactions of OspB proteins with a rabbit antibody against the OspB of the American-type strain B31 (PAB OspB/B31) (FIG. 9). Except for the human US isolates and the European CSF isolate PKa, the other 17 human strains were negative. Eleven strains were tested with H3TS (TABLE 4, FIG. 8) and the reactivity was concordant with PAB OspB/B31 and MAB LA 2 (as thus far tested,

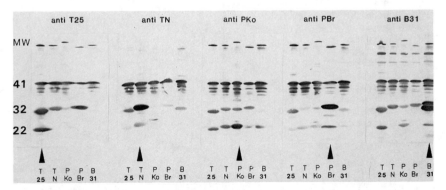

FIGURE 7. Reactivity of five *Borrelia burgdorferi* isolates (T25, TN, and B31 from ticks; PKo from human skin; and PBr from human CSF) tested by Western blot with homologous and heterologous immune sera from i.p. immunized mice (1 : 1000). Homologous reactions are marked by *arrows*. Most reactive proteins have molecular weights of approximately 40, 30 (OspA), and 20 (pC) kilodaltons.

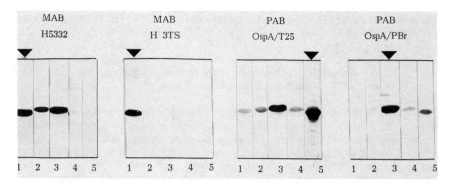

FIGURE 8. Reactivity with OspA-specific polyclonal antibodies (PAB) compared to reactivity with monoclonal antibodies. *B. burgdorferi* strains that are not reactive with MAB show strong reactivity with homologous PAB, heterologous reactions being weaker or negative. PAB Osp/T25 was previously absorbed with *B. burgdorferi* B31 and TN and tested in dilution 1 : 2000; PAB Osp/Br was previously absorbed with *B. burgdorferi* B31, TN, and T25; the serum dilution in the blot was 1 : 2000. Strains tested are indicated as follows: *1*, PKa; *2*, PSpe; *3*, PBr; *4*, PBi; *5*, T25.

TABLE 4. Antigenic Characterization of Human *B. burgdorferi* Isolates by Immunochemical Analysis in the Western Blot

Strain	Source	MAB OspA H5332	H3TS	PAB[a] OspB B31	PKo	Identical Patterns[b] for OspA, OspB with:	Serotype	Serogroup
272	US skin	+	+	+	nd[c]			
297	US CSF	+	+	+	—	anti-PKa	1	I
PKa	Europe CSF	+	+	+	—			
PSpe	Europe CSF	+	—	—	+			
PKle	Europe CSF	+	—	—	+			
PGau	Europe skin	+	—	—	+			
PRi	Europe skin	+	—	—	+			
PW1	Europe skin	+	—	—	+	anti-PSpe		
PSto	Europe skin	+	—	—	+	or	2	II
PJu	Europe skin	+	—	—	+	anti-PKo		
PLe	Europe skin	+	nd	—	+			
PKo	Europe skin	+	—	—	+			
PRui	Europe skin	+	nd	—	+			
ACAI	Europe skin	+	—	—	+			
PBr	Europe CSF	+	—	—	—	anti-PBr	3	II
PFei	Europe CSF	—	—	—	—	anti-PBl	4	III
PBi	Europe CSF	—	—	—	—			
W12	Europe CSF	—	—	—	—	anti-W12	5	III

[a]Protein-specific polyclonal antibody.
[b]See FIGS. 10 and 11, different patterns with strains of different serotype.
[c]Not done.

TABLE 2). As shown in FIGURE 10a, an antibody against the OspB of skin isolate PKo (PAB OspB/PKo) was not reactive with serotype 1. PAB OspB/PKo was reactive with all 11 European skin isolates and with two European CSF isolates. A polyclonal serum against PKo gave identical patterns of reactivity with the OspA and OspB of the PAB OspB/PKo-positive strains (FIG. 10b). This serum further recognizes 41-kDa–, 60-kDa–, and 100-kDa–range protein (with variable MW and without apparent differences in reactivity). If present, pC of skin isolates were strongly reactive with anti-PKo in contrast to lower reactivity of pC from three CSF isolates. Based on common characteristics of OspA and especially OspB, all skin isolates and two of the CSF isolates (PSpe and PKle) were designated serotype 2 (TABLE 4). As shown by SDS-PAGE and Western blot with anti-PKo (FIG. 10b), CSF isolates seem to be more heterogeneous than skin isolates in their OspA and OspB proteins. To investigate this

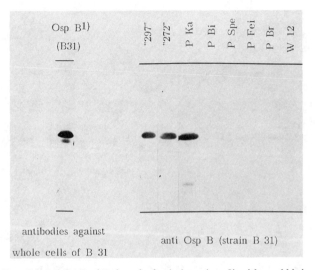

FIGURE 9. Reactivity of OspB of *B. burgdorferi* isolates ($n = 8$) with a rabbit immune serum against the OspB of strain B31. The serum was previously absorbed with skin isolate PRi and was diluted 1 : 500 for the blot. Left lane shows test of the OspB preparation for purity.

topic in more detail, antisera against five of the CSF isolates were produced in rabbits (TABLE 3, sera 8–12). Rabbits were immunized only two times (according to the good differentiating properties of immune sera of shortly immunized mice in serotyping of *B. hermsii*, described by Stoenner *et al.*[15] FIGURE 11 shows the Western blot of the CSF strains (including B31 as control) tested with the five immune sera. Only the region of OspA and OspB is presented in the figure. As expected, PKa, 297, and B31 gave identical patterns (serotype 1). PSpe and PKle were also identical (serotype 2). According to obvious differences in the reactivity of OspB and/or OspA, three further serotypes were defined. PBr was designated serotype 3. OspA from PBr was different from the other *B. burgdorferi* isolates except for similar reactivity in the Western blot with OspA from PFei and PBi with the homologous immune serum anti-PBr, but differences were clearly shown using the heterologous immune serum anti-PBi. Furthermore, PAB OspA/PBr and a panel of OspA-specific MAB (especially LA 5)

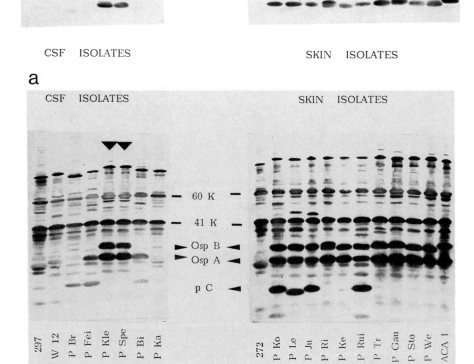

FIGURE 10. Reactivity of 20 human *B. burgdorferi* isolates tested in the Western blot with rabbit immune sera against OspB and whole cells of skin-isolate PKo. (**a**) Western blot with OspB-specific antibody (PAB OspB/PKo). PAB OspB/PKo serum was previously absorbed with *B. burgdorferi* B31 and diluted 1 : 500 for the blot. (**b**) Western blot with whole cell antiserum (anti-PKo). The serum was diluted 1 : 500 for the blot. Two CSF isolates showing the same strong reactivity of OspA and OspB as the European skin isolates are marked by *black arrows*.

also gave different patterns of reactivity compared to the other strains (FIG. 9, TABLE 2). W12 and PBi cannot be differentiated by the available MAB, but according to differences in the Western blot with anti-W12 and anti-PBi (FIG. 11), they were designated as two different serotypes (type 4 and type 5). PFei and PBi gave identical patterns with the five immune sera, and therefore PFei was also designated as type 4.

No further attempts were made to serotype the tick isolates, but obviously the tick strains TN and T25 represent other serotypes not represented among the patient's strains. They are designated serotype 6 and 7, respectively (see TABLE 2 and FIG. 8).

In different subcultures of some strains we observed changes between the amount of OspA and OspB on the one side and of pC on the other side: PKo (FIG. 2), PBi, and

PRui (results not shown). No changes in antigenicity were detected with the homologous antiserum in preparations of different subcultures of PKo. OspA was even detected in a subculture appearing OspA negative by SDS-PAGE. A finding indicating that phenotypic changes may play a role in pathogenesis of the disease is shown in FIGURE 12. Analysis of the IgM response of a patient with neuroborreliosis revealed reactivity of the pC of heterologous strains and nonreactivity with the patient's isolate.

DISCUSSION

Analysis for MW pattern by SDS-PAGE provides valuable information for the characterization of *B. burgdorferi* and for the differentiation of *B. burgdorferi* from other spirochetes. All *B. burgdorferi* except the Swedish tick isolate FI and the skin isolate PRui had major OspB and/or OspA (FIG. 1). As shown here and also in a previous publication,[8] different subcultures of some strains may vary considerably in the amount of OspA and OspB on one side and pC on the other side. We propose to define the OspA and OspB positive stage as the "specific phase" and the OspA and

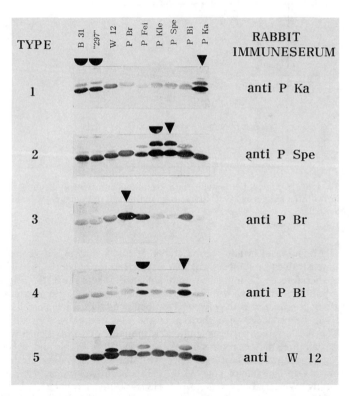

FIGURE 11. Typing of CSF isolates (*"297"–PKa*) with homologous and heterologous rabbit immune sera (strain B31 served as control); ▼ = homologous reaction; ● = heterologous reactions with identical patterns.

OspB negative stage as the "unspecific phase" of an individual strain, analogous to salmonella flagella antigens. Only specific-phase *B. burgdorferi* can be reliably serotyped by OspA- or OspB-specific antibodies. Attempts to select borreliae with major OspA and OspB by cultivating the spirochetes in medium containing pC-specific antibodies were not successful (data not shown). The circumstances leading to changes between OspA/OspB and pC remain unclear. A possible explanation might be that the production of these proteins in the *Borrelia* cell is regulated by plasmids, and that plasmids may be lost or undergo rearrangement. Plasmids coding for the OspA and OspB of strain B31 have been detected in the cytoplasm of *B. burgdorferi* cells.[16]

The OspA and the pC of *B. burgdorferi* have common epitopes recognized by the OspA-specific antibody PAB OspA/PKo and the pC-specific antibody PAB pC/PKo. PAB OspA/PKo detected also traces of OspA-like proteins in *B. turicatae, B. parkeri,* and *B. duttoni.* This cross-reactivity can be eliminated by absorption with a mixture of

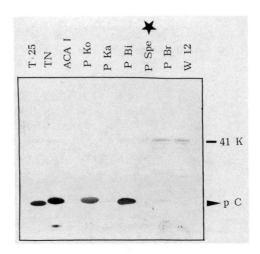

FIGURE 12. IgM response of a patient with lymphocytic meningoradiculitis Bannwarth. Western blot with the autologous CSF isolate (marked by *asterisk*) and eight heterologous *B. burgdorferi* isolates.

the three RFB, however, while the reactivity of OspA and pC of *B. burgdorferi* remains demonstrable (data not shown). *B. burgdorferi* strains nonreactive with MAB H5332 can therefore be distinguished immunologically from RFB. Bearing in mind that *B. burgdorferi* strains show a considerable heterogeneity, our strategy was to characterize *B. burgdorferi* with polyclonal antibodies against whole borreliae, as such antibodies can be produced in a short time and may recognize a broad range of proteins. The Western blot patterns obtained with mouse antisera against whole cells revealed that all three major proteins may be antigenically variable and, as a rule, the homologous sera show the best reactivity with the corresponding strain. Strong reactivity with OspA of homologous MAB H3TS negative strains (T25, PBr) and weak or negative Western blots with a MAB H3TS positive strain (PKa, FIG. 9) were demonstrated using OspA-specific polyclonal antibodies, once more pointing to the antigenic polymorphism and strain-specific epitopes of OspA from European strains. Using OspB-specific polyclonal antibodies, we were able to show that all European skin isolates so far tested ($n = 11$) have common epitopes on their OspB which were not detected in North American isolates and which were detected only in two of seven European CSF isolates. The four North American isolates tested and one European CSF isolate (all belonging to serotype I after the criteria of Barbour) were positive, with a polyclonal antibody against the OspB of the North American type strain B31. This suggests that North American strains may have common epitopes not shared by most of the European strains located not only on the OspA[4] but also on the OspB. According to these findings, we defined strains positive for MAB H3TS and PAB OspB/B31 as serotype I (corresponding to serogroup I of Barbour) and isolates positive for PAB OspB/PKo as serotype 2 (subgroup of serogroup II of Barbour). Attempts at further differentiation performed by checkerboard testing of eight CSF isolates (including one isolate of serotype 1 and two isolates of serotype 2) with five immune sera led to the definition of three further serotypes: 3, 4, and 5. Two tick isolates represent two further serotypes (6 and 7) not represented among the isolates from patients. The other European tick isolates are not yet fully characterized, and it is still an open question whether all *B. burgdorferi* infecting ticks are also pathogenic for humans. We believe that our serotyping system, even if preliminary, may help to select individual strains from the broad panel of *B. burgdorferi* isolates for the production of appropriate monoclonal antibodies.

From a more clinical point of view, we want to point out that the obvious antigenic differences between North American skin isolates and European skin isolates may be responsible for differences in the clinical picture of skin manifestations on both sides of the Atlantic. Such clinical differences concern erythema migrans (multiple skin lesions in the United States versus predominantly single lesions in Europe) and acrodermatitis (a common disease in Europe, very rarely observed in the US).[17]

Phenotype changes of OspA/OspB to pC (as observed in culture) may also play a role *in vivo*. The observation of an OspA-specific IgM immune response detectable only with a heterologous strain and not with the autologous CSF isolate[8] in one patient with neuroborreliosis and of a pC-specific IgM immune response in another patient with neuroborreliosis, also detected only with heterologous strains and not with the autologous CSF isolate (FIG. 12), may be explained by such phenotypic changes. Another indication that *B. burgdorferi* might change its phenotype during chronic infection was obtained by experiments performed by Willy Burgdorfer in rabbits.[18] In these animals the infection with *B. burgdorferi* via ticks caused relapsing spirochetemia, a phenomenon related to antigenic variations (Barbour, Burgdorfer, unpublished data) similar to those described for the relapsing fever spirochetes.[14] It still remains to be investigated whether the antigenic heterogeneity is of importance for the selection of antigens used for diagnostic tests. The considerable heterogeneity of CSF isolates is especially of interest, and may explain "seronegative" cases of neuroborreliosis.

SUMMARY

Borrelia burgdorferi strains (six isolates from North America and 28 isolates from Europe) were analyzed by physicochemical and immunological methods. By SDS-PAGE, all *Borrelia burgdorferi* strains tested had two major proteins with constant molecular weights of 60 and 41 kDa and one, two, or three variable low molecular weight proteins (OspA = 30–32 kDa, OspB = 34–36 kDa, pC = 21–22 kDa). All combinations—except OspB alone or OspB/pC—were observed. *Borrelia burgdorferi* strains were different from relapsing fever borreliae by strong reactivity with OspA- and/or pC-specific polyclonal antibodies, whereas relapsing fever borreliae were only weakly reactive. Among 25 *Borrelia burgdorferi* isolates, seven different serotypes of

Borrelia burgdorferi were defined according to their reactivity in the Western blot with three monoclonal OspA-specific antibodies (H5332, H3TS, and LA5), four OspA- or OspB-specific polyclonal antibodies, and 12 polyclonal antibodies against whole borreliae. Antigenic differences between European CSF and skin isolates were observed, all skin isolates (*n* = 11) belonging to serotype 2 in contrast to only two out of seven CSF isolates. CSF isolates were antigenically heterogenous (serotypes 1, 2, 3, 4, and 5). Serotypes 6 and 7 were represented by two tick isolates, and the other European tick isolates are not yet fully characterized. Antigenic differences between European and North American strains may play a role in differences in the clinical picture of Lyme borreliosis.

ACKNOWLEDGMENT

We thank Waltraud Gueye and Gabi Liegl for expert technical assistance; Drs. Eva Åsbrink (Stockholm, Sweden), Willy Burgdorfer (Hamilton, MT), Russell C. Johnson (Minneapolis, MN), Heinz E. Krampitz (Munich, FRG), H. Peters (Marburg, FRG), Arno Schönberg (Berlin), Gerold Stanek (Vienna, Austria), Alan C. Steere (New Haven, CT) for providing spirochetal strains; and Dr. Willy Burgdorfer for valuable discussion.

REFERENCES

1. BURGDORFER, W., A. G. BARBOUR, S. F. HAYES, J. L. BENACH, E. GRUNWALD & J. P. DAVIS. 1982. Lyme disease—a tick-borne spirochetosis? Science **216:** 1317–1319.
2. ACKERMANN, R. 1986. Erythema-migrans-Borreliose und Fruehsommer-Meningoenzephalitis. Dtsch. Aerztebl. **83:** 1765–1774.
3. WILSKE, B., R. STEINHUBER, H. BERGMEISTER, V. FINGERLE, G. SCHIERZ, V. PREAC-MURSIC, E. VANEK & B. LORBEER. 1987. Epidemiologische Daten zum Auftreten von Erkrankungsfällen sowie zur Durchseuchung von Zecken (*Ixodes ricinus*) mit *Borrelia burgdorferi*. Dtsch. Med. Wochenschr. **112:** 1730–1736.
4. BARBOUR, A. G., S. L. TESSIER & W. J. TODD. 1983. Lyme disease spirochetes and *Ixodes* tick spirochetes share a common surface antigenic determinant as defined by a monoclonal antibody. Infect. Immun. **41:** 795–804.
5. BARBOUR. A. G., S. L. TESSIER & S. F. HAYES. 1984. Variation in a major surface protein of Lyme disease spirochetes. Infect. Immun. **45:** 94–100.
6. WILSKE, B., V. PREAC-MURSIC & G. SCHIERZ. 1985. Antigenic heterogeneity of European *Borrelia burgdorferi* strains isolated from patients and ticks. Lancet i: 2099.
7. BARBOUR, A. G., R. A. HEILAND, M. E. SCHRUMPF & S. L. TESSIER. 1985. Heterogeneity of major proteins of Lyme disease borreliae: A molecular analysis of American and European isolates. J. Infect. Dis. **152:** 478–484.
8. WILSKE, B., V. PREAC-MURSIC, G. SCHIERZ, K. V. BUSCH. 1986. Immunochemical and immunological analysis of European *Borrelia burdorferi* strains. Zbl. Bakt. Hyg. A **263:** 92–102.
9. BARBOUR, A. G. 1986. A proposal for a serotyping system based upon major outer surface proteins of *Borrelia burgdorferi*. Lyme Borreliosis Newsletter **2:** 7–9.
10. WILSKE, B., G. SCHIERZ, V. PREAC-MURSIC, K. WEBER, H.-W. PFISTER & K. EINHAEUPL. 1984. Serological diagnosis of Erythema migrans disease and related disorders. Infection **12:** 331–337.
11. BARBOUR, A. G., S. F. HAYES, R. A. HEILAND, M. E. SCHRUMPF & S. L. TESSIER. 1986. A *Borrelia* genus-specific monoclonal antibody binds to a flagellar epitope. Infect. Immun. **52:** 549–554.
12. BRADFORD, M. M. 1976. A rapid and sensitive method for the quantitation of microgram

quantities of protein utilizing the principle of protein-dye binding. Anal. Biochem. **72:** 248–254.

13. WILSKE, B., G. SCHIERZ, V. PREAC-MURSIC, K. V. BUSCH, R. KUEHBECK, H.-W. PFISTER & K. EINHAEUPL. 1986. Intrathecal production of specific antibodies against *Borrelia burgdorferi* in patients with lymphocytic meningoradiculitis (Bannwarth's syndrome). J. Infect. Dis. **153:** 304–313.

14. BARBOUR, A. G. & S. F. HAYES. 1986. Biology of *Borrelia* species. Microbiol. Rev. **50:** 381–400.

15. STOENNER, H. G., T. DODD & C. LARSEN. 1982. Antigenic variation of *Borrelia hermsii*. J. Exp. Med. **156:** 1297–1311.

16. BARBOUR, A. G. & C. F. GARON. 1987. Linear plasmids of the bacterium *Borrelia burgdorferi* have covalently closed ends. Science **237:** 409–411.

17. ÅSBRINK, E., A. HOVMARK & B. HEDERSTEDT. 1984. The spirochetal etiology of acrodermatitis chronica atrophicans Herxheimer. Acta Derm. Venereol. (Stockholm) **65:** 506–512.

18. BURGDORFER, W. & K. L. GAGE. 1986. Susceptibility of the black-legged tick, *Ixodes scapularis,* to the Lyme disease spirochete *Borrelia burgdorferi*. Zbl. Bakt. Hyg. A **263:**15–20.

19. BARBOUR, A. G. & M. E. SCHRUMPF. 1986. Polymorphisms of major surface proteins of *Borrelia burgdorferi*. Zbl. Bakt. Hyg. A **263:** 83–91.

20. PREAC-MURSIC, V., B. WILSKE & G. SCHIERZ. 1986. European *Borreliae burgdorferi* isolated from humans and ticks—culture conditions and antibiotic susceptibility. Zbl. Bakt. Hyg. A **263:** 112–118.

The Genes Encoding Major Surface Proteins of *Borrelia burgdorferi* Are Located on a Plasmid[a]

ALAN G. BARBOUR

Division of Infectious Diseases
Departments of Medicine and Microbiology
University of Texas Health Science Center
San Antonio, Texas 78284

CLAUDE F. GARON

Laboratory of Pathobiology
National Institute of Allergy and Infectious Diseases
National Institutes of Health
Rocky Mountain Laboratories
Hamilton, Montana 59840

INTRODUCTION

Whereas the spirochetes causing Lyme borreliosis were discoverd only this decade, the *Borrelia* spp. that causes epidemic and endemic relapsing fever were discovered more than a century ago (reviewed in ref. 1). Despite this long familiarity of microbiologists with these microorganisms, very little is known about the genetics of this genus of eubacteria. In comparison to what is understood about gram-negative and gram-positive bacteria, knowledge of the hereditary mechanisms of borreliae is meager. An important reason for this paucity of information has been the difficulty in growing this group of pathogenic organisms *in vitro*. They grow slowly in broth medium and are reluctant to form colonies on solid media.[2] With the increasing impact of Lyme borreliosis as a human and domestic animal disease in North America, Europe, and Asia, there are compelling reasons to decipher the unique features of borrelial genetics.

Our own interest in spirochetal genetics dates from a series of investigations into antigenic variation of the relapsing fever *Borrelia* species *hermsii*. We had found that the change in serotype in a population of borreliae infecting a mouse was attributable to the replacement of the predominant coat protein of the spirochetes by another, antigenically distinct, coat protein.[3] This variation appeared to be determined at the level of transcription.[4,5] Consequently, we asked whether there were any detectable changes in the genome. It turned out that there were. Expression-linked and silent copies of the genes encoding the coat proteins were to be found in the genome. Change in serotype was associated with the transposition of a silent copy of a gene to an expression site.[6] In the course of these studies, we found that the genes for the serotype-specific surface proteins were located on extrachromosomal elements in *B. hermsii*.[7]

[a]This work was supported in part by the National Institute of Allergy and Infectious Diseases (grant no. RO1AI24424).

144

The OspA and OspB proteins of *B. burgdorferi* resemble the variable coat proteins of *B. hermsii* in several ways: (1) All of these abundant borrelial proteins are between 23 and 40 kilodaltons (kDa) in apparent molecular weight.[3] The OspA and OspB proteins of strain B31 of *B. burgdorferi* are 31 kDa and 34 kDa, respectively.[8-10] (2) They are exposed on the surface of the borrelia and are cleavable *in situ* by proteases.[9,11] (3) Monoclonal antibodies directed against these proteins can be used to type strains of *B. hermsii* and *B. burgdorferi*.[3,9,12]

Knowing these similarities, we wondered whether *ospA* and *ospB*, the genes encoding the OspA and OspB proteins, are also arrayed on plasmids. A number of studies were carried out to determine this. Some of these experiments are reported elsewhere[13] and will be reviewed here. Other results are reported in depth here.

MATERIALS AND METHODS

DNA Extraction

A cell lysate was partitioned into plasmid-rich and chromosome-rich DNA fractions by the following procedure.[13] *B. burgdorferi* strain B31 (ATCC 35210) was grown in BSK II medium.[2] A harvest of 5×10^{10} cells was suspended in 2.4 ml of TES (50 mM tris, pH 8.0; 50 mM EDTA; 15% w/v sucrose). To the suspension was added 1.2 mg of lysozyme (Sigma Chemical Co., St. Louis, MO) in 0.6 ml of water. After a 15-minute incubation at 4°C, the following reagents were added to the sample: 3 ml of 1% sodium deoxycholate in TES and 70 μl of diethyl pyrocarbonate (DEPC; Sigma). The tube was shaken in a horizontal position for 10 minutes on a rotary shaker set at 150 revolutions per minute. To the resultant lysate was added 2.5 ml of 7.5-M ammonium acetate, and the resultant precipitate was centrifuged (10,000 g for 20 minutes at 20°C). The pellet (chromosome-rich fraction) was sequentially treated with ribonuclease A, proteinase K in the presence of SDS, and phenol and chloroform.[6] The supernatant (plasmid-rich fraction) was filtered through a Millex-GV 0.2-μm filter (Millipore). The nucleic acids in the supernatant were precipitated with cold isopropanol. The precipitate was suspended in 3 ml of TE (10 mM tris, pH 7.8; 1 mM EDTA) and then treated with ribonuclease A at a final concentration of 0.1 mg/ml (37°C for 30 minutes). DEPC (11 μl) was added, and the mixture was shaken for 5 minutes. Residual proteins were removed by precipitation with 7.5-M ammonium acetate (0.5 ml) and centrifugation (5 minutes in a microcentrifuge). The plasmid-rich DNA in supernatant was recovered by ethanol precipitation and then fractionated by CsCl-ethidium bromide gradient centrifugation (70,000 rpm for 16 hours in a Beckman VTi80 rotor). Two bands were consistently observed in the centrifuge tubes: one, of higher density, contained supercoiled DNA when examined by electron microscopy; the other, of lower density, consisted of linear duplexes. Chromosomal DNA was separated from a small amount of plasmid material contaminating the chromosome-rich fraction by electroeluting (see below) from agarose gels DNA with an apparent size of greater than 60 kilobases.

Low-Percent Agarose Gel Electrophoresis

DNA samples (approximately 2 μg) were applied to 9 cm long, 0.2% agarose gels (Seakem GTG; FMC, Rockland, MN). The electrophoresis was run using either recirculated 10 mM sodium phosphate buffer (pH 6.5) or nonrecirculated tris (90 mM) borate (90 mM) EDTA (2 mM) buffer (TBE). For both buffers the electrophoresis conditions were: 5.5 V/cm for 30 min and 1.4 V/cm for another 15 h (or until the bromphenol blue marker reached the end of the gel). The DNA in the gel was then stained with ethidium bromide and photographed. Size markers in the gels were the high molecular weight, linear double-stranded DNA standards of Bethesda Research Laboratories (BRL), Gaithersburg, MD.

Bal31 Exonuclease Digestion

Six micrograms of plasmid-rich DNA were incubated with 3 units of Bal31 exonuclease (Boehringer-Mannheim, Indianapolis, IN) at 30°C in a buffer containing 20 mM tris (pH 7.2), 0.5 M NaCl, 12.5 mM $MgCl_2$, 12.5 mM $CaCl_2$, and 2 mM EDTA. Samples were removed at 0, 2, 5, 10, 20, and 30 min after addition of the enzyme; the exonuclease reactions were stopped in these aliquots by addition of EDTA (50 mM final concentration).

Direct Gel Hybridization

After being destained in water, the gel was placed first in 0.5 N NaOH/0.15 M NaCl for 30 min at room temperature and then 0.5 M tris, pH 7.6 for 30 min at 4°C. The gel was subsequently dried under vacuum (Hoefer, San Francisco, CA) onto a nylon membrane (1.2-μ pore size, Biotrans; ICN Radiochemicals, Irvine, CA) at 60°C. The solution for hybridization and prehybridization was 50% formamide, 6X SSC (standard saline citrate), 5X Denhardt's, 0.5% sodium dodecyl sulfate (SDS), 0.1 mg/ml of denatured, sonicated herring sperm DNA, and 0.1% sodium pyrophosphate. The dried, mounted gel was prehybridized for 4 h and hybridized with the probe for 18 h. The incubation temperature was 37°C. After hybridization the blots were washed at 65°C in a Turbo-Blot apparatus (American BioNuclear, Emeryville, CA) first with 1X SSC containing 0.1% SDS and 1 mM EDTA and finally with 0.1X SSC/0.1% SDS/1 mM EDTA. The mounted gel was placed between sheets of Saran Wrap and exposed to X-ray film with an intensifying screen.

Southern Blot

Total DNA and the three fractions of extracted DNA (chromosome, supercoiled plasmid, and linear plasmid) were digested with HindIII. The resultant restrictions were electrophoretically separated in a 1.0% agarose gel in TBE buffer at 50 V. The fragments were transferred to a nylon membrane by capillary action using methods previously described. The hybridization and washing conditions were those described above.

DNA Probes

A 0.7 kb HindIII-HindIII fragment of recombinant plasmid pTRH45 contains 0.4 kb of the ospB gene.[14] This HindIII fragment was cloned into the vector pBR322 and served as a probe for the ospB gene. The 1 kb EcoRI-HaeIII fragment of plasmid pTRH44 contains the majority of DNA sequence of the ospA gene of B31 as well as 25 bases of the vector pBR322[14]; this fragment was the probe for the ospA gene. (Preliminary studies had shown that pBR322 does not hybridize to B. burgdorferi

DNA.) The probes were radiolabeled with ^{32}P-ATP with a nick translation kit (BRL).

Electroelution of DNA

DNA molecules of greater than 40 kb apparent size were recovered from agarose gels by electroelution into a salt sink of 3-M sodium acetate in an electroeluter (model UEA; International Biotechnologies, Inc., New Haven, CT). The buffer was 20 mM tris (pH 8.0), 5 mM NaCl, 0.2 mM EDTA; the elution was carried out for 2 hours at 100 V. (A preliminary study with *B. burgdorferi* DNA that had been labeled with ^{3}H-thymidine showed that about 30% of the DNA in a plasmid band was recovered from the agarose gel.) DNA to be used in electron microscopy and denaturation studies was not stained with ethidium bromide prior to electroelution. Pipette tips with large bores at their ends were used in all nucleic acid manipulations to minimize shearing of the DNA.

Electron Microscopy and Heteroduplexing

DNA was mounted for electron microscopy by means of the Kleinschmidt aqueous technique.[15,16] Adenovirus 2 DNA (BRL) was the standard used to calibrate contour length measurements. Grids were examined in a JEOL 100B electron microscope at 40 kV accelerating voltage. Electron micrographs were taken on Kodak Electron Image plates at a magnification of 7000X. The magnification was calibrated for each set of plates with a grating replica (E. F. Fullam), and contour lengths were measured with a Numonics Graphics calculator interfaced with a Tektronik 4052A computer. The mean ± standard deviation (SD) of the measured lengths are given. "Percent error" was the mean divided by the standard deviation.

Electroeluted borrelial plasmid DNA was heteroduplexed with recombinant plasmid pTRH44, which had been digested with *Sal*I. This digestion yielded a linear molecule with the intact *ospA* insertion flanked by unequally sized arms of the vector. The methods for heteroduplexing have been described previously.[15,16]

RESULTS

The DNA of *B. burgdorferi* cells was separated first into plasmid-rich and chromosome-rich fractions. The plasmid-rich fraction was then further resolved with ethidium bromide CsCl density ultracentrifugation into its supercoiled and linear DNA components. (Electron microscopy of the plasmid-rich fraction before ultracentrifugation showed that approximately 10–20% of the molecules were supercoiled; there were only rare nicked circles. The majority of the plasmids were linear molecules.) The three resultant DNA preparations were designated "chromosome" (C), "supercoiled plasmid" (S), and "linear plasmid" (L).

Samples of the three fractions were examined by electrophoresis in a low concentration of agarose (FIG. 1A). Four bands in the supercoiled plasmid fraction were discernible in the gel. (From the point of the initial DNA extraction, the supercoiled plasmid sample was approximately 10 times more concentrated than the linear plasmid sample.) By electron microscopy there were both supercoiled and nicked circles in the circular DNA fraction after recovery of the DNA from the ultracentrifuge tubes and removal of the ethidium bromide. There appeared to be more than one

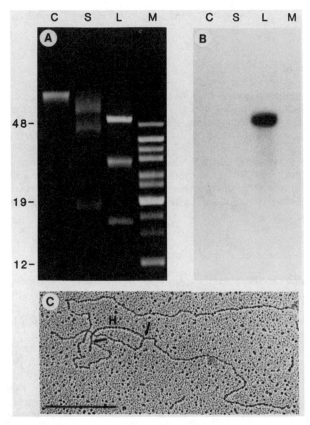

FIGURE 1. The *osp* genes of *B. burgdorferi* are located on a 49-kb linear plasmid. (**A**) Agarose gel electrophoresis. (**B**) Direct gel hybridization. The three forms of extracted DNA—chromosome (lanes C), supercoiled plasmid (lanes S), and linear plasmid (lanes L)—were applied to a 0.2% agarose gel, which was run with sodium phosphate buffer. Molecular size standards (in kilobase pairs) were in the M lanes; the numbers at the left give the sizes of selected standards in kilobase pairs. The DNA in the gel was stained with ethidium bromide (**A**) and then denatured. After neutralization, the gel was dried onto a nylon membrane. The DNA in the dried, mounted gel was directly hybridized with radiolabeled probe (**B**). In this experiment the *ospB* gene probe was used. (**C**) Heteroduplex of the 49-kb linear plasmid and *Sal*I-cut pTRH44 recombinant plasmid. The extent of the region of heteroduplex formation *(H)* is indicated by the two *arrows*. The short and long nonhybridizing arms of the linearized plasmid are seen extending from the left and right arrows, respectively. *Scale bar* = 1.0 μm.

size species of circular plasmid by electron microscopy. The average contoured circumference of 20 measured circular molecules was 28.0 ± 1.9 kb (SD). This amount of variance, *i.e.,* a percent error of 7%, is indicative of heterogeneity. Thus, the four bands in the gel probably represent the supercoiled and nicked versions of at least two differently sized circular plasmids in *B. burgdorferi* B31.

By agarose gel electrophoresis the linear plasmid fraction contained three plasmids with apparent lengths of 49, 29, and 16 kb (FIG. 1A). When the electrophoresis was carried out for 48 h instead of 18 h, the "49 kb" plasmid was located at the bottom of the gel, but still only one band was seen.

The gel shown in FIGURE 1A was dried onto a nylon membrane and incubated with a labeled DNA probe in a direct gel hybridization. Contained in the hybridization probe was a 0.4-kb fragment of the *ospB* gene. A 49-kb band in the linear plasmid lane of the gel hybridized under high stringency conditions with the probe (FIG. 1B). There was no detectable hybridization of the probe to the 29- or 16-kb linear plasmids, to the supercoiled plasmid bands, or to the chromosome fraction with even 20-fold longer exposures of the autoradiographs. The *ospA*-specific DNA probe also hybridized to the 49-kb plasmid under the same conditions in a direct gel hybridization (data not shown).

The topmost linear plasmid band with an apparent size of 49 kb was recovered from unstained gels by electroelution. The presence of *ospA* sequences in this plasmid was confirmed directly by heteroduplex analysis with *Sal*I-digested recombinant vector pTRH44. A 1.3-kb region of homology, corresponding to the *ospA* gene and flanking regions, could be identified near the middle of the 49-kb molecule (FIG. 1C). The "arms" of the probe that did not hybridize with the borrelial plasmid are sequences of the pUC8 vector.

To test whether the sequences in the plasmid that hybridized with the *ospA* and *ospB* probes in the direct gel hybridizations truly represented the *osp* genes themselves and not simply cross-hybridizing sequences, we digested total B31 DNA (T) and the C, S, and L fractions with *Hind*III and performed a Southern blot analysis (FIG. 2). The blot was hybridized with both the *ospA* and *ospB* probes under high stringency conditions. From the restriction map of recombinant plasmid pTRH32, which contains both *osp* genes,[14] we would predict that radio-emitting bands of 2.5 kb and 1.1 kb would be seen in the blot, if the hybridizing sequences in the linear plasmid corresponded to the cloned *osp* genes. Only in the total DNA and linear plasmid (L) lanes were bands observed in the autoradiograph. The hybridizing fragments were 2.5 and 1.1 kb in length.

To determine the true size of the linear plasmids containing the *osp* genes, contour length measurements of the linear duplex molecules were made by electron microscopy. Adenovirus 2 molecules with a known length of 35,937 base pairs served as the standard.[17] The size distributions of the measured molecules are shown in FIGURE 3. When 50 molecules of adenovirus were measured, the percent error was 3%. The mean size of 50 molecules of the isolated linear plasmid band was 48.8 ± 1.6 kb; the percent error was 3%. The 49-kb linear plasmid band was as homogenous in the size distribution of its constituent molecules as a population of adenovirus molecules.

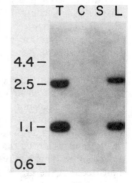

FIGURE 2. Southern blot analysis. Total DNA (T) and chromosome (C), supercoiled plasmid (S), and linear plasmid (L) DNA fractions of *B. burgdorferi* B31 were digested with *Hind*III. The restriction fragments were separated on an agarose gel and transferred to a nylon membrane. The fragments were hybridized under high stringency conditions with the *ospA* and *ospB* gene probes. The sizes of the hybridizing fragments and of molecular size standards in kilobase pairs are shown.

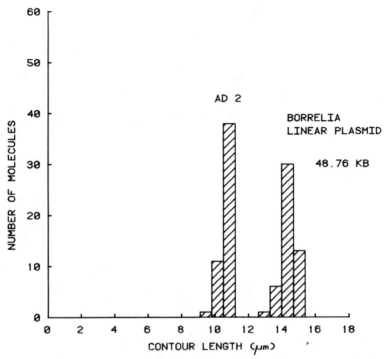

FIGURE 3. Contour length of a *B. burgdorferi* linear plasmid. Fifty molecules each of the size standard adenovirus 2 (*AD 2*) and the electroeluted "49 kb" linear plasmid of strain B31 were measured using electron microscopy. The size distributions of the molecules are shown. With a multiplier factor of 3.39 the mean length of the linear plasmids was estimated to be 48.76 kb.

*Bal*31 exonuclease digestions of the plasmid fraction served not only to confirm the linear nature of the *osp* gene-bearing plasmids but also provided another estimate of the location of the *osp* genes on the plasmid. *Bal*31 exonuclease progressively shortens linear DNA molecules from both ends[18]; it does not act on duplex circular DNA. If the *osp* genes were located on linear plasmids, the hybridizing band would become shorter and eventually disappear with continued *Bal*31 digestion. On the other hand, if the hybridizing sequences in the 49-kb plasmid band were actually from nicked circular plasmid DNA "contaminating" the band, the hybridizing band would not get shorter with *Bal*31 exposure. FIGURE 4 shows the result of the *Bal*31 digestion of a plasmid-rich fraction of B31 DNA and subsequent direct gel hybridization with radiolabeled *ospB* gene probe. The three predominant linear plasmids were shortened by *Bal*31 (left panel). The hybridizing band also became shorter with longer and longer incubation times (right panel). Extrapolating from the reduction in size of the 16 kb and 25 kb plasmids, we estimate that approximately 10 kb had been removed from the 49 kb plasmid after 30 minutes of digestion. Yet the *ospB* probe still bound to the shrinking topmost band. This experiment provided further evidence that the *osp* genes are located on linear molecules and not on circular plasmids in the preparation. In addition, it showed that the *ospB* gene must be at least 5 kb internal to either end of the plasmid. The heteroduplex analysis with the *ospA* gene probe (FIG. 1C) also indicated that the *osp* genes are not to be found at or near the ends of the plasmid.

DISCUSSION

The present study and a previous study[13] have shown that the genes encoding the major surface proteins of *B. burgdorferi*, OspA and OspB, are located on a linear extrachromosomal element in the cell. The plasmid has a length of 49 kb, and the *osp* genes are at least 5 kb from a terminus of the plasmid. A previous report demonstrated that the 49-kb plasmid of *B. burgdorferi* strain B31 has covalently closed ends, most likely in the form of a hairpin.[13] A plasmid or bacteriophage with an architecture like that had not previously been noted in a prokaryotic organism. The best characterized replicon with a similar structure is the vaccinia virus, a pox virus.[19]

In *B. hermsii*, a closely related spirochete and an agent of relapsing fever, the genes for the major surface proteins are likewise positioned on linear plasmids.[7] In the case of strain HS1 of *B. hermsii* the protein-encoding genes are on plasmids with contour lengths of approximately 23 kb (ref. 7 and unpublished obserations, A. G. Barbour and C. F. Garon). For a relapsing fever borrelia, which depends on an extensive antigenic variation to avoid the immune response, there may be an advantage in having its collection of surface antigen genes on plasmids and not in the chromosome. In an extrachromosomal location and as one of presumably multiple copies, a surface coat gene would likely evolve at a faster rate than if it was to be found as a single copy in the chromosome. Base changes, insertions, deletions, duplications, and inversions could occur among the plasmids with only a low risk of being a lethal mutation for the cell. If a major disruption of, for instance, the plasmid's origin of replication occurred as a result of a mutational event such as an insertion, other copies of the plasmid still carry the critical hereditary information needed to retain a gene for a surface protein in the cell.

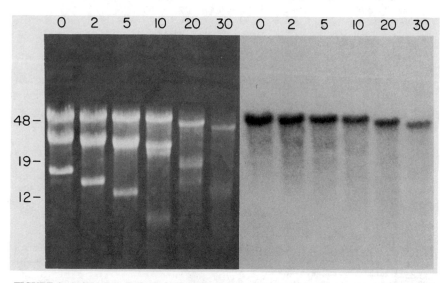

FIGURE 4. *Bal*31 exonuclease digestion of *B. burgdorferi* plasmids. The plasmid-rich fraction of strain B31 DNA was incubated with *Bal*31 for 0, 2, 5, 10, 20, or 30 min. The DNA was separated on a 0.2% agarose gel with TBE buffer. The *left panel* shows the ethidium bromide stain of the gel; the 49 kb, 25 kb, and 16 kb plasmids are shortened. The *right panel* shows the direct gel hybridization of the gel with the *ospB* gene probe.

Antigenic variation may also occur in a Lyme borreliosis infection. If it does, *B. burgdorferi* seems to use a less extensive antigenic repertoire than the relapsing fever borreliae employ. The number of serotypes that can be distinguished among different isolates of *B. burgdorferi* using monoclonal antibody reactivities is limited compared to even a single strain of *B. hermsii*.[20] Nevertheless, there is evidence that the OspB proteins in a population of *B. burgdorferi* cells in a host can change during the course of an infection[21] and during *in vitro* cultivation.[22] The finding by Craft *et al.* that a patient with chronic Lyme borreliosis for several months can suddenly produce an anti-OspB antibody that had not been detected previously suggests that antigenic variation of OspB proteins may occur in humans as well.[23] A putative variation in the expression of OspB protein in *B. burgdorferi* may not be on the basis of expression-linked and silent versions of the *ospB* gene, however. As shown here in the Southern blot analysis, there appears to be only one environment for *ospA* and *ospB* genes. If there were both silent and active environments for an *osp* gene—as there are for a variable major protein of *B. hermsii*[6,7]—one would expect to find more hybridizing fragments in the Southern blot than were observed.

REFERENCES

1. BARBOUR, A. G. & S. F. HAYES. 1986. Biology of *Borrelia* species. Microbiol. Rev. **50:** 381–400.
2. BARBOUR, A. G. 1984. Isolation and cultivation of Lyme disease spirochetes. Yale J. Biol. Med. **57:** 71–75.
3. BARBOUR, A. G., S. L. TESSIER & H. G. STOENNER. 1982. Variable major proteins of *Borrelia hermsii*. J. Exp. Med. **156:** 1312–1324.
4. BARBOUR, A. G., O. BARRERA & R. JUDD. 1983. Structural analysis of the variable major proteins of *Borrelia hermsii*. J. Exp. Med. **158:** 2127–2140.
5. BARSTAD, P. A., J. E. COLIGAN, M. G. RAUM & A. G. BARBOUR. 1985. Variable major proteins of *Borrelia hermsii:* Epitope mapping and partial sequence analysis. J. Exp. Med. **161:** 1302–1314.
6. MEIER, J. T., M. I. SIMON & A. G. BARBOUR. 1985. Antigenic variation is associated with DNA rearrangements in a relapsing fever borrelia. Cell **41:** 403–409.
7. PLASTERK, R. H. A., M. I. SIMON & A. G. BARBOUR. 1985. Transposition of structural genes to an expression sequence on a linear plasmid causes antigenic variation in the bacterium *Borrelia hermsii*. Nature (London) **318:** 257–263.
8. BARBOUR, A. G., S. L. TESSIER & W. J. TODD. 1983. Lyme disease spirochetes and *Ixodes* tick spirochetes share a common surface antigenic determinant as defined by a monoclonal antibody. Infect. Immun. **41:** 795–804.
9. BARBOUR, A. G., S. L. TESSIER & S. F. HAYES. 1984. Variation in a major surface protein of Lyme disease spirochetes. Infect. Immun. **45:** 94–100.
10. HOWE, T. R., L. W. MAYER & A. G. BARBOUR. 1985. A single recombinant plasmid expressing two major outer surface proteins of the Lyme disease spirochete. Science **227:** 645–646.
11. BARBOUR, A. G. 1984. Clonal polymorphisms of surface antigens in a relapsing fever *Borrelia* species. *In* Bayer Symposium VII: The Pathogenesis of Bacterial Infections. G. G. Jackson & H. Thomas, Eds.: 235–245. Springer-Verlag. Heidelberg.
12. BARBOUR, A. G., R. A. HEILAND & T. R. HOWE. 1985. Heterogeneity of major proteins of Lyme disease borreliae: A molecular analysis of North American and European isolates. J. Infect. Dis. **152:** 478–484.
13. BARBOUR, A. G. & C. F. GARON. 1987. Linear plasmids of the bacterium *Borrelia burgdorferi* have covalently closed ends. Science **237:** 409–411.
14. HOWE, T. R., F. W. LAQUIER & A. G. BARBOUR. 1986. Organization of genes encoding two outer membrane proteins of the Lyme disease agent *Borrelia burgdorferi* within a single transcriptional unit. Infect. Immun. **54:** 207–212.

15. GARON, C. F. 1982. Electron microscopy of nucleic acids. *In* Gene Amplification and Analysis, Vol. 2. J. G. Chirikjian & T. S. Papas, Eds.: 573–585. Elsevier. New York.

16. GARON, C. F. 1986. Electron microscopy of nucleic acids. *In* Ultrastructure Techniques for Microorganisms. H. C. Aldrich & W. J. Todd, Eds.: 161–181. Plenum. New York.

17. GINGERAS, T. R., D. SCIAKY, R. F. GELINAS, J. BING-DONG, C. E. YEN, M. M. KELLY, P. A. BULLOCK, B. L. PARSONS, K. E. O'NEILL & R. J. ROBERTS, 1982. Nucleotide sequences from the adenovirus-2 genome. J. Biol. Chem. **257:** 13475–13491

18. WILLIAMS, R. O., J. R. YOUNG & P. A. O. MAJIWA. 1982. Genomic environment of *T. brucei* VSG genes: Presence of a minichromosome. Nature (London) **299:** 417–419.

19. MERCHLINSKY, B. & B. MOSS. 1986. Resolution of linear minichromosomes with hairpin ends from circular plasmids containing virus concatemer junctions. Cell **45:** 879–884.

20. STOENNER, H. G., T. DODD & C. LARSEN. 1982. Antigenic variation of *Borrelia hermsii.* J. Exp. Med. **156:** 1297–1311.

21. BURGDORFER, W. & K. L. GAGE. 1986. Susceptibility of the lack-legged tick, *Ixodes scapularis,* to the Lyme disease spirochete, *Borrelia burgdorferi.* Zbl. Bakt. Hyg. A **263:** 15–20.

22. SCHWAN, T. G. & W. BURGDORFER. 1987. Antigenic changes of *Borrelia burgdorferi* as a result of in vitro cultivation. J. Inf. Dis. **156:** 852–853.

23. CRAFT, J. E., D. K. FISCHER, G. T. SHIMAMOTO & A. C. STEERE. 1986. Antigens of Borrelia burgdorferi recognized during Lyme disease: Appearance of a new immunoglobulin M response and expansion of the immunoglobulin G response late in the illness. J. Clin. Invest. **78:** 934–939.

Serologic Diagnosis of Lyme Disease

LOUIS A. MAGNARELLI

Department of Entomology
The Connecticut Agricultural Experiment Station
P.O. Box 1106
New Haven, Connecticut 06504

With the discovery and cultivation of *Borrelia burgdorferi*,[1,2] diagnostic tests were developed to detect serum immunoglobulins to this bacterium in persons who were suspected of having Lyme disease or related disorders.[3-8] Initially, indirect fluorescent antibody (IFA) procedures were used to confirm clinical diagnoses,[1-4] but in laboratories where large numbers of serum samples were being tested, enzyme-linked immunosorbent assays (ELISA) were implemented.[5-7] Both methods continue to be used on an experimental basis.

Serologic tests for Lyme disease are particularly helpful in distinguishing this malady from other illnesses that also include neurologic or arthritic disorders. During the early stage of Lyme disease, the characteristic skin lesion (erythema migrans) can be atypical or absent,[9] and the resulting clinical picture may be unclear. In these instances, serologic tests are often requested to aid in diagnoses. However, neither the IFA nor ELISA methods are standardized among laboratories, and if there are differences in sensitivities, there are likely to be discrepancies in test results. In view of this potential problem and of the progress that has been made in the past 5 years, it is appropriate to briefly review the current status of immunologic testing for Lyme disease in humans.

POLYVALENT AND CLASS-SPECIFIC ASSAYS

A variety of tests are available for quantitative determinations of total immunoglobulins (Ig) or class-specific antibodies to *B. burgdorferi*. The method of choice usually depends on the expertise of personnel, demands for testing, equipment available, budgetary restrictions, and physicians' needs. For example, at the Connecticut Agricultural Experiment Station, more than 6000 serum samples were tested for antibodies to *B. burgdorferi* during 1983–85. An IFA test with polyvalent, fluorescein isothiocyanate-labeled conjugates was applied during 1983,[10] a year when only 649 samples were assayed. Physicians then requested specific information on titers of IgM and IgG antibodies, and soon thereafter these tests were developed. As the number of specimens rose sharply during 1984, the laborious IFA method became impractical, and an ELISA with polyvalent reagents was utilized.[7] Subsequently, enzyme-linked procedures for class-specific IgM and IgG antibodies were applied to monitor changes in immune responses in treated and untreated patients over extended periods. Other investigators relied on either polyvalent or class-specific reagents in IFA or ELISA systems to confirm *B. burgdorferi* infections.[3-6,11-18] In ELISA, anti-human immunoglobulins conjugated to either alkaline phosphatase or horseradish peroxidase are satisfactory.[5-7,18,19]

There are advantages to performing either or both polyvalent and class-specific assays. For routine screening of large numbers of serum samples, such as in clinical laboratories of hospitals, the former is cost effective and preferred. However, since

154

levels of total serum IgM antibody reflect disease activity[20] and correlate with specific IgM titers,[6,21] detection of these antibodies may be used to predict subsequent neurological, cardiac, or joint involvement. Although IgM antibody usually does not persist,[3] Craft et al.[22] recently detected a resurgence of IgM antibody in some patients who had arthritis. Using immunoblotting techniques, they showed that the initial and late IgM antibody responses were directed against different antigenic components of B. burgdorferi—the 41-kilodalton (kDa) and 34 kDa polypeptides, respectively. Information on IgG antibody titers has been especially useful in separating Lyme disease from aseptic meningitis, unexplained cranial or peripheral nerve palsies, rheumatoid arthritis, juvenile arthritis, and Reiter's syndrome.[3,6]

TEST SENSITIVITY

Differences in sensitivities of IFA methods and ELISA for the diagnosis of Lyme disease probably exist among private, state, and federal laboratories. Standardized tests conducted within institutions, however, clearly indicate reproducibility and comparable sensitivities for these assays.[5-7] In general, the probability of successful confirmation of Lyme disease is highest when blood samples are collected from untreated patients who were experiencing neurologic or arthritic disorders. Even though both procedures are suitable for diagnostic testing, the more objective manner of obtaining results and the ability to perform many more analyses make ELISA the preferred method.

Failure to detect antibodies during the early stage of Lyme disease is an obvious limitation. If blood samples are obtained within 3 weeks after onset of erythema migrans, serologic results are likely to be negative,[5,23] regardless of the assay method or conjugates used. According to Moffat et al.,[24] spontaneous suppressor cell activity is increased during the initial weeks of infection, and under these conditions antibody response may be limited to only the most immunogenic polypeptides. Consequently, it may take several weeks for antibody titers to rise to detectable levels. There is also considerable variability in immune response among patients with erythema migrans,[22,23] and if antibiotics are administered during early illness, antibody production can be aborted or curtailed.[3,18] Thus, depending on the circumstances, serologic confirmation may not be made for some patients who have been clinically diagnosed as having Lyme disease.[25]

Cut-off titers can be lowered to increase test sensitivity. However, this decreases the specificity of assays and can result in a greater number of false positives, especially if antibodies have been produced to related spirochetes, such as Treponema pallidum.[5,8,16] Moreover, different criteria are being used in diagnostic laboratories to define a positive result.[5-7] This, coupled with lower test sensitivity during early disease,[5,19,23] may result in misinterpretations of results and could ultimately affect the accuracy of seroepidemiologic studies designed to monitor changes in prevalence of Lyme disease.

Different strains of B. burgdorferi exist worldwide.[26-28] Therefore, it was important to determine if serologic results vary with antigen preparations that consisted of different strains of this bacterium. Based on comparative IFA analyses of human sera in Sweden[16,29] and in West Germany,[8] there were no significant differences in antibody titers when isolates of B. burgdorferi from North America were compared with those from Europe. Even though immunoglobulins may be directed to different antigenic components of B. burgdorferi,[4,22,28,30] there seems to be consistency in IFA results. Similar studies need to be performed with ELISA.

TABLE 1. Reciprocal Antibody Titers for Serum Samples Analyzed by ELISA with Whole-Cell or Sonicated *B. burgdorferi*

	Total Immunoglobulins	
Patients	Whole-Cell Antigens[a]	Sonicated Antigen[b]
MM	20,480	40,960
JS	1280	640
ES	40,960	40,960
BS	640	640
LG	1280	1280
JL	1280	2560
AG	640	1280
JS	1280	1280
BB	2560	2560
MK	10,240	10,240
ML	10,240	20,480
RH	20,480	10,240
MO	10,240	10,240
RR	20,480	20,480
ST	neg	neg
RS	neg	neg

[a]Washed, whole-cell *B. burgdorferi* (Ct. strain 2591).
[b]Sonicated *B. burgdorferi* (Ct. strain 2591) prepared as described by Craft *et al.*[6]

Cultures of *B. burgdorferi* have been processed differently to produce working antigen for ELISA. Some investigators sonicate washed whole cells before coating the solid phase,[5,6] while others use washed whole cells directly.[7] To determine if these methods of antigen preparation result in different serologic test findings, parallel tests were conducted with human sera. Details on the production of whole-cell and sonicated antigens, on standardization for protein content, and on the use of ELISA have been reported.[6,7] Titration end points for 14 positive samples were within the normal test variability of ≤twofold changes (TABLE 1). Similar tests were conducted to determine if antigen-coated, polystyrene plates could be frozen and used at a later date. Following overnight incubation at 37°C, plates were wrapped in aluminum foil and stored at −60°C for a maximum of 48 days. Results for frozen plates and normal testing procedures (*i.e.,* coating overnight and use on the following day) varied by twofold or less (TABLE 2). With no loss of sensitivity, the use of stored (frozen) plates during periods of extensive work load should facilitate the testing of large numbers of samples.

TEST SPECIFICITY

Of the spirochetes that can cause human illness, the treponemes are more closely related to the *Borrelia* than the leptospires are.[31,32] Accordingly, serologic cross-reactivity between *B. burgdorferi* and *T. pallidum* can occur.[5,6,8,16,33,34] Antisera to other *Borrelia* spirochetes, such as *B. hermsii* and *B. recurrentis,* will also cross-react with the Lyme disease agent in IFA tests and ELISA.[6,33] In the western United States *B. hermsii, B. parkeri,* and *B. burgdorferi* may coexist,[35] and because these organisms are so closely related, efforts to block cross-reactive antibodies by adsorption have been relatively unsuccessful.[6,33] Therefore, without supportive clinical or epidemiological data, serologic results for relapsing fever and Lyme disease infections are likely to be inconclusive.

Serologic cross-reactivity between *B. burgdorferi* and *T. pallidum* is well-documented.[4,5,8,16,33,34] False positives occur most frequently when homologous antibody titers are elevated. Consequently, Russell *et al.*[5] established higher cutoff levels ($\geq 1:256$) in IFA tests for Lyme disease, but 11 of 18 (61%) serum samples from patients with syphilis still reacted at or above this dilution to *B. burgdorferi*. Sera from persons with Lyme disease, however, are usually nonreactive in the rapid reagin card test (RPR)[5,34] or VDRL assays.[6] If these tests are performed along with an IFA method or ELISA for Lyme disease as needed, these diseases can usually be distinguished serologically. According to Russell *et al.*,[5] their IFA test and ELISA for Lyme disease were highly specific (97–100% reliable) when sera from patients with treponemal diseases were excluded from their analyses. In Europe, investigators remove cross-reactive antibodies to treponemes by adsorbing with *Treponema phagedenis*.[8,11,13,17]

In addition to the spirochetal infections, sera from patients with autoimmune diseases, infectious mononucleosis, Rocky Mountain spotted fever (RMSF), and other illnesses also reacted in tests for Lyme disease.[3,36] It is unclear whether these persons had prior, unknown exposure to *B. burgdorferi* or if there were broadly reacting, nonspecific immunoglobulins present. Subclinical infections of *B. burgdorferi* do occur. Steere *et al.*[37] detected IgG antibodies in 10 of 121 asymptomatic residents of Great Island, Massachusetts. Titers sometimes remained elevated for 4 or more years and paralleled those of patients with active arthritis. If persons develop disorders that are similar to those of Lyme disease and are tested for antibodies to *B. burgdorferi,* positive test results for these "residual" antibodies could be misinterpreted. Alternatively, in some illnesses, such as infectious mononucleosis, there may be polyclonal activation of B lymphocytes, which may also result in low-level cross-reactivity.[3]

Seroreactivity to two unrelated disease agents may be the result of dual infections

TABLE 2. Reciprocal Antibody Titers for Serum Samples Analyzed by ELISA with Normal and Frozen Plates

| | Total Immunoglobulins | | | | |
| | Normal Plates | Frozen Plates[a] | | | |
Patients	Overnight at 37°C	7 Days	14 Days	24 Days	48 Days
ED	2560	2560	1280	640	2560
DL	20,480	20,480	20,480	20,480	20,480
JH	5120	5120	5120	2560	5120
DS	1280	1280	1280	1280	1280
GA	40,960	20,480	20,480	20,480	nt[b]
MP	5120	5120	5120	2560	2560
AS	20,480	10,240	20,480	20,480	nt
JK	2560	1280	1280	1280	nt
MP	5120	5120	5120	nt	nt
RH	640	1280	640	nt	nt
LG	640	640	320	nt	nt
JL	1280	1280	2560	nt	nt

[a]Stored at $-60°C$ and warmed to room temperature before use.
[b]Not tested.

rather than cross-reactivity. The primary tick vector of Lyme disease, *Ixodes dammini*,[1,3] also transmits *Babesia microti*.[38,39] Since this protozoan can occur along with *B. burgdorferi* in the same rodent,[40] engorging larval ticks could acquire both agents, and after molting to nymphs could transmit these organisms when they feed on humans or other hosts. Serologic studies, conducted on Long Island, New York,[41] verified the presence of antibodies to both pathogens in patients who were from areas where babesiosis and Lyme disease had been previously reported. Based on clinical and serological findings, these authors concluded that persons were concurrently exposed to both agents by doubly infected ticks.

GENERAL COMMENTS

Serologic tests for *B. burgdorferi* are the most practical means of confirming clinical diagnoses for Lyme disease. Isolation of spirochetes from human tissues is laborious and, thus far, has been a low-yielding process.[3,42] Furthermore, the reliability of detecting *B. burgdorferi* in biopsy tissues by IFA or silver-staining methods has not been fully evaluated. With sufficient clinical and epidemiological information, IFA tests and ELISA are useful aids for antibody detection, and in time, simpler assay methods (*i.e.*, commercial test kits) should become available and improve routine analyses.

Low test sensitivity for samples obtained during early Lyme disease may complicate serodiagnoses, especially when there is no evidence of skin lesions. In serologic studies of syphilis,[43,44] use of flagellar-associated protein rather than sonicated antigen on the solid phase of ELISA improved the sensitivity for IgM and IgG antibodies. Similar applications of fractionated *B. burgdorferi* should be evaluated. When erythema migrans is atypical or does not occur, the associated symptoms can be confused with those of virus infections.[23] An antigen test for urine or blood specimens is needed to help verify *B. burgdorferi* infections.

In patients with neurologic disorders, reactivity of IgG antibody in cerebrospinal fluid (CSF) was stronger than that of serum antibodies.[18,45] Therefore, including CSF specimens in IFA tests for ELISA may help identify undiagnosed central nervous system disorders.[45-48]

Lyme disease can usually be clinically separated from other spirochetal infections. With adequate analyses (RPR, VDRL, and microagglutination tests), the cross-reactivity problems that occur with the treponemes or leptospires should be of minor concern. If needed, adsorption with *T. phagedenis* may help increase specificity. Separating tick-borne relapsing fever from Lyme disease, however, should be based on clinical and epidemiological findings.

Finally, Lyme disease and related disorders occur in North America, Europe, and Australia.[3] Among the arthropod-transmitted pathogens, *B. burgdorferi* is now most prevalent in the United States, and people with outdoor occupations or who live in endemic areas for Lyme disease may be at greater risk.[49] With increased public concern over this spirochetosis, there will be demands to make Lyme disease a reportable illness and to monitor prevalence of human infections. To accomplish this, epidemiological and serological studies should be conducted, and to accurately determine attack rates nationally or in more specific regions, serologic assays should be standardized among state, federal, and private laboratories. When this is accomplished, discrepancies in test results among laboratories, like those reported by Hedberg *et al.*,[50] should be resolved.

SUMMARY

Indirect fluorescent antibody tests and enzyme-linked immunosorbent assays are being used as laboratory aids for the diagnosis of Lyme disease and related disorders. Depending on the needs, polyvalent or class-specific reagents can be used to detect total immunoglobulins (Ig) or IgM and IgG antibodies. The sensitivities of these assays are relatively low when serum samples are obtained from patients within 3 weeks after onset of erythema migrans and are tested by either the IFA method or ELISA. During neuritis or arthritis, IgG antibody levels are usually elevated, and serologic verification is more easily achieved. Cross-reactivity occurs when sera from patients with Lyme disease, relapsing fever, or treponemal infections are screened against heterologous antigens, but these diseases can usually be separated clinically or by further seroanalyses. Although IFA tests and ELISA are both suitable for confirming Lyme disease, the objective results and the ability to perform many more analyses make ELISA the preferred method.

REFERENCES

1. BURGDORFER, W., A. G. BARBOUR, S. F. HAYES, J. L. BENACH, E. GRUNWALDT & J. P. DAVIS. 1982. Lyme disease—a tick-borne spirochetosis? Science **216:** 1317–1319.
2. BARBOUR, A. G. 1984. Isolation and cultivation of Lyme disease spirochetes. Yale J. Biol. Med. **57:** 521–525.
3. STEERE, A. C., R. L. GRODZICKI, A. N. KORNBLATT, J. E. CRAFT, A. G. BARBOUR, W. BURGDORFER, G. P. SCHMID, E. JOHNSON & S. E. MALAWISTA. 1983. The spirochetal etiology of Lyme disease. N. Engl. J. Med. **308:** 733–740.
4. BARBOUR, A. G., W. BURGDORFER, E. GRUNWALDT & A. C. STEERE. 1983. Antibodies of patients with Lyme disease to components of the *Ixodes dammini* spirochete. J. Clin. Invest. **72:** 504–515.
5. RUSSELL, H., J. S. SAMPSON, G. P. SCHMID, H. W. WILKINSON & B. PLIKAYTIS. 1984. Enzyme-linked immunosorbent assay and indirect immunofluorescence assay for Lyme disease. J. Infect. Dis. **149:** 465–470.
6. CRAFT, J. E., R. L. GRODZICKI & A. C. STEERE. 1984. Antibody response in Lyme disease: Evaluation of diagnostic tests. J. Infect. Dis. **149:** 789–795.
7. MAGNARELLI, L. A., J. M. MEEGAN, J. F. ANDERSON & W. A. CHAPPELL. 1984. Comparison of an indirect fluorescent-antibody test with an enzyme-linked immunosorbent assay for serological studies of Lyme disease. J. Clin. Microbiol. **20:** 181–184.
8. WILSKE, B., G. SCHIERZ, V. PREAC-MURSIC, K. WEBER, H.-W. PFISTER & K. EINHAUPL. 1984. Serological diagnosis of erythema migrans disease and related disorders. Infection **12:** 331–337.
9. STEERE, A. C., N. H. BARTENHAGEN, J. E. CRAFT, G. J. HUTCHINSON, J. H. NEWMAN, D. W. RAHN, L. H. SIGAL, P. N. SPIELER, K. S. STENN & S. E. MALAWISTA. 1983. The early clinical manifestations of Lyme disease. Ann. Intern. Med. **99:** 76–82.
10. ANDERSON, J. F., L. A. MAGNARELLI, W. BURGDORFER & A. G. BARBOUR. 1983. Spirochetes in *Ixodes dammini* and mammals from Connecticut. Am. J. Trop. Med. Hyg. **32:** 818–824.
11. WEBER, K., G. SCHIERZ, B. WILSKE & V. PREAC-MURSIC. 1984. European erythema migrans disease and related disorders. Yale J. Biol. Med. **57:** 465–471.
12. RYBERG, B. 1984. Bannwarth's syndrome (lymphocytic meningoradiculitis) in Sweden. Yale J. Biol. Med. **57:** 499–503.
13. ACKERMAN, R., J. KABATZKI, H. P. BOISTEN, A. C. STEERE, R. L. GRODZICKI, S. HARTUNG & U. RUNNE. 1984. *Ixodes ricinus* spirochete and European erythema chronicum migrans disease. Yale J. Biol. Med. **57:** 573–580.
14. HANRAHAN, J. P., J. L. BENACH, J. L. COLEMAN, E. M. BOSLER, J. C. GRABAU & D. L.

MORSE. 1984. Epidemiologic features of Lyme disease in New York. Yale J. Biol. Med. **57:** 643–650.

15. OSTERHOLM, M. T., J. C. FORFANG, K. E. WHITE & J. N. KURITSKY. 1984. Lyme disease in Minnesota: Epidemiologic and serologic findings. Yale J. Biol. Med. **57:** 677–683.

16. ASBRINK, E., A. HOVMARK & B. HEDERSTEDT. 1984. The spirochetal etiology of acrodermatitis chronica atrophicans Herxheimer. Acta Derm. Venereol. (Stockholm) **64:** 506–512.

17. PFISTER, H.-W., K. EINHAUPL, V. PREAC-MURSIC, B. WILSKE & G. SCHIERZ. 1984. The spirochetal etiology of lymphocytic meningoradiculitis of Bannwarth (Bannwarth's syndrome). J. Neurol. **231:** 141–144.

18. STIERNSTEDT, G. T., M. GRANSTROM, B. HEDERSTEDT & B. SKOLDENBERG. 1985. Diagnosis of spirochetal meningitis by enzyme-linked immunosorbent assay and indirect immunofluorescence assay in serum and cerebrospinal fluid. J. Clin. Microbiol. **21:** 819–825.

19. WILKINSON, H. W. 1984. Immunodiagnostic tests for Lyme disease. Yale J. Biol. Med. **57:** 567–572.

20. STEERE, A. C., J. A. HARDIN, S. RUDDY, J. G. MUMMAW & S. E. MALAWISTA. 1979. Lyme arthritis: Correlation of serum and cryoglobulin IgM with activity, and serum IgG with remission. Arthritis Rheum. **22:** 471–483.

21. CRAFT, J. E., R. L. GRODZICKI, M. SHRESTHA, D. K. FISCHER, M. GARCIA-BLANCO & A. C. STEERE. 1984. The antibody response in Lyme disease. Yale J. Biol. Med. **57:** 561–565.

22. CRAFT, J. E., D. K. FISCHER, G. T. SHIMAMOTO & A. C. STEERE. 1986. Antigens of *Borrelia burgdorferi* recognized during Lyme disease: Appearance of a new immunoglobulin M response and expansion of the immunoglobulin G response late in the illness. J. Clin. Invest. **78:** 934–939.

23. SHRESTHA, M., R. L. GRODZICKI & A. C. STEERE. 1985. Diagnosing early Lyme disease. Am. J. Med. **78:** 235–240.

24. MOFFAT, C. M., L. H. SIGAL, A. C. STEERE, D. H. FREEMAN & J. M. DWYER. 1984. Cellular immune findings in Lyme disease: Correlation with serum IgM and disease activity. Am. J. Med. **77:** 625–632.

25. MAGNARELLI, L. A. & J. F. ANDERSON. 1986. Early detection and persistence of antibodies to *Borrelia burgdorferi* in persons with Lyme disease. Zbl. Bakt. Hyg. A **263:** 392–399.

26. BARBOUR, A. G., R. A. HEILAND & T. R. HOWE. 1985. Heterogeneity of major proteins in Lyme disease borreliae: a molecular analysis of North American and European isolates. J. Infect. Dis. **152:** 478–484.

27. BARBOUR, A. G. & M. E. SCHRUMPF. 1986. Polymorphisms of major surface proteins of *Borrelia burgdorferi.* Zbl. Bakt. Hyg. A **263:** 83–91.

28. WILSKE, B., V. PREAC-MURSIC, G. SCHIERZ & K. V. BUSCH. 1986. Immunochemical and immunological analysis of European *Borrelia burgdorferi* strains. Zbl. Bakt. Hyg. A **263:** 92–102.

29. ASBRINK, E., B. HENDERSTEDT & A. HOVMARK. 1984. The spirochetal etiology of erythema chronicum migrans Afzelius. Acta Derm. Venereol. (Stockholm) **64:** 291–295.

30. BARBOUR, A. G. 1984. Immunochemical analysis of Lyme disease spirochetes. Yale J. Biol. Med. **57:** 581–586.

31. JOHNSON, R. C. 1977. The spirochetes. Annu. Rev. Microbiol. **31:** 89–106.

32. HYDE, F. W. & R. C. JOHNSON. 1984. Genetic relationship of Lyme disease spirochetes to *Borrelia, Treponema,* and *Leptospira* spp. J. Clin. Microbiol. **20:** 151–154.

33. MAGNARELLI, L. A., J. F. ANDERSON & R. C. JOHNSON. 1987. Cross-reactivity in serologic tests for Lyme disease and other spirochetal infections. J. Infect. Dis. **156:** 183–188.

34. HUNTER, E. F., H. RUSSELL, C. E. FARSHY, J. S. SAMPSON & S. A. LARSEN. 1986. Evaluation of sera from patients with Lyme disease in the fluorescent treponemal antibody-absorption test for syphilis. Sex. Trans. Dis. **13:** 232–236.

35. BARBOUR, A. G. & S. F. HAYES. 1986. Biology of *Borrelia* species. Microbiol. Rev. **50:** 381–400.

36. MERTZ, L. E., G. H. WOBIG, J. DUFFY & J. A. KATZMANN. 1985. Ticks, spirochetes, and new diagnostic tests for Lyme disease. Mayo Clin. Proc. **60:** 402–406.

37. STEERE, A. C., E. TAYLOR, M. L. WILSON, J. F. LEVINE & A. SPIELMAN. 1986.

Longitudinal assessment of the clinical and epidemiological features of Lyme disease in a defined population. J. Infect. Dis. **154:** 295–300.

38. SPIELMAN, A., C. M. CLIFFORD, J. PIESMAN & M. D. CORWIN. 1979. Human babesiosis on Nantucket Island, USA: Description of vector, *Ixodes* (*Ixodes*) *dammini*, n. sp. (Acarina: Ixodidae). J. Med. Entomol. **15:** 218–234.

39. SPIELMAN, A., M. L. WILSON, J. F. LEVINE & J. PIESMAN. 1985. Ecology of *Ixodes dammini*-borne human babesiosis and Lyme disease. Annu. Rev. Entomol. **30:** 439–460.

40. ANDERSON, J. F., R. C. JOHNSON, L. A. MAGNARELLI, F. W. HYDE & J. E. MYERS. 1986. *Peromyscus leucopus* and *Microtus pennsylvanicus* simultaneously infected with *Borrelia burgdorferi* and *Babesia microti*. J. Clin. Microbiol. **23:** 135–137.

41. BENACH, J. L., J. L. COLEMAN, G. S. HABICHT, A. MACDONALD, E. GRUNWALDT & J. A. GIRON. 1985. Serological evidence for simultaneous occurrences of Lyme disease and babesiosis. J. Infect. Dis. **152:** 473–477.

42. BENACH, J. L., E. M. BOSLER, J. P. HANRAHAN, J. L. COLEMAN, G. S. HABICHT, T. F. BAST, D. J. CAMERON, J. L. ZIEGLER, A. G. BARBOUR, W. BURGDORFER, R. EDELMAN & R. A. KASLOW. 1983. Spirochetes isolated from the blood of two patients with Lyme disease. N. Engl. J. Med. **308:** 740–742.

43. PEDERSEN, N. S., C. S. PETERSEN, M. VEJTORP & N. H. AXELSEN. 1982. Serodiagnosis of syphilis by enzyme-linked immunosorbent assay for IgG antibodies against the Reiter treponeme flagellum. Scand. J. Immunol. **15:** 341–348.

44. PEDERSEN, N. S., C. S. PETERSEN & N. H. AXELSEN. 1982. Enzyme-linked immunosorbent assay for detection of immunoglobulin M antibody against the Reiter treponeme flagellum in syphilis. J. Clin. Microbiol. **16:** 608–614.

45. WILSKE, B., G. SCHIERZ, V. PREAC-MURSIC, K. VON BUSCH, R. KUHBECK, H.-W. PFISTER & K. EINHAUPL. 1986. Intrathecal production of specific antibodies against *Borrelia burgdorferi* in patients with lymphocytic meningoradiculitis (Bannwarth's syndrome). J. Infect. Dis. **153:** 304–314.

46. SUCHANEK, G., W. KRISTOFERITSCH, G. STANEK & H. BERNHEIMER. 1986. Anti-myelin antibodies in cerebrospinal fluid and serum of patients with meningopolyneuritis Garin-Bujadoux-Bannwarth and other neurological diseases. Zbl. Bakt. Hyg. A **263:** 160–168.

47. KRISTOFERITSCH, W., A. J. STECK, N. MURRAY, G. STANEK & H. LANSCHUTZER. 1986. Oligoclonal antibodies in CSF of patients with meningopolyneuritis, Garin-Bujadoux-Bannwarth: Ig class, light chain type and specificity. Zbl. Bakt. Hyg. A **263:** 307–313.

48. STIERNSTEDT, G., M. GRANSTROM, B. HEDERSTEDT & B. SKOLDENBERG. 1986. Serological diagnosis of *Borrelia* meningitis. Zbl. Bakt. Hyg. A **263:** 420–424.

49. BOWEN, G. S., T. L. SCHULZE, C. HAYNE & W. E. PARKIN. 1984. A focus of Lyme disease in Monmouth County, New Jersey. Am. J. Epidemiol. **120:** 387–394.

50. HEDBERG, C. W., M. T. OSTERHOLM, K. L. MACDONALD & K. E. WHITE. 1987. An interlaboratory study of antibody to *Borrelia burgdorferi*. J. Infect. Dis. **155:** 1325–1327.

Immunoglobulin G Subclasses Specific to *Borrelia burgdorferi* in Patients with Lyme Disease

KARIM E. HECHEMY,[a] HERVIE L. HARRIS,[a]
MICHAEL J. DUERR,[a] JORGE L. BENACH,[b]
AND CHARLES B. REIMER[c]

[a]*Wadsworth Center for Laboratories and Research*
New York State Department of Health
Albany, New York 12201

[b]*Bureau of Communicable Disease Control*
New York State Department of Health
Stony Brook, New York 11794

[c]*Division of Host Factors, Center for Infectious Diseases*
Centers for Disease Control
Atlanta, Georgia 30333

INTRODUCTION

One of the parameters in the study of disease pathogenesis and immune protection is the analysis of the IgG subclass-specific antibody produced during the immune response.[1] Four subclasses of human IgG are currently recognized. Each subclass is defined by unique primary structure of the constant region of the heavy chain molecule, and by characteristic biologic and functional properties.[2] A subclass-restricted response to microbial antigens has also been demonstrated by a number of investigators.[3-5] For example, many carbohydrate antigens preferentially elicit an IgG2 response. In contrast, IgG1 and IgG3 are the dominant response to many protein antigens. Lyme disease,[6] a tick-borne illness, has become a newly recognized nosologic entity caused by a spirochete *Borrelia burgdorferi*.[7] It is characterized by a distinctive skin lesion (stage 1) that may be followed by cardiac and/or neurologic (stage 2), or arthritic (stage 3) sequelae. The immunoglobulin G response to the various antigens of *B. burgdorferi* during the various stages of Lyme disease has recently been reported.[8] In this report, we investigate the composition of the IgG subclass specific to *B. burgdorferi* and to *Treponema phagedenis* biovar. Reiter for the three stages of the disease. *T. phagedenis* was used as a specificity control because of previously reported[9] cross-reactivity with sera from Lyme disease patients.

MATERIALS AND METHODS

Antigen Preparation

B. burgdorferi was grown in BSK II[10] at 35°C for 3 to 4 days and centrifuged at 9000 ×g at 25°C for 30 min. The pellet was washed by centrifugation in phosphate-buffered saline (PBS), pH 7.2. The pellet was then resuspended in PBS to a Klett 66

TABLE 1 Distribution of Sera from Lyme Disease Patients According to Disease Stage

Stage	Symptoms	No. of Sera
1	ECM	9
2	neurologic and/or cardiac	13
3	arthritic	56

reading of 500, layered on a 25% w/w sucrose solution, and centrifuged as above at 4°C. The pellet obtained consisted of two layers, one upper cream color layer and a narrow gray layer. The upper layer was resuspended carefully, decanted and recentrifuged at 4°C. The pellet was then resuspended in PBS and the centrifugation on sucrose repeated until the pellet was uniformly colored. The final pellet was then resuspended in distilled water (DW) and lyophilized.

Treponema phagedenis biovar. Reiter was grown for 5 days as described,[11] and processed as for *B. burgdorferi*.

Antisera

Sera from patients clinically diagnosed as having Lyme disease (TABLE 1) and serologically confirmed were used in this study.

Monoclonal Antibodies

The procedure for preparation, characterization, and specificity evaluation of the monoclonal antibodies (mAbs) used in this study (TABLE 2) were previously presented in detail by Reimer *et al.*[12]

Serum Absorption

Lyophilized *T. phagedenis* was resuspended in saline (4 mg/ml). Serum was mixed with the suspension (1 : 9) and incubated with shaking (50 rpm) at 37°C for 3 h and then overnight at 4°C. The suspension was then centrifuged at $15,000 \times g$ for 15 min, and the supernatant filtered through a 0.45 μm filter. The filtrate was then frozen at -80°C until further use. As absorption control, sera were mixed with saline instead of the *T. phagedenis* suspension and treated as for the absorbed sera.

TABLE 2. Quality Control: Specificity of Monoclonal Antibodies

Class of Antibodies	Mouse Anti-Human IgG Clone	Epitope Location	OD_{490}, Myeloma			
			IgG1	IgG2	IgG3	IgG4
IgG1	HP 6001	Fc	.19	.03	.04	.01
IgG2	HP 6002	Fc	.04	.50	.05	.04
IgG3	HP 6047	hinge	.05	.03	.76	.02
IgG4	HP 6025	Fc	.06	.07	.07	.34
IgG	HP 6000	Fc	.51	.46	.48	.37

Enzyme-linked Immunosorbent Assay

The enzyme-linked immunosorbent assay (ELISA) was performed to detect IgG (refers to total specific IgG antibodies) and IgG subclasses produced as a result of *B. burgdorferi* infection. Two series were performed, one with the homologous *B. burgdorferi* and the other with the heterologous *T. phagedenis*. The antigens were suspended (0.08 mg dry wt/ml) in 0.06 M carbonate buffer (pH 9.6) and the suspensions were sonicated for 10 seconds. Each antigen suspension was added (2 μg/well) to a series of microtiter plates. The antigens were then force-precipitated[13] with 0.1 ml of 0.05% sodium acetate in 95% ethanol for 20 h at 4°C. The next day the wells were washed three times with PBS-Tween and then blocked for 20 min at 25°C with PBS containing 1% bovine albumin. Patient sera (dilutions 1 : 20 to 1 : 160) were added to the wells and incubated in duplicate for 20 h at 4°C. Plates were washed six times in PBS-Tween. Monoclonal antibodies to human IgG (TABLE 2, dilutions 1 : 100 to 1 : 400) were added. The second incubation was carried out for 2 h at 37°C, washed, and the plates were developed with peroxidase-labeled sheep anti-mouse IgG (no cross-reaction to human IgG; Organon Teknika-Cappel, Malvern, PA). The color reaction (*o*-phenylenediamine) was allowed to develop for 30 min and then read in a microtiter reader.

Electrophoresis and Electroblotting

Antigens (*B. burgdorferi* and *T. phagedenis*) in solubilizing buffer (1.5 to 2 mg dry wt/ml) were incubated in a water bath at 37°C for 5 minutes. The solubilized antigens were subjected to SDS-PAGE electrophoresis with the Laemmli buffer system.[14]

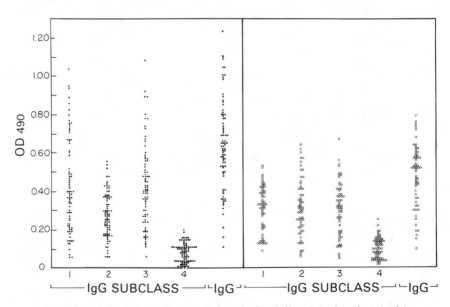

FIGURE 1. IgG subclass patterns to *B. burgdorferi (left)* and *T. phagedenis (right)*.

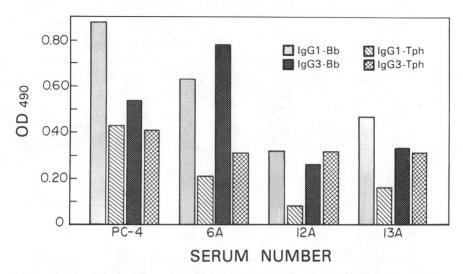

FIGURE 2. IgG1 and IgG3 to *B. burgdorferi* and *T. phagedenis* in four sera.

Electrophoresis was carried out at a constant current of 30 mA with 0.025 M Tris/0.192 M glycine in 0.1% SDS for 3–4 hours. Electroblotting was done on nitrocellulose paper (NCP) with 25 mM phosphate buffer, pH 7.4. The transfer conditions were 250 mA for 18 h at 4°C. The NCP were then blocked with 10% non-fat dry milk in PBS and cut into lanes. Eight lanes (four per antigen) were incubated with patient sera diluted at 1 : 80 in blocking buffer for 24 h at 4°C. The lanes were then washed six times in PBS containing 0.01% Tween 20 (PBS-T). Two lanes (one per antigen) were incubated with one of the IgG subclasses (TABLE 2), incubated for 2 h at 37°C, and washed six times. All lanes were then incubated with horseradish-peroxidase-labeled sheep anti-mouse IgG for 2 h at 37°C and washed with PBS. The enzyme substrate for color development was 4-chloro-1-naphthol.[15]

RESULTS

IgG Subclass Composition

The profile of IgG subclass antibodies to *B. burgdorferi* and *T. phagedenis* in 78 patients diagnosed with Lyme disease is shown in FIGURE 1. *B. burgdorferi* antigen reacted predominantly with IgG1 and IgG3 subclasses and to a lesser extent with IgG2 and least with IgG4. In contrast, *T. phagedenis* reacted almost equally with IgG1, IgG2, and IgG3 subclasses. The reactivity with IgG4 was also minimal. A representative pattern of reactivity of the IgG subclasses with both antigens is shown in FIGURES 2 and 3. In virtually all sera, the IgG1 measured higher with *B. burgdorferi* than with *T. phagedenis*. This was not true with IgG3. In a number of sera (30%), IgG3 measured the same with both antigens or somewhat higher with *T. phagedenis* (*e.g.*, serum 12A and 13A). The extent of reactivity of IgG2 and IgG4 with either antigen was mixed so that no definite pattern was observed. The average optical density (OD)

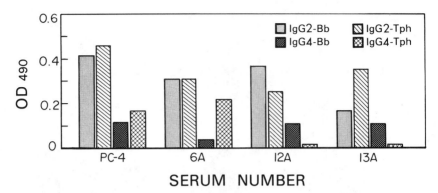

FIGURE 3. Representative pattern of IgG2 and IgG4 to *B. burgdorferi* and *T. phagedenis* in the same four sera.

test results with both antigens according to disease stage (TABLE 3) shows that at each stage the average reactivity of IgG1 and IgG3 was higher with *B. burgdorferi* than with *T. phagedenis* and the reactivity of IgG2 and IgG4 was similar.

Serum Absorption

Because of the significant reactivity of the IgG subclasses from Lyme disease patients with *T. phagedenis,* we absorbed the sera with *T. phagedenis* and retested the sera for the IgG subclasses to *B. burgdorferi*. Based on 80% reduction of IgG antibody (TABLE 4) activity when the absorbed sera was tested with *T. phagedenis,* the antibody reactivity of the IgG1, IgG2, and IgG3 to *B. burgdorferi* was reduced by 13%, 67%, and 36%, respectively. The test results for IgG4 on the absorbed and unabsorbed were too low to calculate the percent reduction in activity.

Immunoblot

A serum from a patient with stage 3 Lyme disease was reacted with the electroblotted antigens. The reaction of IgG1 with *B. burgdorferi* revealed a minimum of 12 bands and with *T. phagedenis* a minimum of 7, and the reaction of IgG3 revealed

TABLE 3. Average OD_{490} Values of the IgG Subclass Antibodies to *B. burgdorferi* (Bb) and *T. phagedenis* (Tph) in Sera from Lyme Disease Patients

	OD_{490}									
	IgG1		IgG2		IgG3		IgG4		IgG	
Stage	Bb	Tph	Bb	Tph	Bb	Tph	Bb	Tph	Bb	Tph
1	.30	.22	.27	.27	.43	.26	.07	.09	.49	.40
2	.27	.20	.24	.28	.39	.26	.07	.08	.49	.42
3	.54	.32	.31	.34	.48	.34	.10	.11	.74	.50
All Stages	.44	.28	.28	.31	.44	.31	.08	.10	.64	.48

TABLE 4. Average Percent Decrease of OD_{490} after Absorption of Sera with *T. phagedenis* and Subsequent Testing with *B. burgdorferi*

Class of Antibodies	Percent Reduction in OD_{490}
IgG1	13
IgG2	67
IgG3	36
IgG4[a]	—
IgG	36, 80[b]

[a]Percent reduction could not be calculated because the OD were too low.
[b]As control, the sera were absorbed with *T. phagedenis* and tested with *T. phagedenis*.

three and five bands, respectively. The reaction of IgG2 revealed two bands with each antigen. With this serum, IgG4 reacted only with *B. burgdorferi* and the relative migration of the two bands detected with IgG4 was similar to the two bands detected with IgG2 reaction with *B. burgdorferi*. Only with IgG1, we observe bands from both antigens that had the same relative migration at 64, 58, and 38 kDa (FIG. 4).

DISCUSSION

The distribution of the IgG subclasses that reacted with *B. burgdorferi* in patients with Lyme disease indicates that IgG1 and IgG3 appeared to be the predominant subclasses. IgG1 and IgG3 dominate the immune response to many protein antigens[4] and IgG2 the immune response to carbohydrate and lipopolysaccharide (LPS).[3,5] It appears, therefore, that the major immunogens in *B. burgdorferi* are proteins. Baugh

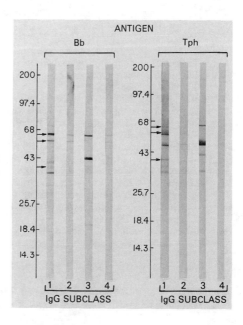

FIGURE 4. Immunoblot of sera from patients with stage 3 Lyme disease. *Arrows* indicate bands with the same relative migration at 64, 58, and 38 kDa.

et al.[16] have shown that in secondary syphilis, a spirochetal infection, patient sera have predominantly IgG1 and IgG3 in the circulating immune complexes.

The reactivity of the IgG2 with *B. burgdorferi* was mostly removed after absorption with *T. phagedenis*. This may indicate that carbohydrates specific to *B. burgdorferi* are not prominent immunogens. The apparent lack of a dominant immune response to *B. burgdorferi* LPS, recently isolated,[17] does not preclude the stimulation of the release of IL-1, which may cause the arthritis characteristic of the third stage as suggested by Habicht *et al.*[18]

The immunoblot test results showed that most *T. phagedenis* bands revealed by the sera of patients with Lyme disease had relative migrations different from the *B. burgdorferi* antigen bands. This suggests that similar or identical epitopes are present in different molecular weight polypeptides in both organisms, or that an anamnestic response to *T. phagedenis,* a nonpathogen which is present in humans, may have occurred as a result of the presumed (since no organisms were isolated from the patient) *B. burgdorferi* infection. Further investigation with sera absorbed with *B. burgdorferi* and testing of the absorbed sera with *T. phagedenis* may help determine if an anamnestic response occurred.

Our preliminary results indicate that IgG1 and IgG3 are the predominant subclasses produced in patients with Lyme disease. It is also obvious that a more extensive study of the specificity and the isolation of these subclasses needs to be done before a study of their role in the pathogenesis of Lyme disease is to be undertaken.

REFERENCES

1. HUSSAIN, R., R. W. POINDEXTER, E. A. OTTESEN & C. B. REIMER. 1986. Use of monoclonal antibodies to quantify subclasses of human IgG. II. Enzyme immunoassay to antigen specific (anti-filarial) IgG subclass antibodies. J. Immunol. Meth. **94:** 73.
2. SHAKIB, F. & D. R. STANWORTH. 1980. Human IgG subclasses in health and disease, Part 1. Ric. Clin. Lab. **10:** 463.
3. YOUNT, W., M. DORNER, H. KUNKER & E. KABAT. 1986. Studies on human antibodies. VI. Selective variations in subgroup composition and genetic markers. J. Exp. Med. **127:** 633–646.
4. SEPPALA, I., A. ROUTONEN, A. SARNESTO, P. MATTILA & O. MAKELA. 1984. The percentages of six immunoglobin isotypes in human antibodies to tetanus oxoid: Standardization of isotype-specific second antibodies in solid phase assays. Eur. J. Immunol. **14:** 868–875.
5. SMITH, D. S. & M. H. NAHM. 1987. IgG subclass deficiency and immunocompetence to carbohydrate antigens. Clin. Immunol. Newsletter **8:** 97–100.
6. STEERE, A. C., S. E. MALAWISTA, D. R. SNYDMAN, R. E. SHOPE, W. A. ANDIMAN, M. R. ROSS & F. M. STEELE. 1977. Lyme arthritis: An epidemic of oligoarticular arthritis in children and adults in three Connecticut communities. Arthritis Rheum. **20:** 7.
7. BURGDORFER, W., A. G. BARBOUR, S. F. HAYES, J. L. BENACH, E. GRUNWALDT & J. P. DAVIS. 1982. Lyme disease: A tick-borne spirochetosis? Science **216:** 1317.
8. CRAFT, J. E., D. K. FISCHER, Y. T. SHIMAMOTO & A. C. STEERE. 1986. Antigens of *Borrelia burgdorferi* recognized during Lyme disease. Appearance of a new immuno-globulin M response and expansion of the immunoglobulin G response late in the illness. J. Clin. Invest. **78:** 934.
9. WILSKE, B., G. SCHIERZ, V. PREAC-MURSIC, K. WEBER, H.-W. PFISTER & K. EINHAUPL. 1984. Serological diagnosis of erythema migrans disease and related disorders. Infection **12:** 331.
10. BARBOUR, A. G. 1984. Isolation and cultivation of Lyme disease spirochete. Yale J Biol. Med. **57:** 521–525.
11. IZZAT, N. N., J. M. KNOX & R. D. WENDE. 1971. Mass cultivation of avirulent *Treponema pallidum* (Nichols). Microbiol. **3:** 247.

12. REIMER, C. B., D. J. PHILIPS, C. H. ALLOISIO, D. D. MOORE, G. G. GALLAND, T. W. WELLS, C. M. BLACK & J. S. MCDOUGAL. 1984. Evaluation of thirty-one mouse monoclonal antibodies to human IgG epitopes. Hybridoma **3:** 263.

13. HECHEMY, K. E. 1983. Forced precipitation method for preparing antigen/antibody particles. U.S. patent no. 4,397,959.

14. LAEMMLI, V. K. 1970. Cleavage of structural proteins during the assembly of the head of bacteriophage T4. Nature (London) **227:** 680.

15. HAWKES, P. C., E. NIDAY & J. GORDON. 1982. A dot-immunobinding assay for monoclonal and other antibodies. Anal. Biochem. **119:** 142.

16. BAUGHN, R. E., M. C. MCNEELY, J. L. GORIZZO & D. M. MUSHER. 1986. Characterization of the antigenic determinants and host components in immune complexes from patients with secondary syphilis. J. Immunol. **136:** 1406.

17. BECK, C. J., G. S. HABICHT, J. L. BENACH & J. L. COLEMAN. 1985. Chemical and biologic characterization of a lipopolysaccharide extracted from the Lyme disease spirochete (*Borrelia burgdorferi*). J. Infect. Dis. **152:** 1.

18. HABICHT, G. S., G. BECK & J. L. BENACH. 1987. Lyme disease. Sci. Amer. **257:** 78.

Introduction

Ecology

DENNIS J. WHITE

Bureau of Communicable Diseases
New York State Department of Health
Albany, New York 12237

Has any past domestic vector-borne disease episode or entity in the last 40 years evoked a multi-national mobilization of personnel and fiscal resources comparable to that which has been directed toward Lyme disease? Perhaps more than any single event occurring during the most recent decade, the discovery of the etiologic agent and the means of transmission of Lyme disease has served not only to rejuvenate the stagnating field of domestic medical entomology, but also to redefine the boundaries of investigation within which traditional medical entomology is conducted. Although many medical entomologists may disagree with these observations, even a cursory comparison of the proceedings of the earlier conferences with this third international conference on Lyme disease confirms the perception that medical entomology has indeed expanded its scope of endeavor. At the very least, the emergence of Lyme disease fortuitously coincided with the availability of technically advanced laboratory tools and procedures that complement the traditional components of medical entomology.

One of the traditional components of medical entomology, the natural history or ecology of the interactions of disease agent, vector, and host, will always remain a steadfast priority of vector-borne disease investigations. Unless one is at least partially aware of the ecological parameters establishing or affecting such a complex association, an individual is forever destined to understand only incompletely the disease process or means to alleviate the disease.

In what follows, a number of prominent investigators, building upon ecological and epidemiological studies, contribute significant new information on the ecology of Lyme disease. These studies ensure that we will have a comprehensive understanding of how *Borrelia burgdorferi* interacts with the ecological components of its natural history.

As reflected in these presentations, scientific inquiry has been directed toward many of these components, namely vector competence studies; cell-, tissue-, and organ-specific spirochetal infection and pathogenesis studies; vertical and horizontal transmission investigations; geographically dependent vector overwintering mechanisms; host/reservoir susceptibility studies; and vector control or transmission reduction investigations. The ecological investigations of Lyme disease and *Borrelia* infections continue to provide valuable information. However, we are still at the point where an ounce of investigation results not only in an ounce of answers, but also in the generation of a pound of further questions.

The ultimate concern of public health agencies is to reduce the incidence of disease morbidity. The continual discovery of distinct *Borrelia* isolates and new vector species, an ever-expanding list of hosts, and the development of a very complex vector natural history render the objective of decreasing Lyme disease incidence ever more difficult to achieve. The data presented in the papers in this part indicate that, although we in public health have acquired vast amounts of information elucidating the reasons for the increasing incidence and geographic distribution of this disease, we are still unable to address the desire on the part of our constituents for a reduction of disease incidence. I am not so naive as to agree with the sentiment most often expressed by the general public that "controlling the vector" is the only, or the best, way to reduce disease incidence given information currently available. However, as a medical entomologist I share the concerns of the general populace facing the emergence of a chronic, debilitating, inadequately recognized vector-borne disease, especially in areas that have not previously faced the realities of an insidious tick-borne disease.

Scientists, clinicians, and public health agencies must begin to address this epidemic, armed with the information now on hand, if we are to prevent further clinical and geographic expansion of this wide-spectrum disease. As certain investigators have said at this conference, we must aggressively pursue novel approaches toward our common objective of reducing (1) the rate of geographical expansion and (2) the rate of the disease incidence. The elusive "weak links" in the complex ecological relationships among disease agent, vector, and host must be found and probed. Methods must be discovered to alter the spirochete's invasive properties or render the spirochete nonpathogenic, even if in just one cell, tissue, or organ host environment. Transmission studies must be designed to determine vertical and horizontal transmission mechanisms and to determine potential genetic, semiochemical, physiologic, and behavioral adaptations of the vector or the spirochete that could alleviate these routes of intra- or interspecific transmission. Are there means of rendering the tick or the spirochete more susceptible to novel biologic, genetic, chemical, or physical control procedures during estivation or overwintering of tick vectors? At what stage of the vector's natural history is it most susceptible to external control approaches? Many investigators report on their success in reducing rates of tick infestation of mice by what appears to be an environmentally acceptable approach. Do other novel approaches exist for any concept of control of any stage of any vector on any host or in the environment? How soon can we prepare and evaluate potential vaccines for protection against *Borrelia* infections?

I recognize that I have presented some hypothetical situations and asked some difficult questions. However, we as health care providers and public health investigators must continue to ask ourselves similar questions. How are we going to abate the continuing migration of this disease into new areas? More importantly, how are we going to decrease the risk of disease transmission in these endemic areas?

The investigators contributing to this part have attempted to open the doors and begin answering these questions. Let us apply this new knowledge to the previous foundation and establish a unified quest for solutions.

Development of *Borrelia burgdorferi* in Ixodid Tick Vectors

WILLY BURGDORFER,[a] STANLEY F. HAYES,[a]
AND JORGE L. BENACH[b]

[a]*Laboratory of Pathobiology*
Rocky Mountain Laboratories
Department of Health and Human Services
Public Health Service
National Institutes of Health
National Institute of Allergy and Infectious Diseases
Hamilton, Montana 59840

[b]*New York State Department of Health*
Health Sciences Center
SUNY at Stony Brook
Stony Brook, New York 11794

INTRODUCTION

Ever since the discovery[1] of a tick-borne borrelia as the causative agent of Lyme disease in the United States and of related disorders in Europe, it has been apparent that this spirochete in its ixodid tick vectors behaves differently than do the closely related tick-borne relapsing fever borreliae in argasid ticks.[2] In the latter, spirochetes are ingested, penetrate the gut wall, enter the hemocele, and from there invade the various tissues including those of the central ganglion, Malpighian tubules, salivary glands, and genital organs. The Lyme disease spirochete, *Borrelia burgdorferi*, is limited in the majority of its tick vectors to the midgut, where it accumulates near the microvillar brush border and in the interstitial spaces between epithelial cells. Thus, in our initial collection of *Ixodes dammini* from Shelter Island, New York,[1] all 77 infected adult ticks had spirochetes in their midgut only. Similarly, of 112 infected *I. ricinus* from the Staatswald on the Swiss Plateau, 106 (95%) had spirochetes in their midgut only; the remaining six ticks showed systemic infections with spirochetes concentrated in the central ganglion and ovarial tissues.[3] Infections limited to the midgut were also recorded for the Western black-legged tick, *I. pacificus;* of 25 infected specimens, 17 had spirochetes in midgut only, while the remaining eight showed generalized infections.[4]

To characterize the relationship of *B. burgdorferi* to its tick vectors, investigations were initiated to evaluate the behavior of this spirochete in both naturally and experimentally infected ticks. The study reported here deals with the occurrence of systemic infections in *Ixodes dammini* and the ability of this tick vector to pass the Lyme disease spirochete transovarially to the progeny.

MATERIAL AND METHODS

Collection and Examination of I. dammini *from Nature*

Adult *I. dammini* were collected by flagging vegetation on Shelter Island, New York in the spring of 1982. The ticks were sent to the Rocky Mountain Laboratories where they were individually dissected for removal of one or several midgut diverticula, the central ganglion, and the genital tissues. These were smeared separately on microscope slides that upon air-drying and fixation in acetone were treated with fluorescein isothiocyanate-labeled antibodies to *B. burgdorferi*,[5] and were examined for spirochetes by fluorescence microscopy. Male and female ticks from foci with high infection rates were also placed for feeding and mating on New Zealand white rabbits. Upon repletion, female ticks were stored individually at room temperature and 95% relative humidity until oviposition. When the females were spent, they were dissected and examined for spirochetes as outlined above. Of females with systemic infections, 80 to 100 eggs and larvae were individually smeared, treated with above coated conjugate, and examined for spirochetes by fluorescence microscopy to determine whether transovarial transmission of *B. burgdorferi* had occurred.

Establishment and Examination of Experimentally Infected I. dammini

To study spirochetal development in experimentally infected ticks, larval *I. dammini* derived from spirochete-free females (Shelter Island, New York) were

TABLE 1. Distribution of *Borrelia burgdorferi* in Naturally Infected *Ixodes dammini* (Shelter Island, NY)

Feeding Status	No. of Ticks Examined	Midgut Infection	Generalized Infection
Starved			
Lot A	126 (29 F, 97 M)	77 (61%) (12 F, 65 M)	0/77
Lot B	151 (62 F, 89 M)	102 (67.5%) (58 F, 44 M)	4/102 (3.9%) (4 F)
Engorged	128 (all F)[a]	113 (88.2%)	22/113 (19.4%)

[a]Examined 50–70 days after placement for feeding.

allowed to feed on white-footed mice *(Peromyscus leucopus)* that had been inoculated intramuscularly with 0.1 ml of a suspension prepared by triturating one fully engorged spirochete-infected *I. dammini* female (Shelter Island, NY) in 5.0 ml of modified Kelly media. Starting the fifth day after inoculation and thereafter at intervals of 3 to 5 days, pools of larval ticks were placed freely on mice contained in wire cages above trays of water. Engorged ticks were recovered from the water and stored in desiccator jars until they had molted to nymphs. At that time, aliquots of each tick pool were examined by direct immunofluorescence to determine rates of infection. Pools with high rates (*i.e.*, 80% and above) were eventually fed on New Zealand white rabbits and were allowed to develop into adults. Four to six months later, 80 unfed females and 50 males were dissected to determine distribution of *B. burgdorferi* in their tissues. In addition, 100 females along with males were placed for feeding and mating on New Zealand white rabbits and were maintained in separate vials until oviposition had occurred. Forty-eight spent females were then dissected to determine the distribution of spirochetes in engorged ticks. Dissection and examination were also performed for 25 repleted females that after 4 months of storage had failed to lay eggs.

To determine transovarial passage of *B. burgdorferi* by experimentally infected *I. dammini*, 60 to 100 eggs and larvae of five females with systemic infections were examined for spirochetes as outlined above for naturally infected ticks. Several hundred larvae from each of these five females were also fed on normal New Zealand white rabbits, and 60 to 100 of them were examined for spirochetes after they had molted to nymphs.

Transmission Electron Microscopy

Development of *B. burgdorferi* in *I. dammini* and interactions between this spirochete and its vector tissues were also followed subcellularly by transmission electron microscopy. For this purpose, selected tick tissues were removed by dissection and processed as described previously.[6]

RESULTS

Borrelia burgdorferi *in Naturally and Experimentally Infected* I. dammini

Although the original pool of unfed, adult *I. dammini* from Shelter Island, New York yielded infected ticks with spirochetes in the midgut only,[1] examination of additional ticks from the same area indicated that systemic infections may occur. Thus, of 151 unfed ticks (lot B) collected in 1982, 102 proved infected. Four (3.9%) of these had a generalized infection with spirochetes not only in the midgut but also in the tissues of central ganglion, Malpighian tubules, salivary glands, and genital system. The percentage of ticks with spirochetes throughout their tissues increased to 19.4% when ticks were examined about 2 months after engorgement and oviposition (TABLE 1). Similar results were recorded for experimentally infected *I. dammini* (TABLE 2). Of 130 unfed adults, 106 had midgut infections but only three (2.8%) of these yielded spirochetes in other tissues, particularly the central ganglion. Examination of spent females 43 to 68 days after engorgement revealed that nine (19.5%) of 46 infected

TABLE 2. Distribution of *Borrelia burgdorferi* in Experimentally Infected *Ixodes dammini*[a]

Feeding Status	No. of Ticks Examined	Midgut Infection	Generalized Infection
Starved	130 (80 F, 50 M)	106 (81.5%) (67 F, 39 M)	3/106 (2.8%) (2 F, 1 M)
Engorged	48 (all F)[b]	46 (95.8%)	9/46 (19.5%)
	25 (all F)[c]	23 (92%)	18/23 (78.2%)

[a]Infected as larvae by feeding on experimentally infected white-footed mice (*Peromyscus leucopus*).
[b]Examined 43–68 days after placement for feeding.
[c]Examined 110–130 days after placement for feeding.

TABLE 3. Transovarial Passage of *Borrelia burgdorferi* in Experimentally Infected *Ixodes dammini*

Tick (Female)	No. of Eggs Examined	No. Positive	No. of Larvae Examined	No. Positive	No. of Nymphs Examined	No. Positive
V-15-5	100	12 (12%)[a]	100	8 (8%)[a]	100	0
V-15-8	100	0	80	0	100	0
VI-18-5	100	25 (25%)[a]	100	12 (12%)[a]	60	1(?)[b]
VII-21-5	100	100 (100%)[a]	80	36 (40%)[a]	60	3(?)[b]
VIII-23-1	100	7 (7%)[a]	80	2 (2.5%)[a]	80	1(?)[b]

[a]Extremely mild infection, 1–3 spirochetes per smear.
[b]Particulate antigen, no spirochetal organisms.

specimens had systemic infections. The longer the time period between engorgement and examination, the greater the number of ticks exhibiting generalized infections. Thus, of 25 females that had failed to oviposit for more than 3 months after feeding, 23 (92.9%) proved infected and 18 (78.2%) of these had a systemic infection.

Transovarial Transmission of B. burgdorferi *in Naturally and Experimentally Infected* I. dammini

Of 58 spent *I. dammini* females from a focus where more than 85% of unfed ticks had been found infected with *B. burgdorferi,* 48 (82.5%) proved infected. Twelve of these had a more or less intensive systemic infection with spirochetes in central ganglion, Malpighian tubules, and ovary. However, from each of these 12 females, 100 eggs and 120 larvae individually evaluated for spirochetes were negative. Also negative, as suspected, was the progeny of five females with spirochetes in their midgut diverticula only.

The passage of *B. burgdorferi* via eggs was also examined for five experimentally infected females that showed a generalized infection with spirochetes in their tissues including those of the ovary. As summarized in TABLE 3, few spirochetes were detected in varying percentages of eggs and larvae derived from four females; the progeny of the fifth female (V-15-8) was negative. Positive smears never contained more than three morphologically typical spirochetes, and the percentage of infected larval ticks for each of the ovarially transmitting females was considerably lower than that for the eggs, suggesting a gradual die-off of spirochetes. Indeed, there was no longer evidence of morphologically typical spirochetes in the F_1 nymphs. Strongly fluorescing particulate material was found in a few specimens, but its relationship to *B. burgdorferi* could not be established.

The presence of *B. burgdorferi* in developing oocytes could also be demonstrated by electron microscopy of ovarial tissues of a spent, naturally infected female, even though there was no evidence of spirochetes in the eggs or larvae of this particular tick. As seen in FIGURES 1 & 2, numerous *B. burgdorferi* were found to occupy the space between the oocyte and tunica propria membranes. This space is normally filled with microvillar processes that extend outward to contact the tunica propria. Infected cells, however, appear to be denuded of vitelline processes and the cuticle deposition normally seen in this space is absent.

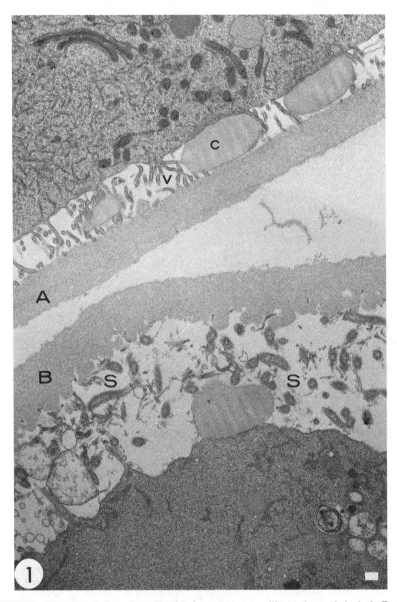

FIGURE 1. Electron micrograph profile of *I. dammini* oocytes, illustrating pathological effect of *B. burgdorferi* on egg development. Oocyte A is free of spirochetes and shows normal development of the microvillar processes (*V*) and cuticle deposits (*C*). Oocyte B is heavily infected with spirochetes (*S*) and is devoid of microvillar processes. *Bar* = 0.2 μ.

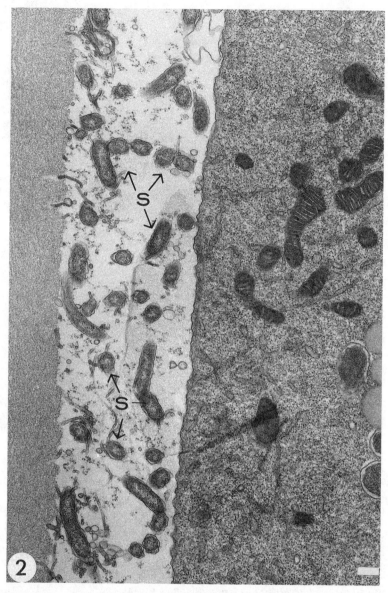

FIGURE 2. Higher magnification of *B. burgdorferi* (*S*) between oocyte and tunica propria membranes. *Bar* = 0.2 μ.

DISCUSSION

Our observations confirm previous findings[1] suggesting that the Lyme disease spirochete, *B. burgdorferi,* in the majority of its vector tick, *I. dammini,* persists and multiplies in the midgut from where it occasionally penetrates the gut wall and initiates a systemic infection of all the tissues, especially those of the central ganglion, Malpighian tubules, and ovary. Ribeiro *et al.*[7] investigated the mode of transmission by adult *I. dammini* and reported that spirochetes disseminate in 57% of gut-infected ticks at 4 days after attachment with spirochetes already in the saliva before rapid engorgement occurs. Correspondingly, infected nymphal *I. dammini* produce spirochete-containing saliva at 3 days postattachment. In a recent histological study, Benach *et al.*[8] presented the hypothesis that multiplication of *B. burgdorferi* takes place shortly after ingestion of blood and that during the midfeeding period some spirochetes enter the hemocele, where they could be detected in hemolymph and in the acellular lamella of the central ganglion. Although *B. burgdorferi* was never found in salivary gland tissues, it was postulated that spirochetes may gain access to salivary gland ducts and are inoculated via mouthparts into the feeding cavity.

Although we did not determine the time of spirochetal dissemination from the midgut, an increased percentage of ticks with systemic infections from less than 4% in unfed to about 19% in engorged ticks are in support of the gut penetration phenomenon, even though our percentages of ticks with systemic infections several weeks after feeding are considerably lower than those reported by Ribeiro *et al.*[7] Our observations suggest that the longer the time between engorgement and examination, the greater the number of more ticks showing systemic infections. The claim that spirochetal dissemination occurs also in nymphal ticks as early as 3 days postattachment needs clarification, for if this mechanism regularly occurred in nature, the prevalence of unfed adult ticks with generalized spirochetal infections would be considerably higher. According to our results, less than 4% of unfed adult *I. dammini* in nature are systemically infected.

The presence of spirochetes in ovarial tissues, particularly in developing oocytes, is a prerequisite for transovarial or vertical transmission. That this phenomenon occurs in *I. dammini* was first demonstrated[9] in unfed larval ticks collected off vegetation on Shelter Island, New York and subsequently also in larval ticks from Lyme disease foci in Massachusetts.[10] In addition, Magnarelli *et al.*[11] recently reported filial infection rates varying from 3.3% to 15% in the progeny of five *I. dammini* females removed from deer, and infection rates of 25% and 27%, respectively, in filial ticks of two females taken off a dog.

Our observations of the progeny of four experimentally infected *I. dammini* females confirm the occurrence of transovarial passage of *B. burgdorferi* to the progeny. Up to 100% of eggs contained spirochetes, but the number of organisms transmitted apparently was too low to establish permanent infections. In fact, decreasing infection rates for larvae and the absence of spirochetes in nymphs suggest a gradual die-off of these organisms. The papers published thus far on transovarial transmission of *B. burgdorferi* by *I. dammini* note the presence of spirochetes either in eggs or larvae. Unfortunately, no information has as yet been presented concerning degree of spirochetal infection, distribution of spirochetes, and transstadial maintenance of *B. burgdorferi* in filial ticks. The only tick vector for which such data are available is the Western black-legged tick, *I. pacificus,* which in one instance has been shown to produce 100% systemically infected progeny that maintained the spirochetes transstadially and in four of five cases passed them via eggs to as many as 97% of F_2 filial ticks.[12]

The lack of transovarial transmission by our naturally infected *I. dammini* females is puzzling because electron microscopy of ovarial tissues of one of these females revealed large quantities of spirochetes in developing oocytes. Either eggs infected with *B. burgdorferi* fail to mature or incorporated spirochetes gradually die-off during oogenesis. Indeed, there is evidence for both phenomena. The latter may explain the survival of only a few morphologically typical organisms in oviposited eggs and in larvae. On the other hand, heavily infected oocytes may fail to mature because spirochetes prevent the formation and deposition of cuticle by destroying the microvillar processes between the vitelline and oocyte membranes.

It is indeed tempting to speculate that transovarial transmission is related to and depends on the pathogenicity of *B. burgdorferi* to tick tissues, particularly oocytes. This interaction may vary from strain to strain as well as among different species of ticks. Studies related to this hypothesis are in progress.

REFERENCES

1. BURGDORFER, W., A. G. BARBOUR, S. F. HAYES, J. L. BENACH, E. GRUNWALDT & J. P. DAVIS. 1982. Lyme disease—a tick-borne spirochetosis? Science **216:** 1317–1319.
2. BURGDORFER, W. 1976. The epidemiology of the relapsing fevers. *In* The Biology of Parasitic Spirochetes. R. C. Johnson, Ed.: 191–200. Academic. New York.
3. BURGDORFER, W., A. G. BARBOUR, S. F. HAYES, O. PÉTER & A. AESCHLIMANN. 1983. Erythema chronicum migrans—a tickborne spirochetosis. Acta Trop. **40:** 79–83.
4. BURGDORFER, W., R. S. LANE, A. G. BARBOUR, R. A. GRESBRINK & J. R. ANDERSON. 1985. The Western black-legged tick, *Ixodes pacificus:* A vector of *Borrelia burgdorferi.* Am. J. Trop. Med. Hyg. **34:** 935–930.
5. BURGDORFER, W. 1984. The New Zealand white rabbit: An experimental host for infecting ticks with Lyme disease spirochetes. Yale J. Biol. Med. **57:** 609–612.
6. HAYES, S. F. & W. BURGDORFER. 1979. Ultrastructure of *Rickettsia rhipicephali,* a new member of the spotted fever group rickettsiae in tissues of the host vector *Rhipicephalus sanguineus.* J. Bacteriol. **137:** 605–613.
7. RIBEIRO, J. M. C., T. N. MATHER, J. PIESMAN & A. SPIELMAN. 1987. Dissemination and salivary delivery of Lyme disease spirochetes in vector ticks (Acari: Ixodidae). J. Med. Entomol. **24:** 201–205.
8. BENACH, J. L., J. L. COLEMAN, R. A. SKINNER & E. M. BOSLER. 1987. Adult *Ixodes dammini* on rabbits: A hypothesis for the development and transmission of *Borrelia burgdorferi.* J. Infect. Dis. **155:** 1300–1306.
9. BOSLER, E. M., J. L. COLEMAN, J. L. BENACH, D. A. MASSEY, J. P. HANRAHAN, W. BURGDORFER & A. G. BARBOUR. 1983. Natural distribution of the *Ixodes dammini* spirochete. Science **220:** 321–322.
10. PIESMAN, J., J. G. DONAHUE, T. N. MATHER & A. SPIELMAN. 1986. Transovarially acquired Lyme disease spirochetes (*Borrelia burgdorferi*) in field-collected larval *Ixodes dammini* (Acari: Ixodidae). J. Med. Entomol. **23:** 219.
11. MAGNARELLI, L. A., J. F. ANDERSON & D. FISH. 1987. Transovarial transmission of *Borrelia burgdorferi* in *Ixodes dammini* (Acari: Ixodidae). J. Infect. Dis. **156:** 234–236.
12. LANE, R. S. & W. BURGDORFER. 1987. Transovarial and transstadial passage of *Borrelia burgdorferi* in the Western black-legged tick, *Ixodes pacificus* (Acari: Ixodidae). Am. J. Trop. Med. Hyg. **37:** 188–192.

Mammalian and Avian Reservoirs for
Borrelia burgdorferi

JOHN F. ANDERSON

Department of Entomology
The Connecticut Agricultural Experiment Station
P.O. Box 1106
New Haven, Connecticut 06504

> This small vile creature [the tick] may, in the future, cause the inhabitants of this land [the present-day United States] great damage unless a method is discovered which will prevent it from increasing at such a shocking rate.
>
> —Pehr Kalm, 1754

Social and environmental changes may alter the prevalence of disease.[1] Lyme disease,[2] which is caused by the tick-vectored spirochete *Borrelia burgdorferi*,[3-5] was first reported in the United States in 1970.[6] By the mid-1980s, hundreds of cases annually were documented in some northeastern states.[7] Reasons for this significant increase in disease will be reviewed here through discussion of the host animals for *Ixodes dammini*, the historical evidence of ticks in northeastern forests, and the vertebrate reservoirs of *B. burgdorferi*. Additionally, I shall report on the borreliae infecting rabbits and their ticks, *Ixodes dentatus*.

HOST ANIMALS FOR *Ixodes dammini*

The vertebrate reservoirs of *B. burgdorferi* in the midwestern and northeastern United States are among those species of animals parasitized by *Ixodes dammini*, a three-host tick with a broad host range.[8-28] Larval and nymphal ticks feed on small-, medium-, and large-sized mammals and on birds (TABLES 1 and 2). Subadults have been recorded from 29 species of mammals within seven orders and from 49 species of ground-inhabiting birds belonging to 17 families. In contrast, adult ticks have been found on 12 species of mammals within six orders. They have not been observed on birds.

Within its geographical range, *Ixodes dammini* may eventually be found to feed on almost every species of land mammal except bats and every species of bird that forages on the ground. Some species, however, are ecologically more important than others.[29] White-footed mice, other rodents, and shrews are important hosts for larvae.[9,17,19-21,25,29,30] Nymphs frequently parasitize white-footed mice, eastern chipmunks, and gray squirrels. Although not as extensively studied, birds also are important hosts for larvae and nymphs.[24,26-28] White-tailed deer are the significant hosts for adults.[9,18,22,24,29-32]

Adequate numbers of host animals for adult ticks and a suitable microclimate for the nonfeeding stages are essential for survival of *I. dammini*. Evidence supporting the hypothesis that white-tailed deer are crucial hosts for adults includes (1) relative numbers of ticks on deer,[9,18,22] (2) the association of increasing numbers of deer with increased abundance of *I. dammini*,[9,22,29,30] (3) correlation of numbers of ticks with numbers of deer,[31] and (4) the abundance of *I. dammini* on islands inhabited with deer and their relatively low populations on islands without deer.[32,33] Deer were reduced to extremely low levels in the 1800s, but have resurged because of enforcement of effective hunting regulations and reforestation of abandoned agricultural land. The increasing prevalence of Lyme disease in eastern North America may be indirectly associated with the rising number of deer.

HISTORICAL EVIDENCE OF TICKS IN NORTHEASTERN FORESTS

Historical evidence of ticks in northeastern forests is limited but provides some information about the prior presence and abundance of ticks. The relatively recent

TABLE 1. Mammalian Hosts for *Ixodes dammini*[8-25]

Order	Common Name	Species	Larva	Nymph	Adult
Marsupialia	Virginia opossum	*Didelphis virginiana*	•	•	•
Insectivora	Short-tailed shrew	*Blarina brevicauda*	•	•	
	Masked shrew	*Sorex cinereus*	•	•	
	Smoky shrew	*Sorex fumeus*	•	•	
	Eastern mole	*Scalopus aquaticus*	•		
Lagomorpha	Eastern cottontail	*Sylvilagus floridanus*	•	•	
Rodentia	Eastern chipmunk	*Tamias striatus*	•	•	
	Woodchuck	*Marmota monax*	•	•	•
	Southern flying squirrel	*Glaucomys volans*	•	•	
	Red squirrel	*Tamiasciurus hudsonicus*	•	•	
	Gray squirrel	*Sciurus carolinensis*	•	•	•
	White-footed mouse	*Peromyscus leucopus*	•	•	
	Deer mouse	*Peromyscus maniculatus*	•		
	Gapper's red-backed mouse	*Clethrionomys gapperi*	•	•	
	Meadow vole	*Microtus pennsylvanicus*	•	•	
	Pine vole	*Microtus pinetorum*	•		
	Beach vole	*Microtus breweri*		•	
	Norway rat	*Rattus norvegicus*	•	•	
	Woodland jumping mouse	*Napaeozapus insignis*	•	•	
	Meadow jumping mouse	*Zapus hudsonius*	•	•	
Carnivora	Long-tailed weasel	*Mustela frenata*	•		
	Raccoon	*Procyon lotor*	•	•	•
	Cat	*Felis catus*	•	•	•
	Gray fox	*Urocyon cinereoargenteus*	•	•	•
	Red fox	*Vulpes vulpes*	•	•	•
	Striped skunk	*Mephitis mephitis*	•	•	•
	Dog	*Canis familiaris*		•	•
	Black bear	*Euarctos americanus*			•
Artiodactyla	White-tailed deer	*Odocoileus virginianus*	•	•	•
Perissodactyla	Horse	*Equus caballus*			•
Primates	Human	*Homo sapiens*	•	•	•

history of *I. dammini* in coastal areas may be found in the publications of Spielman *et al.*[8,29,30] and Anastos.[16] (Many of the specimens Anastos referred to as *I. muris* and *I. scapularis* probably were *I. dammini*.) More recently, the tick has been collected in northern New England and upstate New York[34] and as far south as Maryland.[35] Possibly the earliest reported identified collection of *I. dammini* is that of Nuttall and

Warburton.[36] They recorded adult female *I. ricinis* var. *scapularis* (Say, 1821; probably *I. dammini*) on humans from Bracebridge, Ontario, Canada in 1904. Even today this tick occurs in Long Point, Ontario.[13]

A clue to the abundance of ticks in virgin forests is found in the diary of the Swedish botanist Pehr Kalm.[37] Near Saratoga, New York on 24 June 1749, he wrote "The woods abound with Woodlice [=ticks], which were extremely troublesome to us." Four days later, on 28 June 1749, at Fort Anne, New York, he recorded "Wood-lice (*Acarus americanus* Linn.) [=*Amblyomma americanum* L.] abound here, and are more plentiful than on any part of the journey. Scarcely any one of us sat down but a whole army of them crept upon his clothes." More than a century later, in 1872, Asa Fitch[38] commented "The most common tick of our country, the wood tick from its inhabiting the woodlands, and not occurring in cleared and cultivated grounds, though formerly abundant throughout the northern and middle states, has now become nearly or quite extinct .... At this day, along the route [Kalm] pursued, not one of

TABLE 2. Avian Hosts for *Ixodes dammini*[8,9,15–17,24,26–28a]

Common Name	Scientific Name	Stage of Tick	
		Larva	Nymph
Meleagrididae			
Wild turkey	*Meleagris gallopavo*		•
Phasianidae			
Common bobwhite	*Colinus virginianus*	•	•
Scolopacidae			
American woodcock	*Philohela minor*		•
Tyrannidae			
Eastern phoebe	*Sayornis phoebe*	•	•
Corvidae			
Blue jay	*Cyanocitta cristata*	•	•
Paridae			
Black-capped chickadee	*Parus atricapillus*	•	•
Tufted titmouse	*Parus bicolor*	•	•
Sittidae			
White-breasted nuthatch	*Sitta carolinensis*	•	•
Certhiidae			
Brown creeper	*Certhia familiaris*		•
Troglodytidae			
House wren	*Troglodytes aedon*	•	•
Carolina wren	*Thyrothorus ludovicianus*	•	•
Mimidae			
Gray catbird	*Dumetella carolinensis*	•	•
Brown thrasher	*Toxostoma rufum*		•
Turdidae			
American robin	*Turdus migratorius*	•	•
Swainson's thrush	*Catharus ustulatus*	•	•
Hermit thrush	*Catharus guttatus*		•
Wood thrush	*Hylocichla mustelina*	•	•
Veery	*Catharus fuscescens*	•	•
Vireonidae			
Red-eyed vireo	*Vireo olivaceus*		•
White-eyed vireo	*Vireo griseus*	•	•

(continued)

TABLE 2. (*continued*)

Common Name	Scientific Name	Stage of Tick	
		Larva	Nymph
Parulidae			
Blue-winged warbler	*Vermivora pinus*	•	•
Pine warbler	*Dendroica pinus*	•	
Northern waterthrush	*Seiurus noveboracensis*	•	
Louisiana waterthrush	*Seiurus motacilla*		•
Common yellowthroat	*Geothlypis trichas*	•	•
Yellow-breasted chat	*Icteria virens*	•	
Canada warbler	*Wilsonia canadensis*	•	
Kentucky warbler	*Oporornis formosus*		•
Hooded warbler	*Wilsonia citrina*		•
Ovenbird	*Seiurus aurocapillus*	•	•
Worm-eating warbler	*Helmitheros vermivorus*	•	•
Yellow warbler	*Dendroica petechia*	•	•
Black-and-white warbler	*Mniotilta varia*		•
Prairie warbler	*Dendroica discolor*		•
Sturnidae			
Starling	*Sturnus vulgaris*		•
Icteridae			
Red-winged blackbird	*Agelaius phoeniceus*	•	•
Common grackle	*Quiscalus quiscula*	•	•
Brown-headed cowbird	*Motothrus ater*	•	•
Ploceidae			
House sparrow	*Passer domesticus*		•
Fringillidae			
Northern cardinal	*Cardinalis cardinalis*	•	•
Rose-breasted grosbeak	*Pheucticus ludovicianus*	•	•
Purple finch	*Carpodacus purpureus*	•	•
Rufous-sided towhee	*Pipilo erythrophthalmus*	•	•
Chipping sparrow	*Spizella passerina*	•	•
Field sparrow	*Spizella pusilla*	•	•
White-throated sparrow	*Zonotrichia albicollis*	•	
Swamp sparrow	*Melospiza georgiana*	•	•
Song sparrow	*Melospiza melodia*	•	•
House finch	*Carpodacus mexicanus*	•	•

*a*Unpublished host species (J. F. Anderson and L. A. Magnarelli).

these insects can probably be found." Fitch further wrote, "In those sections of the country which were settled little over a century ago, tradition still speaks of the annoyances which our American wood ticks were." Ticks were abundant in our pristine forests, but some species in large part disappeared with the clearing of the land for agriculture and the marked reduction of certain species of animals (e.g., the white-tailed deer).

Both Kalm and Fitch referred to the species of tick as *A. americanum,* but Bequaert[12] argues convincingly that it was a different species. He suggested that the tick might be a *Dermacentor,* but he was unaware of the woodland-inhabiting *I. dammini.*[8] Although we may never know what species of tick attacked Kalm and his group in the mid 1700s, *I. dammini* is becoming increasingly abundant in forests where deer are proliferating again.

TABLE 3. Mammalian Hosts for *Borrelia burgdorferi* as Confirmed by Isolation

Common Name	Scientific Name
White-footed mouse[a]	*Peromyscus leucopus*[24,25,32,39,40,45-53]
Meadow vole[a]	*Microtus pennsylvanicus*[32,40,50]
Eastern chipmunk[a]	*Tamias striatus*[45]
Raccoon[a]	*Procyon lotor*[39]
Human[a]	*Homo sapiens*[54-57]
Woodland jumping mouse	*Napaeozapus insignis*[24]
White-tailed deer	*Odocoileus virginianus*[40,46]
Dog	*Canis familiaris*[53,58]

[a]Borreliae characterized by PAGE, DNA homology or serologically.

VERTEBRATE RESERVOIRS FOR *Borrelia burgdorferi*

Borrelia burgdorferi was first isolated from wild mammals (white-footed mice and a raccoon) in 1982.[39,40] These isolates were subsequently characterized by polyacrylamide gel electrophoresis (PAGE) and shown to be indistinguishable from the initial B-31 strain and from isolates from humans.[41] These early attempts to isolate spirochetes from bloods of wild mammals resulted in few isolations. Subsequent improvement of the culture medium,[42,43] the successful isolation of borreliae from tissues of inoculated hamsters,[43] and the addition of selective antibiotics[44] to the medium enabled Anderson *et al.*[45] to culture borreliae from tissues of wild-caught white-footed mice and other rodents relatively easily.[45]

Borreliae have been isolated from five mammals, including humans, in the eastern and midwestern United States and identified as *B. burgdorferi* by PAGE, serologic tests, or DNA homology studies (TABLE 3). Additionally, borreliae have been detected, though not characterized, in white-tailed deer, dogs, and a woodland jumping mouse.

Further evidence of exposure of wild and domestic animals to borreliae in Lyme disease foci has been obtained from serologic surveys. Antibodies to these spirochetes have been detected in four species of domestic animals and eight species of wild mammals (TABLE 4). Prevalence rates have been as high as 100% in clinically ill dogs,[62] 83% in white-tailed deer,[67] and 99% in wild sheep.[64] Because species of *Borrelia* share common antigens,[70] none of the studies report specific antibody to *B. burgdorferi*.

Borrelia burgdorferi persists in rodents for relatively long periods of time, possibly from the time of infection until death. They have been isolated from hamsters[71] and white-footed mice 9 months and 7 months[72] after inoculation, respectively; white-footed mice were spirocheturic for 13 months.[73] In Connecticut, mice are naturally infected during all seasons, though infection rates in winter (≤33%) are at least twofold less than in summer (≥66%).[74] Absence of severe inflammation of tissues in rodents[71] and possible antigenic variation[75] may enhance survivorship of these borreliae.

Prevalence of infected mice may be relatively high in the northeastern[32,45,49,50,73] and midwestern[48] United States. In southern Connecticut and on Prudence Island, Rhode Island, where *Ixodes dammini* and Lyme disease are prevalent, *B. burgdorferi* was isolated from 21 of 24 rodents and from 18 of 23 white-footed mice tested, respectively.[32,45] Spirochetes were not isolated from mice captured in northern Connecticut or on islands where the tick and the disease were rare.[32,49] Similarly, in southwestern Wisconsin, where the tick and the disease are common, *B. burgdorferi* was cultured from 15 of 17 white-footed mice.[48] These high rates of infection in host animals are inexorably linked to the large number of infected ticks in Lyme disease foci (TABLE 5). Although infection rates of *I. dammini* varied among sites and studies, they were relatively high at all locations and contrast with the lower rates reported for *Ixodes scapularis*[67] (0.4%) and *Ixodes pacificus*[81-83] (≤3.0%) that occur where the disease is less prevalent.

Birds also harbor borreliae; the type species *Borrelia anserina* infects birds. Borreliae were first detected in six species of birds from a Lyme disease focus in 1983, but inability to sustain spirochetal growth prevented specific identifications.[24] Subsequently, borreliae were isolated from the liver of a veery, *Catharus fuscescens*, captured at the same site, and were identified as *B. burgdorferi* by serology and DNA homology.[27] This isolate was infectious to hamsters and chicks. Like mammals, birds also are reservoirs for Lyme disease spirochetes and would likely be a natural means of distributing the spirochete long distances, possibly even between continents.

The PAGE profiles and the reactions to monoclonal antibodies of isolates from ticks and from mammals in North America are relatively homogeneous. Isolates from *I. dammini*, white-footed mice, humans, a raccoon, and *I. pacificus* all had major proteins with similar molecular weights and responded similarly to various antibodies, though there was variation to antibody H6831.[41,48,81,84-86] In contrast to the mammalian isolates, *B. burgdorferi* from the veery had a slightly smaller molecular weight outer surface protein A.[85]

TABLE 4. Prevalence of Borreliae Antibody in Wild and Domestic Mammals

Common Name[a]	Collection Site (State)	Percent with Antibodies
Dog	Connecticut	≤100[59-62]
Dog	New Jersey	35[63]
Dog	New York	76[60]
Dog	Wisconsin	54[53]
Dog	Texas	20[64]
Horse	Northeast United States	≤12[65,66]
Bovine	Texas	50[64]
Cat	Texas	36[64]
White-tailed deer	Rhode Island	53[47]
White-tailed deer	Connecticut	≤28[59,67,68]
White-tailed deer	North Carolina	11[67]
White-tailed deer	New York	≤83[46,67]
White-tailed deer	Texas	14[64]
White-footed mouse	Rhode Island	41[47]
White-footed mouse	Connecticut	≤10[59,69]
White-footed mouse	Wisconsin	16[25]
Raccoon	Connecticut	≤23[59,67]
Eastern chipmunk	Connecticut	17[59]
Eastern chipmunk	Wisconsin	5[25]
Gray squirrel	Wisconsin	60[25]
Gray squirrel	Connecticut	50[59]
Virginia opossum	Connecticut	17[59]
Jackrabbit	Texas	20[64]
Wild sheep (Anodid)	Texas	99[64]

[a]Scientific names: dog, *Canis familiaris;* horse, *Equus caballus;* bovine, *Bos;* cat, *Felis catus;* white-tailed deer, *Odocoileus virginianus;* white-footed mouse, *Peromyscus leucopus;* raccoon, *Procyon lotor;* eastern chipmunk, *Tamias striatus;* gray squirrel, *Sciurus carolinensis;* Virginia opossum, *Didelphis virginiana;* jackrabbit, *Lepus;* wild sheep, *Ammotragus lervia.*

RABBIT BORRELIAE

While the protein profiles of *B. burgdorferi* among isolates from rodents, humans, a raccoon, *I. dammini,* and *I. pacificus* are similar, recent isolates by J.F. Anderson, R.C. Johnson, L.A. Magnarelli, and J.B. McAninch from eastern cottontail rabbits, *Sylvilagus floridanus,* and their associated tick, *Ixodes dentatus,* are distinctly different. Although all isolates ($n = 61$) reacted to the flagellin antibody (H9724), their reactions to other antibodies varied (i.e., one group of isolates reacted with H5332; another group did not react with this antibody), and none of the isolates had major proteins with approximate molecular weights of 31,000 and 34,000.

Crucial questions concern the infectiousness of rabbit borreliae to humans and domestic animals and the possible role of *I. dammini* and other ticks in transmitting these spirochetes to humans and domestic animals. To determine if humans had

TABLE 5. Prevalence of *Ixodes dammini* Infected with Borreliae

Collection Site (State)	Physiological Age of Ticks	No. Ticks Tested	% Ticks Infected
Connecticut	feeding larvae and nymphs	766	23[24]
Connecticut	feeding larvae and nymphs, questing adults	147	35[39]
Connecticut	questing nymphs and adults	110	21[54]
Connecticut	feeding adults	1193	10[67]
Connecticut	feeding adults	133	14[68]
Rhode Island (Prudence Is.)	feeding larvae, nymphs, adults	172	12[47]
New York (Shelter Is.)	questing adults	126	61[3]
New York (Shelter Is.)	feeding larvae and nymphs	306	41[46]
New York (Long Is.)	questing adults	535	47[46]
New York (Westchester County)	questing nymphs and adults	207	56[67]
Massachusetts (Naushon Is.)	questing nymphs	408	19[76]
Mass. (Nantucket, Naushon Is.)	questing nymphs	395	27[77]
Massachusetts	questing nymphs, adults	422	37[78]
New Jersey	questing adults	19	79[79]
New Jersey	questing adults	492	46[80]
Wisconsin	replete larvae and nymphs	82	66[48]

antibody to these antigens, we screened sera from 50 persons diagnosed with Lyme disease against our standard white-footed mouse isolate (CT. 2591), two *I. dentatus,* and two rabbit kidney isolates by ELISA.[87] Humans with and without ECM had titers within fourfold variation to the five antigens. These findings were not unexpected since species of borreliae share common antigens,[70] and sera from humans infected with borreliae react with homologous and heterologous antigens.[88] Although these studies do not clarify the infectiousness of rabbit borreliae to humans, they do suggest that current methods of detecting antibodies in human sera may not be specific, even though the *B. burgdorferi* serotype has been isolated from *I. dammini,* humans, white-footed mice, other rodents, and a raccoon.

Tick species that could transmit rabbit borreliae to humans are unknown. *Ixodes dentatus* feeds on rabbits and birds[89] and rarely on humans.[90] *Ixodes dammini, I. pacificus,* and *I. scapularis* feed on both lagomorphs and humans and possibly could be competent vectors.

CONCLUSIONS

In conclusion, wild and domestic animals have considerable exposure to *B. burgdorferi* because of the increasing abundance and catholic feeding habits of juvenile *Ixodes dammini,* and because this tick is a competent vector. While the spirochetes isolated from humans in eastern United States are similar to those isolated from rodents, a raccoon, and *I. dammini,* differences in proteins have been shown in a *B. burgdorferi* isolate from a bird and in borreliae from eastern cottontail rabbits and *Ixodes dentatus.* The medical and veterinary importance of borreliae in birds and rabbits needs to be clarified.

ACKNOWLEDGMENT

I thank Carol Lemmon for her assistance.

REFERENCES

1. HUBBERT, W. T., W. F. McCULLOCH & P. R. SCHNURRENBERGER. 1975. Diseases Transmitted from Animals to Man. 6th edit. Charles C Thomas. Springfield, IL.
2. STEERE, A. C., S. E. MALAWISTA, D. R. SNYDMAN, R. E. SHOPE, W. A. ANDIMAN, M. R. ROSS & F. M. STEELE. 1977. Lyme arthritis: An epidemic of oligoarticular arthritis in children and adults in three Connecticut communities. Arthritis Rheum. **20:** 7–17.
3. BURGDORFER, W., A. G. BARBOUR, S. F. HAYES, J. L. BENACH, E. GRUNWALDT & J. P. DAVIS. 1982. Lyme disease—a tick-borne spirochetosis? Science **216:** 1317–1319.
4. JOHNSON, R. C., G. P. SCHMID, F. W. HYDE, A. G. STEIGERWALT & D. J. BRENNER. 1984. *Borrelia burgdorferi* sp. nov.: Etiologic agent of Lyme disease. Int. J. Syst. Bacteriol. **34:** 496–497.
5. STEERE, A. C., T. F. BRODERICK & S. E. MALAWISTA. 1978. Erythema chronicum migrans and Lyme arthritis: Epidemiologic evidence for a tick vector. Am. J. Epidemiol. **108:** 312–321.
6. SCRIMENTI, R. J. 1970. Erythema chronicum migrans. Arch. Dermatol. **102:** 104–105.
7. CENTERS FOR DISEASE CONTROL. 1985. Lyme disease and cases occurring during pregnancy—United States. Morbid. Mortal. Weekly Rep. **34:** 376–378, 383–384.
8. SPIELMAN, A., C. M. CLIFFORD, J. PIESMAN & M. D. CORWIN. 1979. Human babesiosis on Nantucket Island, USA: Description of the vector, *Ixodes (Ixodes) dammini,* n. sp. (Acarina: Ixodidae). J. Med. Entomol. **15:** 218–234.
9. ANDERSON, J. F. & L. A. MAGNARELLI. 1980. Vertebrate host relationships and distribution of ixodid ticks (Acari: Ixodidae) in Connecticut, USA. J. Med. Entomol. **17:** 314–323.
10. HYLAND, K. E. & J. A. MATHEWSON. 1961. The ectoparasites of Rhode Island mammals. I. The tick fauna. Wildl. Dis. **11:** 1–14.
11. JACKSON, J. O. & G. R. DEFOLIART. 1970. *Ixodes scapularis* Say in northern Wisconsin. J. Med. Entomol. **7:** 124–125.
12. BEQUAERT, J. C. 1945. The ticks, or Ixodoidea, of the northeastern United States and eastern Canada. Entomol. Am. **25:** 73–235.
13. WATSON, T. G. & R. C. ANDERSON. 1976. *Ixodes scapularis* Say on white-tailed deer (*Odocoileus virginianus*) from Long Point, Ontario. J. Wildl. Dis. **12:** 66–71.
14. GOOD, N. E. 1973. Ticks of eastern Long Island: Notes on host relations and seasonal distribution. Ann. Entomol. Soc. Am. **66:** 240–243.
15. GOOD, N. E. 1972. Tick locality and host records from Long Island and southeastern New York State. Entomol. News **83:** 165–168.
16. ANASTOS, G. 1947. Hosts of certain New York ticks. Psyche **54:** 178–180.

17. MAIN, A. J., A. B. CAREY, M. G. CAREY & R. H. GOODWIN. 1982. Immature *Ixodes dammini* (Acari: Ixodidae) on small animals in Connecticut, USA. J. Med. Entomol. **19:** 655–664.
18. MAIN, A. J., H. E. SPRANCE, K. O. KLOTER & S. E. BROWN. 1981. *Ixodes dammini* (Acari: Ixodidae) on white-tailed deer (*Odocoileus virginianus*) in Connecticut. J. Med. Entomol. **18:** 487–492.
19. CAREY, A. B., W. L. KRINSKY & A. J. MAIN. 1980. *Ixodes dammini* (Acari: Ixodidae) and associated ixodid ticks in southcentral Connecticut, USA. J. Med. Entomol. **17:** 89–99.
20. CAREY, M. G., A. B. CAREY, A. J. MAIN, W. L. KRINSKY & H. E. SPRANCE. 1981. *Ixodes dammini* (Acari: Ixodidae) in forests in Connecticut. J. Med. Entomol. **18:** 175–176.
21. PIESMAN, J. & A. SPIELMAN. 1979. Host-associations and seasonal abundance of immature *Ixodes dammini* in southeastern Massachusetts. Ann. Entomol. Soc. Am. **72:** 829–832.
22. PIESMAN, J., A. SPIELMAN, P. ETKIND, T. K. RUEBUSH, II & D. D. JURANEK. 1979. Role of deer in the epizootiology of *Babesia microti* in Massachusetts, USA. J. Med. Entomol. **15:** 537–540.
23. WALLIS, R. C., S. E. BROWN, K. O. KLOTER & A. J. MAIN. 1978. Erythema chronicum migrans and Lyme arthritis: Field study of ticks. Am. J. Epidemiol. **108:** 322–327.
24. ANDERSON, J. F. & L. A. MAGNARELLI. 1984. Avian and mammalian hosts for spirochete-infected ticks and insects in a Lyme disease focus in Connecticut. Yale J. Biol. Med. **57:** 627–641.
25. GODSEY, M. S., JR., T. E. AMUNDSON, E. C. BURGESS, W. SCHELL, J. P. DAVIS, R. KASLOW & R. EDELMAN. 1987. Lyme disease ecology in Wisconsin. Distribution and host preferences of *Ixodes dammini*, and prevalence of antibody to *Borrelia burgdorferi* in small mammals. Am. J. Trop. Med. Hyg. **37:** 180–187.
26. SCHULZE, T. L., J. K. SHISLER, E. M. BOSLER, M. F. LAKAT & W. E. PARKIN. 1986. Evolution of a focus of Lyme disease. Zbl. Bakt. Hyg. A **263:** 65–71.
27. ANDERSON, J. F., R. C. JOHNSON, L. A. MAGNARELLI & F. W. HYDE. 1986. Involvement of birds in the epidemiology of the Lyme disease agent *Borrelia burgdorferi*. Infect. Immun. **51:** 394–396.
28. BATTALY, G. R., D. FISH & R. C. DOWLER. 1987. The seasonal occurrence of *Ixodes dammini* and *Ixodes dentatus* (Acari: Ixodidae) on birds in a Lyme disease endemic area of southeastern New York State. J. N. Y. Entomol. Soc. **95:** 461–468.
29. SPIELMAN, A., J. F. LEVINE & M. L. WILSON. 1984. Vectorial capacity of North American *Ixodes* ticks. Yale J. Biol. Med. **57:** 507–513.
30. SPIELMAN, A., M. L. WILSON, J. F. LEVINE & J. PIESMAN. 1985. Ecology of *Ixodes dammini*-borne human babesiosis and Lyme disease. Annu. Rev. Entomol. **30:** 439–460.
31. WILSON, M. L., G. H. ADLER & A. SPIELMAN. 1985. Correlation between abundance of deer and that of the deer tick, *Ixodes dammini* (Acari: Ixodidae). Ann. Entomol. Soc. Am. **78:** 172–176.
32. ANDERSON, J. F., R. C. JOHNSON, L. A. MAGNARELLI, F. W. HYDE & J. E. MEYERS. 1987. Prevalence of *Borrelia burgdorferi* and *Babesia microti* in mice on islands inhabited by white-tailed deer. Appl. Environ. Microbiol. **53:** 892–894.
33. SPIELMAN, A., P. ETKIND, J. PIESMAN, T. K. RUEBUSH II, D. D. JURANEK & M. S. JACOBS. 1981. Reservoir hosts of human babesiosis on Nantucket Island. Am. J. Trop. Med. Hyg. **30:** 560–565.
34. ANDERSON, J. F., L. A. MAGNARELLI & J. B. MCANINCH. 1987. *Ixodes dammini* and *Borrelia burgdorferi* in northern New England and upstate New York. J. Parasitol. **73:** 419–421.
35. COAN, M. E. & D. STILLER. 1986. *Ixodes dammini* (Acari: Ixodidae) in Maryland, USA, and a preliminary survey for *Babesia microti*. J. Med. Entomol. **23:** 446–453.
36. NUTTALL, G. H. F. & C. WARBURTON. 1911. Ixodidae. *In* Ticks: A Monograph of the Ixodoidea. G. H. F. Nuttall, C. Warburton, W. F. Cooper & L. E. Robinson, Eds.: 105–348. Cambridge University Press. London.
37. KALM, P. 1771. Travels into North America, Vol. 2. J. R. Forster. London.
38. FITCH, A. 1872. Fourteenth report on the noxious, beneficial and other insects of the state of New York. Trans. N. Y. State Agric. Soc. (1870). pp. 355–381.
39. ANDERSON, J. F., L. A. MAGNARELLI, W. BURGDORFER & A. G. BARBOUR. 1983. Spirochetes in *Ixodes dammini* and mammals from Connecticut. Am. J. Trop. Med. Hyg. **32:** 818–824.

40. BOSLER, E. M., J. L. COLEMAN, J. L. BENACH, D. A. MASSEY, J. P. HANRAHAN, W. BURGDORFER & A. G. BARBOUR. 1983. Natural distribution of the *Ixodes dammini* spirochete. Science **220:** 321–322.

41. BARBOUR, A. G., S. L. TESSIER & W. J. TODD. 1983. Lyme disease spirochetes and ixodid tick spirochetes share a common surface antigenic determinant defined by a monoclonal antibody. Infect. Immun. **41:** 795–804.

42. BARBOUR, A. G. 1984. Isolation and cultivation of Lyme disease spirochetes. Yale J. Biol. Med. **57:** 521–525.

43. JOHNSON, R. C., N. MAREK & C. KODNER. 1984. Infection of the Syrian hamster with Lyme disease spirochetes. J. Clin. Microbiol. **20:** 1099–1101.

44. JOHNSON, S. E., G. C. KLEIN, G. P. SCHMID, G. S. BOWEN, J. C. FEELEY & T. SCHULZE. 1984. Lyme disease: A selective medium for isolation of the suspected etiological agent, a spirochete. J. Clin. Microbiol. **19:** 81–82.

45. ANDERSON, J. F., R. C. JOHNSON, L. A. MAGNARELLI & F. W. HYDE. 1985. Identification of endemic foci of Lyme disease: Isolation of *Borrelia burgdorferi* from feral rodents and ticks (*Dermacentor variabilis*). J. Clin. Microbiol. **22:** 36–38.

46. BOSLER, E. M., B. G. ORMISTON, J. L. COLEMAN, J. P. HANRAHAN & J. L. BENACH. 1984. Prevalence of the Lyme disease spirochete in populations of white-tailed deer and white-footed mice. Yale J. Biol. Med. **57:** 651–659.

47. ANDERSON, J. F. & L. A. MAGNARELLI. 1983. Spirochetes in *Ixodes dammini* and *Babesia microti* on Prudence Island, Rhode Island. J. Infect. Dis. **148:** 1124.

48. ANDERSON, J. F., P. H. DURAY & L. A. MAGNARELLI. 1987. Prevalence of *Borrelia burgdorferi* in white-footed mice and *Ixodes dammini* at Fort McCoy, Wisconsin. J. Clin. Microbiol. **25:** 1495–1497.

49. ANDERSON, J. F., R. C. JOHNSON, L. A. MAGNARELLI & F. W. HYDE. 1986. Culturing *Borrelia burgdorferi* from spleen and kidney tissues of wild-caught white-footed mice, *Peromyscus leucopus*. Zbl. Bakt. Hyg. A **263:** 34–39.

50. ANDERSON, J. F., R. C. JOHNSON, L. A. MAGNARELLI, F. W. HYDE & J. E. MYERS. 1986. *Peromyscus leucopus* and *Microtus pennsylvanicus* simultaneously infected with *Borrelia burgdorferi* and *Babesia microti*. J. Clin. Microbiol. **23:** 135–137.

51. LEVINE, J. F., M. L. WILSON & A. SPIELMAN. 1985. Mice as reservoirs of the Lyme disease spirochete. Am. J. Trop. Med. Hyg. **34:** 355–360.

52. LOKEN, K. I., C. WU, R. C. JOHNSON & R. F. BEY. 1985. Isolation of the Lyme disease spirochete from mammals in Minnesota. Proc. Soc. Exp. Biol. Med. **179:** 300–302.

53. BURGESS, E. 1986. Natural exposure of Wisconsin dogs to the Lyme disease spirochete. Lab. Anim. Sci. **36:** 288–290.

54. STEERE, A. C., R. L. GRODZICKI, A. N. KORNBLATT, J. E. CRAFT, A. G. BARBOUR, W. BURGDORFER, G. P. SCHMID, E. JOHNSON & S. E. MALAWISTA. 1983. The spirochetal etiology of Lyme disease. N. Engl. J. Med. **308:** 733–740.

55. BENACH, J. L., E. M. BOSLER, J. P. HANRAHAN, J. L. COLEMAN, G. S. HABICHT, T. F. BAST, D. J. CAMERON, J. L. ZIEGLER, A. G. BARBOUR, W. BURGDORFER, R. EDELMAN & R. A. KASLOW. 1983. Spirochetes isolated from the blood of two patients with Lyme disease. N. Engl. J. Med. **308:** 740–742.

56. BERGER, B. W., M. H. KAPLAN, I. R. ROTHENBERG & A. G. BARBOUR. 1985. Isolation and characterization of Lyme disease spirochetes from the skin of patients with erythema chronicum migrans. J. Am. Acad. Dermatol. **13:** 444–449.

57. RAWLINGS, J. A., P. V. FOURNIER & G. J. TELTOW. 1987. Isolation of *Borrelia* spirochetes from patients in Texas. J. Clin. Microbiol. **25:** 1148–1150.

58. LISSMAN, B. A., E. M. BOSLER, H. CAMAY, B. G. ORMISTON & J. L. BENACH. 1984. Spirochete-associated arthritis (Lyme disease in a dog). J. Am. Vet. Med. Assoc. **185:** 219–220.

59. MAGNARELLI, L. A., J. F. ANDERSON, W. BURGDORFER & W. A. CHAPPELL. 1984. Parasitism of *Ixodes dammini* (Acari: Ixodidae) and antibodies to spirochetes in mammals at Lyme disease foci in Connecticut, U.S.A. J. Med. Entomol. **21:** 52–57.

60. MAGNARELLI, L. A., J. F. ANDERSON, A. B. SCHREIER & C. M. FICKE. 1987. Clinical and serologic studies of canine borreliosis. J. Am. Vet. Med. Assoc. **191:** 1089–1094.

61. MAGNARELLI, L. A., J. F. ANDERSON, A. F. KAUFMANN, L. L. LIEBERMAN & G. D.

WHITNEY. 1985. Borreliosis in dogs from southern Connecticut. J. Am. Vet. Med. Assoc. **186:** 955–959.

62. KORNBLATT, A. N., P. H. URBAND & A. C. STEERE. 1985. Arthritis caused by *Borrelia burgdorferi* in dogs. J. Am. Vet. Med. Assoc. **186:** 960–964.

63. SCHULZE, T. L., E. M. BOSLER, J. K. SHISLER, I. C. WARE, M. F. LAKAT & W. E. PARKIN. 1987. Prevalence of canine Lyme disease from an endemic area as determined by serosurvey. Zbl. Bakt. Hyg. A **263:** 427–434.

64. RAWLINGS, J. A. 1987. Lyme disease in Texas. Zbl. Bakt. Hyg. A **263:** 483–487.

65. MARCUS, L. C., M. M. PATTERSON, R. E. GILFILLAN & P. H. URBAND. 1985. Antibodies to *Borrelia burgdorferi* in New England horses: Serologic survey. Am. J. Vet. Res. **46:** 2570–2571.

66. MAGNARELLI, L. A., J. F. ANDERSON, E. SHAW, J. E. POST & F. C. PALKA. 1988. Borreliosis in equids in northeastern United States. Am. J. Vet. Res. **49:** 359–362.

67. MAGNARELLI, L. A., J. F. ANDERSON, C. S. APPERSON, D. FISH, R. C. JOHNSON & W. A. CHAPPELL. 1986. Spirochetes in ticks and antibodies to *Borrelia burgdorferi* in white-tailed deer from Connecticut, New York State, and North Carolina. J. Wildl. Dis. **22:** 178–188.

68. MAGNARELLI, L. A., J. F. ANDERSON & W. A. CHAPPELL. 1984. Antibodies to spirochetes in white-tailed deer and prevalence of infected ticks from foci of Lyme disease in Connecticut. J. Wildl. Dis. **20:** 21–26.

69. MAGNARELLI, L. A., J. F. ANDERSON & W. A. CHAPPELL. 1984. Geographic distribution of humans, raccoons, and white-footed mice with antibodies to Lyme disease spirochetes in Connecticut. Yale J. Biol. Med. **57:** 619–626.

70. BARBOUR, A. G., S. F. HAYES, R. A. HEILAND, M. E. SCHRUMPF & S. L. TESSIER. 1986. A *Borrelia*-specific monoclonal antibody binds to a flagellar epitope. Infect. Immun. **52:** 549–554.

71. DURAY, P. H. & R. C. JOHNSON. 1986. The histopathology of experimentally infected hamsters with the Lyme disease spirochete, *Borrelia burgdorferi*. Proc. Soc. Exp. Biol. Med. **181:** 263–269.

72. DONAHUE, J. G., J. PIESMAN & A. SPIELMAN. 1987. Reservoir competence of white-footed mice for Lyme disease spirochetes. Am. J. Trop. Med. **36:** 92–96.

73. BOSLER, E. M. & T. L. SCHULZE. 1986. The prevalence and significance of *Borrelia burgdorferi* in the urine of feral reservoir hosts. Zbl. Bakt. Hyg. A **263:** 40–44.

74. ANDERSON, J. F., R. C. JOHNSON & L. A. MAGNARELLI. 1987. Seasonal prevalence of *Borrelia burgdorferi* in natural populations of white-footed mice, *Peromyscus leucopus*. J. Clin. Microbiol. **25:** 1564–1566.

75. BARBOUR, A. G. & S. F. HAYES. 1986. Biology of *Borrelia* species. Microbiol. Rev. **50:** 381–400.

76. MATHER, T. N., J. PIESMAN & A. SPIELMAN. 1987. Absence of spirochetes (*Borrelia burgdorferi*) and piroplasms (*Babesia microti*) in deer ticks (*Ixodes dammini*) parasitized by chalcid wasps (*Hunterellus hookeri*). Med. Vet. Entomol. **1:** 3–8.

77. PIESMAN, J., T. N. MATHER, S. R. TELFORD III & A. SPIELMAN. 1986. Concurrent *Borrelia burgdorferi* and *Babesia microti* infection in nymphal *Ixodes dammini*. J. Clin. Microbiol. **24:** 446–447.

78. PIESMAN, J., T. N. MATHER, J. G. DONAHUE, J. LEVINE, J. D. CAMPBELL, S. J. KARAKASHIAN & A. SPIELMAN. 1986. Comparative prevalence of *Babesia microti* and *Borrelia burgdorferi* in four populations of *Ixodes dammini* in eastern Massachusetts. Acta Trop. **43:** 263–270.

79. SCHULZE, T. L., G. S. BOWEN, M. F. LAKAT, W. E. PARKIN & J. K. SHISLER. 1985. The role of adult *Ixodes dammini* (Acari: Ixodidae) in the transmission of Lyme disease in New Jersey, USA. J. Med. Entomol. **22:** 88–93.

80. SCHULZE, T. L., M. F. LAKAT, W. E. PARKIN, J. K. SHISLER, D. J. CHARETTE & E. M. BOSLER. 1986. Comparison of rates of infection by the Lyme disease spirochete in selected populations of *Ixodes dammini* and *Amblyomma americanum* (Acari: Ixodidae). Zbl. Bakt. Hyg. A **263:** 72–78.

81. BURGDORFER, W., R. S. LANE, A. G. BARBOUR, R. A. GRESBRINK & J. R. ANDERSON. 1985. The western black-legged tick, *Ixodes pacificus:* a vector of *Borrelia burgdorferi*. Am. J. Trop. Med. Hyg. **34:** 925–930.

82. LANE, R. S. & W. BURGDORFER. 1986. Potential role of native and exotic deer and their associated ticks (Acari: Ixodidae) in the ecology of Lyme disease in California, USA. Zbl. Bakt. Hyg. A **263:** 55–64.

83. LANE, R. S. & W. BURGDORFER. 1987. Transovarial and transstadial passage of *Borrelia burgdorferi* in the Western black-legged tick, *Ixodes pacificus* (Acari: Ixodidae). Am. J. Trop. Med. Hyg. **37:** 188–192.

84. BARBOUR, A. G., S. L. TESSIER & S. F. HAYES. 1984. Variation in a major surface protein of Lyme disease spirochetes. Infect. Immun. **45:** 94–100.

85. BARBOUR, A. G., R. A. HEILAND & T. R. HOWE. 1985. Heterogeneity of major proteins in Lyme disease borreliae: a molecular analysis of North American and European isolates. J. Infect. Dis. **152:** 478–484.

86. BARBOUR, A. G. & M. E. SCHRUMPF. 1986. Polymorphisms of major surface proteins of *Borrelia burgdorferi*. Zbl. Bakt. Hyg. A **263:** 83–91.

87. MAGNARELLI, L. A., J. M. MEEGAN, J. F. ANDERSON & W. A. CHAPPELL. 1984. Comparison of an indirect fluorescent-antibody test with an enzyme-linked immunosorbent assay for serological studies of Lyme disease. J. Clin. Microbiol. **20:** 181–184.

88. MAGNARELLI, L. A., J. F. ANDERSON & R. C. JOHNSON. 1987. Cross-reactivity in serological tests for Lyme disease and other spirochetal infections. J. Infect. Dis. **156:** 183–188.

89. KEIRANS, J. E. & C. M. CLIFFORD. 1978. The genus *Ixodes* in the United States: A scanning electron microscope study and key to the adults. J. Med. Entomol. Suppl. **2:** 149.

90. SOLLERS, H. 1955. *Ixodes dentatus* (Marx) collected from man. Proc. Entomol. Soc. Wash. **57:** 120.

Lyme Borreliosis in California

Acarological, Clinical, and Epidemiological Studies[a]

ROBERT S. LANE AND PAUL E. LAVOIE

Department of Entomological Sciences
University of California at Berkeley
Berkeley, California 94720
and
Pacific Presbyterian Medical Center
San Francisco, California 94115

In the western United States, Lyme borreliosis (LB) was first reported as a distinct clinical entity in 1978 in a hiker bitten by an *Ixodes* tick in Sonoma County, California.[1] Details of four additional cases among northern California residents with onsets between 1977 and 1980 were described in 1983,[2] and since then the number of cases diagnosed from this region has risen steadily.[3] Elsewhere in the Far West, sporadic cases of LB have been reported from Nevada, Oregon, and Utah.[3,4]

In California and Oregon, the western black-legged tick, *Ixodes pacificus,* has been identified as the primary vector of *Borrelia burgdorferi,* the etiologic agent of LB, and passage of the spirochete via eggs and from stage-to-stage has been demonstrated in this tick.[5,6] Moreover, native Columbian black-tailed deer and exotic axis and fallow deer were found to serve as hosts of *B. burgdorferi* or related spirochetes.[7]

Since 1977, one of us (PEL) has diagnosed LB in numerous patients presenting with a variety of rheumatic and neurologic disorders. Following 10 patient interviews (including one patient seen by another physician), we selected eight exposure sites in northern California that could be pinpointed with reasonable certainty for subsequent acarological follow-up studies. We hypothesized that spirochetal infection rates in adults of *I. pacificus* would be positively associated with the relative abundance of this tick vector. The acarological and epidemiological findings gleaned from these investigations, as well as brief clinical notes on all 10 patients interviewed, are the subject of this report.

MATERIALS AND METHODS

The 10 patients in our series were selected for possible acarological follow-up investigations on the basis of their exposure and travel histories, which were sufficiently detailed in most cases to enable us to locate the specific sites (clinical-case areas) where they contracted their infections. Their infections were acquired in rural or suburban areas of the San Francisco Bay region or immediately north of it in the counties of Contra Costa ($n = 2$), Marin ($n = 3$), Mendocino ($n = 1$), and Sonoma ($n = 4$). More specifically, the cases were acquired adjacent to the Briones Reservoir

[a]This work was supported in part by grant no. RR07006 from the Biomedical Research Support Program, Division of Research Resources, National Institutes of Health (NIH); Public Health Service grant no. AI22501, NIH; and a grant from the Northern California Chapter of the Arthritis Foundation to RSL.

and nearby in central Contra Costa County; in Lagunitas, Mill Valley, and the Point Reyes National Seashore in Marin County; in Yorkville in Mendocino County; and in the Cloverdale, Guerneville, Rio Nido, and possibly Geyserville areas of Sonoma County. The precise locations of the Guerneville and Geyserville exposure sites could not be determined with certainty, and therefore acarological follow-up studies were not undertaken in those areas. Two rural agricultural sciences research field stations of the University of California located near Hopland in Mendocino County (the Hopland Field Station, HFS) and in Browns Valley in Yuba County (the Sierra Foothill Range Field Station, SFRFS) were selected for comparative study. Although human cases apparently have not been contracted at either facility, cases of LB have been reported from similar environments in both geographical areas.

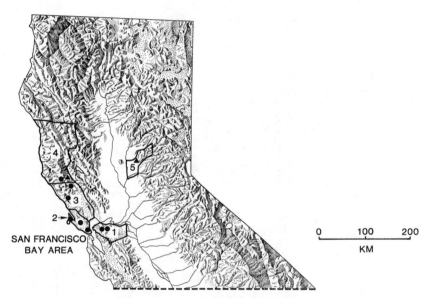

FIGURE 1. Distribution of Lyme borreliosis case (*solid circles*) and comparison study sites (*triangles*) investigated by county in northern California: *1*, Contra Costa County; *2*, Marin County; *3*, Sonoma County; *4*, Mendocino County; *5*, Yuba County.

In the eight clinical-case areas selected for acarological investigations (FIG. 1), the predominant vegetation flagged for ticks was woodland-grass in the Briones Reservoir area, chaparral and woodland-grass at Cloverdale, backyard grass and adjacent woodland-grass at Lagunitas and Mill Valley, grassland at Point Reyes, dense woodland with a grass/forb understory at Rio Nido, and grassland bordering a vineyard and a pond at Yorkville. In comparison areas (FIG. 1), chaparral was flagged at HFS and woodland-grass and riparian vegetation at SFRFS.

Patients were questioned as to their date of onset, travel history, activity resulting in exposure, type of exposure (*e.g.*, tick or other arthropod bite), signs and symptoms, pet ownership, and presence of deer in exposure areas. Convalescent serum samples from seven and acute sera from two of the 10 patients were assayed for antibodies to *Borrelia burgdorferi* by indirect immunofluorescence using the B31 strain as antigen and fluorescein isothiocyanate (FITC) labeled goat anti-human IgG immunoglobu-

TABLE 1. Epidemiologic Characteristics of 10 Lyme Borreliosis Cases Contracted in Northern California, 1975 to 1985

Case No.[a]	Age and Sex	County of Probable Acquisition	Date of Onset	Activity Resulting in Exposure	Pet Ownership Dog(s)	Pet Ownership Cat(s)	History of Tick Bite
1	70 (F)	Sonoma	summer 1975	home environment (resort area)	+	−	+
2	49 (F)	Sonoma	August 1976	vacationing (beach resort)	+[b]	+	−
3	34 (M)	Marin	August 1977	home environment	+	−	−
4	53 (M)	Sonoma	summer 1980	field work	−	−	+
5	52 (F)	Contra Costa	5 August 1983	clearing brush	+	−	−
6	42 (M)	Marin	23 January 1984	hiking	+	+	+
7	?[c] (F)	Contra Costa	8 December 1984	hiking/picking mushrooms	+	−	+
8	46 (F)	Mendocino	January 1985	working in vineyard	+	−	+
9	42 (M)	Marin	July 1985	home environment	+	+	+
10	51 (F)	Sonoma	summer 1984	gardening	+	−	−

[a] All patients were diagnosed on clinical grounds; with one exception (case 7), acute- or convalescent-phase sera were assayed for antibodies to *B. burgdorferi* by indirect immunofluorescence, and patients 2–4 and 9 were found to be seropositive ($\geq 1 : 256$).
[b] Patient boarded son's hunting dogs occasionally.
[c] This patient refused to reveal her age; thus the median age at onset of illness for this series was calculated from only nine patients.

lins. Appropriate positive and negative controls were run with each test. A reciprocal titer of equal to or greater than 256 is considered diagnostic in patients having signs and symptoms compatible with LB. On the other hand, most cases of LB in California are diagnosed solely on clinical grounds as many patients with active disease lack significant serum antibody titers.

Tick collecting was timed to coincide with the seasonal activity of adult *I. pacificus*. Thus, ixodid ticks were obtained by flagging vegetation diurnally in both clinical-case and comparison areas from late fall to early spring, 1984–87. Flagging was accomplished with tick drags consisting of 0.93-m^2 pieces of white flannel attached to wooden handles. Each site was visited an average of 5 (range 1–29) times. Species and developmental stage of all ticks were determined. Ticks were held in desiccators with relative humidities of ca. 85% (*Dermacentor* spp.) or 98% (*I. pacificus*) before dissection.

A rough estimate of relative tick abundance was made by calculating the mean number of ticks collected hourly at each site. Although the basic sampling unit usually consisted of individual hourly collections, in a few instances collecting did not end precisely on the hour and therefore the range was computed by extrapolating from the available data. No attempt was made to quantify the density (*i.e.,* number of individuals per unit area) of ticks because the collection sites varied considerably with respect to vegetational type and extent of habitat available for sampling.

Prior to dissection, ticks were surface sterilized with 3% hydrogen peroxide and 70% ethanol, and washed in phosphate-buffered saline (pH 7.4). Smears prepared from the midgut of each tick (and frequently the central ganglion as well) were examined for presence of spirochetes by direct immunofluorescence with a FITC-labeled, anti-*B. burgdorferi* polyvalent conjugate prepared in rabbits.[5,8] If a tick was found to contain spirochetes, other tissues were examined similarly, including Malpighian tubules, reproductive organs (ovary or testis), and salivary glands. Spirochetes in midgut smears of each infected tick were tested for their reactivity against monoclonal antibodies specific for members of the genus *Borrelia* (H9724)[9] and *B. burgdorferi* (H5332)[10] by indirect immunofluorescence. Isolation was attempted from 13 spirochete-infected ticks by triturating all remaining tissues in 1 ml of BSK II medium, inoculating the suspension into 9 ml of BSK II medium with or without rifampin (50 μg/ml), and maintaining the cultures at 34.5°C for 1 month. Isolates recovered from tick tissues were tested also with the aforementioned *Borrelia*- and *B. burgdorferi*-specific monoclonal antibodies.

Tick infection rates within and between clinical-case areas and comparison areas were compared with Fisher's exact test (two-tailed). The Spearman rank correlation coefficient (r_s) was used to test the hypothesis that spirochetal infection rates in *I. pacificus* adults would be associated with the abundance of this tick. A 5% level of probability was selected for rejection of the null hypothesis.

RESULTS

Clinical and Epidemiological Findings

All 10 patients exhibited erythema migrans, six experienced arthritis/arthralgia, six had neurologic abnormalities, and two had cardiac involvement. Four of nine patients whose sera were tested had significant indirect immunofluorescent titers ranging from ≥1 : 320 to 1 : 5120 (TABLE 1); the remainder had titers of equal to or less than 1 : 40. Two of the patients were treated with penicillin (one oral, one intravenously), four with tetracycline, one with dexamethasone and naproxen, one with ceftriaxone (i.v.) and penicillin (i.v.), one with cefadroxil (i.v.), erythromycin, indomethacin, prednisone, tetracycline, and vibramycin, and one patient received no treatment.

The age distribution of cases ranged from 34 to 70 years, and the sex ratio (male : female) was 2 : 3 (TABLE 1). The median age at onset was 49 years. Seven patients became ill in summer, two in winter, and one in fall. Activities resulting in exposure including working outdoors (40%), recreation (30%), and others that involved the home environment (30%). Three-fifths of the patients reported a history of tick bite. Eight patients owned one or more dogs, and another occasionally boarded her son's hunting dogs. Seven of the nine patients harboring dogs reported that they had found ticks on them, as did one of three patients who owned cats. One of the dogs acquired LB at the same site as its owner. Columbian black-tailed deer (*Odocoileus hemionus columbianus*) occurred in the areas where all 10 patients presumably acquired their infections.

TABLE 2. Mean Number of Ixodid Ticks Flagged Hourly from Vegetation in Lyme Borreliosis Case Areas in Northern California

Case No.	No. Hours Flagging	$\bar{x}$ No. Ticks per Hour (range)		
		D. occidentalis	*D. variabilis*	*I. pacificus*
1	8	2.6 (0–8)	0	6.6 (3–11)[a]
3	2	0	0	0
5	10	10.4 (0–61)	0	41.5 (5–174)
6	18	0.2 (0–3)	0	42.2 (14–119)
7	15	7.1 (0–29)	0.07 (0–1)	27.0 (1–119)
8	4	2.8 (0–6)	0	1.0 (0–2)
9	4	0.3 (0–1)	0.25 (0–1)	1.5 (0–3)
10	8	1.5 (0–5)	0	20.6 (5–55)

[a]Includes 3 larvae and 19 nymphs; all other ticks collected from this site and the other case areas were adults.

Acarological Findings

Two or three species of ixodid ticks were obtained from vegetation in seven of the eight clinical-case areas (TABLE 2). Although ticks were not collected during 2 hours of sampling around the home of patient 3, dogs owned by this patient were found to be tick-infested periodically. At exposure sites yielding specimens, the mean number of *I. pacificus* collected hourly varied between 1.0 and 42.2, and this tick was the most abundant species at 6 of the 7 sites. The Pacific Coast tick, *Dermacentor occidentalis*, ranked second in overall abundance and was the most prevalent tick at one site. Only two individuals of the American dog tick, *Dermacentor variabilis*, were collected.

In comparison areas, *D. occidentalis* and *I. pacificus* were the only ticks collected, with the former ranking first in abundance at the Hopland Field Station (TABLE 3). The relative abundance of *I. pacificus* at both sites was similar to the abundance of this tick in clinical-case areas (TABLES 2 and 3).

A total of 1048 adults of *D. occidentalis* and *I. pacificus* from clinical-case areas were examined for spirochetes (TABLE 4). Of these, none of the 191 *D. occidentalis* was found to contain spirochetes, whereas 1.4% of 857 *I. pacificus* was infected. Positive ticks were detected in four exposure sites with the highest infection rates (5.4% and 5.9%) recorded from the Cloverdale area and Rio Nido in Sonoma County. Multiple

TABLE 3. Mean Number of Ixodid Adults Flagged Hourly from Vegetation in Lyme Borreliosis Comparison Areas in Northern California

Locality	No. Hours Flagging[a]	$\bar{x}$ No. Ticks per Hour (Range)	
		D. occidentalis	I. pacificus
Mendocino County	44	20.6 (0–58)	7.8 (0–23)
Yuba County	11	4.8 (0–13)	23.3 (6–52)

[a]Rounded off to nearest hour.

tissues from 11 of the 12 positive *I. pacificus* were examined and, of these, seven ticks had spirochetal infections that were restricted to the midgut, whereas four had generalized infections involving all tissues. The degree of spirochetal infections in the midguts of these ticks was light (<1 spirochete per several 400× fields) in seven individuals, moderate (1–10 spirochetes per 400×) in three and heavy (>10 spirochetes per 400×) in two. Spirochetes in midgut-tissue smears from 8 of the 12 positive ticks reacted with *B. burgdorferi*-specific monoclonal antibodies (H5332) and those in two of the remainder reacted with the *Borrelia*-specific monoclonal antibodies (H9724). The overall prevalence of spirochete-infected *I. pacificus* in comparison areas (1.0%) did not differ significantly from that in the clinical-case areas (TABLES 4 and 5). Further, spirochetes were detected in the midgut diverticula of two (0.8%) of 253 *D. occidentalis* adults from the HFS and none of 53 from the SFRFS. The distribution of spirochetes in the infected *D. occidentalis* was apparently limited to the midgut, and the degree of spirochetal infection in both ticks was light. In contrast, three of the infected *I. pacificus* from SFRFS had generalized infections and only one had a restricted (midgut) infection. Spirochetes in midgut-tissue smears from both infected *D. occidentalis* and in one of the four positive *I. pacificus* from comparison areas reacted with *B. burgdorferi*-specific monoclonal antibodies (H5332). Spiro-

TABLE 4. Prevalence of Spirochete-infected Ixodid Adults from Lyme Borreliosis Case Areas in Northern California

Case No.	No. Ticks Examined (Sex)		No. Ticks Infected (%)	
	D. occidentalis	I. pacificus	D. occidentalis	I. pacificus
1[a]	20 (10M, 10F)	34 (17M, 17F)	0	2F (5.9)
5	43 (26M, 17F)	252 (118M, 134F)	0	0
6	0	213 (79M, 134F)	—	1M (0.5)
7	105 (51M, 54F)	219 (98M, 121F)	0	1M, 1F (0.9)
8	11 (5M, 6F)	4 (2M, 2F)	0	0
9	1 (F)	5 (2M, 3F)	0	0
10	11 (6M, 5F)	130 (51M, 79F)	0	3M, 4F (5.4)
Total	191 (98M, 93F)	857 (367M, 490F)	0	5M, 7F (1.4)

[a]Two nymphs of *D. occidentalis* and two larvae and 19 nymphs of *I. pacificus* from this site were also tested for spirochetes, with negative results.

chetes in tissues of two of the three positive *I. pacificus* that failed to react with H5332 did bind to the *Borrelia*-specific monoclonal antibodies (H9724).

Spirochetal-infection rates in *D. occidentalis* from clinical-case vs. comparison areas, and in *D. occidentalis* vs. *I. pacificus* within clinical-case and comparison areas, did not differ significantly.

The correlation between spirochetal infection rates detected in adults of *I. pacificus* and the relative abundance of this tick from all areas was not statistically significant ($r_s = 0.15$, $p = 0.85$, one-tailed).

Efforts to isolate spirochetes in BSK II media from 11 of the 16 spirochete-infected *I. pacificus* adults and both infected *D. occidentalis* adults from clinical-case and comparison areas (TABLES 4 and 5) yielded five isolates from *I. pacificus* including four from the Cloverdale area and one from SFRFS. These isolates were identified as *B. burgdorferi* with specific monoclonal antibodies (H5332). Prior to isolation, spirochetes present in midgut-tissue smears prepared from four of the ticks that subsequently yielded isolates had also bound with the *B. burgdorferi*-specific monoclonal antibodies; spirochetes in the tick from SFRFS reacted only with the genus-specific (*Borrelia*) monoclonal antibodies (H9724).

TABLE 5. Prevalence of Spirochete-infected Ixodid Adults from Lyme Borreliosis Comparison Areas in Northern California

	No. Ticks Examined (Sex)		No. Ticks Infected (%)	
Locality	*D. occidentalis*	*I. pacificus*	*D. occidentalis*	*I. pacificus*
Mendocino County	253 (99M, 154F)	188 (113M, 75F)	2M (0.8)	0
Yuba County	53 (30M, 23F)	195 (88M, 107F)	0	4F (2.1)
Total	306 (129M, 177F)	383 (201M, 182F)	2M (0.7)	4F (1.0)

DISCUSSION

The western black-legged tick, *I. pacificus,* is a three-host tick that has been recorded from about 80 species of reptiles, birds, and mammals.[11,12] It occurs along the Pacific Slope from California to British Columbia and in Idaho, Nevada, and Utah.[12] *Ixodes pacificus* is the only tick to have been associated with a case of LB (reported as erythema chronicum migrans) in the far western United States, and recent studies have established that it is the primary tick vector of LB in this region.[5,7] Our findings do not suggest that there is an association between spirochetal infection rates in and the relative abundance of adults of *I. pacificus.* That tick abundance varied up to 40-fold between clinical-case areas suggests that the amount of time that people spend outdoors in tick-infested areas, rather than tick abundance per se, may be a significant risk factor for LB. In Connecticut and New Jersey, however, the incidence of LB has been correlated with the density of *Ixodes dammini* ticks on white-footed mice and on white-tailed deer.[13,14]

Patient interviews revealed that pet ownership may increase the risk of exposure to LB. Of nine patients in our series who owned or harbored dogs, seven reported that they found ticks on their pets occasionally. Moreover, one patient stated that her daughter had been bitten by ticks transported into the home by her dog. Another patient reported that both she and her dog contracted LB at the same ranch. The dog had a clinical history compatible with LB and a diagnostic serum antibody titer to *B. burgdorferi* (J. E. Madigan, pers. commun.). In the eastern United States, exposure to LB is augmented by outdoor activities,[15–17] though the presence of animals, especially cats, also appears to be a significant risk factor for the disease.[18] In our limited series, however, dogs seemed to be a more important risk factor than did cats. Also, deer living in the vicinity of human dwellings may constitute a risk factor, at least indirectly, by seeding an area with replete female ticks whose progeny may infest humans or pets engaged in outdoor activities.

In the Hopland area, spirochetes were not detected in 188 adult *I. pacificus* (TABLE 5), though in an earlier tick and spirochete survey conducted there, 1.35% of the adult *I. pacificus* examined (*n* = 518) was infected.[5] Likewise, only 1 of 213 (0.5%) *I. pacificus* adults from the Point Reyes National Seashore (case 6, TABLE 4) contained spirochetes, whereas 9 of 210 (4.3%) *I. pacificus* adults collected at the same site previously[7] were infected. An isolate of *B. burgdorferi* was recovered subsequently from one of the nine ticks (R. S. Lane, unpubl. data). These findings demonstrate that there can be considerable year-to-year variation in tick infection rates within foci of LB.

We found *B. burgdorferi* for the first time in adults of another human-biting ixodid tick having a broad host range, namely, the Pacific Coast tick, *D. occidentalis*. The degree of spirochetal infection in both positive ticks was light and apparently restricted to the midgut. Moreover, spirochetes were not distributed uniformly within the midgut diverticula of either tick since immunofluorescent examination of multiple midgut smears yielded negative as well as positive tissue specimens. In some populations of *I. pacificus*, the degree of spirochetal infection in the midguts of many infected adults is heavy,[7] and *B. burgdorferi* seems to be distributed more evenly throughout this tissue. In the indirect immunofluorescence test, however, the apparent lack of reactivity of spirochetes in tissue smears prepared from some lightly or moderately infected *I. pacificus* adults (see RESULTS) with both genus-specific (*Borrelia*) and species-specific monoclonal antibodies probably reflects an absence of spirochetes in individual smears rather than the presence of spirochetes belonging to another genus. Further, the staining reactivity of *B. burgdorferi* to specific monoclonal antibodies has been demonstrated to vary significantly (*i.e.*, from none to moderate fluorescence) following prolonged passage in tissues of *I. pacificus*.[6]

Spirochetes in the midgut of each infected *D. occidentalis* bound with monoclonal antibodies specific for *B. burgdorferi*, which suggests that *D. occidentalis* may occasionally serve as a secondary vector of this spirochete in California. The low spirochetal-infection rate, the sparse distribution of spirochetes within the two infected ticks, and the absence of spirochetes in 312 *D. occidentalis* adults examined from Hopland before[7] and in this tick from other localities (TABLES 4 and 5), however, indicate that the vector potential of *D. occidentalis* for *B. burgdorferi* may be low. Besides *I. pacificus*, the only other ixodid tick from the Far West demonstrated to contain *B. burgdorferi* is *Ixodes neotomae* (R. S. Lane and W. Burgdorfer, unpubl. data), which principally parasitizes lagomorphs and wood rats in California and New Mexico.[12,19]

The consistently low prevalence of spirochetal-infection found in *I. pacificus* and other human-biting ixodid ticks from California and Oregon (≤5.9%) during this study and earlier investigations may account for the sporadic occurrence of LB in the Far West.[3,5,7] In the northeastern United States, spirochetal-infection rates in *Ixodes dammini* ticks are generally much higher and may exceed 60–70% in some endemic areas.[16,20,21] Consequently, it is not surprising that cumulative frequencies of LB ranging as high as 4–16% of the population have been reported from some communities in the Northeast, and that in certain "high risk" sites of the United States up to 10% of residents may become infected each year.[17,22-24]

In northern California, the Midwest, and the Northeast, LB is similar epidemiologically with regard to the seasonal occurrence (year-round, but predominantly late spring and summer) and nearly equal sex ratio of cases. However, the age distribution of cases in our small sample (median 49 years) is older, as was reported in earlier clinical accounts from California (range 30 to 58 years).[1,2] In contrast, two-thirds of 210 cases in Westchester County, New York, involved persons less than 40 years of age; children under 19 years made up nearly 43% of the total, and the median age was 27 years (range 1 to 77 years).[25] Similarly, nearly half of the patients in a separate New York study involving 679 cases were 19 years of age or younger.[26] Elsewhere, 30% of 82 patients in Texas with titers of $\geq 1 : 64$ to *B. burgdorferi* were 10 years of age or younger,[27] and the median age at onset ranged from a low of 16 years in Connecticut to a high of 39 years in Minnesota and Wisconsin, and nationally it was only 34 years in 1983 and 1984.[3,18,28,29] It is not known whether the older age distribution of cases seen by us is a bona fide phenomenon or reflects an age-biased sample since children or young adults suffering from LB might be less likely to consult a rheumatologist than would middle-aged or elderly persons.

Three-fifths of our patients presented with a history of tick bite, which is commensurate with earlier reports from Minnesota (75%), New Jersey (63%), and New York (40–86%), but considerably higher than the 21% reported for Connecticut during the initial period of recognition of the disease.[16,18,25,26,29,30] Two patients in our series removed the tick that infected them within less than 8 to 12 hours of attachment. Therefore, transmission of *B. burgdorferi* to humans by some ticks in California is more rapid than is delivery of spirochetes to rodents or rabbits (and by inference humans?) by feeding *I. dammini*.[31-33] Nymphal *I. dammini* usually require 2 to 3 days to transmit *B. burgdorferi* to rodents,[31,32] whereas adults of this tick take somewhat longer to pass on spirochetes to rabbits.[32,33] The mechanism of spirochetal transmission by *I. pacificus* is unknown, but the high prevalence (32–36%) of unfed, infected *I. pacificus* adults having generalized infections (ref. 5 and present study) suggests that salivary delivery by such ticks would be rapid indeed. In contrast, generalized spirochetal infections are encountered rarely in unfed, infected *I. dammini,* and the delay in transmission to vertebrates by this tick presumably is attributable to the time it takes spirochetes to reach the saliva following dissemination from the midgut.[32]

Although none of our patients that reported a tick bite saved the specimen, one of them identified the tick that bit her as male *I. pacificus* when shown both sexes of *D. occidentalis* and *I. pacificus*. In the absence of a voucher specimen, her determination must be viewed with skepticism since males of *I. pacificus* apparently feed little or not at all following placement on suitable laboratory animals (R. S. Lane, pers. observ.). Moreover, the male of the related *I. dammini,* which bites humans infrequently, is not considered to be a significant vector of *B. burgdorferi*.[34]

Since the summer peak in prevalence of LB in California occurs when adult *I. pacificus* and *D. occidentalis* are largely inactive,[12] transmission then may be due to attachment by immatures of one or both of these ticks, or by other species of ticks. Spirochetal-infection rates are similar in all three parasitic stages of *I. pacificus* and immatures of this tick are active in spring and summer (R. S. Lane, unpubl. data). On the other hand, immatures of *D. occidentalis,* which are active also in late spring and summer in the Hopland area, have been found infected naturally only twice (R. S. Lane and J. E. Loye, unpubl. data). Other bloodsucking arthropods such as deer flies, horse flies, mosquitoes, and possibly fleas may occasionally transmit spirochetes to humans in summer, as has been suggested previously.[18,26,35,36]

Lyme borreliosis in California does not differ noticeably from the disease in other parts of the United States. Clinical details of four of the patients presented here have been reported before (*i.e.,* cases 1–3 and 5).[2,37,38] Only two of these patients (cases 2 and 3) were also seropositive (TABLE 1). One patient developed sudden, then permanent and complete, heart block. The neurologic signs included transverse myelitis, meningoencephalitis, memory defects, and facial palsies (bilateral in two cases). Erythema migrans is the best clinical marker here as it is elsewhere in the country.[4] All of the cases in our series and those reported previously from California[1,2,37,38] were characterized by the presence of one or more erythematous skin lesions. The somewhat high prevalence (60%) of cardiac and neurologic manifestations among our patients probably reflects the fact that the diagnosis of LB was made late in the course of illness. Notably, one of our patients (case no. 2) had active LB for at least 11 years, during which time she developed acrodermatitis chronica atrophicans, the first such case to be associated with LB in the United States.[37] To our knowledge, this is the longest symptomatic case reported from the Far West, though recently a case originating on Great Island, Massachusetts reportedly had manifested symptoms of the disease for 18 years.[23] Finally, the fact that five of the nine cases that we assayed for antibodies to *B. burgdorferi* were seronegative, including three patients with late manifestations, is not surprising inasmuch as nearly two-thirds of the clinically diagnosed LB cases from California do not have significant antibody titers to this spirochete.[38]

SUMMARY

The relative abundance of, and spirochetal-infection rates in, adult ixodid ticks from eight Lyme borreliosis clinical-case areas and two comparison areas were investigated in northern California from late fall to early spring, 1984–87. The western black-legged tick (*Ixodes pacificus*) was the most abundant species at seven of nine sites yielding specimens as determined with a tick drag method. The Pacific Coast tick (*Dermacentor occidentalis*) was the most abundant species at two sites, and lesser numbers of this tick and the American dog tick (*D. variabilis*) were obtained from seven and two sites, respectively. Abundance of *I. pacificus* adults varied in clinical-case areas as well as in the comparison areas, and was not correlated significantly with spirochetal infection rates in this tick. Overall, spirochetes were detected in 1.4 and 1.0% of the adult *I. pacificus* collected from clinical case (*n* = 857) and comparison sites (*n* = 383), respectively, and in 0.8% of adult *D. occidentalis* (*n* = 253) from one comparison area. An additional 244 *D. occidentalis* adults from all other sites were tested with negative results. Five spirochetal isolates recovered from *I. pacificus* adults were identified as *Borrelia burgdorferi* with specific monoclonal antibodies. Seven of 10 patients interviewed reportedly contracted their infections in summer, and six presented with a history of tick bite. Nine patients owned or occasionally harbored one or more dogs, and at least one of the dogs contracted Lyme borreliosis at the same site as its owner. Clinical manifestations of the disease in human patients included erythema migrans (100%), arthritis/arthralgia (60%), neurologic abnormalities (60%), and cardiac involvement (20%). Four of nine patients whose sera were assayed by indirect immunofluorescence contained significant antibody titers to *B. burgdorferi*.

[NOTE ADDED IN PROOF: Perry F. Smith *et al.* (this volume) have assessed the frequency of and risk factors for infection with *B. burgdorferi* primarily in outdoor workers from six employee groups in southeastern New York. Consistent with our tentative findings, they found that infection (as measured by seropositivity) was associated with the amount of time people spent outdoors in endemic areas. Seropositivity was found to be significantly associated with leisure activities, whereas the evidence for an association with work-related exposure was less conclusive.]

ACKNOWLEDGMENTS

We thank A. H. Murphy, M. Connor, J. L. Sansing, and S. E. Abbors for permission to conduct studies at the University of California (UC) Hopland Field Station, UC Sierra Foothill Range Field Station, Point Reyes National Seashore, and Briones Watershed, respectively; W.C. Reeves and R. A. Murray for their helpful reviews of the manuscript; W. Burgdorfer and A. G. Barbour for polyclonal and monoclonal antibodies; and M. Hoben, S. A. Manweiler, J. Pascocello, R. N. Brown, J. Leung, R. Leen, and J. E. Loye for technical assistance.

REFERENCES

1. NAVERSEN, D. N. & L. W. GARDNER. 1978. Erythema chronicum migrans in America. Arch. Dermatol. **114:** 253–254.
2. CAMPAGNA, J., P. E. LAVOIE, N. S. BIRNBAUM & D. P. FURMAN. 1983. Lyme disease in northern California. West. J. Med. **139:** 319–323.
3. CENTERS FOR DISEASE CONTROL. 1985. Update: Lyme disease and cases occurring during pregnancy—United States. Morbid. Mortal. Weekly Rep. **34:** 376–378, 383–384.
4. STEERE, A. C. & S. E. MALAWISTA. 1979. Cases of Lyme disease in the United States: Locations correlated with distribution of *Ixodes dammini.* Ann. Intern. Med. **91:** 730–733.
5. BURGDORFER, W., R. S. LANE, A. G. BARBOUR, R. A. GRESBRINK & J. R. ANDERSON. 1985. The western black-legged tick, *Ixodes pacificus:* A vector of *Borrelia burgdorferi.* Am. J. Trop. Med. Hyg. **34:** 925–930.
6. LANE, R. S. & W. BURGDORFER. 1987. Transovarial and transstadial passage of *Borrelia burgdorferi* in the western black-legged tick, *Ixodes pacificus* (Acari: Ixodidae). Am. J. Trop. Med. Hyg. **37:** 188–192.
7. LANE, R. S. & W. BURGDORFER. 1986. Potential role of native and exotic deer and their associated ticks (Acari: Ixodidae) in the ecology of Lyme disease in California, USA. Zbl. Bakt. Hyg. A **263:** 55–64.
8. LANE, R. S., W. BURGDORFER, S. F. HAYES & A. G. BARBOUR. 1985. Isolation of a spirochete from the soft tick, *Ornithodoros coriaceus:* A possible agent of epizootic bovine abortion. Science **230:** 85–87.
9. BARBOUR, A. G., S. F. HAYES, R. A. HEILAND, M. E. SCHRUMPF & S. L. TESSIER. 1986. A *Borrelia*-specific monoclonal antibody binds to a flagellar epitope. Infect. Immun. **52:** 549–554.
10. BARBOUR, A. G., S. L. TESSIER & W. J. TODD. 1983. Lyme disease spirochetes and ixodid tick spirochetes share a common surface antigenic determinant defined by a monoclonal antibody. Infect. Immun. **41:** 795–804.
11. ARTHUR, D. R. & K. R. SNOW. 1968. *Ixodes pacificus* Cooley and Kohls, 1943: Its life-history and occurrence. Parasitology **58:** 893–906.
12. FURMAN, D. P. & E. C. LOOMIS. 1984. The ticks of California (Acari: Ixodida). Bull. Calif. Insect Surv. **25:** 1–239.
13. WALLIS, R. C., S. E. BROWN, K. O. KLOTER & A. J. MAIN, JR. 1978. Erythema chronicum migrans and Lyme arthritis: Field study of ticks. Am. J. Epidemiol. **108:** 322–327.
14. SCHULZE, T. L., G. S. BOWEN, M. F. LAKAT, W. E. PARKIN & J. K. SHISLER. 1984. Geographical distribution and density of *Ixodes dammini* (Acari: Ixodidae) and relationship to Lyme disease transmission in New Jersey. Yale J. Biol. Med. **57:** 669–675.
15. BOWEN, G. S., T. L. SCHULZE & W. L. PARKIN. 1984. Lyme disease in New Jersey, 1978–1982. Yale J. Biol. Med. **57:** 661–668.

16. BOWEN, G. S., T. L. SCHULZE, C. HAYNE & W. E. PARKIN. 1984. A focus of Lyme disease in Monmouth County, New Jersey. Am. J. Epidemiol. **120:** 387–394.

17. HANRAHAN, J. P., J. L. BENACH, J. L. COLEMAN, E. M. BOSLER, D. L. MORSE, D. J. CAMERON, R. EDELMAN & R. A. KASLOW. 1984. Incidence and cumulative frequency of endemic Lyme disease in a community. J. Infect. Dis. **150:** 489–496.

18. STEERE, A. C., T. F. BRODERICK & S. E. MALAWISTA. 1978. Erythema chronicum migrans and Lyme arthritis: Epidemiologic evidence for a tick vector. Am. J. Epidemiol. **108:** 312–321.

19. KEIRANS, J. E. & C. M. CLIFFORD. 1978. The genus *Ixodes* in the United States: A scanning electron microscope study and key to the adults. J. Med. Entomol. Suppl. **2:** 149.

20. BURGDORFER, W., A. G. BARBOUR, S. F. HAYES, J. L. BENACH, E. GRUNWALDT & J. P. DAVIS. 1982. Lyme disease—a tick-borne spirochetosis? Science **216:** 1317–1319.

21. BURGDORFER, W. 1984. The New Zealand white rabbit: An experimental host for infecting ticks with Lyme disease spirochetes. Yale J. Biol. Med. **57:** 609–612.

22. STEERE, A. C., R. L. GRODZICKI, A. N. KORNBLATT, J. E. CRAFT, A. G. BARBOUR, W. BURGDORFER, G. P. SCHMID, E. JOHNSON & S. E. MALAWISTA. 1983. The spirochetal etiology of Lyme disease. N. Engl. J. Med. **308:** 733–740.

23. STEERE, A. C., E. TAYLOR, M. L. WILSON, J. F. LEVINE & A. SPIELMAN. 1986. Longitudinal assessment of the clinical and epidemiological features of Lyme disease in a defined population. J. Infect. Dis. **154:** 295–300.

24. MATUSCHKA, F. R. & A. SPIELMAN. 1986. The emergence of Lyme disease in a changing environment in North America and central Europe. Exper. Appl. Acarol. **2:** 337–353.

25. WILLIAMS, C. L., A. S. CURRAN, A. C. LEE & V. O. SOUSA. 1986. Lyme disease: Epidemiologic characteristics of an outbreak in Westchester County, NY. Am. J. Public Health **76:** 62–65.

26. BENACH, J. L. & J. L. COLEMAN. 1986. Clinical and geographic characteristics of Lyme disease in New York. Zbl. Bakt. Hyg. A **263:** 477–482.

27. RAWLINGS, J. A. 1986. Lyme disease in Texas. Zbl. Bakt. Hyg. A **263:** 483–487.

28. DAVIS, J. P., W. L. SCHELL, T. E. AMUNDSON, M. S. GODSEY, JR., A. SPIELMAN, W. BURGDORFER, A. G. BARBOUR, M. LAVENTURE & R. A. KASLOW. 1984. Lyme disease in Wisconsin: Epidemiologic, clinical, serologic, and entomologic findings. Yale J. Biol. Med. **57:** 685–696.

29. OSTERHOLM, M. T., J. C. FORFANG, K. E. WHITE & J. N. KURITSKY. 1984. Lyme disease in Minnesota: Epidemiologic and serologic findings. Yale J. Biol. Med. **57:** 677–683.

30. HANRAHAN, J. P., J. L. BENACH, J. L. COLEMAN, E. M. BOSLER, J. C. GRABAU & D. L. MORSE. 1984. Epidemiologic features of Lyme disease in New York. Yale J. Biol. Med. **57:** 643–650.

31. PIESMAN, J., T. N. MATHER, R. J. SINSKY & A. SPIELMAN. 1987. Duration of tick attachment and *Borrelia burgdorferi* transmission. J. Clin. Microbiol. **25:** 557–558.

32. RIBEIRO, J. M. C., T. N. MATHER, J. PIESMAN & A. SPIELMAN. 1987. Dissemination and salivary delivery of Lyme disease spirochetes in vector ticks (Acari: Ixodidae). J. Med. Entomol. **24:** 201–205.

33. BENACH, J. L., J. L. COLEMAN, R. A. SKINNER & E. M. BOSLER. 1987. Adult *Ixodes dammini* on rabbits: A hypothesis for the development and transmission of *Borrelia burgdorferi*. J. Infect. Dis. **155:** 1300–1306.

34. SHOPE, R. E. 1984. Epidemiologic studies. Yale J. Biol. Med. **57:** 707–709.

35. ANDERSON, J. F. & L. A. MAGNARELLI. 1984. Avian and mammalian hosts for spirochete-infected ticks and insects in a Lyme disease focus in Connecticut. Yale J. Biol. Med. **57:** 627–641.

36. MAGNARELLI, L. A., J. F. ANDERSON & A. G. BARBOUR. 1986. The etiologic agent of Lyme disease in deer flies, horse flies, and mosquitoes. J. Infect. Dis. **154:** 355–358.

37. LAVOIE, P. E., A. J. WILSON & D. L. TUFFANELLI. 1986. Acrodermatitis chronica atrophicans with antecedent Lyme disease in a Californian. Zbl. Bakt. Hyg. A **263:** 262–265.

38. LAVOIE, P. E., R. S. LANE & R. A. MURRAY. 1987. Seronegative Lyme borreliosis in three Californians with late manifestations. Arthritis Rheum. 30 (Suppl. 4): S36.

Vector Tick Populations and Lyme Disease

A Summary of Control Strategies

TERRY L. SCHULZE,[a] WILLIAM E. PARKIN,[a]
AND EDWARD M. BOSLER[b]

[a]*New Jersey State Department of Health*
Trenton, New Jersey 08625

[b]*New York State Department of Health*
Health Sciences Center
SUNY at Stony Brook
Stony Brook, New York 11794

INTRODUCTION

Over the past decade, the study of Lyme disease has proceeded in a logical and orderly fashion. Concurrent investigations into the clinical spectrum, treatment, pathology, microbiology, epidemiology, and ecology of Lyme disease have added substantially to our knowledge of this disease in a relatively short period of time. Although continued research in these disciplines is essential, increased awareness by the public regarding Lyme disease has resulted in a demand for information on the more pragmatic aspects of controlling the disease, specifically the control of tick vectors. Dr. Robert Shope, in his summation of epidemiological studies presented at the First International Symposium on Lyme Disease and Related Disorders, recognized the importance of control and thought it highly significant that this question had not been adequately addressed.[1] In the ensuing four years published information on the control of *Ixodes dammini,* the principal tick vector, has been limited. In this paper the available information on control of *I. dammini* is discussed in relation to high-risk areas for disease transmission.

TICK HABITAT AND DISEASE FOCI

The success of any control attempt is predicated on a complete understanding of not only the biology and behavior of the target organism, but also its habitat. *Ixodes dammini* are found primarily in wooded habitats.[2,3] Research conducted in New Jersey and New York has shown that *I. dammini* is most abundant in mixed hardwood forests with extensive shrub layers. Fields are rarely exploited by *I. dammini* until they progress into secondary woody succession. *I. dammini* are not uniformly distributed within typical wooded habitats. Ticks are most abundant in areas of vegetational transition, ostensibly as a result of increased host numbers and diversity associated with this "edge" effect.

In more general terms, Lyme disease is considered endemic in Suffolk and Westchester Counties in New York[4] and throughout the southern two-thirds of New Jersey (Fig. 1).[5] Recent tick and canine surveillance data from these states suggest that Lyme disease is spreading into new areas. Lyme disease cases are more frequently observed in suburban environments, and more specifically, in regions experiencing dramatic increases in residential populations. Individual communities located within or near wooded areas are at greater risk. Established disease foci invariably are associated with large tracts of undeveloped woodland, typically, federal, state, and county parks and wildlife refuges as well as military installations.[6]

CONTROL STRATEGIES

Host Reduction

The first published investigation to address control of *I. dammini* ticks evaluated the effect of deer reduction on tick abundance.[7] Attempts to reduce the number of white-tailed deer (*Odocoileus virginianus*), the principal host of *I. dammini* adults, through the use of several trapping techniques and rifle-fire tranquilizers proved impractical. Subsequently, the destruction of approximately 70% of the deer did not markedly reduce tick abundance during the first year. While it can be argued that this study was terminated before the effects of deer reduction were fully manifest, this technique will be difficult to implement. Even if successful, a policy of deer destruction can be expected to draw opposition from such divergent groups as hunters and animal rights activists.

Earlier, the hypothetical reduction in white-footed mouse (*Peromyscus leucopus*) populations, the principal reservoir of *Borrelia burgdorferi*[8] and *Babesia microti*,[9] was thought to enhance transmission by a corresponding increase in density of *I. dammini* larvae and nymphs on the remaining mice.[10] Rodent reduction methods were not discussed.

Habitat Modification

The sole study involving habitat modification evaluated the effects of mowing and burning vegetation on populations of *I. dammini* adults.[11] Burning reduced adult tick populations by 70.0–88.3%. This reduction persisted for up to one year, but was site-dependent. Mowing resulted in similar reduction (70.0%) for a 1-year period. These techniques would only have local application and be limited to nonresidential areas.

Chemical Control

The use of acaricides to control *I. dammini* has been attempted through two divergent techniques. The first involved the dispersal of plastic tubes containing permethrin-treated cotton batting.[12] The treated cotton would be actively harvested by white-footed mice for nesting material. *Ixodes dammini* larvae and nymphs exposed to this nesting material subsequently would be controlled. The study showed that 72% of mice in treated areas were free of ticks, compared to only 1% in untreated areas. No adverse effects on mice were reported. This technique appears to be promising, but data regarding retreatment intervals, impacts of weather on the residual effectiveness of permethrin, and the long-term success of the method need to be obtained.

The second technique employing the use of acaricides involved the application of carbaryl (0.84 kg AI/ha) and diazinon (1.68 kg AI/ha) via high-pressure hydraulic sprayer to wooded areas to control fall populations of *I. dammini* adults.[13] Tick populations were simultaneously monitored at one untreated and two treatment blocks 3 times prior to application (TABLE 1). Postapplication population levels were surveyed 24 and 72 hours after the treatments (TABLE 2). After 24 hours, 86.8% and 74.8% reduction in tick populations was observed in the carbaryl- and diazinon-treated blocks, respectively. At 72 hours postapplication, the population of *I. dammini* adults

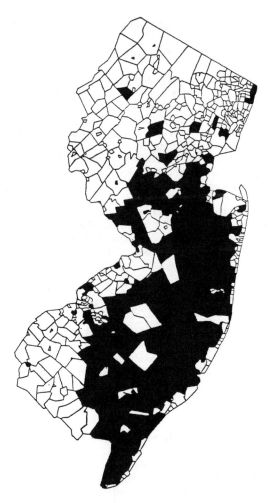

FIGURE 1. Distribution of Lyme disease cases in New Jersey by municipality, 1978–1986.

was reduced 97.1% in the carbaryl-treated blocks and 100% in the diazinon-treated block. As expected, the effects of these applications were observed the following spring, with adults questing during March and April being survivors of the overwintering fall population (TABLE 3). In fall 1986, *I. dammini* population levels in the treated blocks were similar to those in the untreated block (TABLE 4). As such, the effectiveness of this single application was limited to one year.

TABLE 1. Preapplication Population Levels of Adult *Ixodes dammini* at the Wayside Training Area, NWS Earle, November 1985

| | Block No. | No. Ticks (15-min Survey) | | | | No. Ticks per Block in 60-min Survey |
		Area 1	Area 2	Area 3	Area 4	
November 1	1	11	9	18	2	40
	2	14	24	10	4	52
	3	12	7	2	6	27
Total						119
November 4	1	29	18	24	5	76
	2	29	27	11	12	79
	3	15	11	13	6	45
Total						200
November 18	1	24	25	34	6	89
	2	33	19	10	6	68
	3	15	12	11	9	47
Total						204

Historically, application of acaricides to control ticks in wooded areas was thought to be impractical because of the difficulty of sprays penetrating the vegetation. The control of *I. dammini* is an exception, since adults quest within the shrub layer in the fall following abscission. At this time, *I. dammini* adults are particularly vulnerable to acaricide sprays. Fall applications, however, have little effect on larvae and nymphs, which are not active at this time. As such, the effectiveness of a single control attempt directed solely toward adult ticks in a limited area will be temporary. These applications had no demonstrable effects on any life stage of *Amblyomma americanum,* a secondary tick vector of *Borrelia burgdorferi* in New Jersey.[14]

DISCUSSION

Tick Habitat and Disease Foci

Individuals residing in communities located in or near large tracts of undeveloped woodland are at greater risk for acquiring Lyme disease. Wooded residential develop-

TABLE 2. Postapplication Population Levels of Adult *Ixodes dammini* at the Wayside Training Area, NWS Earle, November 1985

| | Block No. (Treatment) | No. Ticks (15-min Survey) | | | | No. Ticks per Block in 60-min Survey (% Reduction)[a] |
		Area 1	Area 2	Area 3	Area 4	
November 19	1 (carbaryl)	2	2	0	5	9 (86.8)
(24 h)	2 (control)	31	16	21	10	78 —
	3 (diazinon)	0	1	3	6	10 (74.8)
November 21	1 (carbaryl)	0	2	0	0	2 (97.1)
(72 h)	2 (control)	80	40	26	22	168 —
	3 (diazinon)	0	0	0	0	0 (100)

[a]Reduction data calculated on mean preapplication population levels.

TABLE 3. Postapplication Population Levels of Adult *Ixodes dammini* at the Wayside Training Area, NWS Earle, Spring 1986

Block No. (Treatment)	No. of Ticks Collected (60-min Survey)			
	Mar. 25	Apr. 14	Apr. 22	$\bar{x}$
1 (carbaryl)	6	1	1	2.3
2 (untreated)	44	19	57	40.0
3 (diazinon)	0	0	3	1.0

ments provide ample habitat for the hosts of all stages of *I. dammini*. Where wooded communities are isolated in more urbanized areas, they may serve as islands of refuge and essentially concentrate hosts and their parasites. The likelihood of disease transmission is increased further by construction practices. Removal of trees for home construction and lawns creates additional edge, which favors an increase in the number of white-footed mice, eastern chipmunks (*Tamias striatus*), and eastern gray squirrels (*Sciurus carolinensis*), important hosts for *I. dammini* larvae and nymphs in New Jersey and New York.[15] Larger mammals such as the raccoon (*Procyon lotor*), Virginia opposum (*Didelphis virginiana*), and striped skunk (*Mephitis mephitis*) readily exploit surburban environments. Populations of these mammals will tend to increase and serve as hosts for *I. dammini* adults, even in the absence of deer. The introduction of canines and other pets will add further to the number of potential hosts.[15] In essence, risk of transmission increases not only by the introduction of people into previously undeveloped tick habitat, but by actually enhancing the habitat for many mammalian hosts.

Control

Previous attempts to control *I. dammini* have met with varying degrees of success. Efficacy, however, is only one consideration in the development of a control strategy. Factors such as site characteristics, practicality, demographics, cost, and even politics must also be addressed. The applicability of the techniques previously used to control *I. dammini* should be evaluated in relation to these factors.

Host Reduction

Reduction of an important host of *I. dammini*, the white-tailed deer, had little short-term effect on tick populations. Several live capture techniques proved impractical and the destruction of deer undoubtedly would be too controversial politically to

TABLE 4. Postapplication Population Levels of Adult *Ixodes dammini* at the Wayside Training Area, NWS Earle, Fall 1986

Block No. (Treatment)	No. of Ticks Collected (60-min Survey)		
	Oct. 31	Nov. 20	$\bar{x}$
1 (carbaryl)	61	18	39.5
2 (untreated)	88	20	54.0
3 (diazinon)	82	22	52.0

receive wide acceptance as a control measure for Lyme disease. Intuitively, however, the number of hosts should have a regulatory effect on the number of tick vectors. While it has been suggested that host reduction may not have the desired effect because of an increase in density of ticks on the remaining hosts, we believe that deer management is an important component of *I. dammini* control. In urban/surburban situations, deer management is essential. Virtually all of the major foci of transmission in New Jersey are associated with areas where deer populations are not adequately managed. Where deer herds are permitted to go unchecked, agricultural interests are adversely impacted and in municipalities in New Jersey where deer management through hunting has been prohibited, deer-car collisions have more than quadrupled.[16] Combined with these interests, the control of Lyme disease as an adjunct to accepted deer management practices will be less controversial.

Habitat Modification

The destruction of vegetation by mowing or burning reduced populations of *I. dammini* adults 70.0% to 88.3%. Whether this level of reduction, particularly at the lower end of the range, will be sufficient to reduce Lyme disease transmission remains to be determined. In many suburban situations where residents pay a premium for wooded properties, it is unlikely that destruction of vegetation would be widely accepted. The destruction of vegetation will temporarily displace hosts, but this destruction will create additional edge and may ultimately increase small mammal populations. Further, this technique is labor-intensive and burning may be prohibited or require permits by local ordinance. This control method may have application in more rural areas.

Chemical Control

The dispersal of acaricide-treated cotton for use as nesting material for white-footed mice is the only control technique directed exclusively against *I. dammini* subadults. Additional field trials are needed to determine the effectiveness of this technique in various habitat settings. It has the added advantages of use by the general public and having no severe and/or controversial environmental impacts.

The more traditional use of acaricide sprays exploited the questing behavior of *I. dammini* adults at times of the year when deciduous foliage is absent. Control was exceptional, but temporary, having no demonstratable effect beyond 1 year. The application method (high-pressure hydraulic sprayer) has logistical limitations and is available only through licensed pest control operators. The use of chemical sprays and, to a lesser extent, the dissemination of acaricide-treated cotton may be considered a potential health hazard. However, the issue surrounding the use of broad-spectrum acaricides is normally less controversial in situations involving disease transmission.

Each of the measures attempted for control of *I. dammini* has its own advantages and disadvantages. However, they share common problems: they have been attempted only in small areas, there has been no long-term follow-up, and they have only been tried individually. Almost without exception, successful control of economically and medically important pests has employed the use of two or more control techniques. Such an integrated approach may include the annual application of acaricides to vegetation to control *I. dammini* adults in the fall and spring, accompanied by the dispersal of acaricide-treated nesting material throughout the late spring and summer to control nymphs and larvae. Control will be enhanced when conducted in areas where deer management techniques are practiced. When implemented in larger areas, the effects of reintroduction of ticks by hosts from untreated areas will be minimized. Once the desired control is achieved, the frequency of application of either or both techniques may be reduced. Avoidance of infested areas, education of the public, and the use of personal and clothing repellents remain important components in the reduction of Lyme disease transmission. While continued development of new control techniques is to be encouraged, research should now evaluate various integrated approaches.

SUMMARY

Although many aspects of Lyme disease have been intensely studied for over a decade, little research has been directed toward control of the principal tick vector, *Ixodes dammini*. Ecological and epidemiological investigations have provided not only an ample understanding of tick biology and behavior, they have also identified the types of areas at risk for disease transmission. The advantages and limitations of previous attempts to control *I. dammini* by host reduction, habitat modification, and acaricide applications have been discussed in relation to overall control strategies for high-risk areas, and an integrated approach to control proposed.

REFERENCES

1. SHOPE, R. E. 1984. Epidemiological studies. Yale J. Biol. Med. **57:** 707–709.
2. CAREY, A. B., W. L. KRINSKY & A. J. MAIN. 1980. *Ixodes dammini* (Acari: Ixodidae) and associated ixodid ticks in south-central Connecticut, USA. J. Med. Entomol. **17:** 89–99.
3. CAREY, M. G., A. B. CAREY, A. J. MAIN, W. L. KRINSKY & H. E. SPRANCE. 1981. *Ixodes dammini* (Acari: Ixodidae) in forests in Connecticut. J. Med. Entomol. **18:** 175–176.
4. BENACH, J. L. & J. L. COLEMAN. 1986. Clinical and geographic characteristics of Lyme disease in New York. Zbl. Bakt. Hyg. A **263:** 477–482.
5. SCHULZE, T. L., M. L. LAKAT, G. S. BOWEN, W. E. PARKIN & J. K. SHISLER. 1984. *Ixodes dammini* (Acari: Ixodidae) and other ixodid ticks collected from white-tailed deer in New Jersey, USA. I. Geographical distribution and its relation to selected environmental and physical factors. J. Med. Entomol. **21:** 741–749.
6. BOWEN, G. S., T. L. SCHULZE, C. HAYNE & W. E. PARKIN. 1984. A focus of Lyme disease in Monmouth County, New Jersey. Am. J. Epidemiol. **120:** 387–394.
7. WILSON, M. L., J. F. LEVINE & A. SPIELMAN. 1984. Effect of deer reduction on abundance of the deer tick (*Ixodes dammini*). Yale J. Biol. Med. **57:** 697–705.
8. BOSLER, E. M., B. G. ORMISTON, J. L. COLEMAN, J. P. HANRAHAN & J. L. BENACH. 1984. Prevalence of the Lyme disease spirochete in populations of white-tailed deer and white-footed mice. Yale J. Biol. Med. **57:** 651–659.
9. SPIELMAN, A., C. M. CLIFFORD, J. PIESMAN & M. D. CORWIN. 1979. Human babesiosis on Nantucket Island, USA: Description of the vector *Ixodes (Ixodes) dammini,* n. sp. (Acarina: Ixodidae). J. Med. Entomol. **15:** 218–234.
10. SPIELMAN, A., M. L. WILSON, J. F. LEVINE & J. PIESMAN. 1985. Ecology of *Ixodes dammini*-borne human babesiosis and Lyme disease. Ann. Rev. Entomol. **30:** 439–460.
11. WILSON, M. L. 1986. Reduced abundance of adult *Ixodes dammini* (Acari: Ixodidae) following destruction of vegetation. J. Econ. Entomol. **79:** 693–696.
12. MATHER, T. N., J. M. C. RIBEIRO & A. SPIELMAN. 1987. Lyme disease and babesiosis: Acaricide focused on potentially infected ticks. Am. J. Trop. Med. Hyg. **33:** 609–614.
13. SCHULZE, T. L., W. M. MCDEVITT, W. E. PARKIN & J. K. SHISLER. 1987. Effectiveness of two insecticides in controlling *Ixodes dammini* (Acari: Ixodidae) following an outbreak of Lyme disease in New Jersey. J. Med. Entomol. **24:** 420–424.

14. SCHULZE, T. L., G. S. BOWEN, E. M. BOSLER, M. F. LAKAT, W. E. PARKIN, R. ALTMAN, B. G. ORMISTON & J. K. SHISLER. 1984. *Amblyomma americanum:* A potential vector of Lyme disease in New Jersey. Science **224:** 601–603.

15. SCHULZE, T. L., G. S. BOWEN, M. F. LAKAT, W. E. PARKIN & J. K. SHISLER. 1986. Seasonal abundance and host utilization of *Ixodes dammini* (Acari: Ixodidae) and other ixodid ticks from an endemic Lyme disease focus in New Jersey. J. Med. Entomol. **23:** 105–109.

16. KUSER, K. E. & L. J. WOLGAST. 1983. Deer roadkill increases with no-firearms-discharge law. Bull. N. J. Acad. Sci. **28:** 71–72.

Prospects for Suppressing Transmission of Lyme Disease[a]

ANDREW SPIELMAN

Department of Tropical Public Health
Harvard School of Public Health
Boston, Massachusetts 02115

HOST ASSOCIATIONS

Not until the last few years has a basic understanding of the mode of transmission and the host relationships of the Lyme disease spirochete in eastern North America begun to emerge. Soon after the first foci of human disease were recognized,[1] epidemiological evidence suggested its zoonotic nature and the role of an *Ixodes* tick vector.[2] Experimental evidence then being reported implicated the tick as the vector of the outbreak of human babesiosis that had recently begun to affect the residents of various nearby islands.[3] This vector, soon to be named *I. dammini*,[4] had previously been known to infest only one of these islands. An extraordinary event was occurring; the health of numerous people had progressively become threatened by two new zoonoses.[5,6] Work on the epidemiology of *Babesia microti* was facilitated by precise knowledge of its etiology[7]; *I. dammini* was demonstrated to be the vector of this tick, deer the definitive host, and white-footed mice the reservoir of the piroplasm. Similar advances in Lyme disease research, however, did not take place until Burgdorfer's seminal discovery of its spirochetal etiology.[8] Although theoretical arguments anticipated that the host relationships of the agent of Lyme disease would be similar to those of the babesial agent,[9] measures designed to prevent this spirochetosis depended upon rigorous and more detailed knowledge.

Vectors

The original demonstration of the spirochetal etiology of Lyme disease was based on the discovery of the agent in the lumen of the gut of *I. dammini,* thereby supporting the epidemiological inference that this tick served as vector.[8] Indeed, prevalence of naturally infected ticks correlated with prevalence of Lyme disease in people.[10-12] Wherever human infections clustered in space and time in the northeastern and north-central part of the United States, *I. dammini* was abundant. The agent was present on nearby islands only where the tick was present. Ultimately, vector competence was demonstrated in the laboratory.[13]

Evidence implicating a variety of vectors in addition to *Ixodes* ticks has been advanced, as has the proposition that there is no vector at all. One such argument depends upon records of the appearance of a characteristic erythema migrans lesion near a point on a person's skin that was bitten by some arthropod. These include suggestions that various ticks, tabanid flies, and mosquitoes may serve as vectors. Of course, the cited bite may merely have served as a point of focal proliferation of

[a]This work was supported in part by NIAID grant no. A1 19693 and a gift from David Arnold.

spirochetes that were inoculated by some less obvious nymphal *I. dammini*. Spirochetes, apparently identical to *B. burgdorferi*, may be found in the heads of insects. No known portal of exit exists for microorganisms sequestered within this body section, however. Vector competence has thus not been demonstrated. Finally, antispirochetal antibody was found in mice caged with other mice that were infected by the spirochete.[14] The epidemiological relevance of this observation has not been established. In any event, nymphal *Ixodes* ticks, which serve as highly effective vectors of the agent, satisfy all known epidemiological requirements for the zoonosis as it exists in nature. Other modes of transmission, if any, might serve some marginal role.

Deer

The presence of numerous deer in eastern and central North America appears to define the distribution of *I. dammini* and of the zoonoses that it transmits.[6] Both Lyme disease and babesiosis are extant solely where these spectacular animals are abundant and have only occurred after the recent onset of their continuing proliferation. Deer, which are parasitized abundantly by all stages of this tick, appear to be the sole hosts to the adult stage in intensely infested island sites where alternative hosts are absent.[15] Although these ticks attach to a variety of mammals, including opposums and fox as well as various domestic animals and people,[4,16] only deer are sufficiently abundant and sufficiently parasitized to explain the intensity of the observed infestations of these ticks. On islands, the abundance of the tick correlates with the abundance of deer,[17] and neither zoonosis nor these ticks occur where deer are absent.[18] These zoonoses are new because deer are new, and reproduction by the vector depends upon deer.

Mice

Various forms of evidence implicate the white-footed mouse, *Peromyscus leucopus*, as the reservoir host for the agent of Lyme disease. Immature *I. dammini* most abundantly parasitize this rodent, and it is far more abundant in zoonotic sites than any other animal.[19] White-footed mice readily became infected after being bitten by infected ticks.[13] They suffered no apparent pathology and remained highly infectious to larval ticks for periods of time that approach their life-span in nature. Virtually all mice in an enzootic site were infected, and prevalence of infection in ticks correlated with frequency of attachment to mice.[20] At this site, 45% of questing nymphs were infected, and spirochetes were found in 65% of nymphs that developed from larvae taken from mice. This prevalence value serves as a benchmark for evaluating the zoonotic contribution of other indigenous animals. Because other "reservoir" animals presumably would infect less than this "benchmark" proportion of ticks, their presence would serve to reduce the force of transmission. Less than 1% of ticks in nature appear to inherit infection.[21] Although a few infected ticks have been taken from ground-feeding birds,[22] their reservoir contribution may be "zooprophylactic," and their vagility might serve to disperse ticks away from zoonotic foci. Thus, as with *B. microti*, transmission of the Lyme disease spirochete appears to depend on the specific association existing between white-footed mice and immature *I. dammini*.

GEOGRAPHICAL LIMITS

Because *I. dammini* has only recently invaded mainland portions of North America, it is difficult to anticipate its eventual geographical limits.[6] The earliest intense infestations that were recognized in the eastern part of the United States were coastal, and this led to speculation that the species range may depend upon some geographical or climatic factor. Of course, the presence of an intense north-central focus, where the climate is particularly harsh, argues persuasively that the tick can withstand conditions existing throughout the East. Indeed, new infestations have recently been reported well inland and to the north of the original sites. As discussed, the presence of abundant deer appears to be a necessary prerequisite for an infestation, but other animals may tend to exclude these ticks if they become sensitized to being bitten.

INTERVENTION METHODS

Personal Protection

Personal protection against the agent of Lyme disease can take the form of avoiding particular sites at certain times of year. In regions in which the infection is known to be endemic in the United States, the presence of deer serves as a useful marker for judging degree of risk.[15,18,22-24] Indeed, their abundance correlates with that of the tick[17] as well as point prevalence of human infection.[41] Daily sighting of deer from a home implies considerable risk to the householders, while few infections occur among residents of nearby homes from which deer rarely are seen. The season of greatest risk is limited to the months in which the nymphal stage of the vector is most abundant. The month of June is most dangerous to the exposed individual.[24,25] Many more people visit infested sites during July and August, however, thereby explaining the somewhat delayed epidemic curve seen in summer communities.[26,27] Certain people may become exposed to infection during fall and winter when exposed to the adult stage of the vector tick. In this manner, casual observation can inform residents of sites and seasons in which precautions should be taken.

Individuals who become aware that they have been exposed to brush-covered, deer-infested sites during the early part of the summer should inspect their bodies periodically in order to detect and remove any attached ticks. The spirochete disseminates from the gut of previously infected nymphs at about 2 days after attachment to a host.[28] They are then salivated into the host during the third day thereafter. If the tick is removed (by gentle traction) before this time, infection is aborted.[29] Once a person has become sensitized to these ticks, itching evident at the point of attachment will tend to aid in their discovery. Thus, daily inspection will provide alert, keen-sighted people with two opportunities to detect infected nymphs before infection has occurred.

Chemical means are available to protect individual residents of deer-infested sites from Lyme disease. Although presumptive drug administration has not yet been evaluated, certain medically qualified residents place their families on prophylactic penicillin during tick season or dose them liberally at first sign of tick bite or illness. The measure may be effective. Less controversial is the use of permethrin to repel ticks that come in contact with treated clothing.[30] This pesticide appears to be more effective than are other known repellants. Clothing must be worn, however, throughout the period of exposure in tick-infested sites. Highly motivated people can gain a measure of personal protection against Lyme disease.

Residual Applications of Acaricide

Broad-scale distribution of residual acaricides has been considered as a measure for reducing the abundance of the ticks that transmit the agent of Lyme disease, and one such application has been reported.[31] Nonfed adult ticks were considered to be the stage most vulnerable to such treatment because they quest exposed on vegetation well above ground level and they may do so over a span of many months. The leaves of deciduous vegetation will have fallen, and little new growth will appear until spring. Nymphal or larval ticks, on the other hand, tend to be concealed within the nests of rodents and to quest during spring and summer beneath foliage that is renewed constantly. Acaricide "aimed at the immature stages will achieve limited success because these stages tend to quest at ground level when foliage is abundant."[31] In any event, a single episode of spraying, applied during November, appeared to reduce the abundance of adult *I. dammini* questing throughout the winter. Although fewer adult ticks would attach to deer in treated sites, engorged ticks detaching from these hosts might be relatively invulnerable to acaricidal applications. The point-specific effect of residual acaricides on subsequent generations of vector ticks and on the intensity of transmission of Lyme disease has not been described. The efficacy of such nonfocused applications, which would be profligate of environmentally objectionable chemical, remains unproved.

Burning and Brush Clearing

Although removal of vegetation remains an option in efforts to protect people against Lyme disease, the effects may be complex. In the event that mice become displaced from denuded land in a manner that permits the immature ticks to remain, episodes of increased transmission may result. Indeed, nymphal *I. dammini* tended to be extraordinarily abundant on freshly mown land on Nantucket Island and in West Yarmouth in Massachusetts (unpublished observation). They readily attached to people's clothing and tended to be unusually numerous on cloth-flags dragged over the ground. Eventually, the force of transmission in such sites would be reduced, but not before a period of increased risk of human exposure might be expected. On the other hand, brush might be burnt in order to destroy the nymphal stage of the vector when it first begins to quest, thereby offering residents of the site an element of prompt protection against Lyme disease.

Springtime burning and mowing of brush in an infested region in coastal Massachusetts recently has been reported.[32] Although the abundance of questing adult ticks in cleared sites appeared subsequently to have been reduced, the effect upon the force of transmission of Lyme disease was not described. One logically might anticipate an improvement in human health where a long-term program of brush-clearing maintains a site free of the vegetation in which mice become numerous. The effect, however, remains to be demonstrated.

Biological Agents

It may be that the abundance of vector *Ixodes* is regulated by predators or parasites. A spider, for example, was seen feeding on a larval *I. dammini* in eastern Massachusetts (Yuval, unpublished observation), and various ants destroy any life-cycle stage when confined together in cages (unpublished). Factors that naturally regulate the abundance of *Ixodes* ticks remain largely unknown.

An early attempt at biological control involved an introduction of a chalcid wasp onto Naushon Island, in eastern Massachusetts.[33] This colony of *Hunterellus hookeri* was established from French *I. ricinus*, reared in the US in *Dermacentor andersoni*, and released with the objective of reducing the abundance of *D. variabilis*. Although these wasps, which are now well established on the island, are presumed to be descended from this original release population, an element of uncertainty remains.[34] In any case, local infestations, both of *D. variabilis* and *I. dammini,* remain intense. Nearly 40% of nymphal *I. dammini* are infected by the wasp, and such ticks die following engorgement. Interestingly, wasp-infected ticks appear not to be infected by spirochetes, and prevalence of the spirochete in ticks is about half that found where the wasp is absent or rare. Barring the possibility that the wasp oviposits solely into ticks that are attached to noncompetent hosts, the wasp may abort development of the spirochete. Perhaps adaptations of Larrousse's experiment provide some hope for locally reducing the intensity of transmission of Lyme disease.

Deprivation of Access to Hosts

The root of the Lyme disease problem in North America may be attacked by measures directed against the deer that serve as the main hosts for the adult stage of the vector tick. Because the present emergence of both *Ixodes*-transmitted zoonoses has its origins in the recent proliferation of these animals,[22] the reciprocal effect should follow local diminution of the deer herd. This supposition was tested in a 6-year experiment conducted on Great Island in West Yarmouth, Massachusetts. Initially, about half of the deer indigenous to this 240-ha peninsula were destroyed.[35] The abundance of larval ticks, however, appeared not to be affected during the summer thereafter. Accordingly, virtually the entire herd was destroyed during the following winter. In all, 54 deer were taken, leaving only one or two survivors. During each of the three successive summers, the abundance of larval *I. dammini* diminished. Nymphal ticks also gradually diminished in number, while there was an apparent increase on nearby Nantucket Island where deer were allowed to proliferate. Interestingly, questing adult *I. dammini* became extraordinarily abundant thereafter in the deer-removal site. The protective effect was somewhat slower than anticipated, but the attempt was successful. A causal relationship between deer abundance and that of vector ticks became evident.

Deprivation of definitive hosts similarly affects the abundance of European *I. ricinus*.[36,37] In a region in which the adult stage of this tick depends entirely on sheep, pasture rotation was followed without delay by a sharp local reduction in the abundance of larvae.

Destruction of deer to protect human health appears to be practical solely under special circumstances. Where the site to be protected lacks deer-proof boundaries, immigration may rapidly renew the deer herd, particularly if the deer are destroyed solely within that site and during a narrow span of time. Unless deer are shot virtually to extinction, the measure may prove insufficient. Then too, such a technically difficult and politically and ethically questionable operation may be difficult to accomplish. Even if the result can not confidently be predicted, a carefully managed deer herd, where feasible, seems prudent.

Acaricide Placed on Hosts

We attempted to place acaricide on the deer that serve as the main definitive hosts of *I. dammini,* but without success. In our initial effort on Great Island, we attached rabon-impregnated plastic disks to the ears of about 20 of these animals. We anticipated that attached adult *I. dammini* would be destroyed in much the same manner as are the various kinds of ticks that feed on similarly treated cattle. Each deer was treated at great expense. They were captured in eight box-traps (3-m long), driven by as many as 99 volunteers into a boma-type corral (28 m in diameter) or into a drop-net (0.5 km in length). Finally, in order to improve efficiency, deer were baited with apples and tranquilized by a staff of three veterinarians using Palmer rifle-fired syringe darts containing M-99. Each dart carried a homing device to assist in finding tranquilized animals. Acaricidal tags and color-coded plastic streamers were placed in both ears of captured deer. Some six of these deer that were recaptured were parasitized by as many ticks as were deer captured for the first time. Unlike those that feed on cattle, these ticks were distributed generally over the deers' bodies and particularly on the ventral surface remote from the ears. The attempt was abandoned. We considered applying systemic acaricide in the form of ivermectin-filled apples, but rejected that alternative because this acaricide was not then licensed for use on animals that might be eaten by people. Destruction of deer by shooting remained the sole option.

Our finding that white-footed mice serve as the main reservoir host both of the Lyme disease and the babesial agents[9,13,19,20,38] encouraged us to attempt to place acaricide on or around mice. The observation that *Ixodes* ticks detach diurnally from their nocturnal hosts caused us to focus on the nests of these rodents, where the infected portion of the tick population presumably concentrates.[39] These mice avidly harvest fiber from their surroundings and would utilize any such acaricide-impregnated cotton as a lining for their nests. Permethrin was chosen to impregnate the cotton because of its powerful acaricidal effect, its environmental acceptability, and its stability and sorbtive properties in cotton. Treated cotton was placed in tubular dispensers and distributed at 1-m intervals in grids placed across the site to be protected. A total of 27.1 g of permethrin would be distributed in some 82 dispensers placed on each hectare of continuously treated land (0.04 lb per acre). Where 1-acre plots had been treated, only a tenth as many ticks infested mice as in nontreated sites. Only a quarter of the treated mice were infested as compared to virtually universal infection in nontreated sites. One year later, less than half as many nymphs could be flagged from the treated sites as from nontreated sites, and of these, less than half as many were infected by the spirochete as in the nontreated sites. In all, risk of human infection had been reduced by 82%, even with the immigration that must have taken place around the edges of the treated plots of land.

Another system had been developed to deliver acaricide to the rodent hosts of immature *D. variabilis*.[40] This modification of the "bait box" system employs diazinone-impregnated fabric placed in tubular holders and baited with peanut derivatives. The fur of any rodents entering these tubes becomes contaminated by the acaricide such that any attached ticks would be destroyed.

The force of transmission was even more markedly reduced where the permethrin-treated cotton had been placed across a larger plot of land.[42] Mouse-resistant margins were provided by the open marshland and road that enclosed the site. During the subsequent season, only 1 of 40 captured mice was infested, and only by three ticks. In contrast, 33 of 34 mice captured in the nontreated site were infested by a mean of 20 ticks per mouse. One year later, only 0.8 infected nymphs could be collected per hour of flagging in the treated site as compared to 21.4 in the nontreated site. The permethrin distribution system appeared to be highly effective.

Cardboard tubes containing permethrin-impregnated cotton[b] have now been approved for distribution in several states in the northeastern United States, and a

---

[b] EDS.' NOTE: The author is an officer of a firm that distributes such a product.

commercial operation has been established that manufactures and markets the device.

PROSPECTS FOR SUPPRESSION

A series of options for suppressing the transmission of Lyme disease have become available. Individuals residing in "high-risk" sites between June and August should remove attached ticks daily and can use permethrin-based clothing impregnants, as well as antibiotics, as appropriate. Where feasible, rigorous management of the local deer herd may be effective. Virtual eradication may be necessary, however, and the protective effect slow in developing. Permethrin-impregnated fiber made available to mice as bedding material appears to reduce transmission markedly.

SUMMARY

A variety of methods have been developed to prevent human infection by the Lyme disease spirochete in the northeastern United States, mainly based on the observations that nymphal *Ixodes dammini* serve as vector, that deer serve as hosts for the reproductive stage of this tick, that white-footed mice serve as the reservoir of infection, and that nymphs are most abundant in early summer and must attach for 2 days before infection is transmitted. Methods for personal protection included seasonal avoidance of infested sites, the use of repellants, and prompt removal of attached ticks. Destruction of mouse habitat, but not of mice, was locally effective. Nondestructive acaricidal treatment of deer proved ineffective, but the elimination of these hosts resulted in reduced transmission after several years. Treatment of mice by means of acaricide-impregnated bedding material effectively reduced transmission.

REFERENCES

1. STEERE, A. C., S. E. MALAWISTA & D. R. SNYDMAN. 1977. Lyme arthritis, an epidemic of oligoarticular arthritis in children and adults in three Connecticut communities. Arthritis Rheum. **20:** 7–17.
2. STEERE, A. C., T. F. BRODERICK & S. E. MALAWISTA. 1978. Erythema chronicum migrans and Lyme arthritis: epidemiological evidence for a tick vector. Am. J. Epidemiol. **108:** 312–321.
3. SPIELMAN, A. 1976. Human babesiosis on Nantucket Island: Transmission by nymphal *Ixodes* ticks. Am. J. Trop. Med. Hyg. **25:** 781–787.
4. SPIELMAN, A., C. M. CLIFFORD, J. PIESMAN & M. D. CORWIN. 1979. Human babesiosis on Nantucket Island, USA: description of the vector, *Ixodes (Ixodes) dammini,* n.sp. (Acarina: Ixodidae). J. Med. Entomol. **15:** 218–234.
5. DAMMIN, G. J., A. SPIELMAN, J. L. BENACH & J. PIESMAN. 1981. The rising incidence of clinical *Babesia microti* infection. Hum. Pathol. **12:** 398–400.
6. SPIELMAN, A., M. L. WILSON, J. F. LEVINE & J. PIESMAN. 1985. Ecology of *Ixodes dammini*-borne human babesiosis and Lyme disease. Ann. Rev. Entomol. **30:** 439–460.
7. WESTERN, K. A., G. D. BENSON, G. R. HEALY & M. G. SCHULZ. 1970. Babesiosis in a Massachusetts resident. N. Engl. J. Med. **283:** 854–856.
8. BURGDORFER, W., A. G. BARBOUR, S. F. HAYES, J. L. BENACH, E. GRUNWALDT & J. P. DAVIS. 1982. Lyme disease–a tick-borne spirochetosis? Science **216:** 1317–1319.
9. SPIELMAN, A., J. F. LEVINE & M. L. WILSON. 1984. Vectorial capacity of North American *Ixodes* ticks. Yale. J. Biol. Med. **57:** 507–513.

10. BOSLER, E. M., J. L. COLEMAN, J. L. BENACH, D. A. MASSEY & J. P. HANRAHAN. 1983. Natural distribution of the *Ixodes dammini* spirochete. Science **220:** 321–322.

11. MAGNARELLI, L. A., J. F. ANDERSON, W. BURGDORFER & A. CHAPPELL. 1984. Parasitism by *Ixodes dammini* (Acari: Ixodidae) and antibodies to spirochetes in mammals at Lyme disease foci in Connecticut, USA. J. Med. Entomol. **21:** 52–57.

12. PIESMAN, J., T. N. MATHER, S. R. TELFORD III & A. SPIELMAN. 1986. Concurrent *Borrelia burgdorferi* and *Babesia microti* infection in nymphal *Ixodes dammini*. J. Clin. Microbiol. **24:** 446–447.

13. DONAHUE, J. G., J. PIESMAN & A. SPIELMAN. 1987. Reservoir competence of white-footed mice for Lyme disease spirochetes. Am. J. Trop. Med. Hyg. **36:** 92–96.

14. BURGESS, E. C., T. E. AMUNDSON, J. P. DAVIS, R. A. KASLOW & R. EDELMAN. 1986. Experimental inoculation of *Peromyscus* spp. with *Borrelia burgdorferi:* evidence of contact transmission. Am. J. Trop. Med. Hyg. **35:** 355–359.

15. PIESMAN, J., A. SPIELMAN, P. ETKIND, T. K. REUBUSH II & D. JURANEK. 1979. Role of deer in the epizootiology of *Babesia microti* in Massachusetts, USA. J. Med. Entomol. **15:** 537–540.

16. MAGNARELLI, L.A., J. F. ANDERSON & A. CHAPPELL. 1984. Antibodies to spirochetes in white-tailed deer and prevalence of infected ticks from foci of Lyme disease in Connecticut. J. Wildl. Dis. **20:** 21–26.

17. WILSON, M. L., G. H. ADLER & A. SPIELMAN. 1985. Correlation between abundance of deer and that of the deer tick, *Ixodes dammini* (Acari: Ixodidae). Ann. Entomol. Soc. Am. **78:** 172–176.

18. ANDERSON, J. F., R. C. JOHNSON, L. A. MAGNARELLI, F. W. HYDE & J. E. MYERS. 1987. Prevalence of *Borrelia burgdorferi* and *Babesia microti* in mice on islands inhabited by white-tailed deer. Appl. Environ. Microbiol. **53:** 892–894.

19. SPIELMAN, A., P. ETKIND, J. PIESMAN, T. K. REUBUSH II, D. JURANEK & M. S. JACOBS. 1981. Reservoir hosts of human babesiosis on Nantucket Island. Am. J. Trop. Med. Hyg. **39:** 560–665.

20. LEVINE, J. F., M. L. WILSON & A. SPIELMAN. 1985. Mice as reservoirs of the Lyme disease spirochete. Am. J. Trop. Med. Hyg. **34:** 355–360.

21. PIESMAN, J., J. G. DONAHUE, T. N. MATHER & A. SPIELMAN. 1986. Transovarially acquired Lyme disease spirochetes (*Borrelia burgdorferi*) in field-collected larval *Ixodes dammini* (Acari: Ixodidae). J. Med. Entomol. **23:** 219.

22. ANDERSON, J. F., R. C. JOHNSON, L. A. MAGNARELLI & F. W. HYDE. 1986. 1984. Involvement of birds in the epidemiology of the Lyme disease agent *Borrelia burgdorferi*. Infect. Immun. **51:** 394–396.

23. MAIN, A. J., K. O. SPRANCE, K. O. KLOTER & S. E. BROWN. 1981. *Ixodes dammini* (Acari: Ixodidae) on white-tailed deer (*Odocoileus virginianus*) in Connecticut. J. Med. Entomol. **18:** 487–492.

24. PIESMAN, J., T. N. MATHER, G. J. DAMMIN, S. R. TELFORD III, C. C. LASTAVICA & A. SPIELMAN. 1987. Seasonal variation of transmission risk of Lyme disease and human babesiosis. Am. J. Epidem. **126.** In press.

25. WILSON, M. L. & A. SPIELMAN. 1985. Seasonal activity of immature *Ixodes dammini* (Acari: Ixodidae). J. Med. Entomol. **22:** 408–414.

26. HANRAHAN, J. P., J. L. BENACH, J. L. COLEMAN, E. M. BOSLER, D. L. MORSE, D. J. CAMERON, R. EDELMAN & R. A. KASLOW. 1984. Incidence and cumulative frequency of endemic Lyme disease in a community. J. Infect. Dis. **150:** 489–496.

27. STEERE, A. C., E. TAYLOR, M. L. WILSON, J. F. LEVINE & A. SPIELMAN. 1986. Longitudinal assessment of the clinical and epidemiological features of Lyme disease in a defined population. J. Infect. Dis. **154:** 295–300.

28. RIBEIRO, J. M. C., T. N. MATHER, J. PIESMAN & A. SPIELMAN. 1987. Dissemination and salivary delivery of Lyme disease spirochetes in vector ticks (Acari: Ixodidae). J. Med. Entomol. **24:** 201–205.

29. PIESMAN, J., T. N. MATHER, R. J. SINKSY & A. SPIELMAN. 1987. Duration of tick attachment and *Borrelia burgdorferi* transmission. J. Clin. Microbiol. **25:** 557–558.

30. SCHRECK, C. E., E. L. SNODDY & A. SPIELMAN. 1986. Pressurized sprays of permethrin or deet on military clothing for personal protection against *Ixodes dammini* (Acari: Ixodidae). J. Med. Entomol. **23:** 396–399.

31. SCHULZE, T. L., W. M. MCDEVITT, W. E. PARKIN & J. K. SHISLER. 1987. Effectiveness of two insecticides in controlling *Ixodes dammini* (Acari: Ixodidae) following an outbreak of Lyme disease in New Jersey. J. Med. Entomol. **24:** 420–424.

32. WILSON, M. H. 1986. Reduced abundance of adult *Ixodes dammini* (Acari: Ixodidae) following destruction of vegetation. J. Econ. Entomol. **79:** 693–696.

33. LARROUSSE, F., A. G. KING & S. B. WOLBACH. 1928. The overwintering in Massachusetts of *Ixodiphagus caucurteri*. Science **67:** 351–353.

34. MATHER, T. N., J. PIESMAN & A. SPIELMAN. 1987. Absence of spirochetes (*Borrelia burgdorferi*) and piroplasms (*Babesia microti*) in deer ticks (*Ixodes dammini*) parasitized by chalcid wasps (*Hunterellus hookeri*). Med. Vet. Entomol. **1:** 3–8.

35. WILSON, M. L., J. F. LEVINE & A. SPIELMAN. 1984. Effect of deer reduction on abundance of the deer tick (*Ixodes dammini*). Yale J. Biol. Med. **57:** 697–705.

36. STEELE, G. M. & S. E. RANDOLPH. 1985. An experimental evaluation of conventional control measures against the sheep tick, *Ixodes ricinus* (L.) (Acari: Ixodidae). I. A unimodal seasonal activity pattern. Bull. Entomol. Res. **75:** 489–499.

37. RANDOLPH, S. E. & G. M. STEELE. 1985. An experimental evaluation of conventional control measures against the sheep tick, *Ixodes ricinus* (L.) (Acari: Ixodidae). II. The dynamics of the tick-host interaction. Bull. Entomol. Res. **75:** 501–518.

38. HEALY, G. R., A. SPIELMAN & N. GLEASON. 1976. Human babesiosis: Reservoir of infection on Nantucket Island. Science **192:** 479–480.

39. MATHER, T. N., J. M. C. RIBEIRO & A. SPIELMAN. 1987. Lyme disease and babesiosis: Acaricide focused on potentially infected ticks. Am. J. Trop. Med. Hyg. **36:** 609–614.

40. SONENSHINE, D. E. & G. HAINES. 1985. A convenient method for controlling populations of the American dog tick, *Dermacentor variabilis* (Acari: Ixodidae) in the natural environment. J. Med. Entomol. **22:** 577–583.

41. LASTAVICA, C. C., M. L. WILSON, V. P. BERARDI & A. SPIELMAN. 1988. Landscape progression of Lyme disease where transmission is intense. This volume.

42. MATHER, T. N., J. M. C. RIBEIRO, S. I. MOORE & A. SPIELMAN. 1988. Reducing transmission of Lyme disease spirochetes in a suburban setting. This volume.

Host Responses to *Borrelia burgdorferi* in Dogs and Horses

EDWARD M. BOSLER,[a] DANIEL P. COHEN,[b]
TERRY L. SCHULZE,[c] CHRISTOPHER OLSEN,[d]
WILLIAM BERNARD,[b] AND BARRY LISSMAN[e]

[a]*New York State Department of Health
Stony Brook, New York 11794*

[b]*University of Pennsylvania Veterinary School
Philadelphia, Pennsylvania 19104*

[c]*New Jersey State Department of Health
Trenton, New Jersey 08625*

[d]*North Fork Animal Hospital
Southold, New York 11971*

[e]*Sachem Animal Hospital
Holbrook, New York 11741*

INTRODUCTION

Since *Borrelia burgdorferi* was originally isolated from the blood of a febrile lame dog residing in an endemic area on Long Island, New York,[1] Lyme borreliosis has been recognized as an emerging disease in dogs and horses. Clinical studies show that dogs develop arthritis with *B. burgdorferi* infection.[2] Both serologic[3] and pathogen isolation studies[4] demonstrate that canines are infected in endemic areas of human disease.[1,5] In these studies between 34% and 42% of asymptomatic dogs were found to be seroreactive to *B. burgdorferi*. Asymptomatic dogs were often found to be more reactive than animals expressing clinical symptoms.[2,4,5]

Antibodies against *B. burgdorferi* have been detected in 12 of 50 (24%) horses sampled in New England[6] and a case of arthritis and panuveitis associated with *B. burgdorferi* infection has been reported.[7] The purpose of this study was to evaluate the host immune response in dogs and horses to *B. burgdorferi*. Humoral antibody levels and spirochetal antigen recognition by immunoglobulins were examined.

MATERIALS AND METHODS

Organisms

The isolate of *B. burgdorferi* used in this study was the Shelter Island, New York strain (ATCC 35210),[8] which has been in continuous passage in our laboratory since 1982. The cultures were maintained in serum-free, modified Kelly's medium[9] incubated at 33°C in 1-liter glass bottles. Spirochete densities reached up to 5×10^8 per milliliter after 4 days of growth. Spirochetes were harvested by centrifugation at 7000 ×g for 20 minutes followed by four washes in phosphate-buffered saline (PBS, pH 7.4) supplemented with 5 mM $MgCl_2$ at the same rate of centrifugation. Protein concentration was estimated and this stock antigen frozen at −70°C until needed.

221

Canine Sera

Serial samples collected over a 4-month period from the initial canine Lyme disease case in New York[1] were tested as reference standards for a known infected animal. This febrile spirochetemic dog presented with migratory lameness, pain and swelling in the carpal joints, and had concurrent humoral IgG antibodies to *B. burgdorferi*. The canine had no previous history of joint problems. Symptoms resolved following a 10-day course of ampicillin (500 mg t.i.d.).

Additional sera were derived from a clinically and temporally characterized serum bank submitted by veterinarians in New York and New Jersey since 1984 for either diagnostic evaluation or as part of serosurveys.[5] In this study symptomatic and asymptomatic animals that were seronegative and seropositive were included. Dogs were diagnosed by veterinarians and considered clinical if the animal had one or more symptoms compatible with Lyme disease. Lameness, pain and swelling of the joints (particularly polyarticular and migratory), and fever were the major symptoms reported. Aggressiveness, inappetance, lethargy, stupor, incontinence, and renal problems prior to or following lameness were also reported in dogs believed to be infected with *B. burgdorferi*. Asymptomatic dogs had no current symptoms of *B. burgdorferi* infection and were sampled in both nonendemic and endemic areas. Asymptomatic dogs from laboratory colonies and nonendemic tick-free areas were considered normal (negative) controls. Canines used by the Suffolk County Police Department (eastern Long Island, NY) are thoroughly examined every 4–5 months. Since these animals work in endemic locations, each was screened for serological reactivity to *B. burgdorferi* in November 1986 and again in March 1987. Serial samples were collected for most individuals.

Equine Sera

Serial samples were collected from a 7-year-old Arabian mare diagnosed as having Lyme disease. The horse presented with depression, partial anorexia, fever and migratory polyarticular pain, and swelling of the fetlock and hock joints on 6/12/85, only 2 months after arriving on Shelter Island from a nonendemic tick-free area in upstate New York. There was no evidence of trauma or history of recent respiratory infection. Serum IgG levels to *B. burgdorferi* were elevated and no humoral antibody was detected to *Leptospira interogans* serovars. Ampicillin was administered (3 g i.v.), followed by penicillin G for 14 days. On 6/15/85 the mare's right hind fetlock, metacarpal region and hock were swollen for 36 hours while on 6/17/85 the right fore fetlock became swollen for 18 hours. No additional episodes of joint involvement or lameness were observed from 6/18/85.

Foals from a breeding farm located in an endemic area of New Jersey were presenting with a newly recognized syndrome involving swelling of the ankles.[10] Serial samples were acquired from certain of these horses from approximately 8 weeks after birth until they were yearlings (1 January).

At the New Bolton Center (University of Pennsylvania School of Veterinary Medicine) a Shetland pony was inoculated with a triturated tick suspension containing live *B. burgdorferi*[10] on 12/9/87. The pony was continuously housed in a tick-free barn. During the first 2 months, daily blood samples were drawn and physical examinations performed. From months 3 to 6 examinations and serial blood collections were done weekly. The pony was reinoculated with a recent tick-derived culture (passage 2) of *B. burgdorferi* and sampled weekly for an additional 2 months. During the course of the study no overt clinical manifestations of *B. burgdorferi* infection were observed.

ELISA

Assays were performed as originally described by Engvall and Perlmann[11] as modified by Russell *et al.*,[12] with the additonal modifications found in Coleman *et al.*[13] Flat-bottomed 96-well polystyrene assay plates (Becton-Dickinson, Oxnard, CA) were coated with 5 μg/ml of whole *B. burgdorferi* sonicated antigen in 0.1-M carbonate buffer (pH 9.6) and held at 4°C for 18 hours. Plates were washed three times with PBS-Tween (phosphate-buffered saline, pH 7.2, containing 0.05% Tween 20) and stored at -70°C until used. Prior to use plates were allowed to thaw for 15 minutes. Serum was diluted 1 : 500 in PBS-Tween containing 0.5% bovine serum albumin. One hundred μl of each sample was aliquoted to duplicate wells and incubated at 37°C for 1 hour, after which each plate was washed three times with PBS-Tween. One hundred μl of alkaline phosphatase or horseradish peroxidase labeled goat derived affinity purified dog or horse IgG (heavy and light chain) or IgM (μ-chain specific) antisera (Kirkegaard and Perry Laboratories, Gaithersburg, MD) was added to each well and incubated at 37°C for 3 hours. Plates were additionally washed three times with PBS-Tween and incubated at 37°C for 1 hour with 100 μl of substrate (*p*-nitrophenyl phosphate; Sigma, St. Louis, MO) at a concentration of 2 mg/ml in 0.05 M carbonate buffer containing 0.001 M $MgCl_2$, pH 9.8. The reaction was stopped by the addition of 50 μl of 5 N NaOH to each well; optical densities (OD) were read on a MR 580 MicroELISA reader (Dynatech, Alexandria, VA) at a wavelength of 410 nm.

A serum was considered positive if its absorbance was above a cutoff value defined as the mean negative control value to which was added three standard deviations of that value.[14] ELISA values are reported as OD of sample/OD cutoff value throughout this paper. Identical enzyme-conjugated antibodies were used in all Western blots and ELISAs on individual samples.

SDS-PAGE and Western Blot Analyses

SDS-PAGE was performed using a Laemmli buffer system on a 10% discontinuous acrylamide gel under reducing conditions according to the method described by Coleman *et al.*[13] Approximately 200 μg of spirochetal proteins were loaded into a single large channel created with a blank Teflon comb in the stacking gel. Each resolving gel was 120 mm high and 0.75 mm thick. Molecular weight standards (Bethesda Research Laboratories, Gaithersburg, MD) were loaded in a separate lane on each gel.

B. burgdorferi proteins were transferred to 0.45-μm nitrocellulose membranes (Bio-Rad Laboratories, Richmond, CA) according to Towbin *et al.*[15] using a Transblot (Bio-Rad) for 18 hours at 200 mA of constant current. Each gel yielded approximately 25 papers 3 mm wide. Strips were incubated in blocking solution (BS)[13] at 25°C for one hour. Strips were drained and overlaid with serum diluted in BS (1 : 50 for IgM and 1 : 100 for IgG) and incubated (4 hours for IgM and 2 hours for IgG). After two 15-minute washes in BS, strips were incubated for 2 hours with either alkaline-phosphatase (AP) or horseradish peroxidase (HRP) conjugated goat antibody to dog or horse affinity purified IgM (μ-chain specific) or IgG (heavy and light chain or γ-chain specific, Kirkegaard and Perry Laboratories). After washing, reactive bands were visualized by the additon of the appropriate enzyme substrates. BCIP (5-bromo-4-chloro-3-indolyl phosphate; Bio-Rad) and NBT (nitro blue tetrazolium; Bio-Rad) were used as AP substrates to obtain purple color development. The HRP substrate was 4-chloro-1-naphthol.

In certain tests biotinylated goat affinity-purified dog and horse IgG (heavy and light chain, Kirkegaard and Perry Laboratories) were used as the secondary antibodies to enhance reactions. After a 2-hour incubation (25°C) and two washes, strips were overlaid with avidin for an additional 2 hours, washed again, and the appropriate substrates added.

All Western blot reactions were stopped by immersing papers in distilled water. ELISA value are reported as OD of sample/OD cutoff value throughout this paper.

RESULTS

Dogs

IgM levels in all samples from our canine index case were considered seronegative with the possible exception of the last specimen. This sample (OD = .187/.137) was taken about 111 days following both antibiotic therapy and resolution of symptoms (TABLE 1).

All specimen IgG levels were seropositive and increased for at least 14 days. After treatment IgG levels at first decreased, then increased and remained at higher levels. Although IgM probes detected between 5 to 10 bound proteins, the 41 kDa (flagellin) was immunodominant and present in all temporal samples. Other reactions were faint and reached maximum numbers 13 days after treatment (FIG. 1). IgG detected more numerous spirochetal proteins. The number of bound proteins appeared to remain constant ($n \geq 30$) in all samples with the exception of an increase at low molecular masses (<18.4 kDa) from the first to second samples. Several days after treatment,

TABLE 1. IgM (μ Chain) and IgG (Heavy and Light Chain) ELISA Values to *B. burgdorferi* in Two IgG Seropositive Canines with Lameness

Date	Symptoms	Optical Density Values	
		IgM	IgG
Reference Case			
05/30/83	yes	.094	.260
06/03/83	yes	.124	.239
06/14/83	no	.103	.636
06/23/83	no	.031	.184
07/08/83	no	.129	.394
09/24/83	no	.187	.306
Recurrent Lameness			
12/03/83	yes	.161	.877
12/24/83	yes	.157	.731
02/24/84	no	.122	.321
10/17/84	yes	.107	.272
03/14/85	no	.146	.345
$\bar{x}$ Negative Control		.083 ± .018	.037 ± .005
Cutoff [$\bar{x} + (3 \times SD)$]		0.137	0.052

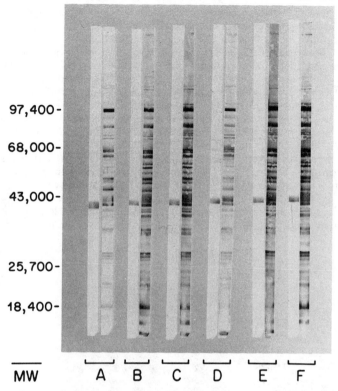

FIGURE 1. Western blots of sera from reference case of canine Lyme borreliosis.[1] For each sample date the paired lanes represent IgM and IgG in sequential order. Lanes: A, 05/30/83; B, 06/03/83; C, 06/14/83, D, 06/23/83, E, 07/08/83, F, 09/24/83.

intensity of reactions decreased with a coincident decrease in detectable humoral IgG. A subsequent rise in IgG was accompanied by an increase in intensity of blot reactions.

A 4-year-old Sheltie with no previous history of lameness or trauma-induced injury experienced acute fever, stupor, and polyarticular pain and swelling of the limbs on 12/3/83. All blood parameters were within normal ranges and a diagnosis of Lyme borreliosis was made. Fever and stupor resolved with tetracycline (250 mg b.i.d. × 10 days) and dexamethasone (250 mg b.i.d. × 1 day), but lameness persisted and treatment was extended for 10 more days. After treatment the dog was asymptomatic for about 7 months, at which time lameness reoccurred; treatment was reinitiated for 20 days. Sera were obtained during periods of acute lameness (12/3/83, 12/24/83, and 10/17/84) and during asymptomatic periods on 2/24/84 and 3/14/85. While IgG immunoglobulins were elevated in all samples, decreasing levels were observed following treatment through the onset of recurrent symptoms. Sera collected 5 months after recurrent lameness demonstrated increased IgG levels. IgM was present in decreasing amounts and once again increased with the onset of recurrent lameness (TABLE 1).

Probing with IgG exhibited a temporal pattern of numerous immunogenic proteins (FIG. 2) similar to the pattern observed in the reference case. The major IgM-bound protein appeared to be flagellin and persisted for at least 15 months after initial symptoms. Between 8 and 10 additional faintly reactive protein bands were detected during the first acute and convalescent samples; these reactions became more faint over time. The majority of less IgM immunogenic proteins were of molecular weights >41.0 kDa; three appeared to correspond to ~43-, ~66-, and ~96-kDa antigens. Very faint binding was detected at kDa's approximating Osp A (31 kDa) and Osp B (34 kDa).

All seropositive dogs with lameness associated with *B. burgdorferi* infection had IgM and IgG blot profiles similar to the reference case.

A dog being evaluated for an ear infection was IgG seroreactive (OD = .559/.029) to *B. burgdorferi*. The animal was asymptomatic (nonlame) at the time of sampling (4/85); routine examinations since 1982 failed to reveal earlier symptoms associated with Lyme disease. During the next year the dog experienced intermittent periods of self-limiting lameness. A sample drawn in 4/86 indicated that IgG levels had increased during the year (OD = .759/.029) and Lyme borreliosis was suspected. A third sample

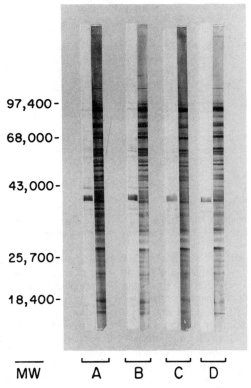

FIGURE 2. Western blots of sera from a lame seropositive dog with recurrent lameness after antibiotic treatment. For each sample date the lanes represent IgM and IgG in sequential order. Lanes: A, 12/03/83; B, 12/24/83; C, 02/24/84; D, 10/17/84.

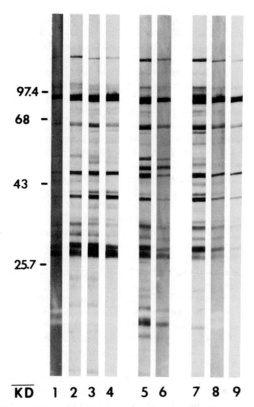

FIGURE 3. IgG Western blots of symptomatic and asymptomatic dog sera. Dog 1: 1, 4/20/85 (nonlame); 2, 05/01/86 (lame); 3, 05/05/87 (nonlame); 4, 07/25/87 (nonlame, posttreatment). Dog 2: 5, 12/27/86 (urinary incontinence); 6, (renal failure). Dog 3: 7, 11/20/86; 8, 03/03/87 (post-prophylactic antibiotics); 9, 08/05/87. No lameness was observed on any sample date yet all were seropositive. OD values: 7, 1.09/.029; 8, .690/.029; 9, .706/.029.

about a year later was increasingly more reactive (OD = 1.110/.029) when the dog was asymptomatic. On 7/7/87 the dog was treated with cortisone and amoxicillin for acute lameness in the front legs accompanied by fever and head tilt. Lameness disappeared by 7/22/87, but the animal remained febrile, was lethargic, and began to pant. Lung radiographs showed generalized pulmonary densities. A lung biopsy was inconclusive; an infection secondary to cancer was suspected. The animal expired on 7/25/87 with persistent IgG levels (OD = .854/.029) to *B. burgdorferi*. Numerous IgG immunogenic proteins were detected by Western blots during all phases of the infection, suggesting persistence of the organism (FIG. 3, lanes 1–4). The highest number of spirochetal immunogens was observed during the asymptomatic period prior to antibiotic therapy.

A 5-year-old spayed mixed breed suddenly became aggressive toward companion dogs in August 1986. Aggressive behavior continued and lameness developed on 12/3/86. Radiographs indicated soft tissue swelling of the left stifle, which was symptomatically ameliorated with injectable cortisone. Within 20 days urinary

incontinence developed and serum drawn 12/23/86 was reactive (IgG OD = .935/
.029) to *B. burgdorferi*. A second serum (1/20/87) was reactive (OD = .683/.029)
and the possibility of concurrent neurological and renal involvement with *B. burgdorferi* was considered. Amoxycillin and DES were initiated. The dog improved and
remained well until 5/7/87, at which time it was hospitalized with renal failure and
euthanized 6 days later. Postmortem examination of the kidney revealed multiple
changes, including glomerular leakage, tubular dilation, increased glomerular and
interstitial fibrosis, and local inflammation for which no etiology could be clearly
defined. Postmortem serum continued to be IgG reactive to *B. burgdorferi* (OD =
.631/.029). Western blots indicated numerous IgG reactive proteins; a decrease in
numbers of bound protein was evidenced from the acute renal phase to the postmortem
sample (FIG. 3, lanes 5 and 6).

A total of 21 asymptomatic canine members of the police force in an endemic area
were tested (10/86); 10 were retested 5 months later (3/87). No animals had a
previous or current lameness. On initial sampling 14 (66%) were IgG reactive
at ≥.576/.111; the remaining seven were seronegative (OD ≤ .068/.111). All reactive
dogs were treated with antibiotics and seven were resampled, all of which had
decreased IgG levels. In contrast, three previously negative dogs seroconverted. Blot
patterns for asymptomatic seropositive animals typically showed numerous reactive
proteins bound by IgG, as illustrated in FIGURE 3, lanes 7–9. After treatment IgG
failed to detect as many proteins, but apparent 31, 34, 41, 66, and 96 kDa entities
persisted. In the three asymptomatic dogs that seroconverted primary IgG response
was to the 41 and 96 kDa proteins, followed by the 31 and 34 kDa proteins
sequentially. One of the three seroconverting animals probed with IgG responded to
the 31 kDa but not the 41 kDa entity in the negative sample. To determine the
sequential pattern of IgG production, larger sample sizes are needed or laboratory
animals must be inoculated.

Thirty-four percent of serosurvey dogs from endemic areas of New Jersey were IgG
reactive in a previous study.[5] IgG probing in a group of these individuals illustrated
numerous bands similar to the reference case. Seven of these dogs developed clinical
Lyme arthritis within a 6-month period. A group of seronegative dogs from the same
study had 1–7 proteins bound by IgG, but no follow-ups were possible.

Normals

Normal animals, either lab reared or seronegatives from nonendemic locations,
demonstrated reactivity to some *B. burgdorferi* proteins. Both IgM and IgG probes
detected the 41 kDa protein while IgG additionally bound to a protein with an
approximate molecular mass of 43 kDa.

Horses

Clinical

The clinically diagnosed Arab mare was IgG reactive in serial samples obtained
over a 5-month period. Based on travel history from nonendemic to endemic area, the
horse was more than likely exposed to *B. burgdorferi* for the first time not more than 2
months earlier. IgG detectable antibody levels steadily declined following treatment
and resolution of symptoms from OD = .573/.052 to .104/.052. Major early IgG
immunogenic proteins appeared to have molecular masses of ~31, ~34, ~41, ~66,

and ~96 kDa. IgG bound to additional proteins for at least 3 weeks (FIG. 4); reactions were less intense after 5 months and the mare had no further episodes of joint problems.

Foals

Two foals with swollen ankles that were suspected to have *B. burgdorferi* infection were selected from another study[10] for detection of immunogens. Both animals were

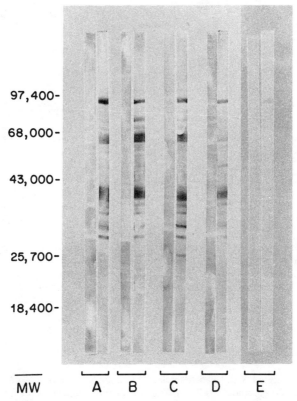

FIGURE 4. IgG Western blots of serial serum samples from a horse with polyarticular pain and swelling of hock and fetlock joints. Lanes: A, 06/13/85, joint pain and swelling; B, 06/18/85, asymptomatic; C, 07/08/85, asymptomatic postantibiotic therapy; D, 11/16/85, asymptomatic; E, normal (negative control), seronegative.

sampled serially after birth and until they reached yearling status. One foal was seroreactive (OD = .225/.051) on acute sampling while the other was only slightly reactive (OD = .074/.051). The seroreactive horse became seronegative and remained so until 6 months later when IgG levels were considered to be positive (OD = .637/.051). FIGURE 5 illustrates a sequential pattern of immunoglobulin development

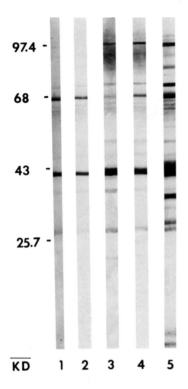

FIGURE 5. IgG Western blot of serial serum samples from a foal with edema. Lanes: 1, 07/25/86 (edema of ankles); 2, 08/04/86; 3, 08/22/86; 4, 08/27/86; 5, 01/29/87 (no edema for lanes 2–5).

in the slightly reactive foal from acute edema through the following 6 months when the animal was asymptomatic. IgM was initially bound weakly to flagellin. IgM affinity to the 41-kDa antigen apparently increases and binding also occurs to proteins of about 66 and 96 kDa. Primary IgG response is to the 41 and ~66 kDa proteins and with increasing time reacts to more immunogens. IgG reactivity sequentially develops, first to Osp A and later to Osp B, in the seropositive foal.

Experimental Inoculation

A pony inoculated with spirochetes failed to elicit any overt symptoms of disease, nor did it mount a significant IgG response until being reinoculated with organisms 6 months later. IgG levels, however, increased slightly above the animal's preexposure OD values by day 10 but were considered negative in relation to the negative cutoff value.[10] Western blots demonstrated IgG binding to about four proteins in the preexposure sample, three of which had molecular masses of approximately 41, 66, and 97 kDa (FIG. 6). Sequential development to Osp A and Osp B was noted over time from the first inoculation; flagellin was detected by IgG in all samples. All reactions were faint immediately prior to the second spirochete injection. Four days after injection IgG probes detected more numerous proteins and significant IgG antibody in the peripheral circulation.[10] These observations could represent an anamnestic response or a response to spirochetes that were sequestered from the peripheral blood.

DISCUSSION

The observed clinical symptomatology associated with the first canine case of Lyme borreliosis (reference case in this study) consisted of fever and lameness.[1] The animal was known to be spirochetemic, produced diagnostic levels of immunoglobulin G, and became symptomless after antibiotic therapy. Other studies have utilized lameness as the major clinical marker of disease activity.[2-5] In these investigations between 34% and 42% of asymptomatic dogs (without lameness) were seropositive and were often more highly reactive than their clinical counterparts.[2,5]

In early human Lyme disease IgM and IgG responses are to the 41-kDa polypeptide, flagellin, which is genus specific.[16] Human IgM responses to flagellin were occasionally found to persist for years and a response can develop to Osp B (34 kDa) outer coat protein during late arthritis.[17] A sequentially expanding IgG response to as many as 11 antigens has been documented in prolonged human illness regardless of symptomatology.[17] Our data indicate that the major IgM response in seropositive canines is to flagellin and persists for over a year even after antibiotic therapy. IgM in dogs also develops to several other immunogens ≥41 kDa and to Osp A and Osp B in both symptomatic seropositive and seroconverting animals. In seropositive symptomatic dogs IgG probing detected more immunogens ($n = \geq 30$) than presently documented for prolonged human illness. As in humans, blot profiles were similar in

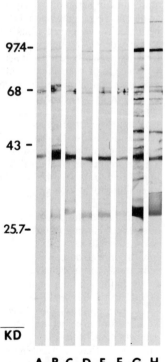

FIGURE 6. IgG Western blot of a Shetland pony inoculated with *B. burgdorferi.* Lanes: A, preinoculation; B, 12/86; C, 1/87; D, 2/87; E, 3/87; F, 6/87; G, 6/87 (reinoculation); H, 8/87.

seropositive dogs with various symptoms of Lyme borreliosis. Consistently IgG dominant immunogenic proteins were Osp A and B, flagellin, and a ~97 kDa MW entity. Our data suggest persistence of the live organism for extended periods of time, allowing antibody production to antigens not recognized in late human disease.

Western blots indicate that IgG responses in (nonlame) asymptomatic seropositive animals are similar to the responses in the reference case and in the clinical seroreactive dogs. Antibody recognition of numerous antigens in nonlame animals for periods of over a year suggests continued *B. burgdorferi* infection. Members of the canine corps were sampled in late November and again in mid-March. Possible reinfection via vectors in these dogs seems unlikely since adult ticks were not abundant and were not detected on the dogs during daily inspection by their handlers between sampling dates. Antibiotic-treated asymptomatic seropositive police dogs demonstrated a decrease in IgG-detectable spirochetal proteins, indicating successful removal of the organism from the host, without subsequent reinfection. In contrast, untreated asymptomatic police dogs developed sequential IgG responses to *B. burgdorferi* antigens even though they remained nonlame, which suggests persistent infection in these dogs. Asymptomatic seropositive dogs can develop lameness. In New Jersey, seven nonlame survey dogs developed joint involvement within 6 months of initial screening.[5] Since these animals were not treated with antibiotics, expression of symptoms may have resulted from persistence of the organism, reinfection via ticks bites, or both.

Lameness is the most commonly reported manifestation of Lyme borreliosis in canines upon presentation to the veterinarian. Based on antigen recognition by antibodies in seropositive asymptomatic dogs, it seems possible that other potential symptoms (*e.g.,* aggression, lethargy, and/or inappetance) during early infection may be clinically overlooked. Consequently, in endemic areas where dogs may be exposed to *B. burgdorferi* frequently from an early age, veterinarians may feel it is prudent to treat serologically reactive dogs even if the animals are apparently symptom free.

Since foals were sampled after maternal antibody levels had depleted, serological responses and Western blot profiles are assumed to represent initial natural infection by *B. burgdorferi* in these animals. IgM detected the 41 kDa antigen during acute symptoms (edema) and the response persisted during convalescence. Additional high molecular weight proteins were detected during convalescence by IgM. In the slightly seropositive foal with swollen ankles, the IgG response was sequential. Initial binding was to the continually present 41-kDa antigen and later to more numerous proteins. The seroreactive foal elicited an initial IgG (acute phase) to ~31 and ~66 kDa proteins in addition to the 41-kDa antigen and later developed responses to numerous proteins, including the 34-kDa antigen. These data also suggest continued presence of the live organism.

The IgG acute phase response in the naturally infected Arab mare was to several antigens, including Osp A and Osp B. Based on the temporal development of IgG in foals, it would seem likely that the mare was infected with the pathogen for several months prior to onset of symptoms. Decreasing IgG detectable proteins and OD values indicate successful removal of the organism.

Even though the inoculated pony remained asymptomatic, sequential development of IgG to the 31- and 34-kDa outer coat proteins was noted after the humoral IgG levels rose slightly above the preexposure values. An anamnestic response could account for the coincident rise in humoral antibody and antigen recognition following reinoculation. It is also possible that the animal was successfully infected with *B. burgdorferi* that persisted in low levels sequestered from the peripheral circulation.

Veterinary serologies should be interpreted with caution. In endemic areas animals are likely to be infected frequently via ticks commencing at an early age. The spectrum of clinical symptomology appears to be expanding in domestic animals as evidenced by humoral antibody recognition of antigen in nonlame individuals. Veterinarians may feel it wise to treat serologically reactive asymptomatic animals, since *B. burgdorferi* appears to be persistent in canine and equine hosts. Detection of circulating antibody in asymptomatic animals may be a predictor of disease. The public health implications with respect to reservoir competency for vector ticks and direct transmission from domestic animal to humans require further investigation.

SUMMARY

By using paired sera the IgM and IgG host responses were analyzed in dogs with ELISA and Western blot techniques. Antibodies in clinical seropositive dogs bound to 4–25 IgM and up to 40 or more IgG antigenic determinants. Early IgM response to the 41-kDa flagellin persisted for at least 9 months and involved as many as seven other peptides. IgG response expanded later in the disease and involved more immunogens than are currently recognized in late human disease. A percentage of asymptomatic dogs that later developed clinical symptoms were seropositive. Immunoblot studies suggested that *B. burgdorferi* is persistent in both asymptomatic and weakly reactive animals and if untreated could lead to disease expression. Clinical seropositive, asymptomatic seronegative, and experimentally infected horses were similarly studied. In experimentally inoculated animals IgG antibodies were initially bound to flagellin and later to the 34- and 31-kDa polypeptides, even though ELISA values were considered only slightly reactive.

REFERENCES

1. LISSMAN, B. L., E. M. BOSLER, H. CAMAY, B. G. ORMISTON & J. L. BENACH. 1984. Spirochete associated arthritis (Lyme disease) in a dog. J. Am. Vet. Med. Assoc. **185:** 219–220.
2. KORNBLATT, A. N., P. H. URBAND & A. C. STEERE. 1985. Arthritis caused by *Borrelia burgdorferi* in dogs. J. Am. Vet. Med. Assoc. **186:** 960–964.
3. MAGNARELLI, L. A., J. F. ANDERSON, A. F. KAUFMANN, L. L. LIEBERMANN & G. D. WHITNEY. 1985. Borreliosis in dogs from southern Connecticut. J. Am. Vet. Med. Assoc. **186:** 955–959.
4. BURGESS, E. C. 1986. Natural exposure of Wisconsin dogs to the Lyme disease spirochete (*Borrelia burgdorferi*). Lab. Anim. Sci. **36:** 288–290.
5. SCHULZE, T. L., E. M. BOSLER, J. K. SHISLER, I. C. WARE, M. K. LAKAT & W. E. PARKIN. 1986. Prevalence of canine Lyme disease from an endemic area as determined by serosurvey. Zbl. Bakt. Hyg. A **263:** 427–434.
6. MARCUS, L. C., M. M. PATTERSON, R. E. GILFILLAN & P. H. URBAND. 1985. Antibodies to *Borrelia burgdorferi* in New England horses: Serologic survey. Am. J. Vet. Res. **46:** 2570–2571.
7. BURGESS, E. G., D. GILLETTE & J. P. PICKETT. 1986. Arthritis and panuveitis as manifestations of *Borrelia burgdorferi* in a Wisconsin pony. J. Am. Vet. Med. Assoc. **189:** 1340–1342.
8. BURGDORFER, W., A. G. BARBOUR, S. F. HAYES, J. L. BENACH & J. P. DAVIS. 1982. Lyme disease—a tick-borne spirochetosis? Science **216:** 1317–1319.
9. BENACH, J. L., H. B. FLEIT, G. S. HABICHT, J. L. COLEMAN, E. M. BOSLER & B. P. LANE. 1984. Interactions of phagocytes with the Lyme disease spirochete: Role of the Fc receptor. J. Infect. Dis. **150:** 123–131.
10. COHEN, D. P., E. M. BOSLER, W. BERNARD, D. M. MEIRS, R. EISNER & T. L. SCHULZE.

1988. Epidemiologic studies of Lyme disease in horses and their public health significance. This volume.

11. ENGVALL, E. & P. PERLMANN. 1971. Enzyme-linked immunosorbent assay (ELISA).
    Quantitative assay of immunoglobulin. Immunochemistry **8:** 871–874.

12. RUSSELL, H., J. S. SAMPSON, G. P. SCHMID, H. W. WILKINSON & B. PLIKAYTIS. 1984.
    Enzyme-linked immunosorbent assay and indirect immunoflourescence assay for Lyme
    disease. J. Infect. Dis. **149:** 465–470.

13. COLEMAN, J. L. & J. L. BENACH. 1987. Isolation of antigenic compounds from the Lyme
    disease spirochete: Their role in early diagnosis. J. Infect. Dis. **155:** 756–765.

14. MAGNARELLI, L. A., J. M. MEEGAN, J. F. ANDERSON & W. A. CHAPPELL. 1984.
    Comparison of an indirect fluorescent antibody test with an enzyme-linked immunosor-
    bent assay for serological studies of Lyme disease. J. Clin. Microbiol. **20:** 181–184.

15. TOWBIN, H., T. STAEHELIN & J. GORDON. 1979. Electrophoretic transfer of proteins from
    polyacrylamide gels to nitrocellulose sheets: Procedure and some applications. Proc. Natl.
    Acad. Sci. USA **76:** 4350–4354.

16. BARBOUR, A. G., S. F. HAYES, R. A. HEILAND, M. E. SCHRUMPF & S. L. TESSIER. 1986. A
    Borrelia genus-specific monoclonal antibody binds to a flagellar epitope. Infect. Immun.
    59: 549–554.

17. CRAFT, J. E., D. K. FISCHER, G. T. SHIMAMOTO & A. C. STEERE. 1986. Antigens of
    Borrelia burgdorferi recognized during Lyme disease. J. Clin. Invest. **78:** 934–939.

Borrelia burgdorferi Infection in Wisconsin Horses and Cows

ELIZABETH C. BURGESS

School of Veterinary Medicine
University of Wisconsin
Madison, Wisconsin 53706

INTRODUCTION

Borrelia burgdorferi infection has been recognized in humans,[1] wild mammals,[2] dogs,[3] and horses[4] living in Wisconsin. The geographic distribution of Lyme borreliosis in humans throughout the state is correlated with the distribution of *Ixodes dammini* and includes primarily the west-central and northwest areas. The one reported case of Lyme borreliosis in a Wisconsin horse was from the west-central part of the state.[4] This animal had arthritis and panuveitis caused by *B. burgdorferi* infection. Dairy and beef cattle farms are located in Lyme endemic areas of Wisconsin and are exposed to *B. burgdorferi*.

The objectives of this study were to determine if *B. burgdorferi* infection occurred in Wisconsin horses and cattle, the geographic distribution and seasonal incidence, and what if any were the clinical signs of disease in each of the species.

MATERIALS AND METHODS

Animals

The horses included a wide variety of breeds and ages. Sexes were male, female, and neutered. Cows were all female of dairy breeds.

Samples

A total of 108 veterinary clinics from 35 of the 72 counties in Wisconsin sent samples for testing. All samples (blood, milk, colostrum, synovial fluid, urine) were sent to this laboratory by Wisconsin veterinary practitioners. Samples were received from July 1986 through June 1987. Records were kept on the date of sampling, the county of origin, and when possible, clinical signs. Samples were sent in response to a request for samples from horses, cows with clinical signs suggestive of borreliosis such as lameness, pain, arthritis, or reproduction failure, or animals that had exposure to *I. dammini*.

Blood samples were taken from the jugular vein and placed in citrated tubes for whole blood culturing or in tubes with no anticoagulant, allowed to clot, and serum removed for antibody testing. Synovial fluid was collected aseptically with needle and syringe with care taken not to contaminate the sample with blood. Urine was collected by catheterization. Colostrum was collected at time of calving and milk samples were taken by hand milking into tubes. All samples were sent by mail to Madison.

Indirect Immunofluorescent Antibody Test (IFA)

Serum, milk, colostrum, and synovial fluid collected from the horses and cows were tested by the IFA test for IgG antibodies to *B. burgdorferi* using standard techniques.[5] The IFA endpoint was the highest serum dilution to show distinct fluorescence of the spirochetes.

B. burgdorferi *Isolation*

Whole blood, milk, synovial fluid, urine or colostrum (0.1 ml) was placed in 7 ml tubes of BSK II medium[6] and incubated at 34°C. A drop of medium from each tube was placed on a slide and examined for the presence of spirochetes by darkfield microscopy. This was done biweekly for 6 weeks. Any spirochetes found were placed on a slide, incubated overnight at 37°C, and then tested by immunofluorescence using a monoclonal antibody (H5532) followed by an FITC conjugated anti-mouse sera to ensure identification.

The total number of samples tested included 430 cow sera, 190 horse sera, 10 cow synovial fluids, 6 horse synovial fluids, 3 cow colostrums, and 1 fetal calf serum for antibody testing and 156 cow bloods, 35 horse bloods, 14 cow synovial fluids, 4 horse synovial fluids, 3 cow colostrums, and 44 cow milk samples for culturing.

Mice

Three Swiss mice were orally inoculated with 0.5 ml of culture media containing approximately 50 urine-cultured spirochetes per milliliter. One mouse was inoculated with spirochetes cultured from the urine of one cow, while the other two mice received spirochetes cultured from the urine of a second cow. All three mice were seronegative to antibodies to *B. burgdorferi* prior to inoculation and no spirochetes were isolated from preinoculation blood. The mice were bled retroorbitally at 7, 21, and 25 days postinoculation, and the serum tested by IFA for *B. burgdorferi* antibodies.

RESULTS

Horses

The geographic distribution of horses with *B. burgdorferi* antibody titers of 1 : 128 or greater is shown on FIGURE 1. The majority of the cases occurred in the northwest and west-central areas of the state. The samples came from a wide geographic distribution in Wisconsin. There is little grazing land in the northernmost countries so few cows or horses are located there. The seasonal incidence of *B. burgdorferi* antibody-positive horses is shown in FIGURE 2. October and May were the peak months for the number of antibody-positive horses tested. Antibody sample results included 118/190 serum samples and 3/6 synovial fluids with *B. burgdorferi* antibody titers of 1 : 128 or greater. Culture results included 2/35 blood and 0/4 synovial fluid samples culture positive for *B. burgdorferi*. The clinical signs and antibody titers of horses from which *B. burgdorferi* was cultured, and horses with antibody-positive synovial fluid, are shown in TABLE 1. Of 83 serum antibody-positive horses with known histories at the time of sampling, 47 had lameness or stiffness, 8 had laminitis, 7 had swollen joints, 6

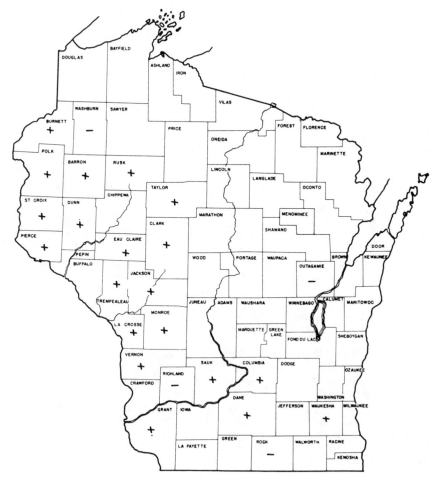

FIGURE 1. Geographic distribution of horses with *B. burgdorferi* antibody titers of 1 : 128 or greater.

were lethargic and had a fever, 8 had unexplained chronic weight loss, and 10 were apparently healthy.

Cattle

The geographic distribution of *B. burgdorferi* antibody-positive cow sera is shown on FIGURE 3. The distribution is similar to that of the horses with the addition of some counties in the east-central area of the state. The seasonal incidence of *B. burgdorferi* antibody-positive cows is shown on FIGURE 4 and was similar to that for the horses. Antibody and culture results are given in TABLE 2.

Of 151 serum antibody-positive cows with known clinical histories at the time of

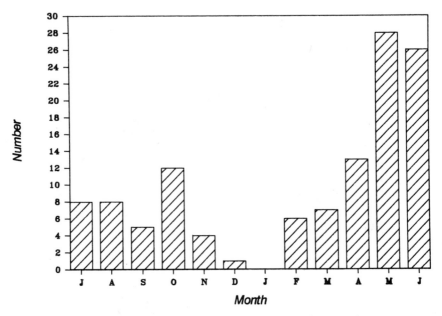

FIGURE 2. Seasonal incidence of *B. burgdorferi* antibody-positive horses.

sampling, 62 had stiffness, swollen joints, or lameness; 36 had abortions, 8 had laminitis; 7 had a fever; 7 had unexplained chronic weight loss; and 30 were apparently healthy. The clinical signs and antibody titers of cows from which *B. burgdorferi* was isolated are shown in TABLE 3.

Of the 36 antibody-positive cows that had abortions, one had a positive blood culture, one had a colostrum antibody titer of 1 : 512, one had a culture positive colostrum, and one aborted calf had an antibody titer of 1 : 256. Of 18 cow herds tested, 16 had 90% of the cows antibody positive at 1 : 128 or above while two herds were antibody negative.

TABLE 1. Clinical Signs in Horses from Which *Borrelia burgdorferi* Was Cultured or That Had *Borrelia burgdorferi* Antibodies in Synovial Fluid (Titers of 1:128 or Greater).

Horse No.	Antibody Titer[a]	*B. burgdorferi* Culture	Clinical Signs
1	9000 serum	+ blood	weight loss
2	1024 serum	+ blood	stiff
3	4096 synovial fluid 1024 serum	− synovial fluid − blood	swollen joint
4	1024 synovial fluid 128 serum	− synovial fluid − blood	swollen joint
5	256 synovial fluid 512 serum	− synovial fluid − blood	swollen joint

[a]Indirect immunofluorescent IgG antibody titer to *Borrelia burgdorferi* titer is given as the reciprocal of the end point dilution.

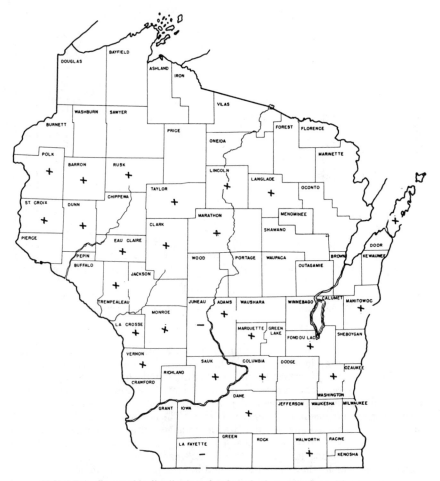

FIGURE 3. Geographic distribution of *B. burgdorferi* antibody-positive cow sera.

Mice

Two of the three urine spirochete inoculated mice developed antibodies by day 25 (1 : 64 and 1 : 128) postinoculation.

DISCUSSION

Borrelia burgdorferi infection occurs in Wisconsin horses and cows and can cause both clinical and subclinical disease. The geographic distribution of *B. burgdorferi* infection in horses corresponds closely to the distribution of Lyme disease in humans in Wisconsin.[7] The geographic range of cows with *B. burgdorferi* infection includes the same areas as for horses and humans but also includes new areas, such as Door county, where no *Ixodes dammini* have been found.[7] *B. burgdorferi* was isolated from three of

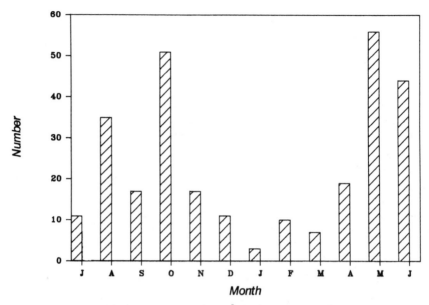

FIGURE 4. Seasonal incidence of *B. burgdorferi* antibody-positive cows.

the cows from Door county. These animals had not traveled out of Door county and no new animals had been introduced to the herd. These findings would suggest that *B. burgdorferi* is being transmitted by means other than by the bite of *I. dammini*. As *B. burgdorferi* was isolated from the urine of two of these cows, it is possible that transmission occurs by the urine-oral route. Oral infection has been demonstrated under experimental conditions in *Peromyscus* sp.[8] The development of *B. burgdorferi* antibodies in the mice orally inoculated with the urine cultured spirochetes indicates that the spirochetes were viable. It is unlikely that the spirochetes would have been absorbed into the blood through the gut if they had not been alive. If these urine spirochetes are viable, they could lead to oral infection. The housing of cows in close association in stanchions on cement where urine can splash from cow to cow could lead to oral transmission. Cows purchased from an endemic area could shed spirochetes in the urine and transmit to the new herd. This could allow for the expanded geographic distribution of *B. burgdorferi* in cows. Other arthropods such as biting flies and

TABLE 2. Results of Cow Samples Tested for Indirect Immunofluorescent Antibodies to *B. burgdorferi* (Titer 128 or Greater) and Samples Cultured for *B. burgdorferi:* Number Positive/Number Tested

B. burgdorferi	Antibody Positive	*B. burgdorferi*	Culture Positive
Serum	282/430	Blood	7/156
Synovial fluid	5/10	Synovial fluid	1/14
Colostrum	2/3	Colostrum	1/3
Fetal calf serum	1/1	Urine	2/10
Milk	0/44	Milk	0/44

mosquitoes may also play a role in transmission in cows in areas where few or no *I. dammini* exist.

The seasonal distribution of clinical cases of *B. burgdorferi* in horses and cows shows a peak in May and June and a second peak in October. This pattern suggests that in highly endemic areas where *I. dammini* are very prevalent, adult *I. dammini* are most likely transmitted to horses and cows. In Wisconsin the adult *I. dammini* emerge in the spring, usually in March and April, and again in September. The clinical cases primarily occur within a month of the adult emergence. This varies from the incidence of clinical cases in humans in Wisconsin, which peaks in the summer months of June and July.[7] Humans are primarily bitten by larval and nymphal forms of the tick.[9] Cases in cows and horses occurred in each month of the year with the exception, in horses, of January. This indicates either a long incubation in some animals, possible urine transmission, or transmission by other arthropods.

The clinical signs reported in the antibody-positive horses and cows do correlate with signs described for borreliosis in dogs, humans and horses.[1,4,10,11]

The isolation of spirochetes and the finding of *B. burgdorferi* antibodies in synovial

TABLE 3. Cows from Which *B. burgdorferi* Has Been Isolated

Cow No.[a]	Antibody Titer[b]	*B. burgdorferi* Culture	Clinical Signs
1	512	+ blood	arthritis
2	neg	+ blood	arthritis
3	512	+ blood	arthritis
4	1024	+ blood	arthritis
5[c]	neg	+ blood	none
6	256	+ blood	none
7	512	+ blood	none
8	1024	+ synovial fluid	swollen carpal joints
9	neg	+ colostrum	abortion
10	512	+ urine	none
11	512	+ urine	none

[a]Cows 1, 2, and 3 all from the same herd.
[b]Indirect immunofluorescent IgG antibody titer given as reciprocal of end point dilution.
[c]Newborn calf.

fluid of animals with swollen joints and lameness provides evidence that *B. burgdorferi* infection is the cause of the lesion. In most cases the synovial fluid antibody titers were higher than the serum antibody titers, indicating that an active infection was occurring in the joints. The finding of *B. burgdorferi* and *B. burgdorferi* antibodies in the synovial fluid of humans with chronic arthritis has been used for diagnosis of Lyme disease.[11]

The finding of spirochetes in the blood of cows with no *B. burgdorferi* antibody and no clinical signs could indicate an early infection. *B. burgdorferi* has been isolated from the blood of humans showing signs of Lyme disease but with no serum antibodies.[12]

Transplacental transmission of *B. burgdorferi* was demonstrated in the cows. *B. burgdorferi* was cultured from the blood of a newborn calf, and an aborted calf had antibodies to *B. burgdorferi*, indicating in utero infection. There is no in utero maternal transfer of antibodies in cows.[13] The findings of spirochetes in the blood of a cow that aborted and the high antibody levels in cows aborting also indicate that *B. burgdorferi* infection may cause reproductive disease in cows. Transplacental transmission of *B. burgdorferi* has been demonstrated in humans and has been associated with abortions, early infant death, and possible heart defects.[14,15] A closely related spirochete of cattle (*B. coriaceus*) is the cause of abortion in cattle in the coastal range mountains of California.[16]

The finding of a large number of cows and horses with evidence of infection with *B. burgdorferi* and especially the isolation of spirochetes from the blood, colostrum, and urine raises the possibility of human infection by contact with these animals. People that live and work in close association with these animals, such as farmers and veterinarians, could be at a higher risk of infection than the general public. Although no spirochetes were isolated from the limited number of milk samples tested, the finding of spirochetes in the colostrum indicates the possibility of infection in the milk. Milk could then be a possible source of infection for humans who drink raw milk.

SUMMARY

Blood samples from Wisconsin horses and cows suspected of having clinical disease due to *Borrelia burgdorferi* infection were submitted by veterinary practitioners. All serum, milk, colostrum, and synovial samples were tested for *B. burgdorferi* antibodies by immunofluorescence. Whole blood, milk, colostrum, and synovial fluid samples were cultured for *B. burgdorferi*. Records were kept on the clinical signs of antibody-positive animals, date of sample, and location of the animal by county. Of the samples tested for antibodies 282/430 cow sera, 118/190 horse sera, 5/10 cow synovial fluids, 3/6 horse synovial fluids, 2/3 cow colostrums, 0/44 cow milk samples and 1 aborted fetus serum were antibody positive at a titer of 1 : 128 or greater. Of samples cultured 7/156 cow bloods, 2/35 horse bloods, 1/14 cow synovial fluids, 0/4 synovial fluids, 1/3 cow colostrums, 0/44 cow milk, and 2/10 cow urine samples were *B. burgdorferi* culture positive. For both cows and horses October and May were the two peak months for the number of antibody-positive samples. The most frequent clinical signs in antibody-positive horses and cows were lameness and swollen joints, but many also had stiffness, laminitis, abortions, and fevers. Not all antibody-positive animals showed clinical signs. These findings show that *B. burgdorferi* infection occurs in horses and cows and can cause clinical illness in some but not all animals. Infection in cows and horses occurs most frequently 1 month after the emergence of adult *I. dammini*. Because spirochetes could be isolated from blood, synovial fluid, colostrum, and urine, these animals could be important in providing an infected blood meal for ticks and bringing *B. burgdorferi* in direct contact with humans.

REFERENCES

1. DRYER, R. F., P. G. GOELLNER & A. S. CARNEY. 1979. Lyme arthritis in Wisconsin. J. Am. Vet. Med. Assoc. **241**(5): 498–499.
2. GODSEY, M. S., T. E. AMUNDSON, E. C. BURGESS, W. SCHELL, J. P. DAVIS, R. KASLOW & R. EDELMAN. 1987. Lyme disease ecology in Wisconsin: Distribution and host preferences of *Ixodes dammini*, and prevalence of antibody to *Borrelia burgdorferi* in small mammals. Am. J. Trop. Med. Hyg. **37**(1): 180–187.
3. BURGESS, E. C. 1986. Natural infection of Wisconsin dogs by the Lyme disease spirochete (*Borrelia burgdorferi*). Lab. Anim. Sci. **36**(3): 288–290.
4. BURGESS, E. C., D. GILLETTE & J. P. PICKETT. 1986. Arthritis and panuveitis as manifestations of *Borrelia burgdorferi* infection in a Wisconsin pony. J. Am. Vet. Med. Assoc. **189**(10): 1340–1342.
5. BOSLER, E. M., J. L. COLEMAN, J. L. BENACH, D. A. MASSEY, J. H. HANRAHAN, W.

BURGDORFER & A. G. BARBOUR. 1983. Natural distribution of the *Ixodes dammini* spirochete. Science **220**: 321–322.

6. JOHNSON, S. E., G. C. KLEIN, G. S. SCHMID, G. S. BOWEN, J. C. FELLY & T. SCHULZE. 1984. Lyme disease: A selective medium for isolation of the suspected etiological agent, a spirochete. J. Clin. Microbiol. **19**(1): 81–82.

7. DAVIS, J. P., W. S. SCHELL, T. E. AMUNDSON, M. S. GODSEY, A. S. SPIELMAN, W. BURGDORFER, A. G. BARBOUR, M. LAVENTURE & R. A. KASLOW. 1984. Lyme disease in Wisconsin: Epidemiologic clinical, serologic, and entomologic findings. Yale J. Biol. Med. **57**: 685–696.

8. BURGESS, E. C. & L. A. PATRICAN. 1987. Oral infection of *Peromyscus maniculatus* with *Borrelia burgdorferi* and subsequent transmission by *Ixodes dammini*. Am. J. Trop. Med. Hyg. **36**(2): 402–407.

9. STEERE, A. C. & S. E. MALAWISTA. 1979. Cases of Lyme disease in the United States: Locations correlated with distribution of *Ixodes dammini*. Ann. Intern. Med. **91**: 730–733.

10. KORNBLATT, A., P. URBAND & A. STEERE. 1985. Arthritis caused by *Borrelia burgdorferi* in dogs. J. Am. Vet. Med. Assoc. **186**(9): 963–965.

11. SYNDMAN, R., D. P. SCHENKEIN, V. P. BERARDI, C. C. LASTAVICA & K. M. PARISER. 1986. *Borrelia burgdorferi* in joint fluid in chronic Lyme arthritis. Ann. Intern. Med. **104**(6): 798–800.

12. RAWLINGS, J. A., P. V. FOURNIER & G. J. TELTOW. 1987. Isolation of *Borrelia* spirochetes from patients in Texas. J. Clin. Microbiol. **25**(7): 1148–1150.

13. TIZARD, I. 1982. Immunity in the fetus and newborn. *In* An Introduction to Veterinary Immunology. 2nd edit. I. Tizard, Ed.: 169. W. B. Saunders Company. Philadelphia, PA.

14. SCHLESINGER, P. A., P. H. DURAY, S. A. BURKE, A. C. STEERE & T. STILLMAN. 1985. Maternal fetal transmission of the Lyme disease spirochete, *Borrelia burgdorferi*. Ann. Intern. Med. **103**(1): 67–68.

15. MARKOWITZ, L. E., A. C. STEERE, J. L. BENACH, J. D. SLADE & C. V. BROOME. 1986. Lyme disease during pregnancy. J. Am. Vet. Med. Assoc. **255**(24): 3394–3396.

16. OSEBOLD, J. W., R. SPEZIALETTI & M. JENNINGS. 1986. Congenital spirochetosis in calves: Association with epizootic bovine abortion. J. Am. Vet. Med. Assoc. **188**: 371–375.

Epidemiologic Studies of Lyme Disease in Horses and Their Public Health Significance

DANIEL COHEN,[a] EDWARD M. BOSLER,[b]
WILLIAM BERNARD,[a] DAVID MEIRS II,[c]
ROBERT EISNER,[d] AND TERRY L. SCHULZE[e]

[a]University of Pennsylvania Veterinary School
Philadelphia, Pennsylvania 19348

[b]New York State Department of Health
Stony Brook, New York 11794-8692

[c]Walnridge Farm
Creamridge, New Jersey 08514

[d]State Department of Agriculture
Trenton, New Jersey 08625

[e]State Department of Health
Trenton, New Jersey 08625

INTRODUCTION

Borreliosis caused by *B. theileri* in horses was first reported from South Africa in 1978.[1] In 1984 serum antibodies to *B. burgdorferi* were detected in Massachusetts by indirect immunofluorescence in 24% and 1% of horses sampled residing in endemic and nonendemic areas, respectively.[2] A subsequent report in 1986 of a case in a Wisconsin pony presented evidence that the agent can be pathogenic for horses, producing signs of uveitis and arthritis.[3] Transmission of Lyme disease from a seropositive horse to a human by means of a bite was reported in 1987 from Belgium.[4] This paper will describe a serologic study of horses on farms in a highly endemic and in less highly endemic areas of New Jersey and Pennsylvania and at the Veterinary Hospital of the University of Pennsylvania and present some clinical and experimental work to support the view of its emerging importance as both an equine and a zoonotic disease problem.

MATERIALS AND METHODS

Serologic Tests

Sera were collected from horses residing on a Standardbred breeding farm (farm A) located in Monmouth County, NJ, a highly endemic area accounting for more than half of all the human Lyme disease cases in the state (FIG. 1).[5] The farm is divided into two sites—Concord (farm 1) and Walnridge (farm 2)—about 3 miles apart. Since the farm is owned and operated by an equine veterinary practitioner, veterinary care and supervision on this farm are of an exceptionally high standard with excellent laboratory support and medical records. Daily veterinary care is provided by the owner

244

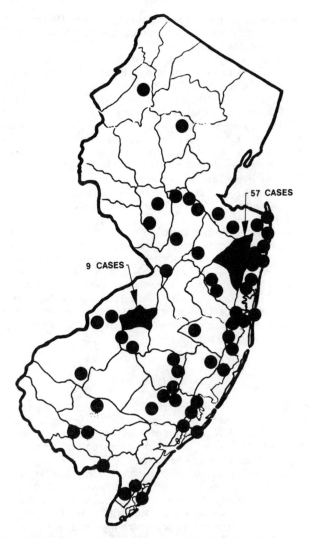

FIGURE 1. Distribution of Lyme disease in New Jersey. *Dark circles* indicate areas in which the disease is endemic. The largest number of cases (57) has been found in Monmouth County.

(DM), and two other veterinarians. They are assisted by a team of veterinary nurses, laboratory technicians, and office and barn personnel. All clinical observations, therapy, routine immunizations, treatments for parasitism, and laboratory findings on each animal are maintained for individual animals. Sera collected from this farm for another purpose in 1983 and held at −70°C at New Bolton Center (NBC), University of Pennsylvania, were also tested. Longitudinal studies were conducted on this farm using specimens collected from yearlings in March, May, July, and September, 1986. Additional serologic surveys were performed on horses hospitalized at NBC for a variety of clinical conditions during the months of June and December, 1986 and on horses from a breeding farm near Mays Landing in southern New Jersey (farm B) and from a stable near Paoli, PA (farm C).

All sera were aseptically collected, coded, and sent to the New York State Department of Health Laboratory at Stony Brook, NY where they were heat inactivated at 56°C for 30 minutes and evaluated by an ELISA as described by Engvall and Perlmann[6] and modified by Russell et al.,[7] with additional modifications described in Coleman et al.[8] Whole spirochetal sonicate was used as antigen and coated to plates at a concentration of 5 μg per well. Known negative and positive controls as determined by Western blot analysis were run on each plate for serosurvey work. When experimentally inoculated animals were tested, each individual's preinoculation sample was used as an additional negative control. Alkaline-phosphatase-labeled anti-horse IgG (heavy and light chain, Kirkegaard and Perry Laboratories, Gaithersburg, MD) was utilized as the secondary antibody in all tests. The optical densities of reactions were read using an MR600 MicroELISA reader (Dynatech, Alexandria, VA) at a wavelength of 410 nm.

The assays on 100 sera were compared to indirect fluorescent antibody (IFA) test results. IFA tests were performed according to the method described by Benach et al.[9] using goat-produced fluorescein isothiocyanate conjugated anti-horse IgG (heavy and light chains; Cooper Biomedical, Malvern, NJ). Selected sera, highly positive for Borrelia, were tested for leptospirosis using the microscopic agglutination test by the Pennsylvania State Department of Agriculture Diagnostic Laboratory at Summerdale. Sera of suspected clinical cases were tested for equine herpes I, equine influenza, and equine arteritis viruses at the New Jersey State Department of Agriculture Diagnostic Laboratory at Trenton.

Animal Inoculations

In November 1986 a group of 10 stabilized ponies were screened for antibodies to B. burgdorferi and six seronegatives were selected. In December 1986 four of the ponies were inoculated with B. burgdorferi from two sources in an attempt to cause infection and disease. Two ponies (1 and 2) were inoculated with adult I. dammini suspensions freshly obtained from endemic areas of New York and New Jersey, where over 50% of the ticks were found to harbor B. burgdorferi. The ticks were triturated in sterile saline, passed through sterile mesh, and inoculated with a total 2 ml suspension as follows: 1 ml intravenously, 0.2 ml intradermally, and 0.8 ml subcutaneously. In early June 1987 the animals were reinoculated with 2 ml of primary cultures of B. burdorferi containing 1.2 million organisms per ml as follows: 1 ml intramuscularly, 0.2 ml intradermally, and 0.8 ml subcutaneously.

Two ponies (3 and 4) were inoculated in December 1986 with primary cultures of B. burgdorferi suspended in modified culture media containing about 800,000 organisms per milliliter and inoculated by the same method as that described above. Two uninoculated ponies (5 and 6) were left between 1 and 3 and between 2 and 4. All ponies were maintained in an inner room of an isolation barn which was fully screened and sprayed with pyrethrin—2,2-dichlorovinyl-dimethyl-phosphate (C-EM-DIE, Rockland Chemical Co., West Caldwell, NJ)—at weekly intervals. No ticks were observed on the animals, nor were any arthropods in the barn during the period of study. Access was limited to the researchers and one caretaker. Blood samples were taken from all animals daily for about 1 month and then biweekly for 4 months and finally weekly until 6 months. All animals were temperatured and physically examined daily.

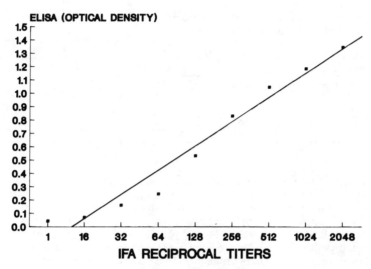

FIGURE 2. ELISA and IFA comparison of equine sera for *B. burgdorferi* antibodies.

RESULTS

Serologic

A comparison between the IFA and the ELISA optical density readings for *B. burgdorferi* IgG antibodies was performed in 1986 on the same 100 equine sera (FIG. 2). There is a direct correlation between the two tests with readings greater than .700 on the ELISA comparable to readings of 1 : 256 and greater on the IFA test. This was considered highly reactive (+ +). The range of .200 to .700 on the ELISA OD scale was selected as being definitely reactive (+). This was equivalent to between 1 : 32 and 1 : 64 to 1 : 256 on the IFA test. Optical readings two standard deviations (SD) from the mean to .200 were considered as equivocal (+ −) and below 2 SD was interpreted as negative (−).

Using the above criteria, the results of the initial survey of the farm in the highly endemic area is seen in TABLE 1. Sixty percent of the resident animals in the highly

TABLE 1. Results of a Survey for *B. burgdorferi* Antibodies in Various Equine Populations

Survey Population	Horses Tested	Percent Positive
Farm A (central NJ):		
residents	180	60.0
visitors	28	14.2
Farm B (southern NJ)	57	12.3
Farm C (Paoli, PA)	20	10.0
University of Pennsylvania Hospital:		
June	111	12.6
October	97	6.2
Total	208	9.6

TABLE 2. Percent Definitely Positive Serologic Titers to Lyme Disease by Age Group on Two New Jersey Farms, 1986

	Farm A		Farm B	
Age Group	% Pos.	No.	% Pos.	No.
Yearlings	59.4	65	4.3	23
2–7	52.6	37	0	3
7–12	55.6	38	33.3	12
12–17	70.3	27	50.0	8
17+	58.3	12	28.6	7

endemic area were positive to *B. burgdorferi*. Animals (visitors) brought for a short time to this farm for breeding purposes were less positive (14.2%). This lower seropositive rate was also observed for farms located in less endemic areas of southern New Jersey (farm B, 12.3%), southeast Pennsylvania (farm C, 10.0%) and the University of Pennsylvania (9.6%). There was a significant lowering of the percentage of seropositive titers observed at the hospital between June and September. The rates were twice as high in June as in September (12.6% and 6.2% respectively).

The age distribution of positive titers to Lyme disease was compared on two New Jersey farms, farms A and B, located within and outside of the highly endemic area (TABLE 2). The major difference in the distribution of the age-specific attack rates is due to the lack of seropositives among the yearlings on farm B. If one were to include the "low positive" or equivocal (+ −) category with the definitely positives in the analysis, the overall positive rates would be 73.1% and 38.6%, respectively (TABLE 3). Once again the greatest disparity would be noted for the yearlings (84.7% and 4.2%, respectively).

Sera from farm A held at − 70°C in a serum bank at the University since 1983 were examined to determine whether the high rates were a recent phenomenon (TABLE 4). This was compared to the March 1986 survey results of 60% for both mares and yearlings. In March 1983 the mares on the farm were 12.2% positive, a rate similar to

TABLE 3. Serologic Results from Two Equine Farms in New Jersey: Horses Tested for *B. burgdorferi* Antibodies, March 1986

	Highly Pos. (++)	Definite Pos. (+)	Equivocal (+ −)	Negative (−)	Total	% Pos.[a]	% Pos.[a] and Equivocal
Farm A							
Yearlings	23	12	15	9	59	59.3	84.7
Mares	41	28	15	31	115	60.0	73.0
Stallions	2	2	1	1	6	66.7	83.3
Residents	66	42	31	41	180	60.0	77.2
Visitors	2	2	9	15	28	14.2	46.4
TOTAL	68	44	40	56	208	53.8	73.1
Farm B							
Yearlings	1	0	0	23	24	4.2	4.2
Adults	4	2	15	12	33	18.2	63.6
TOTAL	5	2	15	35	57	12.3	38.6

[a]Highly positive + definite positive.

TABLE 4. Comparison of Farm A in 1983 and 1986 for Lyme Antibody Titers

Age Group	Year	Positive Titers	Negative Titers	Total	% Pos.	Relative Change
Yearlings	1983	13	24	37	35.1	1.7
	1986	35	24	59	59.3	
Mares	1983	5	36	41	12.2	4.9
	1986	69	46	115	60.0	
Total	1983	18	60	78	23.1	1.9
	1986	104	70	174	59.8	

that seen in the surrounding area and at the Veterinary Hospital of the University of Pennsylvania. The yearlings were almost three times that rate (35.1%).

To determine the rate of antibody decline, a longitudinal survey was undertaken of yearlings in March, July, and September of 1986. FIGURE 3 shows the overall status of the positive and negative titers. The most radical shift is the decline of "highly positive" titers between July and September and the subsequent increase primarily of negative titers. The results of a comparison of paired sera available in March and September is presented in TABLE 5. Sixty percent registered no change in titer, 5.7%

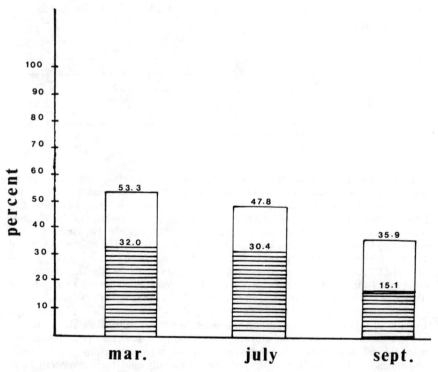

FIGURE 3. Results of a serologic survey in yearlings, 1986: *hatched + nonhatched areas,* positive; *hatched areas,* highly positive.

increased, probably as a result of exposure, and 34% declined during this 6-month period.

Of the 4 ponies inoculated experimentally with infectious material, only pony 1 demonstrated a clear antibody response. Pony 1 was the first pony to be inoculated and received mascerated tick material. Six months later the pony was reinoculated with primary culture material. The serologic results are presented in FIGURE 4. The primary response appeared 9 to 10 days after inoculation. The response remained at a low level, in the equivocal zone, for about 3 weeks. It then dropped and remained close to the level of the two SDs until reinoculation at 6 months. The response to the reinoculation with primary culture was dramatic. Within 4 days there was a definitely positive titer (+) which within a few days approached a highly positive titer (++). Ponies 3 and 4, which had originally received primary culture material in the first inoculation, did not noticeably respond serologically. Pony 2, which had received similar tick material, also did not serologically respond to either primary inoculation or reinoculation.

Clinical Signs

In 1985 and 1986 farm A reported a new clinical syndrome occurring in their foals and yearlings. The syndrome was described by one of us (DM) as edema of the limbs,

TABLE 5. A Comparison of Paired Sera for Lyme Antibody Titers: Farm A, March to September 1986

		SEPTEMBER			
		− −	+	+ +	TOTAL
	− −	24	2	1	27
MARCH	+	7	1	0	8
	+ +	3	8	7	18
	TOTAL	34	11	8	53

No change, 60.4%; increased, 5.7%; decreased, 34.0%.

usually of four legs. It is sometimes associated with conjunctivitis, nasal discharge, or cough, and sometimes accompanied by a dermatitis of the white areas of the lower leg similar to a photosensitivity reaction (TABLE 6). Affected foals frequently seemed to have an elevated percentage of lymphocytes, although the total white blood cell counts were usually within normal limits. The syndrome could not be ascribed, after laboratory testing, to any other known viral or bacterial agent. The syndrome affected 15 out of 78 foals born that year (19.2%). In 1986, there were 14 cases out of 96 foals born (14.6%) and a cluster of cases of polyarthritis in four of the affected animals was observed (TABLE 7). Two of the cases persisted for a long period of time. One had to be destroyed and the second still showed signs of arthritis in the fall of 1987.

The edema may persist for only 1 or 2 days and has been noted for as long as 8 days. Initially all animals were treated with antibiotics and it was believed the short duration of signs was attributable to the efficacy of the therapy. More recently treatment was withheld and no difference in duration of signs was noted, suggesting a self-limiting phenomenon. Although the disease syndrome is generally mild, there is concern about the possible increase in severity indicated by the occurrence of polyarthritis in 1986.

In 1985, foals were raised on two separate locations of the farm. The first group,

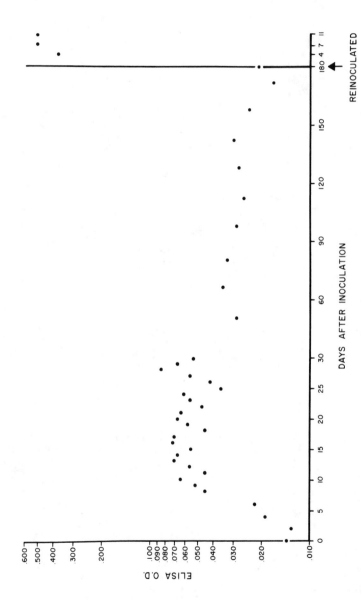

FIGURE 4. ELISA OD for pony no. 1, inoculated with 2 ml of *Borrelia*-infected tick material and reexposed 6 months later to primary culture.

TABLE 6. Clinical Signs and Serologic Results: 1986

No.	Date of Onset	% Lymphocytes	WBC	Signs from Date of Onset[a]																	
				1	2	3	4	5	6	7	8	9	10	11	12	13	14	15	16	17	43
1	7/25		15,200	A	A	A	A	A	A	A	A	A	A	A	A	A	A	A	A	A	A
2	8/5		14,200	A	A	A	A	A	A	A	A	A	A	A	A	A	A	A	A	A	
3	8/11		23,300	A	A	A	A	A	A	A	A	A	A	A	A	A	A	A	A	A	A
4	8/11	41	1600	A	A	A	A	A													
5	7/17	62	7400	S	S	S	A	A													
6	7/17	59.2		S	S	S															
7	7/23	38		S	P	P															
8	7/23	50	13,700	S	S	S															
9	8/20		7700	S	S	S	S														
10	9/8	37	8300	S																	
11	9/19	57	9300	S																	
12	9/19	68	8600	S																	

[a]Key: A, arthritis/pulmonary; P, pulmonary; S, edema of four legs.

TABLE 7. Clinical Signs and Serologic Results: 1985

Site	No.	Date of Onset	% Lymphocytes	WBC	Signs from Date of Onset[a] 1	2	3	4	5	6	7	8	9	10	11	12	13	14	15
Concord	1	9/8			E	E	E	E	E										
	2	9/8	56	5300	D	D	D	D	D	D	D	D	D						
	3	9/23			E	E	E	E	E										
	4	9/24		14,400	P	P	P	P							E				
	5	10/4			E	E													
	6	10/13			D	D	E	E											
Walnridge	7	10/21		19,900	P	P	P	P	P	E	E	E	E	E	E	E	E	E	E
	8	10/24	55	5100	C	C	C	C		E	E	E	E	E	E	E	E	E	E
	9	10/24	62	7600	C	C	C	C	C	E	P	E	E	E	E	E	E		
	10	10/29	56	6100	C		E	E	E	E				E	E				
	11	10/29	77	8700	E		E	E											
	12	10/29	79	7100	E	E	E	E											
	13	10/31	60	5400	E	E	E	E											
	14	10/31	54	10,700	E	E	C	C	C										
	15	11/1		6000	E			E											

[a]Key: E, edema of legs; D, dermatitis; P, pulmonary; C, conjunctivitis.

held at farm 1, foaled earlier in the year, in the spring, and were put out to pasture as weanlings. Cases in this group occurred sporadically over a 2-month period in September and October and involved six foals. The second group at farm 2 were born in the summer and initially placed in a small compound and holding shed to start their feeding after they were weaned in the fall and only later were placed in pasture. This group seemed to have a concentration of cases within a 1- or 2-week period (FIG. 5). This concentration of cases suggested a common source of infection other than by ticks. Serologically all but one animal in each group eventually showed a titer (months later) to Lyme disease, although an initial check of acute and convalescent sera at the time of occurrence failed to show any specific titers to *B. burgdorferi*.

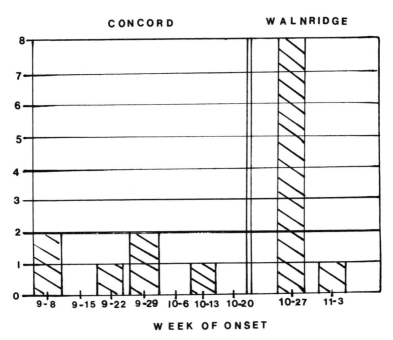

FIGURE 5. Number of cases of edema of the legs in foals at two sites, showing a concentration of cases in a 1- to 2-week period.

In 1986, 2 of the 12 foals serologically tested positive to *B. burgdorferi* at the time they were clinically affected, one in the acute and the other in the convalescent sera 2 weeks later. All other animals tested negative on both acute and convalescent sera. However, when tested in January, 4 to 7 months later, of the 10 sera available for testing nine showed some degree of positivity. In 1985 the first cases were reported in September, in 1986 in late July, and in 1987 early in July.

Rhinopneumonitis (equine herpes virus I) apparently occurred on one of the two sites of farm A but could not account for the cases on the second site. In 1986 the animals were again tested, and despite the continued presence of the syndrome there were no signs of the presence of equine herpes virus I, equine arteritis virus, or leptospirosis. Sera were also subsequently checked and found to be negative for equine infectious anemia. All of the cases occurred in foals and yearlings and none of the cases occurred in older animals, either in mares or in stallions.

A check of the farm in November 1986 by the State Medical Entomologist of the New Jersey State Department of Health (TLS) indicated that the ecologic area was compatible with that for the infection of horses by *I. dammini,* particularly in the pastures bordering on wooded areas. *I. dammini* adults were collected from pastures at farm 1 and farm 2 and *B. burgdorferi* were detected in them in 53.3% and 66.7%, respectively.

DISCUSSION

This report demonstrates the usefulness of the ELISA test for the purposes of conducting large serologic surveys of equine populations for *B. burgdorferi* antibodies. Comparison with the IFA test established a direct relationship between the two. Experimental inoculation of a pony made interpretation of antibody levels clearer. The definitely reactive and highly reactive titers observed are probably the result of repeated exposure. Primary exposure may give a much lower response, perhaps occurring in an equivocal zone, which may be hard to interpret.

The serosurveys conducted established that approximately 10% of the horses in the New Jersey-Pennsylvania area (6–15%) possess definitely reactive antibodies to *B. burgdorferi.* Within this area, however, there exists a focus of infection, indicated by farm A, wherein 60% of the horses tested in 1986 were definitely seropositive. On both sites of this farm (1 and 2), 53–66.7% of the ticks collected in November, 1986 were found to be carrying *B. burgdorferi,* a situation consistent with that found in other highly endemic areas.[10] If one includes lower titers possibly due to primary exposure, then there are a substantial number of equines in our geographic areas that have had contact with this spirochete. This high percentage of antibodies in horses, especially in the highly endemic areas, severely complicates the identification of disease signs associated with the spirochete and requires that we proceed with caution in making associations of clinical signs with the presence of specific antibodies.

The evolution of the equine involvement in the highly endemic area has probably taken place during the last few years. The survey of 1983 established a rate in the mares comparable to that found in less highly endemic areas. However, even in 1983 the yearlings on farm A already had a rate of positivity three times that of the mares, indicating a heavier rate of exposure but not reaching the 60% level found in yearlings by 1986. The longitudinal, paired studies conducted in 1986 further established that a small number of individuals increased their titer (5–7%) during the spring and summer months, suggesting exposure or reexposure to the agent. However, 34% of the pairs declined significantly in titer during the 6-month interval of the study.

Just as the evolution of equine involvement in the serologic pattern is relatively recent, so perhaps is the evolution of clinical signs. The paucity of clinical signs in the presence of such a vast number of seropositive animals is striking. We have not seen cases such as the one described in the literature in a Wisconsin pony. Only a vague syndrome involving transitory edema of the legs has been noted in 3 successive years. However, the occurrence in 1986 of four cases of polyarthritis in this group, two of which required extensive therapy, suggests the possibility that this syndrome may also be evolving into a more debilitating disease pattern that will have important implications for the equine industry in the future.

In 1985 some dermatitis was noted to affect the white areas of the lower limbs. Cottral[11] in 1978, before the identification of *B. burgdorferi,* wrote of an investigator in

England: "Spirochetes were constantly present in every case of canker of the foot and 'greasy heels' of the horses examined by him." Cottral attributed this to *B. theileri*.

Similarly, this evolving pattern may have great significance for the public health aspects of this disease. The role of the horse in maintaining infection as an animal reservoir in closer proximity to man than deer or field mice is yet to be evaluated. The extensive national and international patterns of movement of horses in the racing and breeding industries make the potential role of the horse in the evolving patterns of Lyme disease an important consideration and worthy of epidemiologic monitoring. It is even possible that the spirochete was introduced into the United States from Europe via the horse, which may introduce the agent into other unaffected global areas in the future.

The possibility of direct spread from animal to animal without an arthropod vector has been already established experimentally in studies of field mice.[12,13] The clinical syndrome identified at farm A, site 2 in 1985 was suggestive of a point source of infection. A letter-to-the-editor that appeared in the *Lancet* has described a human case derived from the bite of an infected horse.[4] Oral transmission is a possibility in our outbreak. If this is correct, then the rapid dissemination of the agent through breeding farms is possible in the absence of ticks and may bode further jeopardy for horses and man.

In his 1984 study conducted in a highly endemic area of New England, Marcus[2] obtained 12 positives by IFA procedures out of the 50 horses he examined (24%). Using our criteria and assuming a similarity in test results, we would have only considered 6 or 7 of these as definitely positive, or 12–14%. The others were 1 : 8 to 1 : 32 on the IFA test. This figure would agree with the results obtained in 1983 in the adult population of farm A and in the less highly endemic areas studied for comparison in 1986. Three years later, the rates were 60% in this same highly endemic area of New Jersey. It would be interesting to repeat the survey in the same highly endemic area of Massachusetts today in order to see to what degree the rate of seropositivity has increased. The probability is that it has. While the significance of wildlife reservoirs in maintaining a nidus of infection and in resisting efforts to eradicate Lyme disease is of great importance, the spread of this disease with a multiplicity of mechanisms of dispersal to a variety of domestic animals (dogs, horses and cattle), many of which move in international channels, may pose a special threat to human and animal health. This newly emerging threat is worthy of special consideration by the scientific and health communities.

SUMMARY

A serologic survey of horses in the New Jersey-Pennsylvania area demonstrated that about 10% (6.2–14.2%) have significant levels of serum antibody to *Borrelia burgdorferi*. However, in a highly endemic area of central New Jersey, up to 60% of the mares and yearlings sampled on one farm were seropositive. In 1983, sera from this same farm exhibited only 12% positives in mares and 35% positives in yearlings. Longitudinal studies of paired sera obtained from individual yearlings over a 6-month period in 1985 showed that 34% of them declined during the period. A new clinical syndrome associated with this farm has been observed in 1985–87. In 1985 only an edema of the legs and a dermatitis were noted, in 19.2% of the foals. There was a clustering of cases on one site, where one peer group of foals was sequestered after weaning, which suggested a point source of infection other than arthropods. In 1986, 14.6% of the foals were affected, four of them with arthritis, two of which resisted antibiotic treatment for over several months' time. Experimental infection of a pony with triturated *B. burgdorferi* infected tick material indicated low specific antibody levels starting about the ninth day that continued for a 3-week period. When this animal was challenged 6 months later with primary *B. burgdorferi* cultures, a rapid and significant booster effect was evidenced within 4 days.

REFERENCES

1. VAN HEERDEN, J. & F. REYERS. 1984. *Borrelia* sp. infection in a horse. J. S. Afr. Vet. Assoc. **55:** 41–43.
2. MARCUS, L. C., M. M. PATTERSON, *et al.* 1985. Antibodies to *Borrelia burgdorferi* in New England horses. Am. J. Vet. Res. **46:** 2570–2571.
3. BURGESS, E. C., D. GILLETTE, *et al.* 1986. Arthritis and panuveitis as manifestations of *Borrelia burgorferi* infection in a Wisconsin pony. J. Am. Vet. Med. Assoc. **189:** 1340–1342.
4. MARCELIS, L., P. DE MARNEFFE, *et al.* 1987. Horse reservoir for *Borrelia burgdorferi*? Lancet **1**(8539): 977.
5. BOWEN, G. S., T. L. SCHULZE, *et al.* 1984. A focus of Lyme disease in Monmouth County, New Jersey. Am. J. Epidemiol. **120:** 387–394.
6. ENGVALL, E. & P. PERLMANN. 1971. Enzyme-linked immunosorbent assay (ELISA): Quantitative assay of immunoglobulin. Immunochemistry **8:** 871–874.
7. RUSSELL, H., J. S. SAMPSON *et al.* 1984. Enzyme-linked immunosorbent assay and indirect immunofluorescence assay for Lyme disease. J. Infect. Dis. **149:** 465–470.
8. COLEMAN, J. L. & J. L. BENACH. 1987. Isolation of antigenic components from the Lyme disease spirochete: Their role in early diagnosis. J. Infect. Dis. **155:** 756–765.
9. BENACH, J. L., E. M. BOSLER, *et al.* 1983. Spirochetes isolated from the blood of two patients with Lyme disease. N. Engl. J. Med. **308:** 740–742.
10. SCHULZE, T. L., M. F. LAKAT *et al.* 1986. Comparison of rates of infection by the Lyme disease spirochete in selected populations of *Ixodes dammini* and *Ambylomma americanum*. Zbl. Bakt. Hyg. A **263:** 72–78.
11. COTTRAL, G. E. 1978. Manual of Standardized Methods of Veterinary Microbiology. Ithaca, NY. Comstock Publishing Assoc., Cornell University. Ithaca, NY. p. 506.
12. BOSLER, E. M. & T. L. SCHULZE. 1987. The prevalence and significance of *Borrelia burgdorferi* in the urine of feral reservoir hosts. Zbl. Bakt. Hyg. A **263:** 427–434.
13. BURGESS, E. C. & L. A. PATRICAN. 1987. Oral infection of *Peromyscus maniculatus* with *Borrelia burgdorferi* and subsequent transmission by *Ixodes dammini*. Am. J. Trop. Med. Hyg. **36:**(2): 402–407.

Experimental Infection of the Hamster with *Borrelia burgdorferi*[a]

RUSSELL C. JOHNSON,[b] CARRIE KODNER,[b]
MARIE RUSSELL,[b] AND PAUL H. DURAY[c]

[b]*Department of Microbiology*
University of Minnesota Medical School
Minneapolis, Minnesota 55455

[c]*Department of Pathology*
Fox Chase Cancer Center
Philadelphia, Pennsylvania 19111

INTRODUCTION

The Syrian hamster can be consistently infected with recent human, animal, and tick isolates of *Borrelia burgdorferi*.[1] This capability, combined with the ability to isolate the spirochete from infected tissues, has provided the means to study host-parasite interaction and to conduct *in vivo* antibiotic susceptibility studies.

MATERIALS AND METHODS

Origin and Cultivation of B. burgdorferi

The origin of the strains of *Borrelia burgdorferi* used in this study were strain 297, a human spinal fluid isolate (Allen Steere, Yale University, New Haven, CT); P/Bi, a human spinal fluid isolate and P/Gu, a human skin isolate (Vera Preac-Mursic, Max von Petenkofer-Institut, Munich, FRG); MM, Minnesota mouse (University of Minnesota, Minneapolis, MN); IPT, *Ixodes pacificus* tick (Robert Lane, University of California, Berkeley, CA). The spirochetes were cultured in Barbour-Stoenner-Kelly (BSK) medium[2] at 30°C. Medium for the isolation of spirochetes from animals was prepared by the addition of 0.15% agarose (SeaKem LE, FMC Corp., Marine Colloids Division, Rockland, ME) to the BSK medium.

Histological Examination

At necropsy all organs including the major limb joints (after HCl, triacetic acid, Na$^+$-K$^+$ tartrate decalcification) were processed for 10% buffered Formalin-fixed, paraffin-embedded tissue sections using the Fisher histomatic tissue processor (266 MP), and stained with H & E and Mallory trichrome stains. Slide imprints of the liver and spleen were made from the cut surfaces of the fresh organs and stained with H &

[a]This investigation was supported by Public Health Service grant no. AR34733 from the National Institutes of Health.

258

E. All sections, including the tissue imprint (touch preparation) slides, were stained for spirochetes using a modification of the Dieterle silver-impregnation method.[3]

Passive Immunization

Rabbits received weekly intravenous injections of 10^8 viable cells of the test isolate washed twice with 0.01-M phosphate-buffered saline (pH 7.5). Serum was harvested 2 to 3 weeks after the final injection, and the antibody titer was determined by the indirect fluorescent-antibody assay. Male and female hamsters, 5 to 10 weeks old, were injected with the test serum subcutaneously 18 hours before challenge. Challenge consisted of the intraperitoneal injection of 10^8 cells of the test isolate. At 14 days postchallenge hamsters were sacrificed, and the kidneys and spleens were cultured. Each hamster organ was placed in 6 ml of BSK medium and homogenized with a Stomacher Lab-Blender (Tekmar Co., Cincinnati, Ohio). After the larger tissue debris was allowed to settle, duplicate 1:10 dilutions of the supernatant were made in the isolation medium. Cultures were examined for spirochetes by dark-field microscopy after 3 weeks of incubation at 30°C.

Antimicrobial Agents

The antimicrobial agents tested were erythromycin and tetracycline hydrochloride (Sigma Chemical Co., St. Louis, MO), ceftriaxone (Rocephin; Hoffmann-LaRoche, Inc., Nutley, NJ), Azithromycin (Pfizer, Inc., Groton, CT), Ciprofloxacin (Miles Pharmaceuticals, West Haven, CT), and penicillin G (E. R. Squibb & Sons, Princeton, NJ).

In Vitro *Antimicrobial Susceptibility Procedure*

The MBCs were determined using the broth dilution method. The antimicrobial agents tested are listed above and the concentrations evaluated ranged from 0.01 to 8.0 μg/ml. BSK medium with and without antimicrobial agents were dispensed in triplicate tubes and inoculated to a final density of 10^5 cells/ml from an actively growing culture. The Petroff-Hausser counting chamber was used to determine cell numbers. After 3 weeks incubation at 30°C the assay tubes were examined by darkfield microscopy for the presence of spirochetes and a 10% (vol/vol) inoculum from each tube was inoculated into BSK medium without antibiotics. These tubes were examined for the presence of spirochetes following 3-week incubation at 30°C. The MBC was the lowest concentration of antimicrobial agent from which spirochetes could not be subcultured.

In Vivo *Antimicrobial Susceptibility Procedure*

Syrian hamsters weighing 100 g or greater were injected intraperitoneally with 1000 50% infective doses of *B. burgdorferi*, 297, the Connecticut human spinal fluid isolate. The 50% infective dose of this isolate was previously determined to be 10,000 cells.[4] Fourteen days later when the spirochete can be isolated from as many as six organs,[1] antimicrobial therapy was initiated. Hamsters received five equal daily subcutaneous injections of the antimicrobial agents tested or saline. Hamsters were sacrificed and the spleen and kidneys were cultured[4] 14 days after the final treatment. An animal was considered infected if one or more organs were culture positive after 3 weeks incubation at 30°C. A minimum of 5 animals were tested per antimicrobial dose.

RESULTS AND DISCUSSION

The primary test organism used in our studies was a human spinal fluid isolate of *B. burgdorferi* strain 297. Intraperitoneally infected hamsters were spirochetemic during the first day of infection, followed by a persistent generalized infection. Spirochetes were isolated from the brain, eyes, liver, kidneys, spleen, and testes 14 days postinfection.[1] The greatest number of isolations were made from the spleen and kidneys and these were the organs in addition to blood that were routinely cultured in the animal studies. Hamsters remained infected for as long as 14 months. No obvious signs of illness were observed in the experimentally infected hamsters.

Initially hamsters infected by the intraperitoneal route were examined by histological techniques at 1 to 9 months postinfection.[5] Hamsters infected by this route and for this time period did not display significant histological changes except for mild splenic follicular hyperplasia and intermittent chronic portal triaditis. Thus, while organ infection was documented both by culture and direct tissue visualization, the presence of *B. burgdorferi* in hamster tissue did not elicit a substantial and constant inflammatory infiltrate. Spirochetes were predominately extracellular, with a rare organism appearing to be partially within a macrophage. It was of interest that spirochetes were present in the blood of the left ventricles of the heart in two animals months postinoculation. Thus, in addition to the spirochete persisting in organs on a chronic basis, it appears that they also retain the capacity for spirochetemia on a relatively long-term basis.

We next examined hamsters infected by the cutaneous route beginning 3 hours postinfection and daily for 15 days. At day 5 postinfection spirochetes persisted in the cutaneous tissues at the site of infection and were present in the gonads, lungs, kidneys and heart (without myocarditis). Intracerebral and ocular spirochetes were not seen before day 7 postinfection. Tissue responses in these hamsters appeared to be confined to mast cell lymphocytic dermatitis, mild to modest portal triaditis, splenic lymphoid follicle stimulation with transformed lymphocytes, variable pulmonary interstitial infiltrates (viral-like), and cerebral microgliosis.

Although the experimentally infected hamsters do not display overt signs of illness, they do consistently develop a generalized persistent infection. Thus, they provide a well studied, inexpensive experimental animal in which to conduct host-parasite relationship studies and to evaluate the *in vivo* antimicrobial susceptibility of *B. burgdorferi*.

Control of tick-borne diseases such as Lyme borreliosis is difficult. Vaccination of persons living or working in high-risk areas and susceptible domestic animals would be a practical method for preventing this illness. To investigate this possibility we performed vaccination trials using the hamster as the initial experimental animal. Hamsters were vaccinated subcutaneously with a single dose of an inactivated whole cell preparation of human spinal fluid (HSF) isolate and challenged 30 days postvaccination. Fourteen days after challenge, the blood, spleen and kidney were cultured. From 86% to 100% of the hamsters receiving 50 to 100 μg dry weight of the vaccine preparation were protected from experimental infection.[6] The amount of vaccine preparation required to provide the hamster with protection against *B.*

burgdorferi infection is at least 10 times that necessary to protect hamsters from infection with *Leptospira interrogans*. These results suggest that the immunogenicity of *B. burgdorferi* is low and that an adjuvant should be incorporated into the vaccine preparation.

Borrelia burgdorferi can persist in the tissues of patients with Lyme borreliosis in spite of high levels of specific antibody.[7,8] This raised the question of whether antibodies play an important role in immunity to this illness. We found that anti-*B. burgdorferi* antibodies (IFA titers 1:256–1:8,192) produced in the rabbit protected passively immunized hamsters from challenge.[4] We were also able to protect hamsters from experimental infection by passive immunization with anti-*B. burgdorferi* antibodies (IFA titer 1:1024) produced in the hamster. As little as 0.0125 ml of the rabbit antisera (IFA titer 1:8,192) protected hamsters from challenge by the same strain with which the rabbit had been immunized. These results indicated that *B. burgdorferi* can elicit the formation of protective antibodies in the rabbit and hamster and suggest that humoral immunity could play an important role in resistance to infection by this spirochete. In our passive immunization experiments the antibodies were administered to the hamsters approximately 17 hours prior to challenge. We next determined whether the antibodies would be protective if administered after the hamsters were challenged. Hamsters were injected with 0.5 ml of antisera (IFA titer 1:8,192) 17 hours after challenge. None of the hamsters were protected from challenge. Thus, with our experimental procedure, antibodies can provide protection from infection if present at the time of challenge but not once the spirochete is already present in the tissues. This suggests that the spirochete can be sequestered in the host tissues in such a manner as to be resistant or inaccessible to the protective activity of antibodies.

On the basis of the IFA or ELISA tests polyclonal antibodies formed against an isolate of *B. burgdorferi* from one geographical area reacts well with isolates from diverse locations. However, through the use of monoclonal antibodies variations in protein antigens have been observed.[9,10] We investigated the possibility that immunity to Lyme borreliosis could be strain specific. We chose as our test organisms: 297, human spinal fluid isolate from Connecticut, P/Gu, a human skin isolate from Munich, FRG, and IPT, an *Ixodes pacificus* tick isolate from California. All three isolates were infectious for the hamster. The antisera was prepared in rabbits and had the following IFA titers: HSF, 1:2048; P/Gu, 1:1024; and IPT, 1:1024. Hamsters, in groups of five, received subcutaneous injections of 0.5 ml of antisera or normal rabbit serum. Approximately 17 hours later the animals were challenged by intraperitoneal injection of 1×10^8 cells of the appropriate isolate of *B. burgdorferi*. The hamsters were sacrificed 14 days later and the blood, spleen, and kidneys cultured. As seen in TABLE 1, all hamsters receiving normal rabbit serum were susceptible to infection by the three isolates. Hamsters challenged with the isolate to which they had previously received antisera were protected from infection. In contrast, antibodies to an isolate from one geographical area did not protect hamsters from challenge by an isolate from a different geographical location. These results suggest that a marked heterogeneity exists in the antigen(s) that elicit the formation of protective antibodies among isolates of *B. burgdorferi* from diverse geographical areas. Additional studies are necessary to determine whether heterogeneity in protective antigens also occurs within a geographical area. Our previous passive protection study[4] indicated a high level of cross-protection between antibodies to strain 297 and a Minnesota mouse isolate.

We have found the hamster to be a satisfactory experimental animal for investigating the *in vivo* susceptibility of *B. burgdorferi* to antimicrobial agents.[11] The results of the *in vitro* susceptibility of *B. burgdorferi* 297 to erythromycin and penicillin G did not correlate well with the *in vivo* studies. The minimal bactericidal concentrations (MBCs) for erythromycin and penicillin G were 0.04 and 6.4 µg/ml, respectively. Both erythromycin and penicillin G displayed low activity *in vivo*. The 50% curative dose (CD_{50}) for erythromycin was 235.3 mg/kg and the CD_{50} for penicillin G was >197.5 mg/kg. Erythromycin has also been less effective than tetracycline and penicillin for the treatment of early Lyme borreliosis.[12] Our *in vivo* results with penicillin G were somewhat surprising. Penicillin has been used successfully for the treatment of early Lyme borreliosis and the meningitis associated with this illness.[12,13] However, only 35% to 55% of patients with established arthritis responded favorably to high-dose penicillin therapy[14] and in cases of another borreliosis, louse-borne relapsing fever, therapy with penicillin G was not effective and resulted in a slow clearance of borreliae and frequent relapses.[15] *Borrelia burgdorferi* 297 was susceptible to tetracycline and ceftriaxone *in vitro* and *in vivo*. The MBCs and CD_{50}s for tetracycline and ceftriaxone were 0.8 μg/ml and 28.7 mg/kg and 0.04 μg/ml and 24.0 mg/kg, respectively.[11] The results of these experimental studies compare favorably with clinical results. Tetracycline is presently the drug of choice for the treatment of early Lyme borreliosis, and ceftriaxone has been used successfully to treat cases of Lyme borreliosis that failed to respond to penicillin or tetracycline therapy.[16]

Although erythromycin is highly active *in vitro* against *B. burgdorferi*, it has not been as effective as tetracycline or penicillin for the treatment of Lyme borreliosis.[12] Azithromycin is a new macrolide that differs structurally from erythromycin by a

TABLE 1. Passive Immunization of Hamsters with Rabbit Serum

B. burgdorferi Challenge Strain	Anti-*B. burgdorferi* Rabbit Serum Strain				
	None	297	P/Gu	IPT	MM
297	4/5[a]	0/5	5/5	5/5	0/5
P/Gu	5/5	5/5	0/5	5/5	
IPT	5/5	5/5	5/5	0/5	
MM	5/5	1/5			0/5

[a]Number of culture positive hamsters over total number of hamsters.

methyl-substituted nitrogen in the macrolide ring. This modification has produced profound alternation in potency, half-life, and tissue distribution for azithromycin as compared to erythromycin. Because of these attractive properties, azithromycin was evaluated for its activity against *B. burgdorferi*. Five isolates of *B. burgdorferi* from various sources and geographical locations were used to determine the MBCs for azithromycin, erythromycin, and tetracycline. These isolates displayed similar susceptibilities to the antimicrobial agents. Azithromycin possessed the highest antispirochetal activity, with an MBC of 0.02 to 0.04 μg/ml, followed by erythromycin (MBC, 0.08–0.16 μg/ml) and tetracycline (MC, 0.8–3.2 μg/ml). The *in vitro* susceptibility of strain 297 to the quinolone, ciprofloxacin, was also determined. The MBC of ciprofloxacin was 4 μg/ml, indicating that strain 297 is resistant to action of this antimicrobial agent and possibly to the quinolones in general. The *in vivo* antimicrobial susceptibility studies of azithromycin, erythromycin, and tetracycline were conducted using *B. burgdorferi* 297 as the test organism. Erythromycin possessed low activity against this spirochete, with a CD_{50} of 122.2 ± 51.9 mg/kg. In contrast, strain 297 was very susceptible to the action of azithromycin, with a CD_{50} of 3.71 ± 1.90 mg/kg. Tetracycline also possessed a high level of antispirochetal activity, with a CD_{50} of 15.6 ± 4.58 mg/kg. The results of this study suggest that azithromycin has the potential of being an effective antimicrobial agent for the treatment of Lyme borreliosis.

REFERENCES

1. JOHNSON, R. C., N. MAREK & C. KODNER. 1984. Infection of Syrian hamsters with Lyme disease spirochetes. J. Clin. Microbiol. **20:** 1099–1101.
2. BARBOUR, A. G. 1984. Isolation and cultivation of Lyme disease spirochetes. Yale J. Biol. Med. **57:** 521–525.
3. DURAY, P. H., A. KUSNITZ & J. RYAN. 1985. Demonstration of the Lyme disease spirochete, *Borrelia burgdorferi* by a modification of the Dieterle stain. **16:** 685–687.
4. JOHNSON, R. C., C. KODNER & M. RUSSELL. 1986. Passive immunization of hamsters against experimental infection with the Lyme disease spirochete. Infect. Immun. **53:** 713–714.
5. DURAY, P. H. & R. C. JOHNSON. 1986. The histopathology of experimentally infected hamsters with the Lyme disease spirochete, *Borrelia burgdorferi*. Proc. Soc. Exp. Biol. Med. **181:** 263–269.
6. JOHNSON, R. C., C. KODNER & M. RUSSELL. 1986. Active immunization of hamsters against experimental infection with *Borrelia burgdorferi*. Infect. Immun. **54:** 897–898.
7. STEERE, A. C., R. L. GRODZICKI, A. N. KORNBLATT, J. E. CRAFT, A. G. BARBOUR, W. BURGDORFER, G. P. SCHMID, E. JOHNSON & S. E. MALAWISTA. 1983. The spirochetal etiology of Lyme disease. N. Engl. J. Med. **308:** 733–740.
8. PREAC-MURSIC, V., B. WILSKE & G. SCHIERZ. 1986. European *Borrelia burgdorferi* isolated from humans and ticks: culture conditions and antibiotic susceptibility. Zbl. Bakt. Hyg. A **263:** 112–118.
9. BARBOUR, A. G., A. H. HEILAND ROMONA & T. R. HOWE. 1985. Heterogeneity of major proteins in Lyme disease borreliae: A molecular analysis of North American and European isolates. J. Infect. Dis. **152:** 478–484.
10. WILSKE, B., V. PREAC-MURSIC, G. SCHIERZ & K. V. BUSCH. 1986. Immunochemical and immunological analysis of European *Borrelia burgdorferi* strains. Zbl. Bakt. Hyg. A **263:** 92–102.
11. JOHNSON, R. C., C. KODNER & M. E. RUSSELL. 1986. *In vitro* and *in vivo* susceptibility of the Lyme disease spirochete, *Borrelia burgdorferi* to four antimicrobials. Antimicrob. Agents Chemother. **31:** 164–167.
12. STEERE, A. C., G. J. HUTCHINSON, D. W. RAHN, L. H. SIGAL, J. E. CRAFT, E. T. DE-SANNA & S. E. MALAWISTA. 1983. Treatment of early manifestations of Lyme disease. Ann. Intern. Med **99:** 22–26.
13. STEERE, A. C., A. R. PACHNER & S. E. MALAWISTA. 1983. Neurological abnormalities of Lyme disease: Successful treatment with high-dose intravenous penicillin. Ann. Intern. Med. **99:** 767–772.
14. STEERE, A. C., J. GREEN, R. T. SCHOEN, E. TAYLOR, G. F. HUTCHINSON, D. W. RAHN & S. E. MALAWISTA. 1985. Successful parenteral penicillin therapy of established Lyme arthritis. N. Engl. J. Med. **312:** 869–874.
15. BUTLER, T., P. K. JONES & C. K. WALLACE. 1978. *Borrelia recurrentis* infection: Single dose antibiotic regimens and management of Jarisch-Herxheimer reaction. J. Infect. Dis. **137:** 573–577.
16. DATTWYLER, R. J., J. J. HALPERIN, H. PASS & J. LUFT. 1987. Ceftriaxone-effective therapy in refractory Lyme disease. J. Infect. Dis. **55:** 1322–1325.

An Animal Model for Lyme Arthritis[a]

STEPHEN W. BARTHOLD,[b] KATHLEEN D. MOODY,[b]
GORDON A. TERWILLIGER,[b] ROBERT O. JACOBY[b]
AND ALLEN C. STEERE[c]

[b]Section of Comparative Medicine
Yale University School of Medicine
New Haven, Connecticut 06510

[c]Department of Rheumatology/Immunology
New England Medical Center
Tufts University School of Medicine
Boston, Massachusetts 02111

INTRODUCTION

Interest in Lyme disease of man has led to extensive surveillance among animals as reservoirs of *Borrelia burgdorferi*. Natural infection with *B. burgdorferi* has been found by culture and serology in insectivores, rodents, carnivores and ungulates, as well as birds.[1-7] Naturally occurring disease due to *B. burgdorferi* has also been recognized in several unrelated animal species. Arthritis, associated with the Lyme spirochete, has been documented in dogs,[8,9] horses,[10] and cattle. Erythematous skin lesions containing spirochetes have been noted in white-footed mice (*Peromyscus leucopus*).[6] Other animal counterparts of the Lyme disease complex may be recognized as awareness of Lyme disease increases.

These observations indicate that man is not uniquely susceptible to either infection or disease caused by *B. burgdorferi*. Nonetheless, development of a laboratory model for Lyme disease has proved elusive. Cutaneous erythema-chronicum-migrans-like lesions developed in rabbits 10 to 12 weeks after feeding of spirochete-infected ticks, but no direct causal relationship was established. Lesions were multifocal and arose at sites other than the site of tick feeding.[11,12] ECM-like lesions have also occurred at the site of inoculation within 2 to 17 days in rabbits injected with spirochete-infected tick homogenates or at the site of tick attachment. Spirochetes were demonstrable in the skin lesions.[13,14] Several groups have found spirochetemia in rabbits after inoculation with *B. burgdorferi* cultures or tick homogenates, or after tick feeding.[11-15] No other manifestations of Lyme disease have been found in experimentally infected rabbits. Various inbred and outbred mice, Sprague-Dawley rats, albino hamsters, and golden Syrian hamsters were inoculated with *B. burgdorferi* cultures by several routes, with no evidence of spirochetemia or illness.[15] *Peromyscus* mice were shown to be susceptible to infection with *B. burgdorferi,* but no disease or lesions were found.[16,17] A human isolate and tick isolates of *B. burgdorferi* were infectious to Syrian hamsters inoculated intraperitoneally. Spirochetes were recovered from blood, kidney, liver, brain, spleen, testis, and eye, but no disease occurred. Infectivity was lost after repeated *in vitro* passage of the spirochetes.[18,19] Difficulties in infecting laboratory animals or inducing disease may be influenced by variation in host susceptibility,

[a]This work was supported by National Institutes of Health grant nos. RR00393 and AM20358 and Biomedical Research Support Grant (BRSG) no. RR05358.

attenuation of *B. burgdorferi* by *in vitro* culture, or variation among *B. burgdorferi* isolates.

We have recently found that rats inoculated as neonates or weanlings with low-passage tick isolates or *in vitro* passaged isolates of *B. burgdorferi* develop spirochetemia, multisystemic infection, and a high prevalence of polyarticular arthritis resembling Lyme arthritis in man.[20] This paper provides a chronology of our progress in development of this potentially valuable model.

INFECTION OF RATS WITH *B. burgdorferi*

Studies in LEW/N Rats

We initially examined the susceptibility of 3-week-old female LEW/N rats to *B. burgdorferi* inoculation. This strain and sex were chosen because of their predisposition to bacterial cell-wall-induced arthritis.[21-23] Because *B. burgdorferi* loses infectivity

TABLE 1. Isolation of *B. burgdorferi* from Tissues of Female Weanling LEW/N Rats[20]

Group	Days after Inoculation	B. burgdorferi Isolation[a]				
		Kidney	Spleen	Liver	Brain	Blood
B. burgdorferi	5	6/6	6/6	6/6	NT[b]	6/6
	14	4/6	5/6	0/6	2/6	0/6
	90	1/6	4/6	0/6	NT	0/6
Control[c]	14	0/2	0/2	0/2	0/2	0/2

[a]Number positive/number cultured.
[b]NT = not tested.
[c]Control = sham-inoculated.

for hamsters after repeated passage in culture,[19] a low-passage isolate was used for inoculation.

Several *B. burgdorferi* isolates were cultured from the midguts of naturally infected *Ixodes dammini* captured in Westchester County, New York.[24] The infectivity of isolate N/40 was established by intraperitoneal (i.p.) inoculation of hamsters and recovery from blood and spleen.

Rats were inoculated i.p. with single-passage N/40 *B. burgdorferi* and control rats received sterile medium. Rats were killed at intervals and selected tissues were cultured and processed for histology (TABLE 1). At 5 days, *B. burgdorferi* was recovered from all organs tested. At 14 and 90 days, infection was not detected in some tissues, but persisted in the spleen. All inoculated rats had elevated IgG antibody to *B. burgdorferi* at day 5, as determined by ELISA.[25] No clinical signs were noted, but the spirochete-inoculated rats developed microscopic evidence of arthritis. None had arthritis at 5 days, but some rats examined at 14 and 90 days developed arthritis in one or more joints. None of the joints were cultured, but spirochetes were observed in periarticular tissue, synovium, and the joint space using silver stain.[26] Histological characteristics of the arthritis are described below. No significant lesions were found in other organs.

The susceptibility of neonatal LEW/N rats was next evaluated. Pups were inoculated at 3 days of age i.p. with N/40 *B. burgdorferi* or sterile medium (controls).

At days 5 and 14, *B. burgdorferi* was isolated from all organs cultured, but clearance of spirochetes appeared to occur from several sites by 90 days (TABLE 2). Infected rats developed elevated *B. burgdorferi* antibody by 14 days.

By 3 weeks after inoculation, all remaining neonatally infected rats had clinical evidence of arthritis. They had difficulty walking, with swelling of tibio-tarsal joints. One of these rats was killed on day 26 and *B. burgdorferi* was cultured from affected tibio-tarsal tissue. Clinical signs of arthritis abated by 90 days in the remaining rats, but all had polyarticular arthritis, with demonstrable spirochetes. No lesions developed in other organs. Control rats remained well, were culture-negative, and developed no microscopic abnormalities. Thus, compared to weanling rats, neonatally inoculated rats had greater spread and persistence of spirochetes and a higher incidence of arthritis.

Inoculation of Nonviable B. burgdorferi

Intraperitoneal injection of peptidoglycan-polysaccharide cell wall fragments of group A, B, or C streptococci or lactobacilli into female LEW/N results in deposition

TABLE 2. Isolation of *B. burgdorferi* from Tissues of Neonatally Inoculated LEW/N Rats[20]

Group	Days after Inoculation	*B. burgdorferi* Isolation[a]				
		Kidney	Spleen	Liver	Brain	Blood
B. burgdorferi	5	3/3	6/6	6/6	2/4	4/5
	14	4/4	5/5	5/5	4/5	NT[b]
	90	3/4	5/5	0/5	0/5	1/5
Control[c]	5	0/3	0/3	0/3	0/3	0/3
	14	0/3	0/3	0/3	0/3	0/3
	90	0/3	0/3	0/3	0/3	0/3

[a]Number positive/number cultured.
[b]NT = not tested.
[c]Control = sham-inoculated.

of cell wall material in synovium and induction of arthritis. Acute arthritis is most pronounced at 4 days after inoculation, and is followed by a chronic T-cell-dependent arthritis.[21-23] In comparison, we did not note arthritis at 5 days, with onset of acute arthritis at around 14 days after inoculation. To further explore the possibility that *B. burgdorferi* cell walls were responsible for induction of arthritis, neonatal LEW/N rats were each inoculated i.p. with formalin-inactivated *B. burgdorferi*. At days 14 and 30, none of the rats developed arthritis and their spleens were culture-negative. The finding that *B. burgdorferi* induced arthritis requires the presence of live spirochetes is supported by isolation of spirochetes from articular tissue and visualization of spirochetes in tissue sections.

Infection with Other B. burgdorferi Isolates

The susceptibility of LEW/N rats to other *B. burgdorferi* isolates was next tested. Confirmation of previous findings and more thorough culture of joints for *B.*

TABLE 3. Incidence of Arthritis and Isolation of *B. burgdorferi* from Tissues after Inoculation of Neonatal LEW/N Rats with Different *B. burgdorferi* Isolates[20]

Isolate	Days after Inoculation	*B. burgdorferi* Isolation[a]				
		Arthritis	Kidney	Spleen	Blood	Joint
N/8	14	3/4	1/4	2/4	0/4	0/3
	30	4/4	3/3	4/4	0/6	3/3
N/13	14	4/4	4/4	4/4	0/4	4/4
	30	4/4	4/4	2/3	0/4	4/4
N/40	14	7/9	9/9	9/9	6/8	6/6
	30	7/7	7/7	6/7	0/7	1/2
Control[b]	14	0/2	0/2	0/2	0/2	0/2
	30	0/2	0/2	0/2	0/2	0/2

[a]Number positive/number examined.
[b]Control = sham-inoculated.

burgdorferi were also accomplished by these studies. Neonatal LEW/N rats were inoculated i.p. with *B. burgdorferi* isolates N/8, N/13 or N/40, or sterile medium (controls). All three isolates were infectious to rats and all groups developed a high incidence of arthritis. Spirochetes were isolated from most joint cultures (TABLE 3). Control rats were negative, and lesions were not found in organs other than joints in infected rats.

These data suggest that random field isolates, albeit all from Westchester County, New York, are pathogenic to rats. They also confirm the high percentage of arthritis induction when rats are inoculated as neonates, and confirm the association of live spirochetes with affected joints.

Studies in Other Rat Genotypes

LEW/N rats are susceptible to induction of arthritis by injection of bacterial cell wall fragments, but F344 rats are resistant.[21-23] Neonatal F344 rats were inoculated i.p. with N/40 *B. burgdorferi*. The rats developed multisystemic infections and arthritis (TABLE 4). Joint lesions resembled those seen in LEW/N rats. At 30 days, spirochetes were recovered from all sites cultured. When outbred Sprague-Dawley (SD) rats were inoculated, similar results were obtained, except that spirochetes were not detected in liver and blood at 30 days (TABLE 4). Thus, unlike the bacterial cell wall arthritis model, arthritis induction with *B. burgdorferi* is not genotype dependent.

TABLE 4. Incidence of Arthritis and Isolation of *B. burgdorferi* from Tissues after Inoculation of Neonatal F344 and SD Rats[20]

Strain	Days after Inoculation	*B. burgdorferi* Isolation[a]						
		Arthritis	Kidney	Spleen	Liver	Brain	Blood	Joint
F344	5	2/3	4/4	4/4	4/4	4/4	3/3	NT[b]
	30	3/3	2/2	3/3	1/1	3/3	1/3	4/4
SD	5	0/4	2/2	1/1	1/1	1/2	2/2	1/3
	30	4/4	3/3	2/2	0/3	3/3	0/3	3/3

[a]Number positive/number examined.
[b]NT = not tested.

TABLE 5. Incidence of Arthritis and Isolation of *B. burgdorferi* from Tissues 30 Days after Inoculation of Neonatal LEW/N Rats with Different *in Vitro* Passages of *B. burgdorferi* (N/40)

| Passage Level | *B. burgdorferi* Isolation[a] | | | | |
	Arthritis	Kidney	Spleen	Blood	Joint
2	4/4	3/3	4/4	3/3	4/4
5	4/4	4/4	3/4	4/4	2/2
11	3/3	3/3	2/3	2/3	NT[b]

[a]Number positive/number examined.
[b]NT = culture results not available.

Effects of in Vitro Passage on B. burgdorferi Pathogenicity

In vitro passage has been shown to reduce infectivity of *B. burgdorferi* to experimentally inoculated hamsters,[19] and may explain difficulties experienced by others in infecting laboratory animals or inducing disease. We are currently examining the susceptibility of LEW/N rats to the N/40 isolate of *B. burgdorferi* following *in vitro* passage. Cultures were passaged weekly and inoculated i.p. into neonatal rats at approximately 10^6 organisms per rat. Tissues were cultured for spirochetes and joints examined for arthritis at 14 and 30 days after inoculation (TABLE 5). Multiple passages reduced *in vitro* clumping of spirochetes, but did not affect infectivity or pathogenicity. At the second, fifth, and eleventh passage, *B. burgdorferi* continued to induce spirochetemia, multisystemic infection, and arthritis. No differences in the

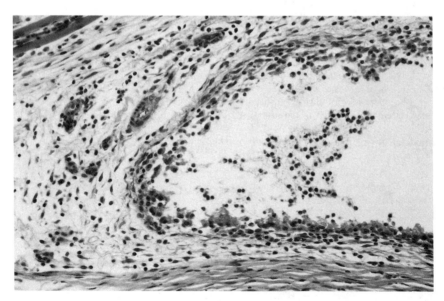

FIGURE 1. Tarsus from a rat, 14 days after inoculation with *B. burgdorferi*, depicting early exudation of fibrin and neutrophils into the synovial space. Magnification: 350×.

quality of arthritis were noted between treatment groups. Thus, multiple *in vitro* passages of *B. burgdorferi* do not diminish infectivity or virulence. Further passaged spirochetes are being evaluated.

FEATURES OF LYME ARTHRITIS IN THE RAT

In the above studies, no appreciable differences in the nature or severity of arthritis were found among rat strains, *B. burgdorferi* isolates, or *B. burgdorferi* passage level. Rats inoculated as neonates had a higher incidence of arthritis than rats inoculated as weanlings, but microscopic features of arthritis did not differ among age groups. The rat Lyme arthritis model differs from the bacterial cell wall model in several ways.

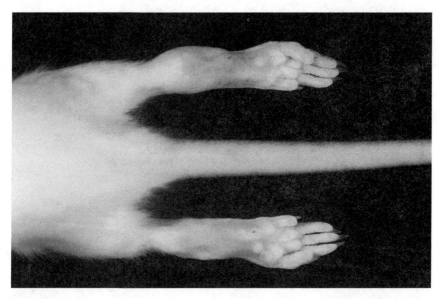

FIGURE 2. Hind limbs of a rat, 30 days after inoculation with *B. burgdorferi*. Note bilateral swelling of tibio-tarsal joints.

Arthritis was not apparent at 5 days after inoculation, a time at which acute arthritis is very evident in LEW/N rats injected with bacterial cell walls.[21–23] Furthermore, *B. burgdorferi* induced arthritis required inoculation of viable organisms, was associated with the presence of spirochetes in joint tissues, and was not rat genotype dependent.

Early arthritic changes were visible in most *B. burgdorferi* infected rats at 14 days after inoculation. One or more joints had edema and hyperemia of synovial tissue, with mild exudation of fibrin and neutrophils into the joint space (FIG. 1). At 30 days this process was more pronounced. Neonatally inoculated rats often had lameness, with swelling of tibio-tarsal joints (FIG. 2). Most rats had arthritis in multiple appendicular joints, including hip, knee, elbow, tarsus, and carpus. Tendonitis was also frequently found, particularly in carpal and tarsal regions. The severity of arthritis varied greatly from site to site, but individual rats usually had severe disease in at least one joint.

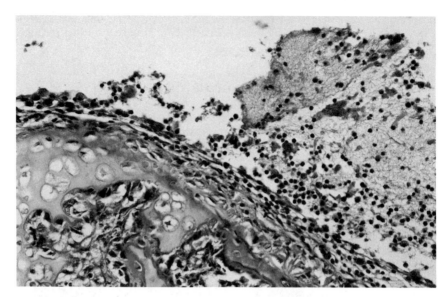

FIGURE 3. Tarsus from a rat, 30 days after inoculation with *B. burgdorferi*. There is intense exudation of fibrin and neutrophils into the joint space, with erosion of the synovial membrane. Magnification: 350×.

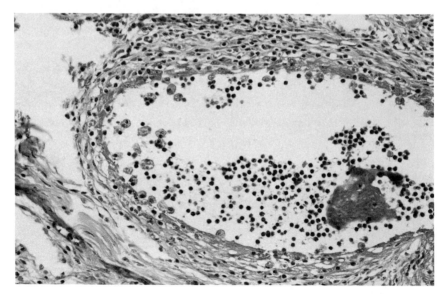

FIGURE 4. Tarsus from a rat, 90 days after inoculation with *B. burgdorferi*. The severity of inflammation has waned, with less fibrin exudation and increasing numbers of mononuclear leukocytes in synovial tissues. Magnification: 350×.

There was intense infiltration of synovial and periarticular tissues with neutrophils and, to a lesser extent, with mononuclear leukocytes. There was severe edema, hyperemia, and fibrovascular proliferation, with synovial epithelial hypertrophy and focal erosion. Exudation of fibrin and neutrophils into the joint space were prominent (FIG. 3). Spirochetes were visible in tissues around the joints, as well as within the joint spaces. By 90 days clinical signs were absent, but arthritis was still present. At this stage, acute inflammation had decreased, with the development of synovial villous hypertrophy and infiltration of mononuclear leukocytes, including macrophages, lymphocytes, and plasma cells (FIG. 4). Spirochetes were still visible in tissue sections and recoverable from joints by culture.

The rat model described here has features similar to Lyme arthritis in man. Synovial biopsies have been available only from patients with arthritis for at least 1 year, but reveal villous hypertrophy, fibrin deposition, infiltrates of mononuclear cells, and presence of spirochetes. Pseudolymphoid follicles and obliterative microangiopathic changes have been reported in man,[27] but have not been observed in rats. Long-term studies of arthritic rats will be necessary to determine if the model mimics chronic arthritis of human Lyme disease. Conversely, the pathogenesis of early Lyme arthritis in man has not been evaluated and thus cannot be compared to the rat. The rat model will be particularly useful in this regard.

SUMMARY

A model of Lyme arthritis has been developed in laboratory rats. Intraperitoneal inoculation of a low-passage tick isolate of *B. burgdorferi* into neonatal and weanling LEW/N rats resulted in multisystemic infection and arthritis. Spirochetes were isolated from blood, liver, kidney, spleen, brain, and joints of inoculated rats. Arthritis, associated with the presence of spirochetes, developed in multiple joints by day 14 and persisted through day 90 after inoculation. Arthritic lesions resembled those found in human Lyme disease lesions. Lesions were not found in other organs, although spirochetes were present. Neonatal F344 and SD rats were also susceptible to infection and induction of arthritis. Three different isolates of *B. burgdorferi* were shown to be pathogenic. Pathogenicity of one isolate was retained after at least 11 *in vitro* passages. Formalin-killed spirochetes were not pathogenic. Other features of the Lyme disease complex have yet to be seen in the rat, but long-term studies are required to completely define the rat model. This highly reproducible model should allow in-depth studies on the pathogenetic mechanisms of this important human disease.

ACKNOWLEDGMENTS

The assistance of Dr. P.H. Duray in examining rat tissues for spirochetes and David Crowder for typing this manuscript is gratefully acknowledged. Ticks used for *B. burgdorferi* isolation were kindly provided by Drs. Durland Fish and Louis Magnarelli.

REFERENCES

1. ANDERSON, J. F. & L. A. MAGNARELLI. 1984. Avian and mammalian hosts for spirochete-infected ticks and insects in Connecticut. Yale J. Biol. Med. **57:** 627–641.

2. ANDERSON, J. F., L. A. MAGNARELLI, W. BURGORFER & A. G. BARBOUR. 1983. Spirochetes in *Ixodes dammini* and mammals from Connecticut. Am. J. Trop. Hyg. **32:** 818–824.
3. BOSLER, E. M., J. L. COLEMAN, J. L. BENACH, D. A. MASSEY, J. P. HANRAHAN, W. BURGDORFER & A. G. BARBOUR. 1983. Natural distribution of the *Ixodes dammini* spirochete. Science **220:** 321–322.
4. LOKEN, K. I., C.-C. WU, R. C. JOHNSON & R. F. BEY. 1985. Isolation of the Lyme disease spirochete from mammals in Minnesota. Proc. Soc. Exp. Biol. Med. **179:** 300–302.
5. MAGNARELLI, L. A., J. F. ANDERSON & W. A. CHAPPELL. 1984. Antibodies to spirochetes in white-tailed deer and prevalence of infected ticks from foci of Lyme disease in Connecticut. J. Wild. Dis. **20:** 21–26.
6. MAGNARELLI, L. A., J. F. ANDERSON & W. A. CHAPPELL. 1984. Geographic distribution of humans, raccoons, and white-footed mice with antibodies to Lyme disease spirochetes in Connecticut. Yale J. Biol. Med. **57:** 619–626.
7. MARCUS, L. C., M. M. PATTERSON, R. E. GILFILLAN & P. H. URBAND. 1985. Antibodies to *Borrelia burgdorferi* in New England horses: Serologic survey. Am. J. Vet. Res. **46:** 2570–2571.
8. LISSMAN, B. A., E. M. BOSLER, H. CAMAY, B. G. ORMISTON & J. L. BENACH. 1984. Spirochete-associated arthritis (Lyme disease) in a dog. J. Am. Vet. Med. Assoc. **185:** 219–220.
9. KORNBLATT, A. N., P. H. URBAND & A. C. STEERE. 1984. Arthritis caused by *Borrelia burgdorferi* in dogs. J. Am. Vet. Med. Assoc. **186:** 960–964.
10. BURGESS, E. C., D. GILLETTE & J. P. PICKETT. 1986. Arthritis and panuveitis as manifestations of *Borrelia burgdorferi* infection in a Wisconsin pony. J. Am. Vet. Med. Assoc. **189:** 1340–1342.
11. BURGDORFER, W., A. G. BARBOUR, S. F. HAYES, J. L. BENACH, E. GRUNWALDT & J. P. DAVID. 1982. Lyme disease: A tick-borne spirochetesis? Science **216:** 1317–1319.
12. BURGDORFER, W. 1984. The New Zealand white rabbit: An experimental host for infecting ticks with Lyme disease spirochetes. Yale J. Biol. Med. **57:** 609–612.
13. KORNBLATT, A. N., A. C. STEERE & D. G. BROWNSTEIN. 1984. Experimental Lyme disease in rabbits: Spirochetes found in erythema migrans and blood. Infect. Immun. **46:** 220–223.
14. KORNBLATT, A. N., A. C. STEERE & D. G. BROWNSTEIN. 1984. Infection in rabbits with the Lyme disease spirochete. Yale J. Biol. Med. **57:** 613–614.
15. BENACH, J. L., E. M. BOSLER, J. L. COLEMAN & J. HABICHT. 1984. Experimental transmission of the Lyme disease spirochete to rabbits (letter). J. Infect. Dis. **150:** 786–787.
16. DONAHUE, J. G., J. PIESMAN & A. SPIELMAN. 1987. Reservoir competence of white-footed mice for Lyme disease spirochetes. Am. J. Trop. Med. Hyg. **36:** 92–96.
17. BURGESS, E. C., T. E. AMUNDSON, J. P. DAVIS, R. A. KASLOW & R. EDELMAN. 1986. Experimental inoculation of *Peromyscus* spp. with *Borrelia burgdorferi:* Evidence of contact transmission. Am. J. Trop. Med. Hyg. **35:** 355–359.
18. DURAY, P. H. & R. C. JOHNSON. 1986. The histopathology of experimentally infected hamsters with the Lyme disease spirochete, *Borrelia burgdorferi.* Proc. Soc. Exp. Biol. Med. **181:** 263–269.
19. JOHNSON, R. C., N. MAREK & C. KODNER. 1984. Infection of Syrian hamsters with Lyme disease spirochetes. J. Clin. Microbiol. **20:** 1099–1101.
20. BARTHOLD, S. W., K. D. MOODY, G. A. TERWILLIGER, A. C. STEERE, P. H. DURAY & R. O. JACOBY. 1988. Experimental Lyme arthritis in rats infected with *Borrelia burgdorferi.* J Infect. Dis. **157:** 842–846.
21. LEHMAN, T. J. A., J. G. ALLEN, P. H. PLOTZ & R. L. WILDER. 1983. Polyarthritis in rats following the systemic injection of *Lactobacillus casei* cell walls in aqueous suspension. Arthritis Rheum. **26:** 1259–1265.
22. WILDER, R. L., J. B. ALLEN, L. M. WAHL, G. B. CALANDRA & S. M. WALL. 1983. The pathogenesis of group A streptococcal cell wall-induced polyarthritis in the rat. Comparative studies in arthritis resistant and susceptible inbred rat strains. Arthritis Rheum. **26:** 1442–1451.
23. WILDER, R. L., G. B. CALANDRA, A. J. GARVIN, K. D. WRIGHT & C. T. HANSEN. 1982.

Strain and sex variation in the susceptibility to streptococcal cell wall-induced polyarthritis in the rat. Arthritis Rheum. **25:** 1064–1072.

24. BARBOUR, A. G. 1984. Isolation and cultivation of Lyme disease spirochetes. Yale J. Biol. Med. **57:** 521–525.

25. CRAFT, J. E., GRODZICKI, R. L. & STEERE, A. C. 1984. Antibody response in Lyme disease: Evaluation of diagnostic tests. J. Infect. Dis. **149:** 289–295.

26. DURAY, P. H., A. KUSNITZ & J. RYAN. 1985. Demonstration of the Lyme disease spirochete by a modified Dieterle stain method. Lab. Med. **16:** 685–687.

27. JOHNSTON, Y. E., P. H. DURAY, A. C. STEERE, M. KASHGARIAN, J. BUZA, S. E. MALAWISTA & P. W. ASKENASE. 1985. Lyme arthritis: Spirochetes found in synovial microangiopathic lesions. Am. J. Pathol. **118:** 26–34.

European Lyme Borreliosis

GEROLD STANEK,[a]

MICHEL PLETSCHETTE,[a]

HEINZ FLAMM,[a]

ALEXANDER M. HIRSCHL,[a]

ELISABETH ABERER,[b]

WOLFGANG KRISTOFERITSCH[c]

AND ERICH SCHMUTZHARD[d]

[a]Hygiene Institute of the University of Vienna
Vienna, Austria

[b]Department of Dermatology
University of Vienna
Vienna, Austria

[c]Department of Neurology
Wilhelminenspital
Vienna, Austria

[d]Department of Neurology
University of Innsbruck
Innsbruck, Austria

INTRODUCTION

Lyme borreliosis is a term introduced to designate a new nosologic entity describing the various disease states of the infection with tick- or insect-borne borrelia. At least part of the Lyme borreliosis spectrum, *e.g.,* erythema chronicum migrans[1,2] and acrodermatitis chronica atrophicans, has been known in Europe for many years although demonstration of the causative infectious agent was made only recently.

ETIOLOGIC AGENT

Consequent to the achievements in the United States in detecting,[3] isolating, and cultivating[4] the etiologic agent of Lyme disease,[5] European researchers were able to demonstrate and cultivate borrelia from ticks, various skin manifestations, and from cerebrospinal fluid.[6–10] European isolates show certain differences with US isolates in the molecular weights of major outer membrane proteins[11] and in reactivity with monoclonal antibodies raised against the outer surface proteins A and B of *Borrelia burgdorferi* type strain.[12] Additionally, a certain amount of heterogeneity of European isolates has been described.[13] Whether this heterogeneity is of some significance for the course of the disease is presently not understood. Despite this, it is now a generally accepted practice to consider spirochetes isolated either from Lyme borreliosis patients or from arthropods to be *Borrelia burgdorferi*.

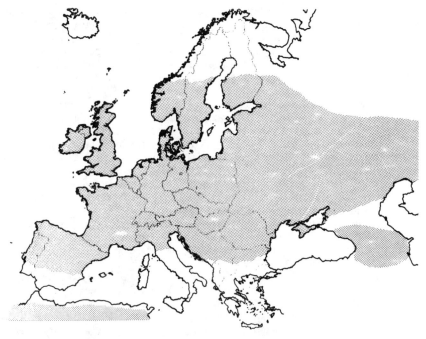

FIGURE 1. Distribution of *Ixodes ricinus* in Europe (data obtained from ref. 32).

VECTORS AND RESERVOIRS

The vector of *Borrelia burgdorferi* that transmits the agent to humans and animals is the sheep tick *Ixodes ricinus*. It is the most frequent species among European Ixodid ticks, occurring in an area covering South Scandinavia, the British Isles, Central Europe, France, Spain, Portugal, Italy, the Balkans, the European part of the USSR, northern Iran, and northern Africa (FIG. 1).

The frequency of ticks infected with *Borrelia burgdorferi* has been studied in many countries, including Austria, Czechoslovakia, Southern Germany, and Switzerland

TABLE 1. European Hard Tick *Ixodes ricinus:* Infection Rate with *Borrelia burgdorferi*[a]

Country	Number and Stage of *Ixodes ricinus*	Infection Rate	
		Mean	Range
Austria	1200 (adults and nymphs)	20%	2.2–40%
Czechoslovakia	570	8%	3–20%
South Germany	2400 adults (20.9%)		11.4–33.8%
	nymphs (10.6%)	13.6%	3.1–25.7%
	larvae (1.1%)		0.0–4.5%
Switzerland	2500 (adults and nymphs)	20%	5.0–34.0%

[a]Determined by Aeschlimann *et al.*, Kmety *et al.*, Wilske *et al.*, and Burger *et al.*

(TABLE 1). A field study in the eastern part of Austria[17] revealed an average infection rate for nymphal and adult ticks of 20%. About 8% of the unengorged ticks from southern Moravia and Slovakia were found to be infected.[16] In Southern Germany, 2403 ticks of various stadia were examined for presence of spirochetes by immuno-fluorescence technique and 13.6% were found positive.[15] The infection rate of adult ticks outnumbered that of nymphal and larval ticks. Between 5% and 34% of ticks collected in the Swiss Plateau were infected with spirochetes.[14]

In addition to the ixodids, *Haemaphysalis* spp. ticks have been examined, but with no positive results. Argas pigeon ticks were considered possible vectors in connection with two particular cases of Lyme borreliosis. Both patients had been bitten by those ticks, which were found in their home. Argas ticks from this location were investigated for presence of borrelia. On three occasions spirochetal organisms could be demonstrated but not cultivated.

Several insect species have been suspected to transmit *B. burgdorferi,* but no isolate from those arthropods exists thus far. Among the vector candidates, tabanids as well as mosquitoes are frequently considered.

Feral animals of the forests as well as certain domestic animals from which ticks obtain blood meals have been considered the major borrelia reservoirs. Yet until recently only a few studies have been conducted in Europe on the role of several such animal species as reservoirs of borrelia.

A serosurvey on 61 wild mice (44 *Clethrionomys glareolus,* 17 *Apodemus* spp.), 72 dogs, and 66 grazing cattle of Southern Germany revealed 20%, 50%, and 33% of the animals to be positive for antibodies to *B. burgdorferi,* respectively.[18] Another such a study has been undertaken by A. Hovmark *et al.*[19] They investigated the serological reaction in cattle and lambs before and after their first grazing period. Of 68 calves, 14 (20.6%) showed seroconversion. At the end of summer, eight of nine lambs with arthritis and 24 of 56 lambs without arthritis showed seroconversion. Arthritic disease of the lambs could be influenced by penicillin. The role of domestic animals as reservoirs of borrelia as well as the veterinary aspect of Lyme borreliosis in Europe are just beginning to come within the scope of epidemiological and diagnostic consideration.

INFECTIVITY FOR HUMANS

What is the incidence of transmission of *Borrelia burgdorferi* to man by the widely distributed, spirochete-bearing tick *Ixodes ricinus?* A field study was undertaken in southwestern Germany to answer this question. Of 41 persons bitten by borrelia-positive ticks, 1 (2%) developed an erythema chronicum migrans and another 19 (46.4%) showed significantly raised antibody titers to *B. burgdorferi.* During a 2-year follow-up none of the latter developed any further manifestation.[20] In our own studies of soldiers exposed to tick bites during outdoor activities, we could demonstrate seroconversion in 22% of late serum samples drawn 6 weeks after exposure. Only 2 (4%) of 50 persons developed an ECM[21] and no further manifestation was recorded.

CLINICAL MANIFESTATIONS OF LYME BORRELIOSIS

The pattern of clinical manifestations of Lyme borreliosis spreads over four organ systems, the skin, the nervous system, the joints, and the heart. Skin manifestations are erythema chronicum migrans (ECM), lymphadenosis cutis benigna (lymphocytoma,

LCB), and acrodermatitis chronica atrophicans (ACA). All these entities are spirochetal infections as proved by culture.[7,8,9,22] The neurological manifestations include
meningopolyneuritis (MPN),[23] cranial neuritis,[24] lymphocytic meningitis, encephalitis,
and myelitis.[25] *Borrelia* could be isolated from cerebrospinal fluid on many occasions in
various European countries. Joint manifestations appear as mono- or oligoarthritis.
Cardiac involvement ranges from various disorders of the conduction system to frank
myocarditis.

GEOGRAPHICAL DISTRIBUTION

The number of cases of Lyme borreliosis that have been recorded in European
countries is extremely variable. Depending on whether and how long a more or less
centralized diagnostic system has been established, the figures may range from a single

TABLE 2. Frequency Distribution (%) of Selected Clinical Manifestations in Lyme
Borreliosis from Eight European Countries

Clinical Diagnosis	Countries[a]							
	A	FRG (South/ North)	CH	F	H	YU	S	UK
n	2.015	373/1.087	481	272	96	250	731	68
ECM[b]	40.7	20.9/44.6	32.8	26.5	56.3	60.0	13.0	48.5
ACA[c]	10.6	9.7/6.6	10.9				0.8	19.2	
LCB[d]	3.0	−/0.5				0.8	1.8	
MPN[e]	42.3	56.6/41.3	18.3	57.1	34.3	36.0	62.1	30.9
Arthritis	1.3	12.9/5.8	22.5	12.9	9.4		4.0	
Carditis	0.2	−/1.2	3.1	3.3				1.5
Systemic symptoms	1.9		12.7			2.4		14.7

[a]Key: A, Austria; FRG, Federal Republic of Germany; CH, Czechoslovakia; F, France; H,
Hungary; YU, Yugoslavia; S, Switzerland; UK, United Kingdom.
[b]ECM = Erythema chronicum migrans.
[c]ACA = Acrodermatitis chronica atrophicans.
[d]LCB = Lymphadenosis cutis benigna.
[e]MPN = Meningopolyneuritis.

case report to several hundreds of cases. In general, physicians in many countries are
becoming more aware of Lyme borreliosis, and therefore the number of diagnosed
cases is continuously increasing. TABLE 2 gives an overview of the frequency distribution of selected clinical manifestations of Lyme borreliosis in Europe. In all the
countries where specific routine serology is done, the skin manifestation ECM and
neurological disorders are regularly found in a proportion ranging from 13.0 to 60.0%,
and 18.3 to 62.1%, respectively, of the cases.[26] Interestingly, acrodermatitis has been
collectively reported from Sweden, Switzerland, the Federal Republic of Germany and
Austria, but not from France, Hungary or the United Kingdom (FIG. 2).[14,15,28-30]
    Epidemiological studies from the latter countries do not mention LCB. Similarly,
cases of arthritis were not reported in the UK and Yugoslavia until 1986. In contrast to
this, Switzerland presents with an arthritis frequency of more than 20% of total cases.
    Lyme borreliosis is often called a summertime hazard. This would be true for the

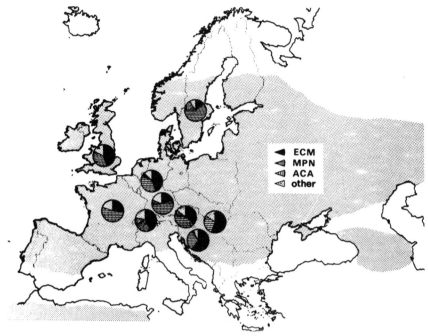

FIGURE 2. Relative frequency of the clinical manifestations erythema chronicum migrans (ECM), meningopolyneuritis (MPN), and acrodermatitis chronica atrophicans (ACA) in eight European countries.

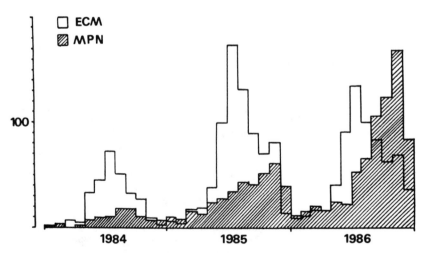

FIGURE 3. Seasonal distribution of erythema chronicum migrans (ECM) and meningopolyneuritis (MPN) in Austria from 1984 to 1986.

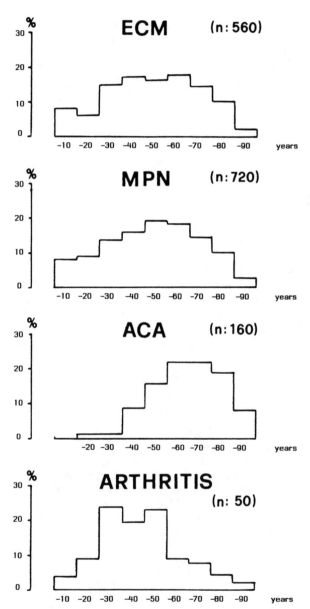

FIGURE 4. Age distribution of Austrian patients with erythema chronicum migrans (ECM), meningopolyneuritis (MPN), acrodermatitis chronica atrophicans (ACA), and arthritis.

early and usually self-limiting manifestations ECM and neuroborreliosis, which appear from 3 to 50 (median: 22) days and from 1 to over 100 (median: 40) days after infection, respectively. Looking at the seasonal distribution over several years, we found a relatively constant pattern of appearance of ECM, with a peak in July despite the doubling of cases in 1985 (FIG. 3). In 1984, the peak of neuroborreliosis records was in August and September. In 1985 and 1986, it shifted to November. Furthermore, in 1986 one can observe an increase in neurological manifestations outnumbering ECM cases. Whether this is due only to increased physicians' awareness or represents a kind of a genuine epidemic spread needs to be followed up in detail.

AGE AND SEX DISTRIBUTION

Lyme borreliosis occurs in all age groups and in both sexes. The early manifestations, ECM and MPN, are nearly equally distributed over all age groups with a median age of 43 (1–89) and 45 (1–83) years. ACA is a condition that frequently occurs in elderly people. A girl 16 years of age was the youngest person we observed with ACA. The median age of ACA patients was 65 (range: 16–85). In contrast to this, the median age of arthritis patients was 31 (range: 7–81) (FIG. 4).

TABLE 3. Sex Distribution of Patients with Selected Clinical Manifestations of Lyme Borreliosis (n = 1700)

Clinical Diagnosis	Sex Ratio (Male/Female)
Erythema chronicum migrans	0.56
Acrodermatitis chronica atrophicans	0.54
Lymphadenosis cutis benigna	0.57
Meningopolyneuritis	1.09
Arthritis	0.90
Carditis	(2.0)
Systemic symptoms	0.54

The skin manifestations ECM, ACA, LCB, and systemic symptoms are more frequently observed in females than in males. Interestingly, patients with neurological manifestations are predominantly males. The sex distribution in patients with arthritis is nearly balanced (TABLE 3). Exposure to ticks is not related to age and sex. The tendency towards an inverted male-female distribution in skin disorders versus neurological affections may reflect a specific reactivity of the host but may also be a consequence of different motivations to seek medical attention.

Although joint disorders are generally a burden of old age, a specific age-related reactivity cannot be seen in Lyme-borreliosis-related arthritis. Here a bias may be brought in by the well-known habit of neglecting joint complaints in the elderly patients. The late appearance of ACA may, however, reflect particular reactivity linked to aging.

CONCLUSION

Although named after an American town, Lyme borreliosis is a European public health reality. It is certainly not a rare disorder. The incidence and substantial number of cases underline the high individual risk of contracting the disease. Lyme borreliosis has been established as an etiology for numerous painful and crippling conditions which, when properly diagnosed, can be relieved by means of a relatively simple treatment.[31] In comparison with other infectious diseases of recent emergence, Lyme borreliosis is indeed less harmful. No fatal outcome has been substantiated.

Long-term case control studies and extensive field research on ecological problems, as well as detailed clinical investigations, are needed to come to a definitively precise picture of the disease in Europe. Yet the features described here and elsewhere do not point to any consistent, fundamental distinction between Lyme borreliosis in Europe and in the United States.

REFERENCES

1. AFZELIUS, A. 1910. Verhandlungen der Dermatologischen Gesellschaft zu Stockholm, October 28. Arch. Derm. Syph. **101:** 404.
2. LIPSCHÜTZ, B. 1913. Über eine seltene Erythemform (Erythema chronicum migrans). Arch. Dermatol. Syph. **118:** 349–356.
3. BURGDORFER, W., A. G. BARBOUR, S. F. HAYES, J. L. BENACH, E. GRUNWALDT & J. P. DAVIS. 1982. Lyme disease—a tick-borne spirochetosis? Science **216:** 1317–1319.
4. BARBOUR, A. G., W. BURGDORFER, S. F. HAYES, O. PETER & A. AESCHLIMANN. 1983. Isolation of a cultivable spirochete from *Ixodes ricinus* ticks of Switzerland. Curr. Microbiol. **8:** 123–126.
5. BARBOUR, A. G. 1984. Isolation and cultivation of Lyme disease spirochetes. Yale J. Biol. Med. **57:** 521–525.
6. ACKERMANN, R., J. KABATZKI, H. P. BOISTEN, A. C. STEERE, R. L. GRODZICKI, S. HARTUNG & U. RUNNE. 1984. *Ixodes ricinus* spirochete and European erythema chronicum migrans-disease. Yale J. Biol. Med. **57:** 123–130.
7. ASBRINK, E., B. HEDERSTEDT & A. HOVMARK. 1984. The spirochetal etiology of erythema chronicum migrans Afzelius. Acta Derm. Venereol. (Stockholm) **64:** 291–295.
8. ASBRINK, E., A. HOVMARK & B. HEDERSTEDT. 1984. The spirochetal etiology of acrodermatitis chronica atrophicans Herxheimer. Acta Derm. Venereol. (Stockholm) **64:** 506–512.
9. PREAC-MURSIC, V., B. WILSKE, G. SCHIERZ, H.-W. PFISTER & K. EINHÄUPL. 1984. Repeated isolation of spirochetes from cerebrospinal fluid of a patient with meningoradiculitis Bannwarth. Eur. J. Clin. Microbiol. **3:** 564–565.
10. STANEK, G., G. WEWALKA, V. GROH & R. NEUMANN. 1985. Isolation of spirochetes from the skin of patients with erythema chronicum migrans in Austria. Zbl. Bakt. Hyg. A **260:** 88–90.
11. WILSKE, B., V. PREAC-MURSIC & G. SCHIERZ. 1985. Antigenic heterogeneity of European *Borrelia burgdorferi* strains isolated from patients and ticks. Lancet **1:** 1099.
12. STANEK, G., G. WEWALKA, V. GROH, R. NEUMANN & W. KRISTOFERITSCH. 1985. Differences between Lyme disease and European arthropod-borne borrelia infections. Lancet **1:** 401.
13. WILSKE, B., V. PREAC-MURSIC, G. SCHIERZ & K. VON BUSCH. 1986. Immunochemical and immunological analysis of European *Borrelia burgdorferi* strains. Zbl. Bakt. Hyg. A **263:** 92–102.
14. AESCHLIMANN, A., E. CHAMOT, F. GIGON, J.-P. JEANNERET, D. KESSELER & CH. WALTHER. 1986. *B. burgdorferi* in Switzerland. Zbl. Bakt. Hyg. A. **263:** 450–458.
15. WILSKE, B., R. STEINHUBER H. BERGMEISTER, V. FINGERLE, G. SCHIERZ, V. PREAC-MURSIC, E. VANEK & B. LORBEER. 1987. Epidemiologische Daten zum Auftreten von Erkrankungsfällen sowie zur Durchseuchung von Zecken (*Ixodes ricinus*) mit *Borrelia burgdorferi*. Dtsch. Med. Wochenschr. **112:** 1730–1736.
16. KMETY, E., J. REHACEK & V. VYROSTEKOVA. 1986. Investigations of ticks for the presence of borrelia in Czechoslovakia. Zbl. Bakt. Hyg. A **263:** 468–470.
17. BURGER, I. 1987. Feldstudien und experimentelle Untersuchungen zur Biologie und Ökologie von *Borrelia burgdorferi*. Dissertation, University of Vienna.

18. KRAMPITZ, H. E. & S. BARK. 1987. Epidemiology of Ixodes-borreliosis in southern Germany. Immun. Infekt. **15:** 141–145.
19. HOVMARK, A., E. ASBRINK, O. SCHWAN, B. HEDERSTEDT, D. CHRISTENSSON. 1986. Antibodies to borrelia spirochetes in sera from Swedish cattle and sheep. Acad. Vet. Scand. **27:** 479–785.
20. PAUL, H., H.-J. GERTH & R. ACKERMANN. 1986. Infectiousness for humans of *Ixodes ricinus* containing *Borrelia burgdorferi*. Zbl. Bakt. Hyg. A **263:** 473–476.
21. SCHMUTZHARD, E., A. PALLUA, R. SCHMITZBERGER, R. SCHLÖGL & G. STANEK. Infections after tick-bite: a prospective epidemiological study from Tirol. Zbl. Bakt. Hyg. A. In press.
22. STANEK, G., G. WEWALKA, V. GROH & R. NEUMANN. 1985. Isolation of spirochetes from the skin of patients with erythema chronicum migrans in Austria. Zbl. Bakt. Hyg. A **260:** 88–90.
23. KRISTOFERITSCH, W., G. SPIEL & P. WESSELY. 1983. Zur Meningopolyneuritis (Garin-Bujadoux-Bannwarth). Nervenarzt **54:** 640–646.
24. SCHMUTZHARD, E., G. STANEK & P. POHL. 1985. Polyneuritis cranialis associated with *Borrelia burgdorferi*. J. Neurol. Neurosurg. Psychiatry **48:** 1182–1184.
25. PFISTER, H.-W., K. M. EINHÄUPL, B. WILSKE & V. PREAC-MURSIC. 1986. Bannwarth's syndrome and the neurological spectrum of arthropod-borne borreliosis. Zbl. Bakt. Hyg. A **263:** 343–347.
26. STIENRNSTEDT, G. 1985. Tickborne borrelia infection in Sweden. Scand. J. Infect. Dis. **45**(Suppl.).
27. LANNER, M., B. HEDERSTEDT, E. ASBRINK, A. HOVMARK & G. STIERNSTEDT. 1987. Serodiagnosis of borrelia infection during 1986 in Sweden. Zbl. Bakt. Hyg. In press.
28. Lyme Disease. 1987. Wkly. Epidemiol. Rec. **34:** 254–255.
29. LAKOS, A. 1988. Lyme disease in Hungary—the first three years. Zbl. Bakt. Hyg. In press.
30. MUHLEMANN, M. F. & D. J. M. WRIGHT. 1987. Emerging pattern of Lyme disease in the United Kingdom and Irish Republic. Lancet **i:** 260–262.
31. KRISTOFERITSCH, W., U. BAUMHACKL, E. SLUGA, G. STANEK & K. ZEILER. 1987. High-dose penicillin therapy in meningopolyneuritis Garin-Bujadoux-Bannwarth. Zbl. Bakt. Hyg. A **263:** 357–364.
32. BLASKOVIC, D. 1967. The public health importance of tick-borne encephalitis in Europe. Bull. W. H. O. **36:** 5–13.

The Geographic Distribution of Lyme Disease in the United States

CAROL A. CIESIELSKI,[a] LAURI E. MARKOWITZ,[a]
ROSE HORSLEY,[b] ALLEN W. HIGHTOWER,[b]
HAROLD RUSSELL,[c] AND CLAIRE V. BROOME[a]

[a]Epidemiology Section, Meningitis and Special Pathogens Branch
[b]Statistical Services Activity
[c]Laboratory Section, Respiratory Diseases Branch
Division of Bacterial Diseases
Center for Infectious Diseases
Centers for Disease Control
Atlanta, Georgia 30333

INTRODUCTION

Erythema chronicum migrans (ECM) was described in Europe and recognized as a dermatologic sequela of *Ixodes ricinus* bites long before it was first reported in the United States.[1] In 1970, the skin lesion characteristic of what is now known as Lyme disease was described in association with a tick bite in central Wisconsin.[2] The next cases were recognized near Lyme, Connecticut in 1975 in association with arthritis,[3] and ECM was reported following a tick bite in California in 1978.[4] Subsequently, a newly discovered spirochete, *Borrelia burgdorferi,* was found to be the etiologic agent, and two ticks were identified as vectors in the United States—*Ixodes dammini* in the Northeast, and *I. pacificus* in the West. The known distribution of these ticks closely corresponded to the location where cases of Lyme disease had been recognized.[5]

To further investigate the epidemiology of Lyme disease in the United States, define geographic regions endemic for the disease, and monitor trends, the Centers for Disease Control (CDC) and the Council of State and Territorial Epidemiologists established national surveillance for Lyme disease in 1982. This report describes the geographic distribution of Lyme disease in the United States, as determined by the national surveillance system.

MATERIALS AND METHODS

Before national surveillance was formally established, the known cases of Lyme disease were tabulated in 1980.[6] Since 1982, reports of all suspected cases of Lyme disease have been solicited from state health departments; these reports are classified using a standardized case definition.

Surveillance reports summarizing clinical, epidemiologic, and serologic data are completed by local physicians or health department officials and forwarded to CDC. The information requested includes demographic data (age, sex, and race of the patient), date of disease onset, symptoms, laboratory results, state and county of residence, geographic location of tick exposure, and travel history in the 30 days preceding illness.

283

Case Definition

Initially, the case definition required that all definite cases have ECM, since it is the most characteristic and best marker for Lyme disease. After the development of serologic tests for *B. burgdorferi* in 1984, laboratory criteria were incorporated into the case definition (TABLE 1). Serologic tests were considered positive if they met the criteria established at the laboratory that performed the tests.

From information on the case report form, we attempted to ascertain where each case was acquired. If the patient was exposed, through place of residence or travel, to an area known to be endemic for Lyme disease, we reported the case as having been acquired in that area. If the patient lived in an area endemic for Lyme disease and there was no history of travel or if the travel history was unknown, the county of residence was classified as the site of acquisition. If the patient did not live in an area previously reporting cases of Lyme disease and there was no history of travel, the

TABLE 1. Case Definition for Lyme Disease

I. Exposure in endemic area[a]
   A. Erythema chronicum migrans (ECM)[b] with exposure in endemic area ≤30 days before onset of ECM.
   B. In the absence of ECM, involvement of at least one organ system[c] and a positive laboratory test for *Borrelia burgdorferi*[d]

II. No exposure in endemic area
   A. ECM with involvement of at least two organ systems
   B. ECM and a positive laboratory test

---

[a]An area within two counties of an area in which at least one definite case of Lyme disease has been previously acquired.

[b]ECM is a skin lesion which begins as a macule or papule and expands in a circular manner to form a large, annular lesion with partial clearing.

[c]Cardiac involvement: atrioventricular conduction defects, myocarditis, or left ventricular dysfunction; neurologic involvement: meningitis, encephalitis, cranial or peripheral neuropathy, cerebellar ataxia, or myelitis; arthritis: red or swollen and painful joints.

[d]A positive serologic test (if performed at CDC, an indirect immunofluorescent assay titer ≥1:256, or an enzyme-linked immunosorbent assay optical density ratio ≥0.2) or isolation of *Borrelia burgdorferi* from a clinical specimen.

county of residence was identified as the acquisition site; if travel history was unknown, we attempted to obtain more information. This was not always possible; the case was then classified as having been acquired in an unknown location.

RESULTS

From 1980 to 1986, 5731 cases of Lyme disease were reported to CDC (TABLE 2). During the years 1982–1986, 491, 600, 1500, 1520, and 1394 cases, respectively, were reported. The number of cases from a state may differ from those reported by individual state health departments due to differences in case definition and because the reporting state, usually the patient's state of residence, may be different from the state of acquisition.

In 1980, Lyme disease was acquired in 11 states: Massachusetts, Connecticut, Rhode Island, New York, New Jersey, Wisconsin, Minnesota, Pennsylvania, Dela-

TABLE 2. Lyme Disease in the United States by State Where Acquired, 1980–1986[a]

Region	Year					
	1980	1982	1983	1984	1985	1986
New England						
New Hampshire			1			7
Maine					1	4
Massachusetts	11	15	13	33	69	163
Rhode Island	3	29	20	20	41	57
Connecticut	52	135	78	483	699	6[b]
Mid-Atlantic						
New York	7	170	267	446	5[b]	482
New Jersey	10	57	70	155	175	219
Pennsylvania	1	2		5	29	31
South Atlantic						
Delaware		1	4	1		
Virginia				1	2	7
Maryland	1	1	5	12	21	14
North Carolina			1	16	14	6
South Carolina				1	3	3
Georgia	1			1	1	2
Florida				1	1	1
North Central						
Wisconsin	25	58	69	176	135	162
Minnesota	8	22	55	86	64	94
Michigan			1		1	
Indiana				1		1
Ohio				1	1	1
Illinois					2	
Missouri					2	
Iowa					1	1
South Central						
Arkansas			1	4		1
Alabama						1
Tennessee			1	1	4	1
Texas			1	18	172	8
Oklahoma						2
Mountain Pacific						
Utah		1	1			1
Nevada	1					
Oregon			1	10	5	10
California			11	24	70	107
Unknown	106			4	2	2
TOTAL	226	491	600	1500	1520	1394

[a]Case definition varies by state. Data are provisional.
[b]Data not available.

ware, Maryland, Georgia, Nevada, and Utah. Forty-seven percent (106/226) of the case reports did not have a state of acquisition specified. However, for most, if not all, illness was acquired in the Northeast.[6] Through 1982, 602 (99%) of the 611 cases reported, where state of acquisition was known, were acquired in seven states: New York, New Jersey, Massachusetts, Rhode Island, Connecticut, Wisconsin, and Minnesota.[7]

Since 1982, the number of states in which Lyme disease has been acquired has increased yearly, from 18 in 1983 to 28 in 1986. Lyme disease has now apparently been acquired in 32 (64%) of the 50 states. Nonetheless, 86% of the 5731 provisional cases reported to CDC were acquired in the same seven states cited above (FIG. 1).

In the past several years, increasing numbers of cases have been reported from areas far removed from the originally described endemic regions of the northeastern

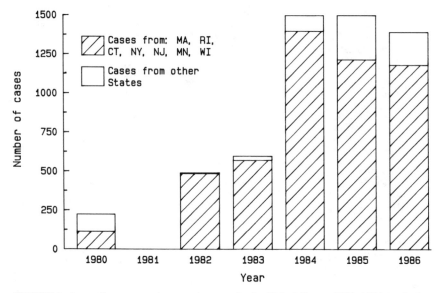

FIGURE 1. Lyme disease cases by reporting year in the United States, 1980–1986 (excluding 1981).

and upper midwestern parts of the country, such as California and the southeastern and south central United States. Lyme disease was acquired in six new states in 1985–1986: Alabama, Maine, Oklahoma, Iowa, Illinois, and Missouri. In three states (Alabama, Maine, and Oklahoma) the basis for classifying the index case was the presence of ECM and positive serologic results. In the other three states, the index cases were classified on the basis of ECM and involvement of at least two organ systems compatible with Lyme disease.

DISCUSSION

The annual number of reported cases of Lyme disease has increased nearly sevenfold between 1980 and 1986. Lyme disease is now the most commonly reported tick-borne illness in the United States.[8] It is unclear to what extent the increased number of cases and reporting areas represent improved recognition of the disease and better reporting rather than an actual increased incidence. Also, the development of serologic testing in 1984[9] increased our ability to detect Lyme disease in patients without ECM. However, Lyme disease may be increasing as studies suggest that the geographic distribution of the *Ixodes* tick population as well as the distribution of Lyme disease cases has expanded locally in some areas.[10,11]

Because of the variability among the states in reporting requirements, case definition, and surveillance methods, these surveillance data should be used to monitor trends, not to represent the true incidence of Lyme disease in the United States. For example, the total number of cases reported has remained relatively constant since 1984 (approximately 1500 per year). However, totals were not available for New York in 1985 and Connecticut in 1986. Had case totals been available for both of these states in the same year, the number of cases reported would have increased substantially.

Reported incidence rates vary among endemic areas. In some regions of the Northeast, incidence rates of Lyme disease as high as 1% have been reported.[12] Differing incidence rates among communities endemic for Lyme disease are probably due to different rates of spirochetal infection in the tick population. Up to 90% of *Ixodes* ticks in some endemic areas along the northern Atlantic coastline have *B. burgdorferi* in their gastrointestinal systems, in contrast to 3% of *Ixodes* ticks on the west coast.[13]

The surveillance system has been useful in identifying new geographic areas where Lyme disease has occurred. Although many states have now reported sporadic cases, the vast majority of cases continue to be acquired in the seven states where Lyme disease was recognized as endemic in 1980. It is difficult to determine the significance of sporadic cases in areas far removed from either the locations of the known tick vectors[14] or locations where previous cases have been described. These cases have been classified as Lyme disease based on the more stringent criteria required for exposure in areas where Lyme disease is not endemic and include both compatible clinical findings and serologic data (TABLE 1). The purpose of this geographic distinction was to improve diagnostic precision. Classifying an area as endemic not only has clinical implications but implies both the presence of *B. burgdorferi* and a suitable tick vector. The recognition of these cases acquired outside of previously endemic areas has led to the search for additional vectors. In 1984, *Amblyomma americanum* was suggested as a potential vector in New Jersey.[15] More recently, *B. burgdorferi* has been isolated from *Ixodes scapularis* ticks in North Carolina.[16] The search for new vectors must incorporate surveillance data, because isolation of the spirochete from other tick species and insects does not necessarily imply transmissibility to humans. Continued surveillance is necessary to precisely define where Lyme disease is acquired in the United States. The findings of additional vectors are important for our understanding of the epidemiology of Lyme disease and for the development of prevention strategies and control measures.

SUMMARY

In 1982, national surveillance for Lyme disease was established by the Centers for Disease Control to monitor trends and determine endemic geographic areas. Initially, the endemic areas corresponded to the known distribution of *Ixodes dammini*, a five-state area of the northeastern seaboard (New York, New Jersey, Connecticut, Rhode Island, and Massachusetts) and Wisconsin and Minnesota. Increasing numbers of cases have been reported outside these areas, however, 86% of the provisional 5731 cases reported to CDC were acquired in these seven states. The number of reported cases increased from 491 in 1982 to approximately 1500 per year in 1984–1986, making Lyme disease the most commonly reported tick-borne illness in the United States. The apparently widening distribution of Lyme disease indicates that physicians in all regions of the country should be familiar with its signs and symptoms. Investigations of the vector in areas endemic for Lyme disease where *Ixodes* ticks are not found are warranted.

REFERENCES

1. AFZELIUS, A. 1921. Erythema chronicum migrans. Acta Derm. Venereol. (Stockholm) **2:** 120–125.
2. SCRIMENTI, R. J. 1970. Erythema chronicum migrans. Arch. Dermatol. **102:** 104–105.
3. STEERE, A. C., S. E. MALAWISTA, D. R. SYNDAM, *et al.* 1977. Lyme arthritis: An epidemic of oligoarticular arthritis in children and adults in three Connecticut communites. Arthritis Rheum. **20:** 1–17.
4. NAVERSEN, D. N. & L. W. GARDNER. 1978. Erythema chronicum migrans in America. Arch. Dermatol. **114:** 253–254.
5. STEERE, A. C. & S. E. MALAWISTA. 1979. Cases of Lyme disease in the United States: Locations correlated with distribution of *Ixodes dammini*. Ann. Intern. Med. **91:** 730–733.
6. CENTERS FOR DISEASE CONTROL. 1981. Lyme disease—United States, 1980. MMWR **30:** 489–492.
7. SCHMID, G. P., R. HORSLEY, A. C. STEERE, *et al.* 1985. Surveillance of Lyme disease in the United States, 1982. J. Infect. Dis. **151:** 1144–1149.
8. CENTERS FOR DISEASE CONTROL. 1985. Update on Lyme disease and cases occurring during pregnancy. MMWR **34:** 376–384.
9. RUSSELL, H., J. S. SAMPSON, G. P. SCHMID, *et al.* 1984. Enzyme-linked immunosorbent assay and indirect immunofluorescent assay for Lyme disease. J. Infect. Dis. **49:** 465–470.
10. DAVIS, J. P., W. L. SCHELL, T. E. AMUNDSON, *et al.* 1984. Lyme disease in Wisconsin: Epidemiologic, clinical, serologic, and entomologic findings. Yale J. Biol. Med. **57:** 685–696.
11. MAIN, A. J., H. E. SPRANCE, K. O. KLOTER, *et al.* 1981. *Ixodes dammini* (Acari:Ixodidae) on white-tailed deer (*Odocoileus virginianus*) in Connecticut. J. Med. Entomol. **18:** 487–492.
12. BENACH, J. L. & J. L. COLEMAN. 1987. Clinical and geographic characteristics of Lyme disease in New York. Zbl. Bakt. Hyg. A **263:** 477–482.
13. HABICHT, G. S., G. BECK & J. L. BENACH. 1987. Lyme disease. Sci. Am. **257:** 78–83.
14. BURGDORFER, W. & J. E. KEIRANS. 1983. Ticks and Lyme disease in the United States. Ann. Intern. Med. **99:** 121.
15. SCHULZE, T. L., G. S. BOWEN, E. M. BOSLER, *et al.* 1984. *Amblyomma americanum:* a potential vector of Lyme disease in New Jersey. Science **224:** 601–603.
16. MAGNARELLI, L. A., J. F. ANDERSON, C. S. APPERSON, *et al.* 1986. Spirochetes in ticks and antibodies to *Borrelia burdorferi* in white-tailed deer from Connecticut, New York State, and North Carolina. J. Wildl. Dis. **22:** 178–188.

Occupational Risk of Lyme Disease in Endemic Areas of New York State

PERRY F. SMITH,[a] JORGE L. BENACH,[b]
DENNIS J. WHITE,[c] DONNA F. STROUP,[a] AND
DALE L. MORSE[c]

[a]*Centers for Disease Control*
Atlanta, Georgia 30333

[b]*New York State Department of Health*
Health Sciences Center
SUNY at Stony Brook
Stony Brook, New York 11794

[c]*New York State Department of Health*
Bureau of Communicable Disease Control
Albany, New York 12237

INTRODUCTION

Since Lyme disease (LD) was first described in 1977,[1] it has become the most commonly reported tick-borne disease in the United States.[2] Although much has been learned about its clinical spectrum, diagnosis, and treatment, we still know little about the prevalence of and specific risk factors for this disease in certain groups that are likely to be at high risk, such as outdoor workers. Outdoor activities are likely to place a person at increased risk since the primary vectors for transmission of *Borrelia burgdorferi,* the causative agent of LD, are *Ixodes* ticks. However, previous studies on the risk from outdoor activities have been contradictory. A study of employees at the Naval Weapons Station, Earle, NJ, found that outdoor workers were nearly five times more likely to have had LD as indoor workers.[3] In contrast, studies in Connecticut, Massachusetts, and New York failed to show a significantly increased risk associated with outdoor leisure activities.[4-6]

In New York, cases of LD have been reported since the late 1970s in the southeastern portion of the state, from Putnam, Suffolk (eastern end of Long Island), and Westchester Counties. Located in these counties are numerous state parks, as well as the Fire Island National Seashore, a federal park located on a 32-mile-long barrier island off the south shore of Long Island. These parks contain areas of woodlands, shrub growth, and grasslands, providing ideal habitats for *Ixodes* ticks and their primary hosts, the white-tailed deer (*Odocoileus virginianus*) and the white-footed mouse (*Peromyscus leucopus*). Cases of LD have been reported among both state and federal park employees, and a 1983 study found that 11% of employees at the Fire Island National Seashore had serologic evidence of infection with *B. burgdorferi* by immunofluorescent antibody assay (Dr. Jorge Benach, unpublished data).

Because of increasing concern about the occupational risk of LD among outdoor employees, we undertook the following serologic study of persons who were employed in areas of New York where LD is endemic. The purpose of the study was to determine the frequency of serologic evidence for infection in an essentially healthy, working population and to assess occupational and leisure outdoor activities as risk factors for infection.

METHODS

We recruited participants for the study from the following groups: state employees of the New York State Office of Parks, Recreation, and Historic Preservation and of the New York State Department of Environmental Conservation who worked in Putnam, Suffolk, or Westchester Counties; federal employees of the National Park Service at the Fire Island National Seashore and of the United States Fish and Wildlife Service in Suffolk County; employees of the Vector Control Bureau, Suffolk County Health Department; and employees of the Greenrock Corporation who worked in and around Rockefeller State Park in Westchester County. All of these organizations are involved primarily in the maintenance of lands in Putnam, Suffolk, or Westchester County. We held meetings with their employees and staff supervisors to provide information about LD and to explain the purpose of the study and to promote voluntary participation in the study. Both indoor and outdoor workers were encouraged to participate.

Following informed consent, participants completed a self-administered questionnaire regarding their current and past employment history, length of time that they spent outdoors each week at work and leisure at the time of the questionnaire, outdoor habitats where they worked or spent leisure time, tick exposure during work and leisure in the previous year, precautions that they usually took to avoid ticks, history of LD and its symptoms, and demographic information. A blood sample was then taken from each participant and tested for antibodies against *B. burgdorferi* at the New York State Department of Health, SUNY at Stony Brook, Stony Brook, New York, by the enzyme-linked immunosorbent assay (ELISA) of Russell.[7] A positive ELISA result was defined as a direct optical density ≥ 0.2. All blood samples that were positive by ELISA underwent further testing for antibodies against polypeptides of *B. burgdorferi* by Western immunoblot assay.[8,9] A negative immunoblot result was evidence for a false-positive ELISA result, and the blood sample was considered to be negative for antibodies againt *B. burgdorferi* in our analysis.

The questionnaires were completed and blood samples were drawn at the participants' worksites from May through July 1986. All participants with symptoms of LD or with serologic reactivity to *B. burgdorferi* were advised to see their physicians for medical evaluation and for consideration of antibiotic treatment.

To calculate participation rates, we used complete employee rosters that were provided by each organization when the blood samples were drawn. We determined participation rates by employee characteristics, using the following information from the rosters: age, gender, outdoor versus indoor work, and permanent versus seasonal job status.

To determine the incidence of seroconversions for antibodies against *B. burgdorferi,* we collected a second blood sample from members of the employee groups from August through November 1986. These samples were tested at the Stony Brook laboratory in the same manner as the first samples. We defined a seroconversion as an increase in the ELISA direct optical density from <0.2 on the first testing to ≥ 0.2 on the second testing.

Some of the samples from the first and second testing were also tested by the Immunology Laboratory, Respiratory Diseases Branch, Division of Bacterial Diseases, Centers for Disease Control (CDC), Atlanta, Georgia by the same ELISA methodology as was used at the Stony Brook laboratory. However, the CDC laboratory used anti-human immunoglobulin conjugates and reference sera that were different from those used at Stony Brook. As a result, the CDC used different criteria to interpret its ELISA results. It reported the results as an optical density ratio of the test serum to a positive control serum, with a positive result defined as an optical density ratio ≥ 0.2.

For comparison with the serologic results of the employees, we tested blood samples from two additional groups. The first group of samples was provided to us by the New York Blood Center in the autumn of 1986 from blood donors in Suffolk and Westchester Counties (endemic counties). The second group was provided by the New York State Department of Health Wadsworth Center for Laboratories and Research, Albany, New York. These samples were taken from persons who attended New York State Department of Health clinics for sexually transmitted diseases in northwestern New York where LD is not endemic. Their blood had been submitted to the state laboratory for serologic testing for syphilis in December 1986 and January 1987 and was nonreactive when tested by the automated reagin test. The samples from both groups had no identifiers, and no information about the donors or about the exact dates of collection was available to us. The samples were tested for antibodies against *B. burgdorferi* in the same manner as the samples from the employee groups.

For univariate analysis of the questionnaire and serologic data, we used the chi-square and Fisher exact tests (two-tailed). Multivariate logistic regression analysis was used to assess the independent effects of multiple risk factors for seropositivity. In the analysis of risk of seropositivity by county, we defined a county with endemic LD as one in which (1) *Ixodes* ticks were known to be present and (2) there had been at least one reported case of physician-diagnosed LD in a person whose most likely place of exposure was within that county. The endemic counties in New York at the time of this study were Putnam, Suffolk, and Westchester.

TABLE 1. Participation Rates of 865 Employees from Six Organizations by Employee Characteristic, New York State, 1986[a]

Employee Characteristic	With Characteristic		Without Characteristic		Relative Participation Rate[b] (95% C.I.)	p Value
	Total	% Participation	Total	% Participation		
Age >30 y	384	56.0	224	44.6	1.3 (1.1–1.5)	.01
Male	647	49.8	218	42.2	1.2 (1.0–1.4)	.06
Outdoor worker	570	52.6	169	24.9	2.1 (1.7–2.7)	<.001
Permanent employee	530	50.8	335	43.3	1.2 (1.0–1.4)	.04

[a]The number of employees with and without each characteristic does not always total to 865 since some information on employees was incomplete.

[b]For employees with the specified characteristic compared to those without the characteristic (*i.e.*, age ≤30 years, female, indoor worker, and seasonal employee, respectively).

RESULTS

Of 865 persons in the employee groups, 414 (48%) participated in the first testing. Analysis of the information from the employee rosters showed that participation rates varied by employee characteristic (TABLE 1). Fifty-six percent of employees over the age of 30 participated, compared with 45% of employees 30 and younger. Males, outdoor workers, and permanent employees had higher rates of participation than females, indoor workers, and seasonal employees, respectively.

Based on the questionnaire information, 322 (78%) of the 414 participants in the first testing were male, and 392 (95%) were white. Participants' ages ranged from 17 to 76 years (mean 37.2, median 35). Ninety-three percent of the participants reported that they worked outdoors on the job at least part of the time. Of the 411 participants

TABLE 2. Prevalence of Antibodies against *Borrelia burgdorferi* by Age, Gender, Ethnicity, Location of Permanent Residence and Employment, New York State, 1986

	Total	Number Seropositive	Percentage Seropositive
Age group (years)			
≤19	29	2	6.9
20–29	110	6	5.5
30–39	113	4	3.5
40–49	73	5	6.8
50–59	61	9	14.8
60–69	22	0	0
70–79	6	1	16.7
Gender			
Male	322	20	6.2
Female	92	7	7.6
Ethnicity			
White	392	25	6.4
Black	8	2	25.0
Hispanic	9	0	0
Other/unknown	5	0	0
Permanent residence			
Putnam County, NY	6	1	16.7
Suffolk County, NY	292	23	7.9
Westchester County, NY	62	3	4.8
Other endemic counties[a]	6	0	0
Nonendemic counties and New York City[b]	45	0	0
Employment			
Putnam County, NY	5	0	0
Suffolk County, NY[c]	328	23	7.0
Westchester County, NY	81	4	4.9

[a]San Diego, CA; Fairfield, CT; Franklin, MA; Bergen, NJ; Burlington, NJ.

[b]Homer, AK; Phillps, AR; Passaic, NJ; Cayuga, Columbia, Dutchess, Nassau, Orange, Rockland, Ulster Counties, NY.

[c]Includes Fire Island National Seashore.

who reported information about their medical history, nine (2%) had a definite past diagnosis of LD, 14 (3%) were uncertain whether or not they had had physician-diagnosed LD, and 388 (94%) denied a previous diagnosis of LD.

Twenty-eight participants had antibodies against *B. burgdorferi* as determined by ELISA at the Stony Brook laboratory. However, one of these did not have a positive confirmatory immunoblot test and was considered to be negative for antibodies specific for LD. Thus, 27 (6.5%) of the 414 participants had serologic evidence of past infection with *B. burgdorferi*.

The prevalence of seropositivity by age group, gender, ethnicity, and location of permanent residence and employment is given in TABLE 2. Older participants tended to have a higher seropositivity rate than younger participants. For example, the rate for all employees over the age of 49 was 11.2%, compared with 5.2% for employees ≤49 years (relative risk = 2.2; 95% confidence interval = 1.0–4.5; p = .07). The rate for males was similar to the rate for females. The rates varied by ethnic background, permanent residence, and county of employment, but many categories had only a few participants. Of the 366 participants with permanent residence in one of the endemic counties, 27 (7.4%) were seropositive, compared with none of the 45 participants with permanent residence in nonendemic counties (relative risk = indeterminant, $p = .06$).

Of the 27 seropositive persons, only three (11.1%) reported a definite past diagnosis of LD. However, seropositive persons were seven times more likely to have had a diagnosis of LD than were seronegative persons (relative rate of diagnosis = 7.1; 95% confidence interval = 2.2–23.0; $p = .02$).

Each of five principal symptoms of LD were reported by only a minority of the 27 seropositive persons (TABLE 3). Seronegative persons reported these symptoms less frequently. Overall, of the 27 seropositive persons, 14 (51.9%) gave a history of one or more of the five symptoms listed in TABLE 3, compared with 109 (28.2%) of the 387 seronegative persons (relative risk of symptoms = 1.8; 95% confidence interval = 1.2–2.9; $p = .02$).

We evaluated exposure to ticks as a risk factor for seropositivity. FIGURE 1 shows the association between the reported number of *Ixodes* tick bites during the past year and the prevalence of seropositivity among the 246 participants who could identify *Ixodes* ticks. Of the seven persons with >4 bites in the past year, four (57.1%) were seropositive compared with eight (3.3%) of the 239 with ≤4 bites (relative risk = 17.1; 95% confidence interval = 7.3–40.2; $p < .001$). Participants were also asked the number of times per week during the past year that they had found ticks on themselves, including all attached and unattached ticks of any species, during work and leisure (FIG. 2). Ticks that were found immediately following time at work were counted with ticks found during work. The prevalence of seropositivity was associated with the number of ticks found during leisure: of the 107 who reported finding >1 tick per week during leisure, 12 (11.2%) were seropositive, compared with 14 (4.7%) of the 299 who reported ≤1 tick per week during leisure (relative risk = 2.4; 95% confidence interval = 1.2–4.9; $p = .03$). This association was not found when we considered the number of ticks found during work or during work and leisure combined. Tick-avoidance precautions, including wearing long pants, tucking pants legs into one's socks, wearing long-sleeved shirts, using insect repellent on one's skin or clothes, and checking oneself for ticks, were not significantly associated with antibody status during either work or leisure (TABLE 4).

TABLE 3. Symptoms of Lyme Disease as Reported by Seropositive and Seronegative Participants in the Employee Study Group, New York State, 1986

History of Symptom	Seropositive Employees ($n = 27$)		Seronegative Employees ($n = 387$)		RR[a] (95% Confidence Interval)	p Value
	Number	(%)	Number	(%)		
Rash[b]	7	(25.9)	40	(10.3)	2.5 (1.2–5.2)	.02
Fever >38°C with severe head-ache and/or stiff neck	3	(11.1)	40	(10.3)	1.1 (0.4–3.3)	.75
Numbness or paralysis	3	(11.1)	16	(4.1)	2.7 (0.8–8.6)	.12
Arthritis	7	(25.9)	45	(11.6)	2.2 (1.1–4.6)[c]	.06[c]
Heart palpitations	4	(14.8)	23	(5.9)	2.5 (0.9–6.7)	.09

[a]Relative risk of symptom for seropositive persons compared with seronegative persons.

[b]Participants were asked if they had had a "red circular expanding skin rash," suggesting erythema chronicum migrans.

[c]The discrepancy between the 95% confidence interval and p value is due to the confidence interval being test-based, whereas the p value is calculated by Fisher's exact test.

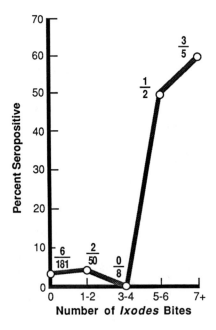

FIGURE 1. Prevalence of seropositivity among study participants by number of *Ixodes* tick bites during the past year, New York State, 1986. Results are based on the responses of the 246 participants who said they could identify *Ixodes* ticks. Numbers shown on the graph indicate the number of seropositive persons per total number of persons in each category.

FIGURE 3 shows the prevalence of seropositivity among the study participants by the amount of time that they reported spending outdoors during work and leisure each week. Participants with long outdoor work hours did not have higher prevalence rates than those reporting less outdoor work time. However, of the 88 persons who spent >30 hours outdoors during leisure, 11 (12.5%) were seropositive, compared with 16 (4.9%) of 325 persons who spent ≤30 hours in outdoor leisure time (relative risk = 2.5; 95% confidence interval = 1.2–5.2; p = .02). When outdoor work and leisure times were combined, there was no consistent association with prevalence of seropositivity (FIG. 3).

We also assessed the risk of seropositivity from time spent in each of the following outdoor habitats: meadows, mowed lawns, paved areas, sand beaches, shrub growth, and woodlands. There was no significantly elevated risk associated with either work or leisure time in any of these areas.

In assessing employment history, we considered the total number of years of outdoor employment in endemic counties, specific job titles, and currently having a second outdoor job. FIGURE 4 shows the prevalence of seropositivity by the number of years of outdoor employment. Of the 256 persons with a history of outdoor work (≥1 year), 22 (8.6%) were seropositive, compared with one of 23 (4.3%) who had no history of outdoor work (relative risk = 2.0; 95% confidence interval = 0.3–13.0; p = .70). Specific job titles and having a second outdoor job were not significantly associated with antibody status.

In a multiple logistic model which included the number of *Ixodes* tick bites during the past year, ticks found during leisure each week, leisure hours spent outdoors each week, and county of residence, seropositivity was significantly and independently associated with both the number of *Ixodes* tick bites (p = .002) and ticks found during leisure (p = .03), but not with outdoor leisure hours (p = 1.0) or county of residence

(p = .78). No additional risk factors were found to be associated with seropositivity in multiple additional regression analyses except for spending time in mowed lawn during leisure (p = .05).

Two hundred forty seronegative participants in the first testing took part in the second testing, with a mean interval between testings of 108 days (median: 113 days; range: 26–171 days). Only one (0.4%) of these 240 seroconverted on the second testing. This person was a 53-year-old man with an estimated 50 hours of outdoor activities each week, equally split between work and leisure. He denied any prior symptoms of LD at the time of his second test in mid-September, but reported being bitten three times by *Ixodes* ticks in July.

Eighty-two of the blood samples from the first and second testing were tested at both the Stony Brook Laboratory and at the CDC laboratory. Discrimination of seropositive from seronegative samples by the two laboratories was identical for 81 (99%) of the specimens.

The comparison group of New York Blood Center donors included 362 persons. Of these, four (1.1%) were positive for antibodies against *B. burgdorferi*. In comparison,

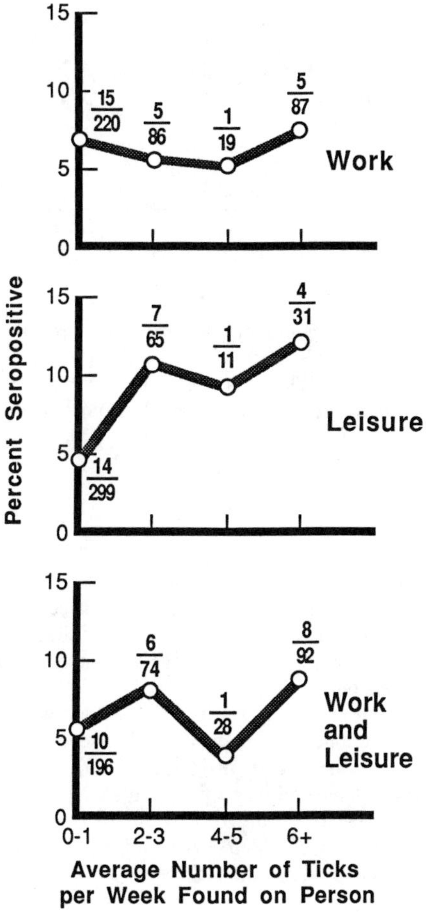

FIGURE 2. Prevalence of seropositivity among study participants by number of ticks per week found on person during work, leisure, and during work and leisure combined, New York State, 1986. Numbers shown on the graphs indicate the number of seropositive persons per total number of persons in each category.

TABLE 4. Evaluation of Seropositivity for Antibodies against *Borrelia burgdorferi* by Tick-Avoidance Precautions at Work and Leisure, New York State, 1986

Tick-Avoidance Precaution	Persons Not Taking Precaution		Persons Taking Precaution		RR[a] (95% Confidence Interval)	p Value
	Total	% Seropositive	Total	% Seropositive		
At Work						
Wear long pants	58	3.4	356	7.0	0.5 (.1–1.9)	.40
Tuck pants legs into socks	388	6.4	26	7.7	0.8 (.2–3.4)	.68
Wear long-sleeved shirt	309	5.8	105	8.6	0.7 (.3–1.5)	.45
Use insect repellent on skin	326	7.4	88	3.4	2.2 (.7–6.7)	.28
Use insect repellent on clothes	328	7.6	86	2.3	3.3 (.9–12.2)	.13
Check oneself for ticks	134	6.0	280	6.8	0.9 (.4–2.0)	.92
At Leisure						
Wear long pants	167	6.0	247	6.9	0.9 (.4–1.9)	.87
Tuck pants legs into socks	396	6.6	18	5.6	1.2 (.2–8.1)	1.00
Wear long-sleeved shirt	346	7.2	68	2.9	2.5 (.6–9.5)	.28
Use insect repellent on skin	330	7.0	84	4.8	1.5 (.5–4.1)	.63
Use insect repellent on clothes	353	7.4	61	1.6	4.5 (.8–26.2)	.15
Check oneself for ticks	146	7.5	268	6.0	1.3 (.6–2.7)	.68

[a]Relative risk of seropositivity for persons not taking the tick-avoidance precaution compared with those taking the precaution.

the participants in the employee groups were almost six times more likely to be seropositive (relative risk = 5.9; 95% confidence interval = 2.4–14.6; $p < .001$).

Of 100 blood samples from persons attending Department of Health clinics in areas of New York where LD is not endemic, all were negative for antibodies against *B. burgdorferi*.

DISCUSSION

In this study we were interested in differentiating leisure activity from occupational activity as risk factors for infection with *B. burgdorferi*, with seropositivity as our measure of infection. We found that seropositivity was associated with leisure-time outdoor exposure, while the evidence for an association with work exposure was less consistent.

For instance, seropositivity was associated with finding ticks on oneself during leisure, but not during work. However, ticks that were acquired during work may not have been noticed until leisure hours after work when the ticks had had time to engorge with blood and when people may have been more likely to find them during bathing. We tried to minimize this effect by counting the ticks that were found immediately following work hours with those found during work, but it was difficult to be certain when and where the ticks were acquired.

The analysis of the amount of time spent outdoors also suggested that outdoor leisure activity was a risk factor for infection with *B. burgdorferi*. We found by univariate analysis that spending >30 hours outdoors during leisure increased a person's risk of being seropositive. Although logistic regression analysis failed to show this association, it did suggest that leisure time spent specifically in mowed lawn increased a person's risk. Spending time outdoors during work was not associated with seropositivity. One reason for this lack of association may be that the reported outdoor work hours were relevant only to the respondent's current job and did not account for prior occupational exposure. In contrast, the reported leisure hours that were spent outdoors may have reflected a long-term pattern of activity and been a better measure of life-long outdoor exposure.

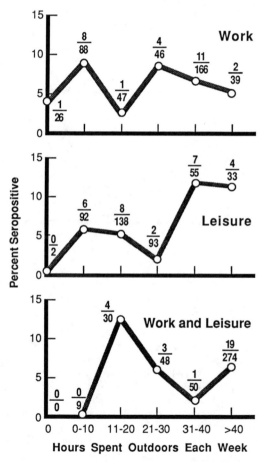

FIGURE 3. Prevalence of seropositivity among study participants by number of hours spent outdoors each week during work, leisure, and during work and leisure combined, New York State, 1986. Numbers shown on the graphs indicate the number of seropositive persons per total number of persons in each category.

Although not shown conclusively by this study, outdoor occupational exposure is probably an important risk factor for infection with *B. burgdorferi*. Employees with a prior history of outdoor jobs were twice as likely to be seropositive as those without such a history. However, this association was not statistically significant, in part because of the low number of indoor workers in the study group. The significantly lower rate of seropositivity in the blood donor group relative to the employee group also suggests an occupational risk. Since we had no information on individual blood donors, we can only speculate about the reasons for their lower seroprevalence rate. Like the employees, the majority of the blood donors were likely to have lived in counties where LD is endemic since we took blood samples from donors only in Suffolk and Westchester Counties. Thus, the risk from leisure activities around their homes may have been similar to that of the employee group. However, the blood donor group was not so likely to have included as high a percentage of outdoor workers as the 93% which occurred in the employee group. This difference could have resulted in a lower occupational exposure to ticks and would account for the lower seroprevalence rate in the blood donors.

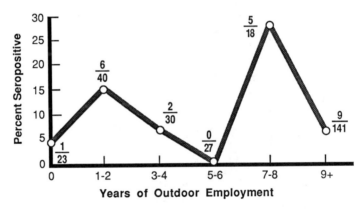

FIGURE 4. Prevalence of seropositivity among study participants by number of years of outdoor employment in endemic counties, New York State, 1986. See text for the definition of endemic counties. Numbers shown on the graph indicate the number of seropositive persons per total number of persons in each category.

Caution is needed when interpreting the results of this study. Since employee participation in this study was voluntary and only 48% of eligible employees volunteered, the results may have been influenced by selection bias. It is reasonable to suspect that some employees, such as indoor workers, might have considered themselves to be at low risk for LD and therefore have been less likely to participate. In fact, we found that indoor workers were less likely to participate than outdoor workers. If the nonparticipants were also less likely to be seropositive, then the prevalence rate of antibodies in the participant group would overestimate the rate for the entire employee group.

However, the antibody prevalence and incidence rates in our study appear consistent with results from previous studies of populations living in areas with high rates of LD. We found that 6.5% of the employee group had serologic evidence of past infection with *B. burgdorferi*. In comparison, a 1982 study, using an indirect immunofluorescent assay to test blood samples from summer residents in a community on Fire Island National Seashore, found that 9.7% of the residents had antibodies at a dilution of ≥1:64 and 6.3% had antibodies at ≥1:128.[6] In 1983, the prevalence rate for employees at the Fire Island National Seashore was 11%, determined by indirect immunofluorescent assay at ≥1:128 (unpublished data of Dr. Jorge Benach). The seroconversion rate for our employee group was 0.4%, which was lower than the 3.1% reported in the 1982 Fire Island study.[6] However, incidence of LD varies greatly by geographic location, as shown by numerous surveillance-based studies of clinical LD that have found peak annual incidence rates ranging from .01% to 3.3%.[3–5,10]

Evidence suggests that there are large numbers of asymptomatic, though previously infected, persons in areas where LD is endemic. In our study, only 52% of the seropositive employees gave a history of symptoms of LD. Steere estimated that 50% of infected persons on Great Island, Massachusetts, were asymptomatic.[5] *B. burgdorferi* is able to cause chronic infection in humans[11,12] and can result in late manifestations of LD without causing early symptoms.[13] It is not known how many asymptomatic persons are currently infected and will later develop complications of LD, although the number is likely to increase because of the geographical spread of LD and the large number of people who are at risk for exposure during outdoor leisure and occupational activities. Because early antibiotic treatment of symptomatic LD helps to prevent later complications[5,14,15] and treatment which is delayed until the late stages of LD may not be as effective as early treatment,[16,17] prompt antibiotic therapy for symptomatic LD is advisable. However, it is not currently known if asymptomatic seropositive persons should also receive treatment. Studies are needed to clarify the long-term natural history of initially asymptomatic infection with *B. burgdorferi* and to determine the role, if any, of antibiotic therapy for asymptomatic seropositive persons. This information would have important implications for serologic testing and treatment of the increasing number of people who are at high risk for LD because of outdoor exposure in areas where LD is endemic.

Although serologic testing for LD has greatly improved the ability to diagnose and study the disease, there are limitations to the current state of the art. Serologic testing is insensitive for diagnosing early LD when erythema chronicum migrans is the only manifestation[7,18] or following early treatment with antibiotics which appear to blunt the antibody response.[19] In addition, there is no current standardization for LD serology. The sensitivity and specificity of the test can vary with the type of assay[20] and with different laboratories performing the test.[21] A standardized test with improved sensitivity for diagnosing early LD is clearly needed. Such a test would promote further understanding of LD by improving the accuracy of seroepidemiologic studies, as well as benefit the practicing physician in the diagnosis of LD.

SUMMARY

Although Lyme disease (LD) is the most common tick-borne disease in the United States, little is known about the frequency of and risk factors for infection with *Borrelia burgdorferi* in occupational groups. In 1986, we recruited primarily outdoor workers from six employee groups in southeastern New York where LD is endemic. Of 414 participants who completed questionnaires and had blood samples tested for antibodies against *B. burgdorferi* by ELISA and Western immunoblot, 27 (6.5%) were seropositive, but only 14 of the 27 reported previous symptoms of LD. Persons who spent more than 30 hours per week outdoors during leisure were 2.5 times more likely to be seropositive than those who did not ($p = .02$). Those with a history of outdoor employment were twice as likely to be seropositive as those without such a history, although this finding was not statistically significant ($p = .70$). However, the seroprevalence rate for the employees was 5.9 times higher than the rate for a comparison group of anonymous blood donors from the same region of New York ($p < .001$). These results suggest that there was a relatively high rate of seropositivity for the employee groups and that infection was frequently asymptomatic and associated with outdoor exposure.

REFERENCES

1. STEERE, A. C., S. E. MALAWISTA, D. R. SNYDMAN, et al. 1977. Lyme arthritis: an epidemic of oligoarticular arthritis in children and adults in three Connecticut communities. Arthritis Rheum. **20:** 7–17.
2. CENTERS FOR DISEASE CONTROL. 1985. Update: Lyme disease and cases occurring during pregnancy—United States. MMWR **34(25):** 376–384.
3. BOWEN, G. S., T. L. SCHULZE, C. HAYNE, et al. 1984. A focus of Lyme disease in Monmouth County, New Jersey. Am. J. Epidemiol. **120:** 387–394.
4. STEERE, A. C., T. F. BRODERICK & S. E. MALAWISTA. 1978. Erythema chronicum migrans and Lyme arthritis: epidemiologic evidence for a tick vector. Am. J. Epidemiol. **108:** 312–321.
5. STEERE, A. C., E. TAYLOR, M. L. WILSON, et al. 1986. Longitudinal assessment of the clinical and epidemiological features of Lyme disease in a defined population. J. Infect. Dis. **154:** 295–300.
6. HANRAHAN, J. P., J. L. BENACH, J. L. COLEMAN, et al. 1984. Incidence and cumulative frequency of endemic Lyme disease in a community. J. Infect. Dis. **150:** 489–496.
7. RUSSELL, H., J. S. SAMPSON, G. P. SCHMID, et al. 1984. Enzyme-linked immunosorbent assay and indirect immunofluorescence assay for Lyme disease. J. Infect. Dis. **149:** 465–470.
8. COLEMAN, J. L. & J. L. BENACH. 1987. Isolation of antigenic components from the Lyme disease spirochete: their role in early diagnosis. J. Infect. Dis. **155:** 756–765.
9. TOWBIN, H., T. STAEHELIN & J. GORDON. 1979. Electrophoretic transfer of proteins from polyacrylamide gels to nitrocellulose sheets: procedure and some applications. Proc. Natl. Acad. Sci. U.S.A. **76:** 4350–4354.
10. HANRAHAN, J. P., J. L. BENACH, J. L. COLEMAN, et al. 1984. Epidemiologic features of Lyme disease in New York. Yale J. Biol. Med. **57:** 643–650.
11. STEERE, A. C., R. L. GRODZICKI, A. N. KORNBLATT, et al. 1983. The spirochetal etiology of Lyme disease. N. Engl. J. Med. **308:** 733–740.
12. SNYDMAN, D. R., D. P. SCHENKEIN, V. P. BERARDI, et al. 1986. *Borrelia burgdorferi* in joint fluid in chronic Lyme arthritis. Ann. Intern. Med. **104:** 798–800.
13. STEERE, A. C., S. E. MALAWISTA, N. H. BARTENHAGEN, et al. 1984. The clinical spectrum and treatment of Lyme disease. Yale J. Biol. Med. **57:** 453–460.
14. STEERE, A. C., G. J. HUTCHINSON, D. W. RAHN, et al. 1983. Treatment of the early manifestations of Lyme disease. Ann. Intern. Med. **99:** 22–26.
15. STEERE, A. C., S. E. MALAWISTA, J. H. NEWMAN, et al. 1980. Antibiotic therapy in Lyme disease. Ann. Intern. Med. **93:** 1–8.
16. STEERE, A. C., A. R. PACHNER & S. E. MALAWISTA. 1983. Neurologic abnormalities of Lyme disease: successful treatment with high-dose intravenous penicillin. Ann. Intern. Med. **99:** 767–772.
17. STEERE, A. C., J. GREEN, R. T. SCHOEN, et al. 1985. Successful parenteral penicillin therapy of established Lyme arthritis. N. Engl. J. Med. **312:** 869–874.
18. WILKINSON, H. W. 1984. Immunodiagnostic tests for Lyme disease. Yale J. Biol. Med. **57:** 567–572.
19. DAVIS, J. P., W. L. SCHELL, T. E. AMUNDSON, et al. 1984. Lyme disease in Wisconsin:

epidemiologic, clinical, serologic, and entomologic findings. Yale J. Biol. Med. **57:** 685–696.

20.   CRAFT, J. E., R. L. GRODZICKI & A. C. STEERE. 1984. Antibody response in Lyme disease: evaluation of diagnostic tests. J. Infect. Dis. **149:** 789–795.

21.   HEDBERG, C. W., M. T. OSTERHOLM, K. L. MACDONALD, *et al.* 1987. An interlaboratory study of antibody to *Borrelia burgdorferi*. J. Infect. Dis. **155:** 1325–1327.

Clinical Manifestations and Epidemiological Characteristics of Lyme Disease in Hailin County, Heilongjiang Province, China

AI CHENGXU,[a] WEN YUXIN,[a] ZHANG YONGGUO,[a]
WANG SHAOSHAN,[a] QIU QUICHENG,[b] SHI ZHIXUE,[c]
LI DEYOU,[b] CHEN DONGQUAN,[c] LIU XIAODONG,[b]
ZHAO JIENHUA[c]

[a]Institute of Microbiology and Epidemiology
P.O. Box 130
Academy of Military Medical Sciences
Beijing, 100850, China

[b]Antiepidemic Station
Mudanjiang Forestry Administration
Mudanjiang, Heilongjiang Province, China

[c]Antiepidemic Station
Hailin Forestry Bureau, Heilongjiang Province, China

SUMMARY

Clinical manifestations and epidemiological characteristics of Lyme disease in Hailin county, Heilongjiang Province, China have been reported. The clinical picture of erythema chronicum migrans (ECM) is variable. ECM in the form of annular erythematous patch is uncommon. It is an extensive and indurated lesion. In some instances, a vesicle or necrosis appears in the center of the lesion. Secondary erythema may present in some patients. The neurologic abnormalities consist of meningitis, facial palsy, and polyneuritis. Cardiac abnormalities are rare. In addition, there were cases with lymphadenosis benigna cutis (LABC), which had heretofore only been reported in Europe. The attack rate of ECM is 8.4%. There was a significant sex difference, and most cases occurred in May and June. All patients had a history of tick bite. The prevalence rates of neurologic abnormalities and arthritis were 4.6% and 6.6%, respectively. Three strains of spirochete that are closely related to *Borrelia burgdorferi* were isolated from *Ixodes persulcatus* ticks and facial palsy patients. From the above results it is concluded that a focus of Lyme disease exists in this region.

INTRODUCTION

Lyme disease is a tick-borne spirochetosis caused by a new species of spirochete, *Borrelia burgdorferi*. The reported vector ticks are *Ixodes dammini, Ixodes pacificus, Ixodes ricinus,* and *Ambylomma americans.* In the United States, the etiological agent has been isolated from wild animals, Ixodid ticks, and patients.

Steere *et al.*[1] first reported the presence of Lyme disease in the town of Lyme, Connecticut in 1975, manifested as epidemic arthritis. Subsequent studies showed that the spectrum of this disease comprises early and late manifestations in skin, nervous system, and joints.

This disease was not reported in China or in other parts of Asia until the summer of 1985, when we encountered cases of erythema chronicum migrans (ECM), facial palsy, and lymphadenosis benigna cutis (LABC) among forest workers in the Hailin forest district. All patients had history of tick bite. This paper reports preliminary results on clinical and epidemiological features of the disease and isolation of spirochetes.

METHODS

Diagnostic Basis

Clinical diagnosis of Lyme disease was based on Bowen's diagnostic criteria,[2] modified according to local conditions. Patients with the following symptoms and history were diagnosed as having Lyme disease:

1. ECM, either alone or with other symptoms, and a history of tick bite.
2. Meningismus or meningitis, episodic headache, neck stiffness, nausea or vomiting, with tick bite history.
3. Facial palsy, with paralysis either at the time of survey or history of paralysis, and either completely or partially recovered, among those living in the forest district.
4. Migratory inflammation of large joints with recurrent attacks and a history of tick bite.
5. LABC, with swelling of tick bite and nodule growing in size but no other symptoms, and a course running from weeks to years.

Detection of Cases

The tick bite experience of the inhabitants was surveyed from house to house monthly between May and August 1987. The site and date of tick bite were recorded. Size and color of the lesion were examined and photographed. The history of malaise, fatigue, headache, and fever were recorded, and lymph gland enlargement and body temperature examined. Some cases were followed up for 1–2 weeks to observe the development of erythema. The presence of recurrent headache, pain caused by peripheral neuritis, facial palsy symptoms, joint pain, and cardiac abnormalities were also recorded. Patients attending the clinic were also included in this survey.

Isolation of Etiologic Agent

Isolation from Ticks

Using Burgdorfer's method,[3] we dissected female adult ticks (*Ixodes persulcatus*) collected from forest district and picked out their midgut tissue, which was smeared and fixed with acetone. Sera of patients with convalescent facial palsy were used to perform indirect immunofluorescent assay for spirochetes. We also ground starved ticks and inoculated the emulsion intraperitoneally to inbred mice (AMMS-13). After

8 and 14 days the inoculated mice were sacrificed and their liver, spleen, kidney, and brain were smeared with anti-Lyme spirochete standard sera (kindly supplied by Dr. Stanek) to perform fluorescent antibody and immunoperoxidase stains to detect spirochete.

Isolation from Patients

Using Steere's method,[4] we collected blood samples from neuropathy patients, inoculated 0.1 ml plasma into BSK medium (generously provided by Dr. Allen Steere), incubated at 33°C, and examined them weekly under dark-field microscopy for 6 weeks. Concurrently, the culture inoculated with patients' plasma was centrifuged at 14,500 rpm for 20 minutes. The sediment was collected and stained with fluorescent antibody for spirochete.

Serological Test

Adopting Wilkinson's method,[5] we used indirect fluorescent antibody assay (IFA) to detect patient's anti-Lyme disease antibody. The antigen used was *B. burgdorferi* B31 (kindly supplied by Dr. Stanek), which was grown in BSK medium at 33°C for 10 days. The medium was centrifuged at 14,500 rpm for 30 minutes. The sediment was dropped on glass slide as antigen. The patients' sera were used for detection of anti-Lyme disease antibody in serial twofold dilution with 1 : 128 as positive titer level.

RESULTS

Clinical Manifestations

Among 1,572 forest workers and their dependents and rural inhabitants in the neighborhood interviewed, 302 cases of Lyme disease with different stages were detected (TABLE 1). Seventeen cases had two or more pathological conditions.

Skin Lesions

ECM. One hundred thirty-two cases (44%) were in the early stage. All patients had tick bite history. Some cases had general malaise, fatigue, and headache accompanying the appearance of ECM. Children usually had intermittent low-grade fever and enlargement of regional lymph node.

Red macule or papule begins at the site of tick bite, 2–5 days after the bite. Erythema gradually expands. The center of lesion appears pale while the border is fresh red. The annular or oval erythema usually measures 3 × 5 or 10 × 18 cm. ECM in the form of annular erythematous patch is uncommon. Lesions are extensive and indurated and usually flat, although some are elevated. There are vesicles or necrosis in the center in some lesions. Subjective symptoms such as itching, pain or burning may be present. The erythema usually lasts for 1–4 weeks.

Two ECM cases had secondary erythema, occurring 8–10 days after primary erythema. They were multiple in number, of different sizes, distributed in other parts of body surface or scalp away from the primary site, and persisted for about 2 weeks.

Lymphadenosis Benigna Cutis. Six cases were observed among 302 cases surveyed. The nodular lesion was commonly seen on earlobe, scalp, chest, and abdomen. No subjective complaint was noted. The longest course lasted 20 years.

Neurological Involvement

Facial Paralysis. Nineteen cases (6%) of facial palsy (3 new cases and 16 old cases) were found during 1966–86. Some completely recovered, some partially. One case had a relapse of paralysis on the contralateral side 1 year after the first attack. Onset occurred suddenly with leakage of water from mouth during morning gargling, failure to close eye on the affected side, mouth angle slanted toward healthy side, and leveled forehead furrows. Fifteen patients remembered tick bite in the past, three had ECM, four had arthritis, two had LABC, and one had chronic meningitis.

Meningitis or Meningismus. Forty-four cases (14%) belonged to this category. Main symptoms were episodic headache, usually in frontal and occipital region, neck stiffness, nausea, or vomiting.

TABLE 1. Clinical Manifestations of Lyme Disease in Forest District, Hailin County, Heilongjiang Province, April–August 1986[a]

Clinical Presentation	No. Cases	%
Erythema chronicum migrans	132	44
Meningitis syndrome	44	15
Facial palsy	19	6
Polyneuritis	10	3
Arthritis	104	34
Carditis	4	1
Lymphadenosis benigna cutis	6	2

[a]No. of persons with Lyme disease was 302.

Polyneuritis. Ten cases (3%) were encountered. One case showed glove and sock distribution of paralysis of hands and feet with pain in toes and fingertips. Another case had sacral nerve pain.

Cardiac Abnormalities

Physical examination without electrocardiogram tracing revealed only four cases having bradycardia or symptoms of palpitation.

Arthritis

Arthritis is a common malady among the forest residents. We found 104 cases (34%) of chronic arthritis, mainly affecting the knee joints, which were asymmetrical in distribution and migratory. Most cases had history of tick bite.

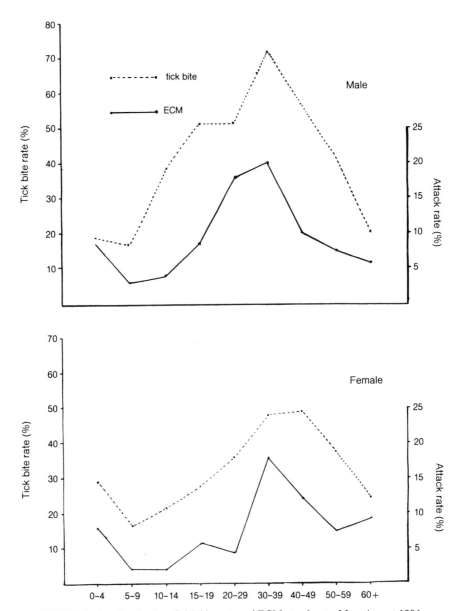

FIGURE 1. Age distribution of tick bite rate and ECM attack rate, May–August 1986.

Treatment

Six cases of ECM with fever and generalized lymphadenopathy were treated by penicillin G, 800,000 units intramuscularly daily for 10 days. Fever and erythema subsided 2–3 days after treatment. Another case of sacral neuritis received the same dose of penicillin therapy, achieving complete recovery. One case of polyneuritis with paralysis and pain of extremities received 5,000,000 units of penicillin G intravenously daily for 10 days. Pain disappeared and paralysis was controlled. After 10 days of rest, a second course of penicillin G, 8,000,000 units intravenously daily, was started; the effect is still under observation. No Herxheimer reaction was noted after large-dose penicillin therapy.

Epidemiological Characteristics

ECM Attack Rate

Inhabitants (n = 1572) of a forest center and a small village were investigated. Among them, 132 cases were observed. The attack rate in 4 months (April to August 1986) was 8.4%. Seventy-six cases (9.9%) occurred among 765 males, and 56 cases (6.9%) among 807 females. The difference in attack rates is significant (χ^2 = 4.5, $p < .05$).

ECM can occur in all ages, but the attack rate rises as age increases, being highest among the same age group (30–39 years) in both sexes (FIG. 1).

FIGURE 2 shows the attack rates of every 10-day interval. Cases begin to appear in the last 10 days of April, reaching a peak in the first 10 days of June, and gradually fall in middle June. Only sporadic cases are seen in the first 10 days of August. Case distribution by 10-day interval shows the same trend as the number of persons who experienced tick bite during the 10-day interval.

Comparison of Outdoor and Indoor Activities

Participants in outdoor activities, especially those taking place in forests, had a significantly higher attack rate than did participants with indoor lifestyles (TABLE 2). Some participants who had indoor lifestyles also participated in tree planting and in picking wild vegetables, mushrooms, or edible fungus. It appears that Lyme disease is an occupational disease of forest workers, because they have constant daily contact with the ticks and are infected repeatedly.

Prevalence Rates of Neurologic Abnormalities and Arthritis

The prevalence rate of neurologic abnormalities is 4.6% (TABLE 3). All age groups were affected and no significant difference between males and females was noted (χ^2 = 0.2, $p > .05$).

TABLE 4 shows the prevalence rate of arthritis. Forest inhabitants had a higher arthritis prevalence rate (6.6%). Prevalence rate of arthritis increased as age increased. The highest was found in the group between 40 and 59 years of age. This category is the late manifestation of the disease. Its presence in subjects past middle age, in contrast to migratory erythema cases, which occur among young adults (20–39), is quite evident. The prevalence rates of arthritis between male and female have no significant difference (χ^2 = 0.9, $p > .05$).

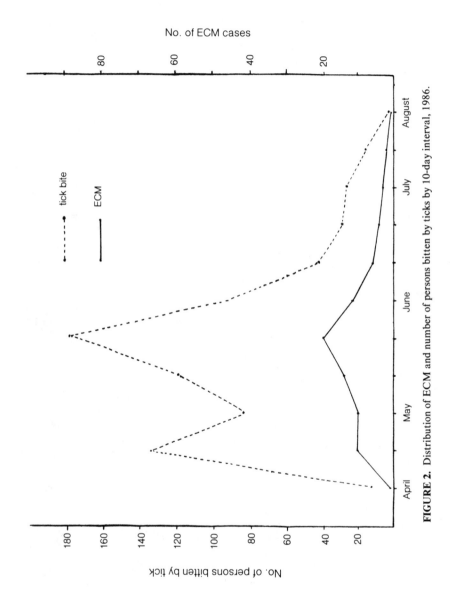

FIGURE 2. Distribution of ECM and number of persons bitten by ticks by 10-day interval, 1986.

Isolation of Etiological Agent

Isolation from Ticks

The midgut tissue from 98 female adults, *Ixodes persulcatus,* was dissected. Indirect immunofluorescent test was performed by using convalescent sera from facial palsy patients to test for reaction with tick tissue. Forty-three percent of ticks were found to be positive. One strain of spirochete was isolated from a pool of six female adults inoculated into inbred mice (AMMS13). The strain of spirochete is immunologically closely related to *Borrelia burgdorferi.*

Isolation from Patients

Fifteen blood and six cerebrospinal fluid specimens from nineteen patients suffering from nervous system involvement were inoculated into BSK medium. Three strains of spirochetes were isolated from the blood of cases with neurologic abnormalities. Two strains (HL86002, HL86003) of spirochete are immunologically closely related to *Borrelia burgdorferi* (TABLE 5).

TABLE 2. ECM Attack Rate by Location of Activity, Hailin County, Heilongjiang Province, May to August 1986

Location of Activity	No. Investigated	Cases	Rate[a]
Indoor[b]	841	35	4.2
Outdoor[c]	731	99	13.5

[a]Cases per 100.
[b]Infants and children, students, office workers.
[c]Forest workers, agricultural workers, dependents.
$\chi^2 = 45, p < 0.001.$

Serological Test

Twenty-one specimens of sera and plasma of neurological involvement patients were tested by indirect immunofluorescent assay to detect Lyme disease antibodies. Eight of them (38%) gave a positive test; the highest titer reached 1 : 512.

DISCUSSION

Erythema chronicum migrans is an early stage of Lyme disease. Clinical diagnosis is not difficult to make because it is based on the specific skin lesions. According to Steere *et al.*,[6] however, basing Lyme disease diagnosis on this lesion alone is insufficient. In some cases skin lesion does not occur, whereas some patients have erythema of different sizes and shape. Only a few cases had typical annular erythema, causing difficulty in clinical diagnosis. Thus knowledge of history of tick bite, season of illness, and living or staying in focus are useful for diagnosis of this disease.

Neurologic abnormalities, including meningitis, cranial neuritis, and peripheral radiculoneuritis constitute the second stage of Lyme disease. Among those presenting with cranial neuritis, facial palsy is most commonly seen. In Europe, 63% of patients

TABLE 3. Prevalence Rate of Lyme Neurologic Abnormalities in Forest Residents, Hailin County, Heilongjiang Province, 1986

Age Group (Years)	Males			Females			Total		
	No. Investigated	Cases	%	No. Investigated	Cases	%	No. Investigated	Cases	%
0–4	38	1	2.6	52	0	0.0	90	1	1.1
5–9	103	2	1.9	129	1	0.7	232	3	1.3
10–14	128	2	1.6	150	2	1.3	278	4	1.4
15–19	115	3	2.6	106	7	6.6	221	10	4.5
20–29	106	5	4.7	101	8	7.9	207	13	6.3
30–39	105	5	4.7	94	8	8.5	199	13	6.5
40–49	69	8	11.5	91	11	12.1	160	19	11.9
50–59	67	5	7.5	51	2	3.9	118	7	5.9
60 and above	34	2	5.9	33	1	3.0	67	3	4.5
TOTAL	765	33	4.3	807	40	4.9	1572	73	4.6

TABLE 4. Prevalence Rate of Lyme Arthritis in Forest Residents, Hailin County, Heilongjiang Province, 1986

Age Group (Years)	Male			Female			Total		
	No. Investigated	Cases	%	No. Investigated	Cases	%	No. Investigated	Cases	%
0–4	38	0	0.0	52	0	0.0	90	0	0.0
5–9	103	1	0.9	129	9	7.0	232	10	4.3
10–14	128	5	3.9	150	8	5.3	278	13	4.7
15–19	115	5	4.3	106	5	4.7	221	10	4.5
20–29	106	3	2.8	101	5	5.0	207	8	3.9
30–39	105	10	9.5	94	6	6.4	199	16	8.0
40–49	69	16	23.2	91	7	7.6	160	23	14.4
50–59	67	12	17.9	51	7	13.7	118	19	16.1
60 and above	34	4	11.7	33	1	3.0	67	5	7.5
TOTAL	765	56	7.3	807	48	5.9	1572	104	6.6

with neurologic abnormalities have unilateral or bilateral facial palsy. Fifty percent of American patients with neurologic abnormalities have facial palsy. These situations are rarely seen in other diseases. Arthritis accompanying or occurring after facial palsy is also not commonly seen in other diseases. We found 19 new and old cases of facial palsy. Diagnostic bases are: (1) cases occurred in the forest area, having Lyme disease at other stages; (2) most cases had history of tick bite, or ECM and arthritis; (3) cases occurred in summer; (4) *Ixodes persulcatus* is the predominant tick species in the area, and a strain of spirochete closely related to *B. burgdorferi* was isolated from these ticks; (5) antibody against *B. burgdorferi* was detected in convalescent patients, reaching a titer of 1 : 512.

Arthritis is a late stage of Lyme disease. Clinically it simulates oligoarticular rheumatoid arthritis in children and adults, but Lyme arthritis runs a shorter course than rheumatoid arthritis. Some Lyme arthritis cases may also exhibit migratory polyarthritis, persisting for 1 year or longer. So, if there is no ECM history and the subject does not live in Lyme disease focus, the clincial diagnosis of Lyme disease cannot be made. In our series, patients all lived in forest district and were frequently bitten by ticks. The majority of patients had ECM and chronic meningitis, so even at

TABLE 5. Identification of Spirochetes Isolated from Blood of Patients with Neurologic Abnormalities of Lyme Disease by Indirect Immunofluorescence Assay

	Spirochete Strain		
Serum	B31	HL86002	HL86003
Reference	1 : 1024	1 : 512	1 : 512
86002[a]	1 : 512	1 : 1024	1 : 1024
Syphilis	1 : 32	1 : 32	1 : 16
Normal human	<1 : 8	<1 : 8	<1 : 8

[a]Serum collected from patient with Lyme disease.

the beginning of the survey, when serological test was not applied, clinical diagnosis was fairly accurate.

The epidemiological survey shows that the characteristics of Lyme disease in the Hailin forest district are essentially similar to those of American cases. For example, ECM attack rate in our survey is 8.4%, quite close to the 7.5% reported by Hanrahan.[7] ECM attack season is highest in Hailin during May and June, whereas in North America it is during June and July. This difference may be related to the difference in rise and fall of tick and human activities. In our series, all ECM cases have history of tick bite, whereas Steere *et al.*[8] reported only 30% of their ECM cases remembered tick bite history. Probably the larvae and nymph of *Ixodes dammini,* which can also bite man, were neglected by the patients.

Based on clinical manifestations, epidemiological characteristics, and isolation of spirochetes closely related to *B. burgdorferi* from ticks and patients, it is concluded that a natural focus of Lyme disease exists in the study area.

REFERENCES

1. STEERE, A. C., S. E. MALAWISTA, D. R. SNYDMAN, *et al.* 1977. Arthritis Rheum. **20:** 7–17.
2. BOWEN, G. S., M. GRIFFIN, C. HAYNE, *et al.* 1984. J. Am. Med. Assoc. **251:** 2236–2240.

3. BURGDORFER, W., A. G. BARBOUR, S. F. HAYES, *et al.* 1982. Science **216:** 1317–1319.
4. STEERE, A. C., R. L. GRODZICKI, A. N. KORNBLATT, *et al.* 1983. N. Engl. J. Med. **308:** 733–740.
5. WILKINSON, H. W. 1984. Yale J. Biol. Med. **57:** 567–572.
6. STEERE, A. C., T. F. BRODERICK &. S. E. MALAWISTA. 1978. Am. J. Epidemiol. **108:** 312–321.
7. HANRAHAN, J. P., J. L. BENACH, J. L. COLEMAN, *et al.* 1984. J. Infect. Dis. **150:** 489–490.
8. STEERE, A. C., S. E. MALAWISTA & N. H. BARTENHAGEN, *et al.* 1984. Yale J. Biol. Med. **57:** 453–460.

Introduction

A Perspective on Therapy of Lyme Infection

HAROLD C. NEU

Departments of Medicine and Pharmacology
College of Physicians and Surgeons
Columbia University
New York, New York 10032

The therapy of spirochetal infection is well established for those organisms that have been known for the past century. Penicillin provided a cure of syphilis caused by *Treponema pallidum* and made possible the elimination of the serious long-term consequences of syphilis, namely cardiac and neurological disease. It is also well established that yaws, pinta, and endemic syphilis respond to penicillin treatment, with clearing of the cutaneous lesions produced by these treponemas. Relapsing fever due to *Borrelia* is appropriately treated with penicillin or tetracycline, which end the bouts of fever.

Therapy of Lyme infection due to *Borrelia burgdorferi* is less clearly understood and established. The rationale for treatment would be to stop the cutaneous reaction erythema chronicum migrans and its associated constitutional symptoms; to prevent late sequelae of infection such as arthritis, neurological disorders, and acrodermatitis chronica atrophicans; and to treat the late arthritis and neurological disease.

The first therapy of an illness analogous to Lyme disease took place in Europe in the 1940s, when penicillin was used to treat erythema migrans.[1-4] Steere and colleagues,[5,6] in the late 1970s, showed that use of penicillin and tetracycline administered four times a day for 10 days was effective in treatment of erythema migrans.[6] The duration of the erythema cutaneous migrans symptoms was 2–4 days compared to 10 days in untreated patients. Erythromycin was less effective than tetracycline or penicillin, and tetracycline was the most efficacious in preventing joint, cardiac, and neurological complications. Of the original 88 patients, all responded. Although they did not have relapse of disease in the 3-year follow-up, musculoskeletal pain and fatigue were common. There has been no evaluation of whether any of the patients will in subsequent years develop any late neurological disease.

In the subsequent studies of Steere *et al.*,[7] use of benzathine penicillin in patients with established arthritis of a large joint resulted in improvement in 43% of patients, and 20 million units of intravenously administered penicillin produced improvement in 45% whereas none of the patients who received placebo resolved. This study would seem to suggest that the high-dose penicillin therapy was no more beneficial than the lower serum levels achieved with weekly benzathine penicillin.

A number of uncontrolled studies of the use of penicillin to treat late neurological symptoms of Lyme disease have been reported. In most patients there has been subjective improvement and also improvement in cerebrospinal fluid findings. In this part, Skoldenberg[8] presents data on 113 patients with neurological disease thought to be related to *Borrelia* infection in which 105 were treated with penicillin at doses of 12 g or 9 g each day. Response was demonstrated by decreased pleocytosis in the cerebrospinal fluid, fall of CSF protein, and changes in neurological findings. Only a few patients were treated with cefuroxime or doxycycline, so the efficacy of these agents is not really established. Steere and colleagues[9] have reported the use of high-dose intravenous penicillin for 12 patients with stiff neck, headache, and radicular pain. All showed clinical improvement in 7 to 10 days, but five of twelve had headaches for several weeks after therapy and three of twelve continued to have pain, arthralgias, and fatigue.

Both Berger[10] and Weber[11] note in this part that 40% of patients with ECM required several courses of therapy. Weber[12] notes that 28% of treated patients had late muscular and arthritis complaints. Weber states that he and his colleagues have recently found that amoxicillin or amoxicillin-clavulanate are as effective as oral penicillin and tetracycline for therapy of cutaneous *Borrelia* infection.

The most recent studies have been those of Luft and colleagues,[13] which evaluate the effect of the aminothiazolyl cephalosporin, ceftriaxone. Luft and colleagues have shown that ceftriaxone kills *B. burgdorferi* more rapidly and at lower concentrations than do penicillin, tetracycline, or minocycline. Luft has suggested that there is a major difference between MICs and MBCs of *B. burgdorfrei* for penicillin, which explains the poor response in some cases.

It is important to realize that we do not have established means of determining the MICs and MBCs of organisms that grow as slowly as *Borrelia*. MIC data has direct relevance to the activity of antimicrobial agents against aerobic and anaerobic bacteria, which divide every 30 to 90 minutes. The relation of *in vitro* studies of an organism such as *B. burgdorferi* to the clinical disease in man is clearly less well established than is the MIC data on an *Escherichia coli* producing a urinary tract infection. Furthermore, MIC data on *Borrelia* is based on a very small number of isolates, making generalization to all parts of the world difficult.

There are a number of important basic questions regarding the chemotherapy of *B. burgdorferi* infections. First, should one treat with an antibiotic such as tetracycline, doxycycline, amoxicillin, or penicillin V when a patient from an area in which the infection is common presents with the cutaneous lesion? The rationale of this approach would be that current serological techniques are far from satisfactory and a positive titer may not develop for 6 weeks, if at all. Indeed, the cost of the chemotherapeutic agent is considerably less than the cost of serological procedures. On the basis of the data presented at this conference and previous publications, it is reasonable and justifiable to treat cutaneous lesions. The data of Steere and colleagues and Weber and colleagues suggest that late complications will be less. Ideally, double-blind comparative studies with longer follow-up should be done to determine that the untreated individuals indeed have more late complications. However, the more rapid resolution of the illness itself is beneficial.

In my evaluation for ECM it would seem that amoxicillin would be preferred to penicillin V since the phenoxymethyl penicillin derivatives generally are less active than penicillin G or amoxicillin. Penicillin G is not suitable due to erratic oral absorption. Doxycycline would be preferred to tetracycline-HCl since it has better serum tissue levels and can be taken twice daily at 100 mg orally with minimal gastrointestinal distress.

How long should patients be treated? Should the therapy be for 7, 10, 14, or 21 days? There is no data on which to base a time period that is most appropriate. A period of 10 to 14 days has been suggested, but this period has been arbitrarily chosen without data. It has also been suggested that patients who are allergic to penicillin and for whom tetracycline is inappropriate receive erythromycin for 15 to 20 days at 30 mg/kg/day. There is no data on which this recommendation is based.

The next problem concerns the therapy of established arthritis and neurological illness. Should the therapy be intravenous penicillin at high dose, such as we now advocate for neurological involvement due to syphilis? Should ceftriaxone be administered intravenously at high dose, namely 2 g twice daily, or could ceftriaxone be administered by the intramuscular route once daily or even every other day? It will be extremely difficult to assemble enough patients allocated to several arms of the above possible protocols to achieve a statistically sound answer. Given the costs of hospitalization and the preliminary results of Luft and colleagues,[10] it would seem reasonable to recommend ceftriaxone as an appropriate agent if high-dose penicillin fails. The data is not sufficient to state unequivocally that ceftriaxone is the first choice of therapy for neurological disease due to *B. burgdorferi*.

Where should therapy of Lyme disease go in the future? The activity of ceftriaxone against *B. burgdorferi* would appear to be related to the acyl side chain of this aminothiazolyl cephalosporin. There will be a number of oral agents with a similar structure available in the next several years. Most of these compounds do not produce high blood levels, but they are much less protein bound than ceftriaxone, so the amount of free drug may be similar, and some of them have long half-lives which would permit twice-daily oral therapy. The activity of these agents should be investigated, and if the *in vitro* data is reasonable, clinical trials undertaken.

Although we have come a long way in our understanding of the chemotherapy of *B. burgdorferi* infections, there is much to be learned. Indeed, this conference has demonstrated that more is unknown than known. The approach to therapy has been hampered by difficulties in diagnosis, uncertainties about serology, and the lack of large-scale controlled therapy studies. Hopefully we are entering a new era in the therapy of *B. burgdorferi* infections in all of their protean forms that will see the establishment of the best agent(s) to use, the optimal length of therapy, and the best forms of retreatment when initial therapy is not fully successful.

REFERENCES

1. SVARTZ, N. 1946. Penicillinbehandling vid dermatitis atroficans Herxheimer. Nord. Med. **32:** 2873.
2. THYRESSON, N. 1949. The penicillin treatment of acrodermatitis chronica atrophicans (Herxheimer). Acta Derm. Venereol. (Stockh.) **29:** 572–621.
3. HOLLSTROM, E. 1951. Successful treatment of erythema migrans Afzelius. Acta Derm. Venereol. (Stockh). **31:** 235–243.
4. HAUSER, W. 1955. Zur Kenntnis der akrodermatitis chronica atrophicans. Arch. Dermatol. Syph. **199:** 350–393.
5. STEERE, A. C., S. E. MALAWISTA, J. NEWMAN, P. N. SPIELER & N. H. BARTENHAGEN. 1980. Antibiotic therapy in Lyme disease. Ann. Intern. Med. **93:** 1–8.
6. STEERE, A. C., G. J. HUTCHINSON, D. W. RAHN, L. H. SIGAL, J. E. CRAFT, E. T. DeSANNA & S. E. MALAWISTA. 1983. Treatment of the early manifestations of Lyme disease. Ann. Intern. Med. **99:** 22–26.
7. STEERE, A. C., J. GREEN, R. T. SCHOEN, E. TAYLOR, G. J. HUTCHINSON, D. W. RAHAN & S. E. MALAWISTA. 1985. Successful parenteral penicillin therapy of established Lyme arthritis. N. Engl. J. Med. **312:** 869–874.
8. SKÖLDENBERG, B., *et al.* 1988. Treatment of Lyme borreliosis with special emphasis on neurological disease. This volume.
9. STEERE, A. C., A. R. PACHNER & S. E. MALAWISTA. 1983. Neurological abnormalities of Lyme disease: Successful treatment with high-dose intravenous penicillin. Ann. Intern. Med. **99:** 767–772.
10. BERGER, B. W. 1988. Treatment of erythema chronicum migrans of Lyme disease. This volume.
11. WEBER, K., *et al.* 1988. Antibiotic therapy of early European Lyme borreliosis and acrodermatitis chronica atrophicans. This volume.
12. WEBER, K., U. NEUBERT & R. THURMAYER. 1986. Antibiotic therapy in early erythema migrans disease and related disorders. Zbl. Bakt. Hyg. A **263:** 377–388.
13. DATTWYLER, R. J., J. J. HALPERN, D. J. VOLKMAN & B. H. LUFT. 1987. Ceftriaxone is superior to high dose penicillin in the treatment of late Lyme borreliosis. Presented at the 22nd Interscience Conference on Antimicrobial Agents and Chemotherapy. New York.

Treatment of Lyme Borreliosis with Emphasis on Neurological Disease

BIRGIT SKÖLDENBERG,[a] GÖRAN STIERNSTEDT,[a]
MATS KARLSSON,[a] BENGT WRETLIND,[b] AND
BO SVENUNGSSON[c]

[a]Department of Infectious Diseases
Danderyd Hospital
S-182 88 Danderyd, Sweden

[b]Department of Bacteriology
Danderyd Hospital
S-182 88 Danderyd, Sweden

[c]Roslagstull Hospital
114 89 Stockholm, Sweden

ERYTHEMA MIGRANS AND EARLY LYME DISEASE

In Sweden, there has been a long tradition of treating patients with erythema chronicum migrans (ECM) and acrodermatitis chronica atrophicans with antibiotics. More than 30 years ago, two Swedish dermatologists, Hollström and Thyresson, described successful treatment with oral penicillin.[1,2] In a follow-up study of phenoxymethylpenicillin, 1 g twice daily for 10 days in 132 patients with uncomplicated ECM, Åsbrink et al. did not find any late major neurological, arthritic, or cardiac complications.[3] In contrast, among 16 untreated patients with ECM, two developed meningitis and one arthritis. In 1980 and 1981, Steere et al. compared antibiotic regimens in adults with early Lyme disease, namely 250 mg four times daily for 10 days of phenoxymethylpenicillin, erythromycin, or tetracycline.[4] Three of 40 penicillin-treated patients and 4 of 29 given erythromycin developed late major complications as compared to none of 39 patients given tetracycline. In 1982, all 49 adult patients were given tetracycline and none developed major complications. However, tetracycline (1 g daily for 10 days) is not uniformly successful in the prevention of late complication of Lyme borreliosis.[5] In 1987, Dattwyler and Halperin described five patients with early Lyme disease who developed late complications after an average of five months, despite receiving tetracycline early in the course of their illness.

SENSITIVITY OF *Borrelia burgdorferi* TO ANTIBIOTICS

One of the main aims of treating Lyme borreliosis is to achieve bactericidal concentrations to the causative agent *B. burgdorferi* in all tissues involved for a sufficient period of time. The susceptibility to different antibiotics of different *B. burgdorferi* strains should be related to the absorption, the tissue distribution, and the pharmacokinetics of the antibiotics concerned. Penicillin is capable of *in vitro* killing of *B. burgdorferi* at concentrations readily obtained *in vivo* if higher oral doses of phenoxymethylpenicillin are used. The mean minimal inhibitory concentration (MIC) values for tetracycline are close to those of the peak plasma concentration after oral dose of 250 mg tetracycline on an empty stomach.

317

Sensitivity testing of *B. burgdorferi* strains have shown *in vitro* susceptibility to erythromycin, tetracycline, ampicillin, and penicillin G with MICs of less than 2 μg/ml as well as to minocycline and doxycycline.[6,7] Two Swedish strains from our own laboratory had MICs of 2 μg/ml for doxycycline. In an experimental infection model of *B. burgdorferi* in hamsters, Johnson *et al.* found a discrepancy between *in vitro* and *in vivo* results.[8] Only ceftriaxone and tetracycline were efficacious in their model, whereas penicillin G and erythromycin were not.

The penetration to the cerebrospinal fluid (CSF) and central nervous system of an antibiotic for Lyme borreliosis should be considered. Penicillin has low lipid solubility and it penetrates the CSF barrier by 1–2%, if meninges are normal, and by 2–6% if meninges are inflamed. Doxycycline has a long half-life and higher lipophilic quality than penicillin. Doxycycline penetrates into CSF by 26% or more.[9] Ceftriaxone also has a long half-life (longer than the half-lives of other cephalosporins of the third generation) and it penetrates readily into the CNS.[10]

Although *in vitro* and experimental trials supply useful guidelines, we need prospective human *in vivo* studies to provide solid recommendations of antibiotics for use in Lyme borreliosis.

LYME NEUROBORRELIOSIS

In 1951, the Swedish dermatologist Hellerström reported on the effectiveness of intravenous penicillin in a patient with meningitis after ECM.[11] From 1976 to 1980, Steere *et al.* studied the effect of prednisone, 40 to 60 mg per day, on 15 patients with neurologic abnormalities of Lyme disease.[12] Later, they studied the effect of intravenous penicillin G, 12 g daily for 10 days, in 12 patients. Compared to patients given prednisone, the duration of meningitic symptoms was significantly shorter in patients given penicillin (1 vs. 29 weeks). However, in both groups, a mean of 7 to 8 weeks was required for complete recovery of motor deficits.

In 1983, we published results describing the beneficial effect of intravenous penicillin G on 21 patients with chronic meningitis, later found to be related etiologically to *B. burgdorferi* infection.[13] In 45 patients with tick-borne *Borrelia* infection of the CNS, we have described the benefit of high-dose intravenous antibiotics (penicillin G in 43 patients and cefuroxime or doxycycline in two patients).[14] There are no placebo-controlled therapeutic studies on neuroborreliosis, but the patients could be considered to have served as their own controls, especially in our previous study.

We have studied 113 patients with neurologic Lyme borreliosis and meningitis who were treated consecutively from 1975 to 1986 with intravenous high-dose antibiotics. The serological diagnosis of *Borrelia* infection of the CNS was made as previously described.[14,15] Forty-seven patients received 12 g daily of penicillin G (45 for 14 days and 2 for 10 days) and 58 patients received 9 g daily of penicillin G (46 for 10 days, 12 for 14 days). Eight patients were treated with either intravenous doxycycline, 200 mg daily, or cefuroxime, 4.5 to 9 g daily, for 10 to 14 days. The treatment groups were analyzed according to clinical characteristics and duration of symptoms before and after treatment as well as the occurrence of other late major complications of Lyme borreliosis.

There was a slight predominance of females (58%). The median age was 43 to 46 years in the treatment groups. Thirty-two patients (28%) described an erythema-migrans-like skin lesion and five of the 32 patients received oral phenoxymethyl-penicillin.

All patients had meningitis with CSF pleocytosis. A total of 79 patients (70%) had peripheral nerve symptoms. Facial-nerve paralysis and radicular pain dominated, but other cranial nerve paralysis or noncranial nerve paralysis was also present. Fifteen patients (13%) had central nervous symptoms, including hemiparesis, spastic paraparesis, ataxia, and encephalitis.

The duration of symptoms before the start of the treatment with antibiotics is illustrated in FIGURE 1. Almost half of the patients (45%) were treated more than 4 weeks after the onset of symptoms. Seventeen patients (15%) had persisting or progressive symptoms between 4 and 11 months. In the patients who received penicillin G, 9 or 12 g, 34 and 40 patients, respectively, were treated 4 weeks or later after the

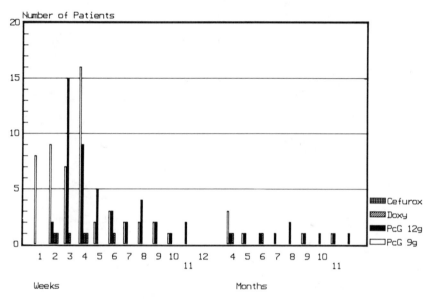

FIGURE 1. Treatment after onset of symptoms with intravenous antibiotics in 113 patients. Treatments were: penicillin G, 12 g, in 47 patients (14 days in 45, 10 days in 2); penicillin G, 9 g, in 58 patients (10 days in 46 patients, 14 days in 12); doxycycline, 200 mg, in 5 patients; and cefuroxime, 4.5–9 g, in 3 patients.

onset of symptoms. However, 41% and 14%, respectively, of the patients were treated earlier.

During treatment, all patients improved or recovered. There was often a fairly rapid improvement of meningeal or general symptoms. The radicular pain diminished or disappeared gradually within weeks. The other peripheral nerve symptoms usually disappeared within a few weeks, although it took a longer time in some patients. Two patients still had facial muscle weakness 1 to 3 years after treatment. In one patient, the facial-nerve paralysis appeared during the third day of treatment. The central nervous symptoms were stopped in their progression. The few patients with encephalitic symptoms improved rapidly. The patients with hemiparesis, spastic paraparesis, or ataxia improved to a greater or lesser extent but still had sequelae for years after

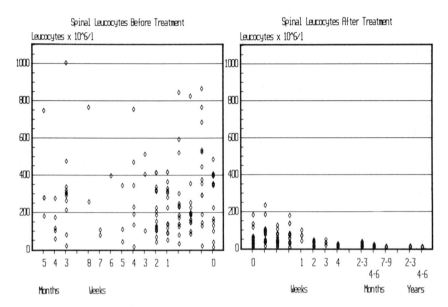

FIGURE 2. Spinal pleocytosis before and after treatment (259 CSF samples; 130 before and 129 after treatment).

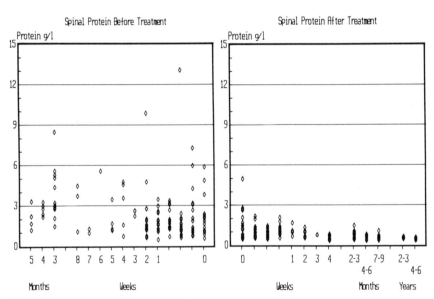

FIGURE 3. Spinal protein before and after treatment (259 CSF samples; 130 before and 129 after treatment).

treatment. No late major neurologic, arthritic, or cardiac complications could be demonstrated in the long-term follow-ups during 9 months to 2.7 years.

The CSF pleocytosis before and after treatment is demonstrated in FIGURE 2. A total of 259 CSF samples are plotted in the diagram. About one-third of the 130 pretreatment samples were collected 4 weeks before treatment and 16% of the samples at 3–5 months before treatment. The CSF leukocytes decreased fairly rapidly. Fifty-one of 129 posttreatment samples were collected between 4 months and 3 years after treatment. As can be seen in FIGURE 3, the spinal protein decreased after treatment, but more slowly at long-term follow-up of some patients.

The dynamics of the specific antibody pattern to *Borrelia* proteins is illustrated in FIGURE 4. It concerns a 49-year-old woman with progressive Lyme borreliosis with spastic paraparesis and fairly severe bilateral hearing defects. The patient improved gradually after treatment with penicillin G, 12 g daily for 14 days, and 5 years after treatment she now has only minor spastic paraparesis. CSF and serum samples, collected before and after treatment, were tested with Western blot technique for IgG and IgM antibodies to SDS-PAGE separated antigens of a Swedish tick strain (152) and of a Swedish CSF strain (20). Before treatment, IgG-antibodies were seen mainly against 60- and 41-kDa *Borrelia* proteins, less against 32–33 kDa proteins. Posttreatment, the IgG bands gradually diminished and were faint at 8 months after treatment. Only weak IgM could be demonstrated. The dynamics of IgG and IgM antibodies in CSF and sera determined by Western blot were similar to those found by ELISA method. The intrathecal synthesis of IgG antibodies gradually decreased but could be detected to a low extent of 3.5 years after treatment. The spinal protein decreased from 5.9 g/l pretreatment to 0.56 g/l at 11 months posttreatment.

CONCLUSION

In a consecutive series of 113 patients with Lyme neuroborreliosis, there seemed to be clinical benefit with either penicillin G, 9 g or 12 g, for 10 to 14 days or in 8 patients with intravenous doxycycline, 0.2 g, or cefuroxime, 4.5 to 9 g. The series included patients with either stage 2 or stage 3 Lyme neuroborreliosis and meningitis. Seventeen patients had symptoms for 4–11 months before treatment and 15 patients had progressive central nervous symptoms. The occurrence of Herxheimer reaction during the first days of treatment with antibiotics, as in neurosyphilis, should be considered, especially in patients with peripheral or central nervous symptoms. We could not demonstrate any major consequences of a Herxheimer reaction in the 113 patients treated. Milder Herxheimer reaction could be indicated in some patients by increased fever, malaise, and nausea during the first days of treatment in some patients.

In general, treatment series of Lyme borreliosis have indicated responders as well as nonresponders to antibiotics. We need to evaluate optimal treatment regimens of Lyme borreliosis in clinically and serologically well-defined patient materials, in early disease as well as in late disease, and include penicillin G, doxycycline and ceftriaxone. In late disease the role of corticosteroids might also be considered in controlled studies.

In other infectious diseases of the CNS, such as pneumococcal meningitis and herpes simplex encephalitis, the prognosis of disease is directly correlated not only to an optimal chemotherapeutic agent but also to the time of start of therapy after onset of disease. It is reasonable to have a similar relationship between start of treatment after the onset of Lyme borreliosis and prognosis of disease.

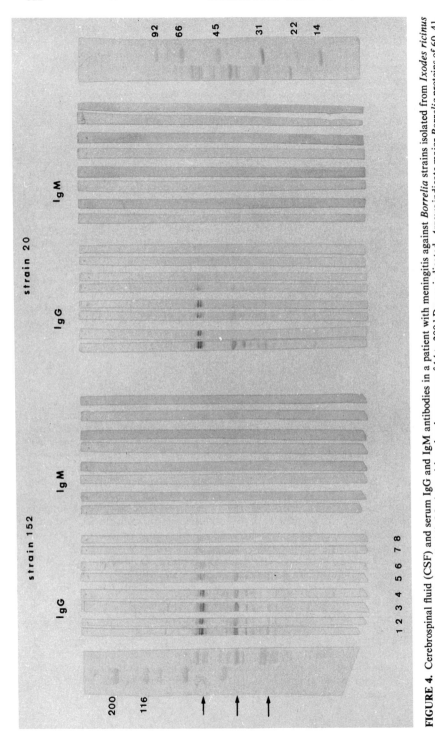

FIGURE 4. Cerebrospinal fluid (CSF) and serum IgG and IgM antibodies in a patient with meningitis against *Borrelia* strains isolated from *Ixodes ricinus* (strain 152) and from human CSF (strain 20). Markers with molecular masses of 14 to 200 kDa are indicated. *Arrows* indicate major *Borrelia* proteins of 60, 41, and 32–33 kDa. The separated tick antigen (strain 152) is seen beside the markers to the left, and the CSF antigen (strain 20) to the right. Paired CSF and serum samples taken before and 2 weeks, 2 months, and 8 months after antibiotic treatment are indicated by 1, 2; 3, 4; 5, 6; and 7, 8 respectively.

SUMMARY

We have studied 113 patients with neurologic Lyme borreliosis and meningitis who were treated with intravenous high-dose antibiotics (penicillin G, 12 g, mostly for 14 days in 47 patients; penicillin G, 9 g, mostly for 10 days in 58 patients; doxycycline, 200 mg, in 5 patients; and cefuroxime, 4.5–9 g, in 3 patients). Seventy percent of the patients had peripheral nerve symptoms and 13% had central nervous symptoms. Almost half of the patients were treated more than 4 weeks after the onset of symptoms and 15% of the patients had persisting or progressive symptoms between 4 and 11 months. There seemed to be clinical benefit as well as a decrease of spinal fluid pleocytosis and spinal proteins. No significant symptoms of Herxheimer reaction were demonstrated.

REFERENCES

1. HOLLSTRÖM, E. 1951. Successful treatment of erythema chronicum migrans Afzelius. Acta Derm. Venereol. **31:** 235–243.
2. THYRESSON, N. 1949. The penicillin treatment of acrodermatitis atrophicans chronica (Herxheimer). Acta Derm. Venereol. **29:** 572–621.
3. ÅSBRINK, E. & I. OLSSON. 1985. Clinical manifestations of erythema chronicum migrans Afzelius in 161 patients. Acta Derm. Venereol. **65:** 43–52.
4. STEERE, A. C., G. J. HUTCHINSON, D. W. ROBIN, L. H. SIGAL, J. E. CRAFT, E. T. DeSANNA & S. E. MALAWISTA. 1983. Treatment of the early manifestations of Lyme disease. Ann. Intern. Med. **99:** 22–26.
5. DATTWYLER, R. J. & J. J. HALPERIN. 1987. Failure of tetracycline therapy in early Lyme disease. Arthritis Rheum. **30:** 448–450.
6. JOHNSON, S. E., G. C. KLEIN, G. P. SCHMID & J. C. FEELEY. 1984. Susceptibility of the Lyme disease spirochete to seven antimicrobial agents. Yale J. Biol. Med. **57:** 99–103.
7. BERGER, B. W., M. H. KAPLAN, I. R. ROTHENBERG & A. C. BARBOUR. 1985. Isolation and characterization of the Lyme disease spirochete from the skin of patients with erythema chronicum migrans. J. Am. Acad. Dermatol. **13:** 444–449.
8. JOHNSON, R. C., C. KODNER & M. RUSSELL. 1987. *In vitro* and *in vivo* susceptibility of the Lyme disease spirochete, *Borrelia burgdorferi,* to four antimicrobial agents. Antimicrob. Agents Chemother. **31:** 164–167.
9. WHITESIDE YIM, C., N. M. FLYNN & F. T. FITZGERALD. 1985. Penetration of oral doxycycline into the cerebrospinal fluid of patients with neurosyphilis. Antimicrob. Agents Chemother. **28:** 347–348.
10. ALLAN, J. D., G. M. ELIOPOULOS & R. C. MOELLERING. 1986. The expanding spectrum of beta-lactam antibiotics. Adv. Intern. Med. **31:** 119–146.
11. HELLERSTRÖM, S. 1951. Erythema chronicum migrans Afzelius with meningitis. Acta Derm. Venereol. **31:** 227–234.
12. STEERE, A. C., A. R. PACHNER & S. E. MALAWISTA. 1983. Neurologic abnormalities of Lyme disease: Successful treatment with high-dose intravenous penicillin. Ann. Intern. Med. **99:** 767–772.
13. SKÖLDENBERG, B., G. STIERNSTEDT, A. GÅRDE, G. KOLMODIN, A. CARLSTRÖM & C. E. NORD. 1983. Chronic meningitis caused by a penicillin-sensitive microorganism. Lancet **ii:** 75–78.
14. STIERNSTEDT, G., B. SKÖLDENBERG, A. GÅRDE, G. KOLMODIN, H. JÖRBECK, B. SVENUNGS-SON & A. CARLSTRÖM. 1987. Clinical manifestations of *Borrelia* infections of the nervous system. Zbl. Bakt. Hyg. A **263:** 289–296.
15. STIERNSTEDT, G., M. GRANSTRÖM, B. HEDERSTEDT & B. SKÖLDENBERG. 1985. Diagnosis of spirochetal meningitis by enzyme-linked immunosorbent assay and indirect immuno-fluorescence assay in serum and cerebrospinal fluid. J. Clin. Microbiol. **21:** 819–825.

Antibiotic Therapy of Early European Lyme Borreliosis and Acrodermatitis Chronica Atrophicans

KLAUS WEBER,[a] VERA PREAC-MURSIC,[b]
UWE NEUBERT,[b] RUDOLF THURMAYR,[c]
PETER HERZER,[b] BETTINA WILSKE,[b]
GÜNTHER SCHIERZ,[b] AND WALTER MARGET[b]

[a] *Rosenstrasse 6*
8000 Munich, Federal Republic of Germany

[b] *Departments of Microbiology, Dermatology, Internal Medicine,*
and Pediatrics
University of Munich
Munich, Federal Republic of Germany

[c] *Institute for Medical Statistics and Epidemiology*
Technical University of Munich
Munich, Federal Republic of Germany

INTRODUCTION

Trials to treat manifestations of the *Borrelia burgdorferi* infection have been carried out since 1946 (literature in refs. 1–3). Early European experience seemed to indicate a favorable effect of penicillin on the early and late cutaneous manifestations of the disease. Similar observations have been made to a much lesser extent in patients treated with tetracyclines, chloramphenicol, and streptomycin.

Recent developments have shown that these early experiences can be corroborated to a certain degree but that they have been incomplete, since the complex nature of the disease was not fully understood until a few years ago. There are only a few comparative therapeutic trials on the early phase that take into account the new concept of the disease.[3-7] Only a preliminary comparative study has been performed for the treatment of patients with acrodermatitis chronica atrophicans (ACA),[3] a third-stage manifestation of Lyme borreliosis. In this paper, we present further details on our comparative nonrandomized therapeutic investigations carried out since December 1978.

PATIENTS AND METHODS

Patients

Patients with Erythema Migrans (EM)

Between December 1978 and July 1987, we treated 118 consecutive, nonselected patients with erythema migrans and three patients with a recent history of the condition. Ninety-two patients were seen in the private office of one of us (K.W.) and

324

22 patients were seen by U.N. in the dermatology department at the University of Munich; among the latter group, 16 patients were treated with oral penicillin and 6 with tetracyclines. We have already reported on the outcome in 65 oral penicillin recipients and 19 tetracycline or 28 minocycline recipients.[1-3,7] Seven amoxicillin–clavulanic-acid recipients were taken care of by several dermatologists using a questionnaire designed and checked by K.W.

Patients with ACA

Between October 1979 and July 1987, we observed 34 patients with ACA. Sixteen patients were treated in the dermatology department of the University of Munich, 12 patients in the private office of one of us (K.W.) and 6 patients in the medical polyclinic, University of Munich (by P.H.). Several of our patients have been described in some detail in previous papers.[2,3,8,9]

Diagnostic Criteria

EM

Most patients had a typical ring-shaped or homogeneous erythema migrans and a few had atypically shaped lesions as previously described.[9] The lesions in two patients were so small—2 cm in diameter—and nonexpanding (in one) or so faint (in another) that we required the successful isolation of *B. burgdorferi* for inclusion. Elevated antibody titers aided occasionally in the diagnosis, but were not regarded as prerequisite.

ACA

Only patients with the typical bluish-red discoloration, present at least on one extremity, and IgG antibody titers of ≥64 were included as ACA patients. Two untreated patients and patients who were lost to follow-up were excluded.

Treatment Regimens

EM

This was a nonrandomized study on patients with erythema migrans. Between December 1978 and December 1984, 23 patients received phenoxymethylpenicillin, 1.2 to 3.6 million units (U) per day, 22 patients phenoxymethylpenicillin, 4.5 million per day, and 20 patients propicillin (a similar type of oral penicillin), 3.0 million U daily, amounting to 65 oral penicillin recipients. The daily dosage was divided in two or three doses and applied for usually 10, sometimes for 14 days.

Twenty-eight patients received minocycline, 100 mg twice daily mostly for 14 days from July 1984 through September 1986. Five patients received tetracycline, 500 mg two to three times daily for 8 to 21 days, and four patients doxycycline, 100 mg twice daily for 10 to 14 days from March 1983 through spring 1985.

Amoxicillin and clavulanic acid in a fixed combination (Augmentin®) was administered to 20 patients between November 1986 and July 1987, 1000 mg amoxicillin and 250 mg clavulanic acid three times daily for the first 3 days, then 500 mg amoxicillin and 125 mg clavulanic acid three times daily for the following 7 days. This fixed combination was previously tested in *in vitro* and *in vivo* experiments.[10]

ACA

This was a nonrandomized study on patients with ACA. Between February 1980 and April 1985, eight patients received phenoxymethylpenicillin, usually 4.5 million U, and six patients propicillin, 3.0 million U, both divided in two to three doses for 2 to 4 weeks. Parenteral penicillin was applied between October 1979 and December 1986: three patients obtained clemizol–penicillin-G, 1 million U daily for 7 to 10 days, four patients benzathinpenicillin, 2.4 million U once weekly for 2 to 3 weeks, and two patients penicillin G intravenously, 10 or 20 million U daily for 7 to 10 days, followed in one man by propicillin, 1 million U three times daily for 3 weeks. Tetracycline, 500 mg twice daily for 3 weeks, was administered to one female. Doxycycline, 100 mg twice daily for 10 to 21 days, was given to three patients, and minocycline, 100 mg twice daily for 7 or 14 days, to two patients. One female received amoxicillin, 500 mg three times daily for 4 weeks. Two men received ceftriaxone, 2 g intravenously daily for 2 weeks, and two patients the amoxicillin–clavulanic-acid combination as described above.

Follow-up

EM

Patients with erythema migrans were prospectively followed up for different periods of time (see TABLE 1). Most oral penicillin recipients were followed up until summer 1985, most tetracycline recipients until spring 1987, and the amoxicillin–clavulanic-acid recipients until May 1988.

ACA

Most patients with ACA were followed up through the summer of 1987 (see TABLE 3).

Criteria for Response

EM

In patients with erythema migrans, clinical criteria and development of IgG and IgM antibody titers were monitored.

ACA

In patients with ACA, clinical criteria, measurements of serum immunoglobulins, erythrocyte sedimentation rate (ESR), and IgG antibody titers were assessed.

TABLE 1. Pretreatment and Outcome Characteristics in Patients with Erythema Migrans ($n = 121$)

	Oral Penicillin ($n = 65$)	Tetracyclines ($n = 36$)	Amoxicillin and Clavulanic Acid ($n = 20$)
Pretreatment characteristics			
Sex: M/F (ratio)	25/40 (0.6)	17/19 (0.9)	9/11 (0.9)
Age (y)	42 (16–75)	47 (19–73)	48 (3–71)
Size of erythema migrans (cm)[a]	15 (2–65)[b]	18 (4–80)	10 (2–50)
Duration of erythema migrans (weeks)	5 (0.5–43)	3 (0.5–28)	3 (0.5–52)
Number of symptoms	1.5 (0–9)	1.3 (0–6)	1.3 (0–5)
Elevated IgM antibody titer[c]	18/45	11/30	5/18
Elevated IgG antibody titer[c]	11/45	5/30	6/18
ESR (normal <10 mm/h)	5 (1–27)[d]	7 (2–35)[e]	6 (2–16)[f]
IgG (normal <1320 mg/dl)	1077 (559–1530)[g]	1100 (743–2550)	1220 (880–1630)[h]
IgM (normal <250 mg/dl)	145 (59–711)[g]	126 (37–395)	165 (94–267)[h]
IgA (normal <350 mg/dl)	201 (93–394)[g]	220 (84–466)	183 (137–451)[h]
Outcome characteristics			
Follow-up (mo)	29 (1–71)	17 (1–70)	7 (4–14)
Resolution of erythema migrans (weeks)	2.1 (1–20)	2.4 (1–10)	1.3 (1–17)
Jarisch-Herxheimer reaction (n patients)	6	1	$5/p < .05$
Number of symptoms within first 3 weeks (except first day)[i]	0.2 (0–6)	0.3 (0–4)	0.3 (0–5)
Number of patients with symptoms >3 weeks[i]	23	8	3
Symptoms >3 weeks[i] Number of symptoms	0.3 (0–6)	0.1 (0–4)	0.1 (0–4)
Longest duration (mo)	0.3 (0–46)	0.3 (0–24)	0.2 (0–13)

Besides follow-up, there was no statistically significant difference among treatment groups. Values are medians (range in parentheses) unless specified otherwise.

[a] Mean of maximum diameters.

[b] $n = 49$.

[c] Number of patients with titers of 1 : 32 to 1 : 256 per number of patients tested (highest values).

[d] $n = 40$.

[e] $n = 27$.

[f] $n = 14$.

[g] $n = 53$.

[h] $n = 11$.

[i] After initiation of therapy.

Laboratory Tests

Antibody titers against *B. burgdorferi* were determined by indirect immunofluorescence (IIF) test, according to Wilske *et al.*[11,12] In short, sera with antibody titers of ≤1 : 16 were not absorbed, whereas sera with titers of ≥1 : 64 were exhaustively absorbed with *Treponema phagedenis*. Sera with IgM antibody titers of ≥64 were pretreated with an anti-IgG antiserum (Behring-Werke) and in a few instances the IgM fraction was used. This was followed in both instances by the absorption with *Treponema phagedenis*. After the performance of these procedures, antibody titers of ≥1 : 64 were regarded as positive and those of 1 : 32 as borderline. According to a recent evaluation, five out of 273 sera of healthy control persons had an IgG antibody titer of ≥1 : 32 (1.8%) and three of ≥1 : 64 (1.1%), whereas two had an IgM antibody titer of ≥1 : 32 (0.7%) and one of ≥1 : 64 (0.4%).[12] The IgG-IFT-Abs test was more sensitive than the IgG-ELISA test, but the IgM-Abs test was less sensitive than the IgM-ELISA tests.[12]

Isolation of *B. burgdorferi* from the skin of patients was attempted as outlined elsewhere.[13,14] Several of our isolates were used for *in vitro* and *in vivo* studies.[10]

The uncorrected Westergren method was used for the determination of the ESR. Serum immunoglobulins were measured in most instances by laser or rate nephelometry, less frequently by the immunodiffusion method of Mancini *et al.* (literature in ref. 1). Other laboratory tests and special procedures were mentioned in previous papers.[1-3,8,9,14]

Statistical Analyses

Differences of qualitative data were examined by Fisher's exact chi-square test and differences of quantitative data by Mann-Whitney or Kruskal-Wallis test.

RESULTS

Patients with Erythema Migrans

Pretreatment and outcome chracteristics are listed in TABLE 1. There was no statistically significant difference among the treatment groups, with the exception that groups were followed up for different times (this difference resulted from the nonrandomized study design) and that more amoxicillin–clavulanic-acid recipients developed a Jarisch-Herxheimer reaction ($p < .05$).

The exact resolution time of the erythema migrans was sometimes difficult to assess. A number of patients reported clearing of the lesion, although the erythema migrans was still present at the follow-up visit.

In several patients, symptoms intensified or new ones appeared within the first 3 weeks after initiation of therapy (this time was chosen somewhat arbitrarily); Jarisch-Herxheimer–like symptoms that appeared within the first 24 hours after initiation of therapy were not counted here; regardless of whether symptoms were new or intensified, we included all symptoms occurring between the second and twenty-first day (TABLE 1).

Seventy-six later symptoms and signs (manifestations) occurring later than 3 weeks after initiation of therapy were noted in 33 (27%) out of 121 patients for a median of 6 (range: 1–46) months (TABLE 2).

Seventeen patients had constitutional symptoms for 3 (1–46) months and 14 had

TABLE 2. Later Manifestations in Patients with Erythema Migrans (n = 121)

Manifestation	n	Duration in Months (Median, Range)
Arthralgia	19 (16%)	13 (1–46)
Headache	7 (6%)	9 (1–46)
Fever	7 (6%)	3 (1–6)
Myalgia	5 (4%)	6 (2–8)
Fatigue	5 (4%)	4 (1–36)
Sleeplessness, irritability	3 (3%)	36 (6–46)
Loss of memory	3 (3%)	20 (6–24)
Difficulty concentrating	3 (3%)	6 (4–9)
Pain within erythema migrans	2 (2%)	20 (12–28)
Paresis	2 (2%)	7 (4–9)
Depression	2 (2%)	4 (3–4)
Radicular pain	2 (2%)	3 (2–4)
Palpitations	2 (2%)	2 (1.5–2)
Single manifestations	14 (12%)	3 (1–24)

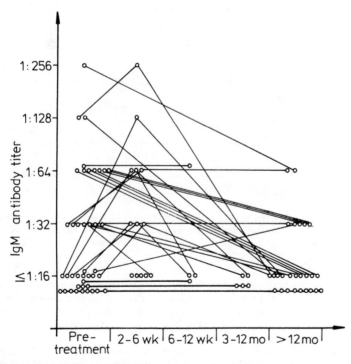

FIGURE 1. IgM antibody titer pairs in 41 erythema migrans patients treated with oral penicillin. Pretreatment and latest posttreatment values are presented. The values after 2–6 weeks are also presented for those patients if they were higher than the pretreatment values. In six patients, pre- and posttreatment titers >12 mo were ≥1 : 32.

neurological signs and symptoms for 6 (2–46) months. Most patients had only one later manifestation, but nine penicillin recipients, three tetracycline recipients, and three amoxicillin–clavulanic-acid recipients had 3 (2–7) later manifestations. The single manifestations referred to in TABLE 2 were the following: lethargy, ear ringing, abdominal pain, eye pressure, dysesthesia, hyperesthesia, neck stiffness, weight loss, elevated heart rate, conjunctivitis, diarrhea, sore throat, tracheolaryngitis, and profuse sweating. We found that most later manifestations started to develop not more than 3 months after therapy. Only three patients taking oral penicillin acquired symptoms 5 to 6 months after therapy.

Only four penicillin recipients, one tetracycline recipient, and one amoxicillin–

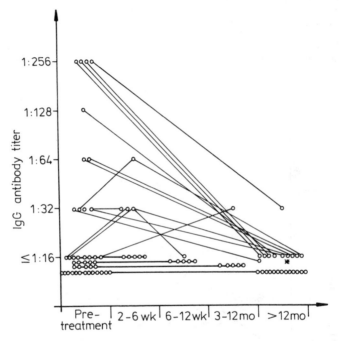

FIGURE 2. IgG antibody titer pairs in 41 erythema migrans patients treated with oral penicillin. Only two patients had a borderline posttreatment value of 1 : 32, one of them still after 3 years. For further explanation, see FIGURE 1; * = titer before absorption of 1 : 256.

clavulanic-acid recipient required retreatment. In the latter two patients and in at least three penicillin recipients there was a suspicion of meningoencephalitis or meningo-radiculitis before, during, or after therapy. These patients either refused more complete workup or the lumbar puncture was possibly done too late (in two patients 6 months after therapy) to prove a complication.

FIGURES 1 to 6 represent the antibody titers of all patients with erythema migrans for whom sera were available for the IIF test according to the method of Wilske *et al.*[11,12] The serological findings obtained in patients seen by Dr. U. Neubert have been reported elsewhere[14] and are not included here. Six out of 21 penicillin recipients with initially elevated IgM antibody titers had IgM antibody titers of 1 : 32 or 1 : 64 more

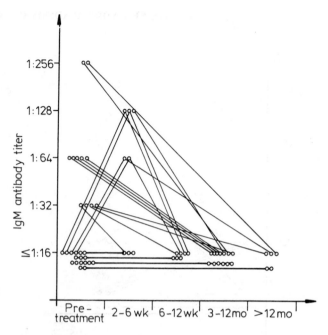

FIGURE 3. IgM antibody titer pairs in 28 erythema migrans patients treated with tetracycline. All posttreatment values were ≤1 : 16. For further explanation, see FIGURE 1.

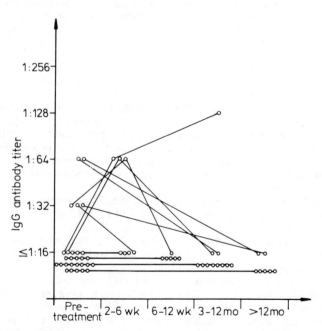

FIGURE 4. IgG antibody titer pairs in 28 erythema migrans patients treated with tetracycline. One patient had an elevated titer after 10 months. For further explanation, see FIGURE 1.

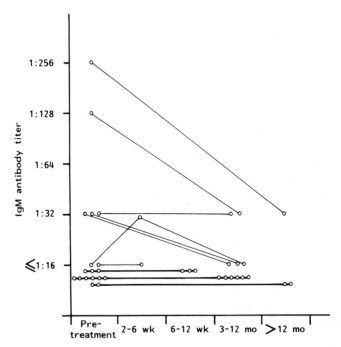

FIGURE 5. IgM antibody titer pairs in 18 erythema migrans patients treated with amoxicillin and clavulanic acid. One patient had a borderline posttreatment value of 1 : 32 >12 mo. For further explanation, see FIGURE 1.

than 1 year after therapy, as compared to zero out of 14 tetracycline recipients (p = 0.06); most patients taking amoxicillin–clavulanic-acid have not yet been followed-up for that long (FIGS. 1, 3, and 5).

Three out of the six penicillin recipients with the prolonged IgM response still had an IgM antibody titer of 1 : 32, 62, 37, and 30 months after therapy, respectively; one of them had no clinical manifestation and two still had arthralgia at that time; in one man who lacked later symptoms, the IgM antibody titer had become negative 45 months after therapy (initial value 1 : 64); sera of two more patients, one with long-lasting headache and one without sequelae, were not available later than 19 months after therapy.

Another 42-year-old female penicillin recipient had intermittent arthralgia of the right elbow for 4 years and an IgG antibody titer of 1 : 256 initially, of 1 : 32 3 years after therapy, and of 1 : 16 5 years after therapy (FIG. 2). A 56-year-old female minocycline recipient had an IgG antibody titer of 1 : 128 10 months after therapy and no complaints at that time; she had two tick bites without apparent illness in the meantime (FIG. 4).

B. burgdorferi was isolated by one of us (V.P.-M.) from seven out of ten erythema migrans lesions and from all five ACA lesions prior to therapy. *B. burgdorferi* could be identified in brain and liver of a newborn whose mother had obtained oral penicillin for an erythema migrans during the first trimester of pregnancy.[9,30] Control cultures of erythema migrans lesions were negative in three amoxicillin–clavulanic-acid recipients.

Patients with ACA

Pretreatment and outcome characteristics are shown in TABLE 3. There was no statistically significant difference among the treatment groups. Complete resolution of ACA skin involvement occurred in 15 patients after a median of 18 (3–44) months, in 7 oral penicillin recipients after 18 (3–44) months, in 6 parenteral penicillin recipients after 9 (5–28) months, and in 2 tetracycline recipients after 14 (7–20) months.

Later extracutaneous manifestations and remnants of the ACA, consisting of 41 signs and symptoms altogether, were present in 28 (82%) out of 34 ACA patients (TABLE 4). Resolution of ACA was incomplete in six oral and two parenteral penicillin recipients, as well as in four tetracycline recipients and in the five patients taking other antibiotics, a median of 10 (1–72) months after therapy. Resolution was called incomplete when a usually slight bluish-red discoloration and occasionally a slight swelling of the skin were still present after therapy; atrophy was not counted in this context. In a 50-year-old female tetracycline recipient, *B. burgdorferi* was isolated from a bluish-red ACA remnant 37 months after initial therapy; at that time, she had a very painful polyarthralgia for 33 months, enlarged lymph nodes in both axillae and in the right supraclavicular region, and an IgG antibody titer against *B. burgdorferi* of 1 : 256 (initially 1 : 512; case 11, TABLE 5). Two cases recovered spontaneously.

Twenty-four later extracutaneous manifestations were present in 16 (47%) out of 34 ACA patients for a median of 18 (1–73) months (TABLE 4). Six patients had intermittent arthralgia (two possibly arthritis) for 27 (15–34) months and six had

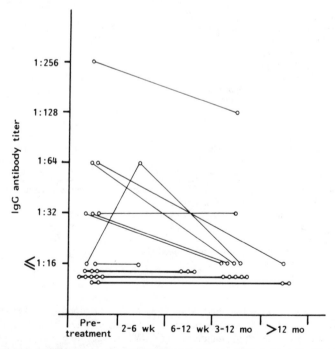

FIGURE 6. IgG antibody titer pairs in 18 erythema migrans patients treated with amoxicillin and clavulanic acid. In three patients, posttreatment values were ≤1 : 16 >12 mo. For further explanation, see FIGURE 1.

TABLE 3. Pretreatment and Outcome Characteristics in Patients with Acrodermatitis Chronica Atrophicans ($n = 29$)

	Oral Penicillin ($n - 14$)	Parenteral Penicillin ($n = 9$)	Tetracyclines ($n = 6$)
Pretreatment characteristics			
M/F ratio	0.4	0.5	0.2
Age (y)	65 (33–77)	58 (41–78)	62 (41–72)
Extent of skin involvement[a]	1.5 (1–5)	1.3 (1–5)	1.2 (1–3)
Duration of skin involvement (mo)	12 (4–60)	25 (4–48)	28 (6–120)
Number of extracutaneous symptoms	1.5 (0–4)	1.2 (0–3)	0.3 (0–3)
IgG antibody titer[b]	512 (64–4000)	1000 (128–2000)	512 (128–4000)
ESR (normal <10 mm/h)	15 (2–80)	12 (4–43)	11 (4–37)[c]
Serum IgG (normal <1320 mg/dl)	1315 (1010–2650)	1310 (935–1842)	1515 (1130–1690)[c]
Serum IgM (normal <250 mg/dl)	216 (37–632)	234 (150–448)	104(74–359)[c]
Serum IgA (normal <350 mg/dl)	332 (181–603)	226 (125–554)	231 (112–378)[c]
Outcome characteristics			
Follow-up (mo)	28 (1–73)	30 (8–93)	8 (2–37)
Resolution of skin involvement (mo)[d]	18 (1–72)	11 (5–34)	8 (2–38)
Jarisch-Herxheimer reaction (n patients)	0	1	1
Extracutaneous symptoms >3 weeks[e]			
Number	0.8 (0–2)	0.9 (0–3)	0.3 (0–3)
Duration (mo)	16 (0–73)	8 (0–34)	1 (0–37)
Retreatment			
Number	0.4 (0–3)	0.4 (0–1)	0.5 (0–2)
Interval after initial therapy (mo)	6 (4–26)	5 (2–66)	4 (1–14)
IgG antibody titer after 12–36 months	256 (64–1000)	128 (32–1000)	256 (32–512)

There was no statistically significant difference among treatment groups. Values are medians (range in parentheses) unless specified otherwise.

[a]1–4, number of extremities affected; 5, additional localization elsewhere.
[b]Reciprocal values.
[c]$n = 4$.
[d]Complete and incomplete resolution taken together.
[e]After initiation of therapy.

musculoskeletal pain other than arthralgia, mainly myalgia, for 7 (4–30) months. The peripheral neuropathy was usually noted in the areas affected by the ACA. Three patients (two oral penicillin recipients and one tetracycline recipient) revealed lymphadenopathy consisting of nontender firm nodules 1 to 1.5 cm in size, found most frequently in the axillar or inguinal region, for 20 (1–73) months. One had sleeplessness and irritability for 73 months, one had palpitations for 25 months (he presumably

TABLE 4. Later Manifestations in Patients with Acrodermatitis Chronica Atrophicans (ACA, *n* = 34)

Manifestation	*n*	Duration (Months, Median)
ACA remnants	17 (50%)	14 (2–73)
Musculoskeletal	11 (34%)	18 (4–34)
Peripheral neuropathy	5 (15%)	12 (8–57)
Lymphadenopathy	3 (9%)	20 (1–73)
Relapse	1 (3%)	4
Other	4 (12%)	22 (8–73)

died due to the sequelae of aortic stenosis), one had occipital headache for 18 months, and one had fatigue (in addition to peripheral neuropathy and biopsy-proven myositis) for 8 months. Some of the later symptoms were difficult to associate with the disease.

A woman died of an undetermined neoplasm (possibly a lymphoma) at the age of 76 years, 53 months after penicillin therapy and 32 months after retreatment with tetracycline. A man developed acute myelogenous leukemia at the age of 60 years, 24 months after therapy, 4 years after the beginning of the ACA (courtesy Dr. O. Prümmer, University of Ulm).

TABLE 5. Retreatment in Patients with Acrodermatitis Chronica Atrophicans

	No.	Sex	Age[a] (y)	Reason for Retreatment	Antibiotic	Interval after Initial Therapy (mo)
Oral penicillin recipients	1	F	72	ACA remnants	tetracycline	21
	2	F	73	ACA remnants	parenteral penicillin	26
	3	M	46	ACA remnants, neuropathy	parenteral penicillin	4
				neuropathy	erythromycin	24
				neuropathy	minocycline	46
	4	F	68	ACA remnants	parenteral penicillin	5
	5	F	59	neuropathy	minocycline	15
	6	F	72	ACA remnants, arthritis	minocycline, ceftriaxone	4 12
Parenteral penicillin recipients	7	M	56	ACA relapse	minocycline	66
	8	F	78	ACA remnants	oral penicillin	12
	9	F	53	neuropathy	doxycycline	4
	10	F	66	ACA remnants, myositis	minocycline	2
Tetracycline recipient	11	F	47	ACA remnants, neuropathy,	minocycline	14
				ACA remnants,[b] arthralgia	ceftriaxone	37
Minocycline recipient	12	F	66	dizziness[c]	oral penicillin	0.2
Augmentin recipient	13	M	38	ACA remnants	tetracycline	2

[a]At time of initial therapy.
[b]*B. burgdorferi* was isolated from a slight bluish-red area of the skin of the left ankle, 3 cm in diameter, prior to second retreatment.
[c]Probably due to minocycline.

A 61-year-old man, previously described,[3,8] developed a relapse of the ACA in exactly the same areas where he had his primary skin involvement, 5½ years after the intramuscular injection of 1 million U clemizol–penicillin-G daily for 9 days (FIG. 7). After retreatment with minocycline, 100 mg twice daily for two weeks, his ACA disappeared again and the IgG antibody titer also declined. (FIG. 7).

Retreatment was necessary in 13 patients for various reasons (TABLE 5). If retreatment occurred early, the outcome of the previous therapy was difficult to assess.

IgG antibody titers showed a slower decline than in patients with erythema migrans when the IgG antibody titers 1 year after therapy were compared (FIGS. 2, 4, 6, 8–10). The development of the IgG antibody titers in ACA is depicted in FIGURES 8 through 10. With the pretreatment values as reference point, a fourfold or greater decline occurred in 18 patients, in three of them before and in six after retreatment (FIG. 9). A fourfold or greater rise was observed in two oral penicillin recipients, one with lymphadenopathy and sleeplessness (patient no. 2 in TABLE 5) and one with ACA remnant and peripheral neuropathy (no. 3 in TABLE 5) after 46 and 42 months, respectively, despite additional retreatment with parenteral penicillin in both instances and in the patient with the relapse (FIGS. 7 and 9).

The ESR declined in 8 out of 9 patients tested within the first 3 months and rose above pretreatment values in 7 out of 22 patients within the next 5 years, although

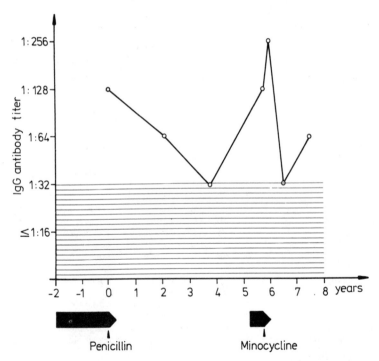

FIGURE 7. Relapse of acrodermatitis chronica atrophicans in a 61-year-old man 5½ years after initial therapy with parenteral penicillin. IgG antibody titers declined after therapy and rose with the relapse. *Bars* indicate presence of skin lesions, *hatched area* the normal range.

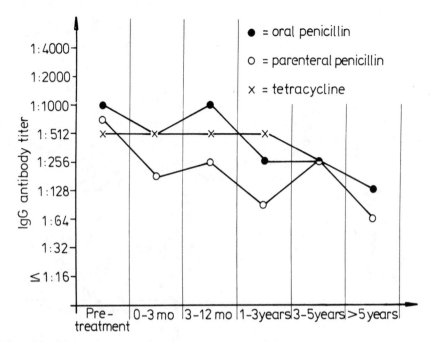

FIGURE 8. Development of IgG antibody titers (medians) in 29 patients with acrodermatitis chronica atrophicans.

other reasons could not always be excluded (FIG. 10). Serum immunoglobulins did not decline significantly 1 to 3 years after therapy (FIG. 10).

DISCUSSION

Our nonrandomized study on 121 consecutive patients with erythema migrans has not provided definite hints for the superiority of any antibiotic tested. Our investigation on patients with ACA has revealed some evidence that oral and presumably even parenteral penicillin are not sufficiently effective to cure patients with third-stage involvement of Lyme borreliosis such as ACA and associated manifestations; our experience with the other antibiotics in a few more ACA patients was too limited to be conclusive.

Recent *in vitro* and *in vivo* experiments have shown that several antibiotics such as tetracycline, ceftriaxone, and amoxicillin perform better than penicillin G.[10,13,15-17] Besides penicillin, only tetracycline and erythromycin have been tested in comparative therapeutic trials in early Lyme borreliosis so far.[3-7] These studies have not been able to clearly demonstrate that tetracycline is superior to penicillin. In the first of these investigations, Steere *et al.* compared penicillin versus nonantibiotic (placebo) therapy and obtained evidence for the beneficial effect of penicillin in clearing of erythema migrans, an observation that had been reported previously in dozens of cases in noncomparative investigations, and in preventing subsequent arthritis.[4] In another study by the same group, some evidence seemed to indicate that tetracycline was

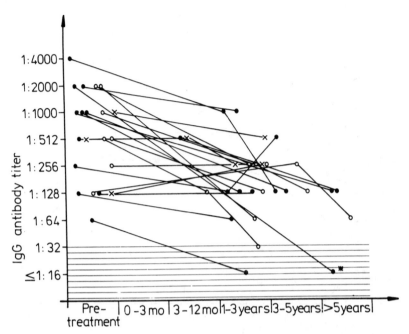

FIGURE 9. Pretreatment and latest posttreatment IgG antibody titers in 21 patients with acrodermatitis chronica atrophicans, with intermediate values in four patients prior to retreatment; ● = oral penicillin; ○ = parenteral penicillin; × = tetracycline; * = titer before absorption was 1 : 256.

superior to penicillin and erythromycin in preventing severe later manifestations.[5] The statistical evaluation, however, revealed a *p* value of .07, and brief attacks of arthritis in two tetracycline recipients were not regarded as a severe late manifestation; the inclusion of only a single tetracycline recipient who developed severe later manifestations would make it even more difficult to demonstrate a significant difference. There have been observations on severe late manifestations following tetracycline therapy[18] (Dr. P. Lavoie, personal communication).

The tetracycline dosage was rather low in the above-mentioned investigation.[5] Recently, we have not been able to demonstrate that minocycline (100 mg twice daily for usually 2 weeks) is better than penicillin; therefore, minocycline appears not to be superior to low doses of tetracycline.[7]

Only clinical criteria for the therapeutic response have been considered in the studies previously mentioned.[3-7] In our present series, we evaluated the antibody response in addition to clinical criteria. There was no statistically significant difference in the decline of the antibody titers, although six penicillin recipients, compared to none of the tetracycline recipients, still had elevated IgM antibody titers 1 year after therapy. But it cannot be ruled out that the penicillin recipients were in danger of developing more severe late disease, although none did. Two of these patients, however, did have long-lasting arthralgia and one had long-lasting headache.

We could not prove severe later manifestations according to an earlier definition,[5] so that the later symptoms and signs observed in our patients have to be classified as minor. The later symptoms and signs observed by us, however, indicate the possibility of more serious manifestations such as meningoencephalitis or meningoradiculitis of Bannwarth in a few of our patients.

In fall 1986 we began to treat erythema migrans patients with amoxicillin–clavulanic-acid. Amoxicillin–clavulanic-acid was chosen for three reasons. First, it is an oral antibiotic. Secondly, its MIC_{90} was 0.25 mg/ml as compared to the MIC_{90} values for penicillin G (4), amoxicillin (0.5), and tetracycline (0.5).[10] Thirdly, experiments in gerbils revealed that a dosage of 50 mg per kg per day of amoxicillin–clavulanic-acid was curative in three animals as compared to a failure rate in four out of five gerbils on 320 mg per kg per day of penicillin G, in one out of four gerbils on 100 mg per kg per day of tetracycline (200 mg per kg per day was curative in 4 animals), and in 1 out of 3 gerbils on 50 mg per kg per day of amoxicillin.[10] Clavulanic acid was found to have an inhibitory effect on *B. burgdorferi,* with an MIC_{90} of 2 mg/ml, although this organism does apparently not produce β-lactamase (Dr. V. Preac-Mursic, personal communication). So far, our preliminary observations with amoxicillin–clavulanic-acid in humans have failed to demonstrate a superiority compared to penicillin, but a Jarisch-Herxheimer reaction occurred more frequently than in the other groups ($p < .05$); the significance of this is unclear.

The effect of various antibiotics on patients with ACA has been quite impressive to most early and present investigators.[19] Patients for whom there had been no treatment available, often for many years previously, quickly benefitted from the antibiotics after they appeared on the market in the late 1940s and early 1950s.

However, three lines of evidence have cast some doubt on the efficacy of the antibiotics tested so far. First, a number of ACA patients have shown remnants of their

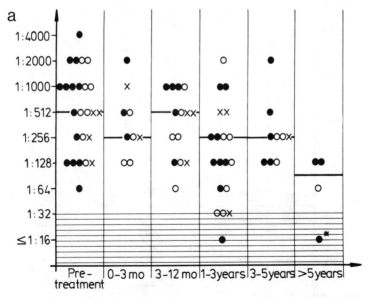

FIGURE 10. Development of (**a**) IgG antibody titers, (**b**) serum IgG, (**c**) serum IgM, (**d**) serum IgA, and (**e**) ESR in our patients with acrodermatitis chronica atrophicans. Posttreatment values were usually lower than pretreatment values but the difference was not statistically significant. *Bars* indicate medians, *hatched areas* the normal range; * = titer before absorption was 1 : 256. ● = oral penicillin; ○ = parenteral penicillin; × = tetracycline. (*Continued on following pages.*)

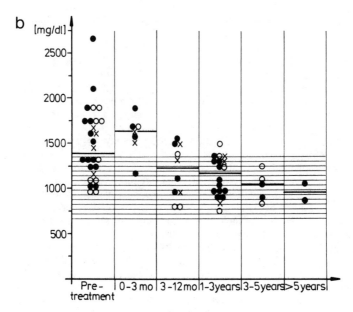

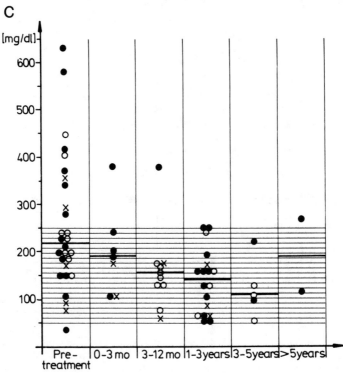

FIGURE 10. *Continued.*

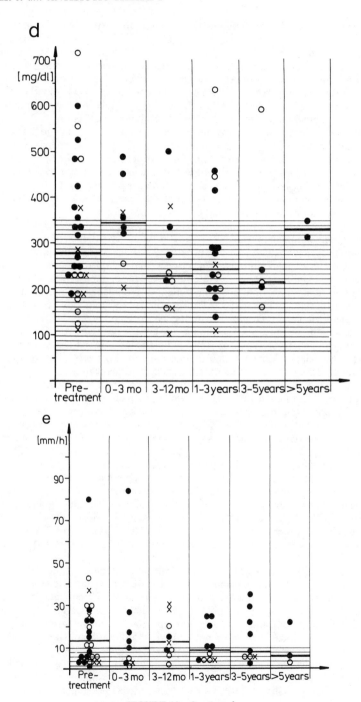

FIGURE 10. *Continued.*

skin involvement at the latest follow-up after therapy with penicillin and tetracycline.[3,8,19-23,25] Some patients did not respond at all.[20,22,23,25] Follow-up in most of these patients was usually up to 2 years. Our findings in 17 patients with ACA remnants, including one in whom *B. burgdorferi* was isolated, support these reports. However, follow-up in our patients with ACA remnants was only for a median of 10 (range: 2–73) months, as compared to the median follow-up of 28 (7–93) months in our 15 patients with complete clearing of the ACA; a longer follow-up would presumably increase the number of patients with complete resolution of the ACA.

Secondly, peripheral neuropathy might continue or may even start to develop anew after antibiotic therapy,[26,27] as was also found in our five patients. Follow-up was for 6 (2–8) years in 7 out of 12 patients with posttreatment peripheral neuropathy in one series.[26] The 92 cases seen by Hopf represent a selected group of patients with neuropathy.[26] Kaiser has described a relapse of the peripheral neuropathy in five out of 120 nonselected patients.[27] The observation of the relapse of the skin involvement in one of our patients corresponds to that finding.

Thirdly, other later manifestations have been noted in ACA patients. Arthralgia has been observed in one previous case[23] and in six of our patients. The occurrence of later musculoskeletal pain in 34% of our 34 ACA patients was even higher than in our patients with erythema migrans. We suspect that lymphadenopathy may be an important sign to indicate activity of later disease; each of our three patients had other concomitant signs and symptoms in addition to lymphadenopathy, such as ACA remnants, arthralgia, or irritability. All three still had IgG antibody titers of $\geq 1 : 128$, and one had viable *B. burgdorferi* in the ACA remnant at the time when the lymphadenopathy was present. We cannot rule out the possibility that the occurrence rate (9%) is an underrepresentation, since lymph nodes were not checked in all of our patients. The relapse found in one of our patients $5\frac{1}{2}$ years after therapy with parenteral penicillin is evidence against the efficacy of this regimen.

Jarisch-Herxheimer–like reactions in ACA do not seem to be common. Götz and Ludwig noted fever of up to 38°C of unknown origin in one of their penicillin recipients (case 10[21]), and our group described an exacerbation of the peripheral neuropathy shortly after initiation of therapy with tetracycline.[3] One of our present patients developed flu-like symptoms for 2 days and an intensification of the color of her ACA skin lesions together with profound fatigue after the first and second injection of benzathin-penicillin, respectively; in addition, the possibility that the pericarditis for which she was admitted to another hospital after the second injection represented a local Jarisch-Herxheimer reaction developing in the heart cannot be ruled out.

ESR and immunoglobulins of our patients did not decline significantly after therapy, although there was a definite decrease in several patients. The decline of ESR values has already been noted in earlier studies,[19,20,24] but Pirilä[20] and Hauser[24] especially have observed, as we did, patients with no decrease or even with an increase of the ESR.

IgG antibody titers declined in some patients and remained at the initial level, as we and others have reported previously[8,28,29] and as we can corroborate now. An at least fourfold decrease could be documented in 18 out of our 29 patients in whom IgG antibody titer controls were available; three of these patients even had an at least fourfold increase 1 year and later after therapy and two of the latter had a decline again after retreatment. We have not followed IgM antibody titers in our ACA patients since we have previously found them to be insignificant.[11]

Retreatment has been more often necessary in our ACA than in erythema migrans patients. Early workers have already tried to improve treatment results by retreatment.[19,,21-23] Our patients recently treated with ceftriaxone, amoxicillin–clavulanic-acid, or amoxicillin still had ACA remnants a few months after therapy, but follow-up was too short to obtain enough information.

In conclusion, comparative therapeutic trials by others and ourselves failed to demonstrate the superiority of tetracycline or—in our pilot study—of amoxicillin–clavulanic-acid over oral penicillin in patients with erythema migrans. In ACA, too, no significant difference has been found in our preliminary investigation comparing oral penicillin, parenteral penicillin, and tetracycline. Since there is a discrepancy between results obtained from recent *in vitro* and *in vivo* experiments and the observations made in therapeutic trials in humans, more work seems to be necessary to improve the treatment of early and late Lyme borreliosis. Presently, our preliminary recommendation would be to treat early Lyme borreliosis and ACA with one of the tetracyclines in appropriate dosage, although penicillin and amoxicillin with or without clavulanic acid may also be of benefit.

SUMMARY

In a study on 121 consecutive patients with erythema migrans, 65 patients obtained oral penicillin, 36 tetracyclines, and 20 amoxicillin–clavulanic-acid. Follow-up was carried out for a median of 29, 17, and 7 months, respectively. In another limited trial on 29 patients with acrodermatitis chronica atrophicans (ACA), 14 patients received oral penicillin, 9 parenteral penicillin, and 6 tetracyclines. There was no statistically significant difference among treatment groups in both therapeutic trials, with the exception of different follow-ups due to the nonrandomized study design and different occurrence of the Jarisch-Herxheimer reaction in patients with erythema migrans. Later extracutaneous manifestations developed in 27% of the patients with erythema migrans and in 47% of the patients with ACA despite antibiotic therapy. We could not prove the superiority of any antibiotic tested in either early or late European Lyme borreliosis.

ACKNOWLEDGMENTS

We are indebted to Dr. C.D. Reimers for his advice and to Dr. T. Becker, Frau U. Perschau, M. Füchtenbusch, and our dermatological colleagues for their helpful contributions.

REFERENCES

1. WEBER, K., A. PUZIK & T. BECKER. 1983. Erythema-migrans-Krankheit: Beitrag zur Klinik und Beziehung zur Lyme-Krankheit. Dtsch. Med. Wochenschr. **108:** 1182–1190.
2. WEBER, K., G. SCHIERZ, B. WILSKE & V. PREAC-MURSIC. 1984. European erythema migrans disease and related disorders. Yale J. Biol. Med. **57:** 463–471.
3. WEBER, K., U. NEUBERT & R. THURMAYR. 1986. Antibiotic therapy in early erythema migrans disease and related disorders. Zbl. Bakt. Hyg. A. **263:** 377–388.
4. STEERE, A. C., S. E. MALAWISTA, J. NEWMAN, P. N. SPIELER & H. N. BARTENHAGEN. 1980. Antibiotic therapy in Lyme disease. Ann. Intern. Med. **93:** 1–8.
5. STEERE, A. C., G. J. HUTCHINSON, D. W. RAHN, L. H. SIGAL, J. E. CRAFT, E. T. DeSANNA & S. E. MALAWISTA. 1983. Treatment of the early manifestations of Lyme disease. Ann. Intern. Med. **99:** 22–26.

6. BERGER, B. W. 1986. Treating erythema chronicum migrans of Lyme disease. J. Am. Acad. Dermatol. **15:** 459–463.
7. WEBER, K. & R. THURMAYR. 1988. Oral penicillin versus minocycline in early Lyme borreliosis. Zbl. Bakt. Hyg. In press.
8. WEBER, K., G. SCHIERZ, B. WILSKE & V. PREAC-MURSIC. 1984. Zur Klinik und Ätiologie der Acrodermatitis chronica atrophicans. Hautarzt **35:** 571–577.
9. WEBER, K. & U. NEUBERT. 1986. Clinical features of early erythema migrans disease and related disorders. Zbl. Bakt. Hyg. A **263:** 209–228.
10. PREAC-MURSIC, V., B. WILSKE, G. SCHIERZ, M. HOLMBURGER & E. SÜSS. 1987. In vitro and in vivo susceptibility of Borrelia burgdorferi. Eur. J. Clin. Microbiol. **6:** 424–426.
11. WILSKE, B., G. SCHIERZ, V. PREAC-MURSIC, K. WEBER, H.-W. PFISTER & K. EINHÄUPL. 1984. Serological diagnosis of erythema migrans disease and related disorders. Infection **12:** 331–337.
12. WILSKE, B., G. SCHIERZ, V. PREAC-MURSIC, H.-W. PFISTER, K. WEBER, K. V. BUSCH & A. BARUSCHKE. 1988. IgM and IgG immune response to Borrelia burgdorferi in erythema migrans and neuroborreliosis. Zbl. Bakt. Hyg. In press.
13. PREAC-MURSIC, V., B. WILSKE & G. SCHIERZ. 1986. European Borrelia burgdorferi isolated from humans and ticks: Culture conditions and antibiotic susceptibility. Zbl. Bakt. Hyg. A **263:** 112–118.
14. NEUBERT, U., H. E. KRAMPITZ & H. ENGL. 1986. Microbiological findings in erythema (chronicum) migrans and related disorders. Zbl. Bakt. Hyg. A **263:** 237–252.
15. JOHNSON, S. E., G. C. KLEIN, G. P. SCHMID & J. C. FEELEY. 1984. Susceptibility of the Lyme spirochete to seven antimicrobial agents. Yale J. Biol. Med. **57:** 549–553.
16. BERGER, B. W., M. H. KAPLAN, I. R. ROTHENBERG & A. G. BARBOUR. 1985. Isolation and characterization of the Lyme disease spirochete from the skin of patients with erythema chronicum migrans. J. Am. Acad. Dermatol. **13:** 444–449.
17. JOHNSON, R. C., C. KODNER & M. RUSSELL. 1987. In vitro and in vivo susceptibility of the Lyme disease spirochete, Borrelia burgdorferi, to four antimicrobial agents. Antimicrob. Agents Chemother. **31:** 164–167.
18. STEERE, A. C., P. H. DURAY, D. J. H. KAUFFMANN & G. P. WORMSER. 1985. Unilateral blindness caused by infection with the Lyme disease spirochete, Borrelia burgdorferi. Ann. Intern. Med. **103:** 382–384.
19. THYRESSON, N. 1949. The penicillin treatment of acrodermatitis atrophicans chronica (Herxheimer). Acta Derm. Venereol. (Stockholm) **29:** 572–621.
20. PIRILÄ, V. 1951. The penicillin treatment of acrodermatitis atrophicans chronica. Acta Derm. Venereol. (Stockholm) **31:** 576–591.
21. GÖTZ, H. & E. LUDWIG. 1951. Die Behandlung der Akrodermatitis chronica atrophicans Herxheimer mit Penicillin. Hautarzt **2:** 6–14.
22. BRUNNER, N. 1951. Zur Penicillinbehandlung bei Sklerodermie und Akrodermatitis atrophicans Herxheimer. Hautarzt **2:** 545–547.
23. LUDWIG, E. 1955. Erfolgreiche Aureomycin- und Terramycinbehandlung als Beitrag zur Klärung der Wirkungsweise von Penicillin bei der Akrodermatitis atrophicans Herxheimer. Dermatol. Wochenschr. **131:** 169–178.
24. HAUSER, W. 1955. Zur Kenntnis der Akrodermatitis chronica atrophicans. Arch. Dermatol. Syph. **199:** 350–393.
25. BETZ, E. 1972. Nachuntersuchungen über den Behandlungserfolg an den Akrodermatitis chronica atrophicans (Herxheimer) Erkrankten der Universitäts-Hautklinik Köln auf Grund von klinischen und histologischen Befunden. Dissertation, Köln.
26. HOPF, H. C. 1966. Acrodermatitis chronica atrophicans (Herxheimer) und Nervensystem. Monographien Gesamtgebiete Neurol. Psychiat. 114. Springer. Berlin and New York.
27. KAISER, M. 1972. Neurologische Komplikationen bei Akrodermatitis chronica atrophicans (Herxheimer) und ihre Beeinflussung durch die Penicillintherapie. Dissertation, Göttingen.
28. ACKERMANN, R., H. P. BOISTEN, J. KABATZKI, U. RUNNE, K. KRÜGER & W. P. HERRMANN. 1984. Serumantikörper gegen Ixodes-ricinus-Spirochäte bei Acrodermatitis chronica atrophicans (Herxheimer). Dtsch. Med. Wochenschr. **109:** 6–10.
29. ASBRINK, E., A. HOVMARK & B. HEDERSTEDT. 1985. Serologic studies of erythema

chronicum migrans Afzelius and acrodermatitis chronica atrophicans with indirect immunofluorescence and enzyme-linked immunosorbent assays. Acta Derm. Venereol. (Stockholm) **65:** 509–514.

30. WEBER, K, H.-J. BRATZKE, U. NEUBERT, B. WILSKE & P. H. DURAY. 1988. *Borrelia burgdorferi* in a newborn despite oral penicillin for Lyme borreliosis during pregnancy. Ped. Infect. Dis. **7:** 286–289.

Treatment of Erythema Chronicum Migrans of Lyme Disease

BERNARD W. BERGER

Department of Dermatology
New York University School of Medicine
New York, New York 10016

INTRODUCTION

Prior to the establishment of Lyme disease (LD) as a distinct clinical entity, the effectiveness of antibiotic treatment of erythema chronicum migrans (ECM) alone or with extracutaneous signs and symptoms had been demonstrated.[1-3] The findings led to the successful use of antibiotics in the treatment of LD.[4] Revisions in antibiotic treatment evolved in concert with a growing understanding of the cause and clinical course of LD,[5,6] which was reflected in the treatment of a similar spirochestosis known in Europe as erythema chronicum migrans Afzelius[7] and erythema migrans disease.[8]

This paper describes the clinical response to antibiotic therapy of 215 patients who presented with ECM of Lyme disease.

PATIENTS AND METHODS

Between June 1981 and July 1987, 197 adults and 18 children with ECM of LD were evaluated and treated. Two hundred thirteen of the patients were initially evaluated and treated within the first 4 weeks of the appearance of the ECM lesions. Four patients were pregnant women in their 12th, 14th, 22nd, and 24th week of gestation.

All patients presented with ECM, which has been clinically defined as a discernible, centrifugally expanding, usually erythematous patch.[5] The intensity of LD was judged to be minor if the patients manifested ECM alone or in association with headache, fatigue, and/or musculoskeletal discomfort that were mild in nature. The intensity of the illness was considered major if ECM appeared in multiplicity or if a solitary ECM lesion was accompanied by fever and marked musculoskeletal pain, fatigue, and headache. Anorexia, chills, lymphadenopathy, sore throat, nausea, vomiting, eye pain, memory lapses, Bell's palsy, supraventricular tachycardia, complete heart block, and myocarditis were present in some of these patients.

From 1981 through 1986 varying antibiotic regimens were used to treat 161 patients (TABLE 1). In 1987, amoxicillin and doxycycline were substituted for penicillin V potassium and tetracycline. Forty-six patients received a combination of amoxicillin (500 mg q.i.d. × 15–30 days) and probenecid (500 mg q.i.d. × 15–30 days). Five patients were treated with doxycycline (100 mg t.i.d. × 15–30 days) and strongly advised to use a sun screen. On the basis of past experience[9] patients manifesting a major form of the illness were treated for 30 days and those with a minor form of the illness, 15 days. Three patients in the 1987 group were treated with intravenous ceftriaxone (2–4 g per day × 14 days), two because of cardiac abnormalities (complete heart block, myocarditis), and one because she could not tolerate oral medication.

TABLE 1. Summary of Findings (1981–86)

No. of Patients	Treatment	Days ECM Present before Treatment	Minor LD (No. Retreated/Total)	Major LD (No. Retreated/Total)
Adults				
13	penicillin V potassium, 250 mg q.i.d. × 10 days	2–21 (median = 9)	0/5	3/8
56	penicillin V potassium, 500 mg q.i.d. × 15 days	1–28 (median = 9)	2/48	3/8
4[a]	penicillin V potassium, 500 mg q.i.d. × 21–30 days	4–10 (median = 6)	0/4	—
17	benzathine penicillin G (Bicillin), 2.4 million units i.m.	2–21 (median = 8)	0/8	2/9
38	penicillin V potassium, 500 mg q.i.d. probenecid, 500 mg q.i.d. × 15 days	1–56 (median = 10)	—	4/38
12	tetracycline, 500 mg q.i.d. × 15 days	2–21 (median = 9)	0/8[b]	1/4
2	erythromycin, 500 mg q.i.d. × 15 days	2–7 (median = 7)	—	1/2
1	minocycline (Minocin), 100 mg q.i.d. × 15 days	14	—	1/1
Children				
13	penicillin V potassium, 50 mg · kg^{-1} · day^{-1} × 15 days	2–28 (median = 9)	0/7	0/6
1	penicillin V potassium, 50 mg · kg^{-1} · day^{-1} × 7 days	2	—	1/1
1	penicillin V potassium, 50 mg · kg^{-1} · day^{-1} × 10 days	74	—	1/1
1	penicillin V potassium, 50 mg · kg^{-1} · day^{-1}; probenecid, 500 mg b.i.d. × 15 days	14	—	0/1
2	erythromycin, 50 mg · kg^{-1} × 15 days	1–7 (median = 4)	—	0/2

Abbreviations: ECM, erythema chronicum migrans; i.m., intramuscular; q.i.d., four times per day; b.i.d., twice per day.

[a] Pregnant women.

[b] Three patients could not tolerate tetracycline after 8 days of treatment and were switched to penicillin, 500 mg four times a day for 7 days.

The efficacy of treatment was based on the prevention of major late manifestations of LD (meningoencephalitis, myocarditis, recurrent attacks of arthritis) as proposed by Steere et al.[6] and the prevention of severe posttreatment fatigue, headache, and musculoskeletal pain. Patients who experienced a recurrence of their LD signs and symptoms following an initial course of therapy were retreated with the original antibiotic.

The patients were seen 10 to 12 days following their first visit and again on an as-needed basis. The patients were contacted by telephone 3 to 6 months following their final office visit.

RESULTS (1981–86)

Lyme Disease of Minor Intensity

Seventy-eight of the eighty patients with LD of minor intensity did not require retreatment (TABLE 1). The duration of time between the onset of treatment and the resolution of all signs and symptoms of LD ranged from 2 to 28 days (median interval, 9 days). The ECM lesions resolved in 4 to 5 days. Postinflammatory hyperpigmentation was noted for an additional 1 to 2 weeks on some patients with crusted ECM lesions or ECM lesions on their lower extremities. Included in this group were the four pregnant women who subsequently delivered full-term, normal infants.

Lyme Disease of Major Intensity

Sixty-four of the eighty-one patients with LD of major intensity responded to their initial course of treatment. Three patients had Bell's palsy and one patient had supraventricular tachycardia prior to treatment. The duration between the onset of treatment and resolution of LD signs and symptoms ranged from 2 to 30 days (median interval, 12 days). Time for resolution of ECM in the LD major group was 4–5 days.

Seventeen of the eighty-one patients (21%) presenting with LD of major intensity required retreatment. Thirteen of these patients responded to their second course of medication. The time between the onset of treatment and the resolution of LD signs and symptoms ranged from 30 to 180 days (median interval = 53 days). Four patients in the penicillin-probenecid group did not respond to retreatment with their original medication. Two of these patients were given intravenous ceftriaxone (2 g/day for 14 days). They both had significant improvement and were able to resume normal activities. One patient was treated with intravenous penicillin (20,000,000 IU/day for 14 days) and was moderately improved. The remaining patient was lost to follow-up.

RESULTS (1987)

It is too early to judge the efficacy of treatment in this group of 54 patients; however, some observations are reportable.

Amoxicillin-Probenecid

This group consisted of 46 patients. Twenty-six had a major form of the illness and 20 a minor form. A Jarisch-Herxheimer-like reaction occurred in 23 (50%) of these patients for varying periods during the first 4 to 5 days of therapy. It occurred more frequently in patients with LD major (16 of 26 patients). Five of the 46 patients developed a generalized pruritic, erythematous, maculopapular eruption during the eighth to tenth day of treatment, which was consistent with a drug eruption.

Doxycycline

Five patients were treated with doxycycline. No Jarisch-Herxheimer-like reactions occurred. A photosensitivity reaction appeared on the sun-exposed skin of one patient not protected by a sun screen.

DISCUSSION

Shresta et al.,[10] in a study of early LD, divided their patients into those with localized disease (ECM, sometimes accompanied by regional lymphadenopathy or minor constitutional symptoms) and those with disseminated infection (clinical evidence of spread of the spirochete to other systems). Ten patients with localized disease responded to a 10-day course of tetracycline or penicillin, but 5 of 26 patients with disseminated infection required an additional 10 days of therapy. None of the patients had subsequent manifestations of the illness.

Similarly, in this study, where ECM of LD was viewed in terms of the variability of its clinical expression, it was apparent that patients manifesting a minor form of the illness usually responded to their initial course of antibiotic therapy and as previously reported, those with a major form of the illness were at greater risk for development of complications that would require retreatment and a prolonged recovery period.[5,6,11,12]

The clinical variability of early LD is probably due in part to the LD spirochete, Borrelia burgdorferi. Studies on fresh isolates obtained from skin biopsy specimens of ECM lesions revealed differences in monoclonal antibody typing[13,14] and culture growth characteristics.[13] Antimicrobial susceptibility studies indicated a variability in vitro as reflected in differing mean inhibitory concentrations and/or mean bactericidal concentrations in the presence of the same antibiotic.[13,15–17]

These in vitro studies support the rationale for the use of antibiotics in the treatment of LD but differ on the effectiveness of penicillin.[13,17] Clinical studies on the treatment of ECM also reflect differences in antibiotic efficacy, leading some authors to prefer tetracycline,[12] some phenoxymethyl penicillin,[7,18] and others minocycline or high doses of parenteral penicillin.[19] The failures of tetracycline,[20] penicillin and erythromycin,[6] and penicillin and probenecid[21] in the treatment of LD have been reported. Intravenous penicillin, as the treatment of choice for major complications of LD,[22,23] may be replaced by intravenous ceftriaxone, which was effective therapy for five patients with late LD who failed to respond to intravenous penicillin.[21] However, ceftriaxone has not been universally effective in the treatment of late LD (Dattwyler and Halperin, personal communication).

The reported treatment failures, as well as those in my own study, demonstrated a need for an oral antibiotic that can be readily absorbed, producing serum and cerebrospinal fluid (CSF) levels sufficient to kill Borrelia burgdorferi organisms. A report by Faber et al.[24] indicated treponemicidal levels of amoxicillin in the serum and CSF were achieved in syphilis patients treated with a combination of amoxicillin and probenecid. This information, and in vitro studies that have shown Borrelia burgdorferi to be susceptible to ampicillin,[15,16] have suggested the use of amoxicillin with probenecid in the treatment of ECM of LD. An objection to this regimen is a report that probenecid may interfere with the accumulation of penicillin in brain tissue.[25]

It is too early to report on the efficacy of this regimen, but it is of interest that the occurrence of Jarisch-Herxheimer–like reactions in 23 of 46 patients treated with amoxicillin and probenecid has a greater frequency than previously reported.[5,12] The appearance of a drug eruption on five of the 46 patients (11%) is consistent with the incidence of ampicillin drug eruptions occurring in the general population,[26] but in my experience is higher than encountered with the treatment regimens used in 1981–86.

Until a preferred antibiotic for the treatment of LD has been conclusively determined, we should alert our patients to the necessity of compliance with treatment protocols and the possibility of reactions to the medications used.

SUMMARY

Between June 1981 and July 1987 the efficacy of antibiotic treatment of 215 patients with erythema chronicum migrans of Lyme disease was evaluated in terms of the necessity for retreatment and the prevention of the late manifestations of Lyme disease. The principal antibiotics utilized to treat 161 patients through 1986 were varying doses of tetracycline, or penicillin alone or in combination with probenecid. Two of 80 patients with a minor form of the illness and 17 of 81 patients with a major form of the illness required retreatment. There were four patients who did not respond to retreatment with their original medication.

A 15- to 30-day course of amoxicillin (500 mg q.i.d.) and probenecid (500 mg q.i.d.) or doxycycline (100 mg t.i.d.), and on three occasions ceftriaxone (2–4 g/day i.v.), were used to treat 54 patients in 1987. Although it is too early to judge the efficacy of treatment in these patients, increases in the incidence of Herxheimer reactions and drug eruptions were observed. Strict compliance with treatment protocols and the possibility of reactions to medications should be thoroughly discussed with patients.

REFERENCES

1. HOLLSTROM, E. 1958. Penicillin treatment of erythema chronicum migrans Afzelius. Acta Derm. Venereol. (Stockholm) **38:** 285–289.
2. SONCK, C. E. 1965. Erythema chronicum migrans with multiple lesions. Acta Derm. Venereol. (Stockholm) **45:** 34–36.
3. SCRIMENTI, R. J. 1970. Erythema chronicum migrans. Arch. Dermatol. **102:** 104–105.
4. STEERE, A. C., S. E. MALAWISTA, J. H. NEWMAN, et al. 1980. Antibiotic therapy in Lyme disease. Ann. Intern. Med. **93:** 1–8.
5. BERGER, B. W. 1984. Erythema chronicum migrans of Lyme disease. Arch. Dermatol. **120:** 1017–1021.
6. STEERE, A. C., G. J. HUTCHINSON, D. W. RAHN, et al. 1983. Treatment of the early manifestations of Lyme disease. Ann. Intern. Med. **99:** 22–26.
7. ÅSBRINK, E. & I. OLSSON. 1985. Clinical manifestations of erythema chronicum migrans Afzelius in 161 patients. Acta Derm. Venereol. (Stockholm) **65:** 43–52.
8. WEBER, K., A. PUZIK & T. BECKER. 1983. Erythema migrans krankheit. Dtsch. Med. Wochenschr. **108:** 1182–1190.
9. BERGER, B. W. 1986. Treating erythema chronicum migrans of Lyme disease. J. Am. Acad. Dermatol. **15:** 459–463.
10. SHRESTA, M., R. L. GRODZICKI & A. C. STEERE. 1985. Diagnosing early Lyme disease. Am. J. Med. **78:** 235–240.

11. KOHLHEPP, W., H. MERTENS & P. OSCHMANN. 1976. Acute and chronic illness after tick-bite *Borrelia burgdorferi* infections. Zbl. Bakt. Hyg. A **263**: 365–371.
12. STEERE, A. C., J. GREEN, G. J. HUTCHINSON, D. W. RAHN, A. R. PACHNER, *et al.* 1986. Treatment of Lyme disease. Zbl. Bakt. Hyg. A **263**: 352–356.
13. BERGER, B. W., M. H. KAPLAN, I. R. ROTHENBERG, *et al.* 1985. Isolation and characterization of the Lyme disease spirochete from the skin of patients with erythema chronicum migrans. J. Am. Acad. Dermatol. **13**: 444–449.
14. BARBOR, A. G. & M. E. SCHRUMPF. 1986. Polymorphisms of major surface proteins of *Borrelia burgdorferi*. Zbl. Bakt. Hyg. A **263**: 83–91.
15. JOHNSON, S. E., G. C. KLEIN, G. P. SCHMID, *et al.* 1984. Susceptibility of the Lyme disease spirochete to seven antimicrobial agents. Yale J. Biol. Med. **57**: 549–553.
16. PREAC-MURSIC, V., B. WILSKE & G. SCHIERZ. 1986. European *Borrelia burgdorferi* isolated from humans and ticks. Zbl. Bakt. Hyg. A **263**: 112–118.
17. JOHNSON, R. C., C. KODNER & M. RUSSELL. 1987. *In vitro* and *in vivo* susceptibility of the Lyme disease spirochete, *Borrelia burgdorferi*, to four antimicrobial agents. Antimicrob. Agents Chemother. **31**: 164–167.
18. NEUMANN, R., E. ABERER & G. STANEK. 1976. Treatment and course of erythema chronicum migrans. Zbl. Bakt. Hyg. A **263**: 372–376.
19. WEBER, K., V. NEWBERT & R. THURMAYR. 1986. Antibiotic therapy in early erythema chronicum migrans disease and related disorders. Zbl. Bakt. Hyg. A **263**: 377–388.
20. DATTWYLER, R. J. & J. J. HALPERIN. 1987. Failure of tetracycline in early Lyme disease. Arthritis Rheum. **30**: 448–450.
21. DATTWYLER, R. J., J. J. HALPERIN, H. PASS & B. J. LUFT. 1987. Ceftriaxone as effective therapy in refractive Lyme disease. J. Infect. Dis. **155**: 1322–1325.
22. STEERE, A. C., A. R. PACHNER & S. E. MALAWISTA. 1983. Neurologic abnormalities of Lyme disease: Successful treatment with high-dose intravenous penicillin. Ann. Intern. Med. **99**: 767–772.
23. STEERE, A. C., J. GREEN, R. T. SCHOEN, *et al.* 1985. Successful parenteral penicillin therapy of established Lyme arthritis. N. Engl. J. Med. **312**: 869–874.
24. FABER, W. R., J. D. BOS, P. J. RIETRA, H. FASS & V. W. VAN ELJK. 1983. Treponemicidal levels of amoxicillin in cerebrospinal fluid after oral administration. Sex. Trans. Dis. **10**: 148–150.
25. FISHMAN, R. A. 1966. Blood-brain and cerebrospinal fluid barrier to penicillin and related organic acids. Arch. Neurol. **15**: 113–124.
26. NAZARETH, I., P. MORTIMER & G. D. MCKENDRICK. 1972. Ampicillin sensitivity in infectious mononucleosis. Scand. J. Infect. Dis. **4**: 229–230.

New Chemotherapeutic Approaches in the Treatment of Lyme Borreliosis[a]

BENJAMIN J. LUFT,[b] DAVID J. VOLKMAN,[c]
JOHN J. HALPERIN,[c] AND RAYMOND J. DATTWYLER[b]

[b]Department of Medicine
[c]Department of Neurology
Health Science Center
SUNY at Stony Brook
Stony Brook, New York 11794

INTRODUCTION AND BACKGROUND

The therapeutic value of penicillins and tetracyclines for treatment of Lyme borreliosis was initially established on the basis of empiric therapeutic trials for erythema chronicum migrans,[1] acrodermatitis chronica atrophicans,[2,3] Lyme arthritis,[4] and meningitis.[5] In controlled studies by Steere and colleagues,[1] the therapeutic value of these chemotherapeutic agents was unequivocally established when compared to patients not treated with antibiotics. *B. burgdorferi* was not isolated from the patients in these studies, and therefore *in vitro* sensitivity data was not available. Furthermore, most of these initial studies were performed before any *in vitro* sensitivity data was available. The development of *in vitro* techniques for the cultivation of *Borrelia burgdorferi*[6] now gives us the opportunity to study factors affecting the bacteriostatic and bactericidal action of various chemotherapeutic agents, including penicillin and tetracycline. By utilizing these findings, new chemotherapeutic approaches to the treatment of Lyme borreliosis may be established. Furthermore, there is a need for animal models of infection in order to establish whether *in vitro* susceptibility studies correlate with *in vivo* efficacy.

Susceptibility of *Borrelia burgdorferi* to various antimicrobial agents has been reported for approximately twenty human and tick isolates.[7-10] The small number of isolate studies may be due to the difficulties experienced in isolating *B. burgdorferi* from clinical specimens. Uniformly, in all studies, the most effective antimicrobial agent *in vitro* was erythromycin.[7-10] Paradoxically, in one clinical study erythromycin was significantly less efficacious then either tetracycline or penicillin.[1] The minimum inhibitory concentration (MIC) of penicillin G for *B. burgdorferi* varied from 0.25 to 2.0 μg/ml[7,9] in two studies with geometric mean concentrations of 0.93 μg/ml and 1.10 μg/ml, respectively, and between 0.005 and 0.08 μg/ml in another study.[8] The minimum inhibitory concentration and minimum bactericidal concentration (MBC) also seemed to vary among the β-lactam antibiotics. In one study, ampicillin was more active than penicillin.[7] In a study by Johnson *et al.*,[10] the minimum bactericidal concentration of penicillin[7] for a clinical isolate from a patient with Lyme meningitis was 6.5 μg/ml, whereas the MBC of ceftriaxone was only 0.04 μg/ml. By using a Syrian hamster model of infection, they also demonstrated that ceftriaxone was more efficacious than penicillin in the treatment of *B. burgdorferi* infection in this experimental model. Tetracycline is also active against *B. burgdorferi* and is

[a]This research was funded in part by a grant from Hoffmann-LaRoche, Inc., Nutley, NJ.

frequently used in the treatment of Lyme borreliosis. *In vitro* studies have demonstrated that the MIC of *B. burgdorferi* to tetracycline varies between ≤0.25 and 2.0 μg/ml.[7,9,10]

It appears from studies of antimicrobial susceptibility that both the minimum inhibitory and bactericidal concentrations of chemotherapeutic agents against a significant number of strains of *B. burgdorferi* are relatively high, especially when the levels of drug achieved in the serum after oral administration are considered (TABLE 1). For instance, after oral administration of 250 mg of tetracycline the peak serum level is approximately 2 μg/ml. However, the absorption of tetracycline is dependent on whether the drug is administered during fasting or with food. In the clinical situation the levels of the drug achieved in the serum may be lower. Increasing the dose of tetracycline to 500 mg increases the serum level to 4 μg/ml.[11] Oral doses of 250 mg and 500 mg of phenoxymethylpenicillin results in peak serum levels of 2–3 μg/ml and 3–5 μg/ml, respectively.[11] Therefore, both the minimum inhibitory and bactericidal concentrations of penicillin and tetracycline for some strains of *B. burgdorferi* are equivalent to or above the concentration of drugs achieved by oral administration. It would appear that higher doses of tetracycline, 500 mg every 6 hours may be useful in

TABLE 1. Pharmacokinetic Profile of Two Chemotherapeutic Agents Used in the Treatment of Early Lyme Borreliosis

Antibiotic	Dose (mg)	Route	Peak Serum[a] Level	CSF Level[a,b] (% Serum)	Half-life (h)
Tetracycline	250	oral	2	0.2–0.4 (10–20)	10
	500	oral	4	0.4–0.8 (10–20)	10
Phenoxymethyl-penicillin	250	oral	2–3	undetectable	1
	500	oral	3–5	undetectable	1

[a]Concentration in μg/ml.
[b]Concentrations found in uninflamed meninges.

the treatment of early Lyme disease. Also, the use of a better-absorbed β-lactam, such as amoxicillin, along with probenecid, which prolongs its half-life needs to be evaluated in the treatment of Lyme borreliosis.

RESULTS AND DISCUSSION

In Vitro *Studies*

In order to gain further insight into various factors that may affect the ability of β-lactam and tetracycline to kill or inhibit the growth of *B. burgdorferi,* we performed studies to determine the effect of various concentrations of organisms on the ability of tetracycline and penicillin to kill or inhibit the growth of *B. burgdorferi.* Furthermore, in addition to ascertaining the effective concentration of various antimicrobials in inhibiting the growth of or killing *B. burgdorferi,* we determined the maximal rate at which the organism can be killed by the drug.

Effect of Spirochete Concentrations on Activity of Antimicrobials

In order to determine whether the concentration of spirochetes in the culture affects the ability of β-lactam antibiotics to exert their antimicrobial effect, three concentrations of spirochetes were subjected to various concentrations of penicillin and ceftriaxone. It is apparent from the percent viability recorded in TABLE 2 that the susceptibility of *B. burgdorferi* to a given concentration of penicillin or ceftriaxone is not influenced by the size of the inoculum, at least in the range of 1×10^6 to 1×10^7 organisms per milliliter.

Rate at Which B. burgdorferi *Are Killed by Antimicrobials*

The rates at which various concentrations of penicillin kill *B. burgdorferi* are presented in FIGURE 1. Six hours of incubation of *B. burgdorferi* with concentrations of penicillin varying between 0.1 mg and 1000 μg/ml had little effect on the viability of the spirochetes. At 24 hours, a 100-fold increase in penicillin concentration from 0.1 μg to 10 μg/ml did not accelerate the rate at which the organisms were killed, and a 2000-fold increase in penicillin concentration to 100 μg/ml only increased the rate of killing threefold (0.1 μg/ml, 58% viability; 100 μg/ml, 20% viability). To kill 99% of the organisms required 72 hours with 0.1 μg/ml penicillin and 48 hours with concentration of 1 μg/ml and above. The slow rate at which spirochetal cultures were killed, compared to other bacterial pathogens, is to be noted.[12,13] It seems that the length of time needed to kill *B. burgdorferi* is prolonged even when compared to other spirochetal infections, including *Treponema pallidum*.[12,13]

The rate at which ceftriaxone killed *B. burgdorferi* was also assessed (FIG. 2). As can be seen, the kinetics of killing by ceftriaxone is similar to that seen with penicillin. However, in contrast to penicillin, at 24 hours 0.1 μg/ml and 100 μg/ml of ceftriaxone killed *B. burgdorferi* in a comparable manner.

The effect of various concentrations of tetracycline on the growth of *B. burgdorferi* was also examined (FIG. 3). The activity of tetracycline contrasted with penicillin and

TABLE 2. Effect of Inoculum Size on Susceptibility of *B. burgdorferi* (B31) to Penicillin and Ceftriaxone[a]

Drug Conc. (μg/ml)	Penicillin Inoculum Size (Organisms/ml)			Ceftriaxone Inoculum Size (Organisms/ml)		
	1×10^6	5×10^6	1×10^7	1×10^6	5×10^6	1×10^7
0.1	20	5	10	0.5	1.0	3.0
1.0	1	3	4	1.0	0.5	0.2
2.0	4	3	1	0	0.5	0.1
4.0	1	2	3	0	0.5	0.2
10.0	0	1	3	0	0	0.1

[a]Effects were measured as percent motility, calculated as follows. *B. burgdorferi* was obtained from 4-day cultures in BSK II medium. Three concentrations of spirochetes, 1×10^6, 5×10^6, and 1×10^7 spirochetes per ml, were cultured with various concentrations of penicillin or ceftriaxone. At 48 hours the percent viability was measured by the following formula: % viability = number of motile organisms in test mixture/number of viable organisms in initial inoculum × 100. Viability of the organism was determined by dark-field microscopy. Motile organisms were considered to be viable.

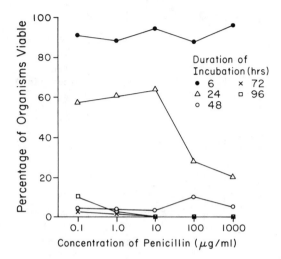

FIGURE 1. Effect of the concentration of penicillin G on the rate at which *B. burgdorferi* were rendered nonmotile *in vitro*. Spirochetes (1×10^7/ml) in 2 ml BSK II were cocultured with various concentrations of penicillin G. At various time points, an aliquot of the cultures was obtained and the number of motile organisms per ml was determined by dark-field microscopy and compared to the initial inoculum. Percent viability was ascertained as described in TABLE 2.

ceftriaxone in several important ways. After as little as 6 hours of incubation of the organisms with tetracycline, there was a significant decrease in *B. burgdorferi* viability at concentrations as low as 0.1 µg/ml. Furthermore, unlike penicillin and ceftriaxone, the spirochetocidal action of tetracycline increased progressively to the highest concentration used in the experiment. However, it was not until 72 hours that 99% of the organisms could be killed with 1.0 µg/ml of tetracycline. Furthermore at 96 hours, there was a regrowth of the organisms at the lower concentrations of 0.1 and 1.0 µg/ml of tetracycline. Thus, although tetracycline has a more rapid rate of action, at low concentration, it does not seem to kill the organism effectively.

Measurement of MIC and MBC of Five Strains of B. burgdorferi

We examined the minimum inhibitory and bactericidal concentrations of penicillin G, ceftriaxone, tetracycline, and erythromycin against five strains of *B. burgdorferi* (TABLE 3) (generously provided by Dr. Jorge Benach and Dr. Alan MacDonald). The five strains consisted of three human isolates and two tick isolates. Ceftriaxone was uniformly more active than penicillin G. The mean MIC for ceftriaxone was 0.03 µg/ml, compared to an MIC of 0.50 µg/ml for penicillin G. Tetracycline and erythromycin also potently inhibited the growth of *B. burgdorferi,* with a mean MIC of 0.14 and 0.04 µg/ml, respectively. Most interesting was the large discrepancy between the MIC and MBC levels, especially for the β-lactam antibiotics. For instance, the mean MIC for penicillin was 0.50 µg/ml, whereas the range of MBC levels was

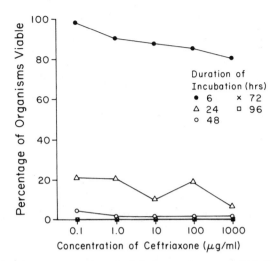

FIGURE 2. Effect of the concentration of ceftriaxone on the rate at which *B. burgdorferi* were rendered nonmotile *in vitro*. Spirochetes (1×10^7/ml) in 2 ml BSK II were cocultured with various concentrations of ceftriaxone. At various time points, an aliquot of the cultures was obtained and the number of motile organisms per ml determined by dark-field microscopy and compared to the initial inoculum. Percent viability was ascertained as described in TABLE 2.

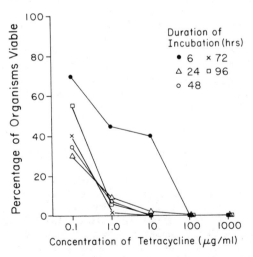

FIGURE 3. Effect of the concentration of tetracycline on the rate at which *B. burgdorferi* were rendered nonmotile *in vitro*. Spirochetes (1×10^7/ml) in 2 ml BSK II were cocultured with various concentrations of tetracycline. At various time points, an aliquot of the cultures was obtained and the number of motile organisms per ml determined by dark-field microscopy and compared to the initial inoculum. Percent viability was ascertained as described in TABLE 2.

between 1 and greater than 50. This probably indicates that time periods beyond 48 hours are necessary to achieve complete eradication of this pathogen from culture.

Clinical Studies of the Treatment of Lyme Borreliosis

In our *in vitro* studies ceftriaxone was shown to have remarkable activity against *B. burgdorferi*. In addition, ceftriaxone with its prolonged half-life of approximately 5½ hours permits the maintenance of high serum levels of the antibiotic for prolonged periods of time. This is in contrast to penicillin G given parenterally, which attains a very high serum level that dissipates quickly. Ceftriaxone also penetrates into the synovial fluid of the inflamed joint, attaining concentrations of between 66% and 100% of the concomitant level in serum.[14]

Ceftriaxone penetrates the central nervous system and maintains cerebrospinal fluid levels, even in the noninflamed meninges, above the MIC that we determined for

TABLE 3. Minimum Inhibitory (MIC) and Minimum Bactericidal Concentration (MBC) for Five Strains of *B. burgdorferi*

| Antibiotic | MIC | | MBC | |
	Mean[a]	Range	Mean[a]	Range
Penicillin G	0.50	0.1–1.0	7.96	2–50+[b]
Ceftriaxone	0.03	0.01–1.0	3.81	1–50+[b]
Tetracycline	0.14	0.01–1.0	4.10	2–6
Erythromycin	0.04	0.01–1.0	2.17	0.1–10

Minimum inhibitory and bactericidal concentrations were measured by incubating 2×10^6 organisms/ml with various concentrations of antibiotics (serial dilutions of 0.01 μg/ml to 50 μg/ml). At 48 hours the cultures were examined for motile spirochetes. The minimum inhibitory concentration was the lowest concentration in which the number of motile organisms was not greater than the initial inoculum. At 48 hours, cultures were centrifuged 10,000 ×g and the pellet was reinoculated into fresh medium. The minimum bactericidal concentration was the lowest concentration of antibiotic at which no growth occurred.

[a]Geometric mean.
[b]Values >50 were ascribed a value of 50 in the calculation of the geometric mean.

B. burgdorferi.[15] These factors may play an important role in treatment of spirochetal infections. For instance, it has been shown in syphilis that prolonged elevation in antibiotic levels is preferable because slowly multiplying organisms may regenerate during the time that the antimicrobial concentrations drop to subinhibitory levels. We therefore evaluated whether ceftriaxone with its unique pharmacological properties may be useful in the treatment of late Lyme borreliosis.

Human Studies

Efficacy of Ceftriaxone in Patients with Lyme Borreliosis Who Failed Penicillin Therapy

In our first study on the efficacy of ceftriaxone,[16] seven patients with severe Lyme borreliosis who had continued to be symptomatic after receiving high-dose penicillin

TABLE 4. Characteristics of Seven Patients with Lyme Disease Treated with Ceftriaxone

Characteristic	Number of Patients
History of ECM	7/7
Treatment of ECM	4/7
Previous penicillin therapy[a]	7/7
Previous intravenous therapy[b]	5/7
Previous oral therapy	2/7
Arthritis	5/7
Peripheral neuropathy	6/7
Fatigue	7/7
Symptoms >1 year	5/7

[a]Penicillin G: 24×10^6 units/day for 10 days.
[b]Phenoxymethylpenicillin: 4 g/day with probenecid 2 g/day for 30 days.

therapy were treated with ceftriaxone (TABLE 4). All patients had a history of a rash consistent with erythema chronicum migrans and all had immunological evidence of infection with *B. burgdorferi*. Oligoarticular arthritis characterized by significant pain and swelling was present in five patients, and six patients complained of paresthesias and had significant peripheral neuropathy documented by neurophysiological testing (TABLE 4). All seven complained of severe fatigue. Five of the patients had been symptomatic for more than 1 year.

Each of the patients received ceftriaxone either intravenously or intramuscularly. Two patients received 1 gram of ceftriaxone twice a day for 14 days and the others received 2 grams twice a day for 14 days. After treatment with ceftriaxone in the five patients with arthritis, all objective and subjective evidence of arthritis resolved between 3 and 5 weeks after the discontinuation of ceftriaxone (TABLE 5). Improvement in limb paresthesias was reported in five of the six patients with neuropathy. Nerve conduction studies confirmed significant improvement in sensory amplitudes and conduction velocities in these five patients ($p < .05$). The subjective feelings of fatigue improved in all patients. In subsequent follow-up, all patients remained clinically well for 6 months to a year after the completion of ceftriaxone therapy.

TABLE 5. Patient's Response to Ceftriaxone Therapy

Arthritis[a]		Fatigue[b]		PNS[c]	
Before	After	Before	After	Before	After
s,e	0	+	improved	+	0
k,h	0	+	improved	+	0
s,k	0	+	improved	+	+
0	0	+	improved	+	0
k,e	0	+	improved	+	0
0	0	+	improved	+	0
k,s	0	+	improved	0	0

[a]Arthritis involvement of the following: s, shoulders; e, elbows; k, knees; h, hips; and 0, no involvement

[b]Fatigue was defined as a debilitating, severe sense of fatigue; +, presence of fatigue.

[c]Involvement of the peripheral nervous system (PNS) was defined as objective abnormalities of nerve conduction; +, presence of involvement; 0, no involvement.

Randomized Trial Comparing Parenteral Ceftriaxone to Parenteral Penicillin

Although the patients in the previous study received ceftriaxone therapy well after the penicillin therapy, it was not entirely clear whether the effect seen was due to ceftriaxone or to a cumulative effect of the previous penicillin therapy plus the ceftriaxone therapy. We therefore performed a randomized study in patients with late Lyme borreliosis that compared this regimen of ceftriaxone, 4 grams daily for 14 days, to 18 million units of penicillin daily (TABLE 6)[17] for 10 days. Patients who had a history of erythema chronicum migrans or immunological evidence of previous Lyme infection and clinical evidence of oligoarticular arthritis, carditis, or neurological dysfunction were randomized to receive either penicillin or ceftriaxone.

Sixteen patients with monoarticular or oligoarticular arthritis were studied in all. In fifteen of the sixteen patients joint pain was accompanied by swelling and in one patient pain was the only symptom of arthritis. This one patient subsequently went on to develop an erosive arthritis after penicillin therapy. In the penicillin group, three of seven patients who originally complained of arthritis resolved their arthritis; however, one patient with carditis who did not complain of arthritis prior to therapy

TABLE 6. Symptoms of Lyme Borreliosis in Randomized Study Comparing Parenteral Penicillin to Ceftriaxone

	Penicillin[a]		Ceftriaxone[b]	
	Before[c]	After[d]	Before[c]	After[d]
Arthritis	7 (70%)	5 (50%)	9 (75%)	0 (0%)
Peripheral neuropathy	3 (30%)	1 (10%)	7 (60%)	0 (0%)
Fatigue	8 (80%)	5 (50%)	10 (85%)	1 (8%)
Carditis	1 (10%)	0 (0%)	0 (0%)	0 (0%)

[a]Ten patients received penicillin G, 3×10^6 units, six times daily for 10 days.
[b]Twelve patients received ceftriaxone, 2 g, twice daily for 14 days.
[c]No. of patients with symptoms (% of patients) prior to therapy.
[d]No. of patients with re-exacerbation of symptoms within 6 months of completion of therapy.

subsequently developed arthritis. In contrast, all nine patients with arthritis who were treated with ceftriaxone had complete resolution of their arthritis. Furthermore, of the five patients with arthritis who failed penicillin therapy, four were retreated with ceftriaxone. Three of these four retreated patients resolved their arthritis. The one patient who had failed retreatment with ceftriaxone had already developed an erosive arthritis of the hip. Thus, it appears that after 6-month follow-up ceftriaxone is significantly ($p < .05$) superior to penicillin in the treatment of arthritis caused by *B. burgdorferi*. However, because of the episodic nature of this illness, further follow-up is necessary to determine whether the differences seen are due to eradication of the organism or to differences in the time intervals before recurrence.

Peripheral neuropathy was also documented in 13 patients. Of these 13 patients, only one failed to resolve peripheral neuropathy as measured by neurophysiological studies. There were no statistically significant differences in electromyograms between patients treated with penicillin and ceftriaxone. Finally, severe fatigue is a prominent complaint of patients with late Lyme borreliosis. Of the eight patients with severe fatigue who were treated with penicillin, only two felt resolution of this symptom compared to all patients treated with ceftriaxone. This study demonstrates that high doses of ceftriaxone had a remarkable and significant impact on the course of this disease and was significantly ($p < .05$) more efficacious than penicillin.

SUMMARY

1. It was demonstrated that while *B. burgdorferi* may be sensitive to relatively small concentrations of penicillin and ceftriaxone, the organism is killed slowly. This implies that, as in syphilis, prolonged blood levels of these drugs may be necessary in order to ensure cure. In contrast, the activity of tetracycline is more rapid in its action but is more dependent on drug concentration achieved. Unfortunately, the MIC and MBC for some strains are at or above the peak level achieved under optimal conditions.
2. Increasing the concentrations of penicillin or ceftriaxone above the MIC for the organism has little effect on the rate of killing. In contrast, the killing by tetracycline can be augmented by increasing concentrations of the drug.
3. Ceftriaxone is more active than penicillin, as measured by MIC, against the five strains of *B. burgdorferi* tested.
4. Ceftriaxone was efficacious in the treatment of Lyme borreliosis, which was recalcitrant to penicillin therapy. In a randomized trial comparing ceftriaxone to high-dose penicillin therapy, ceftriaxone was significantly more efficacious than penicillin in the treatment of the late complications of Lyme borreliosis.

REFERENCES

1. STEERE, A. C., G. J. HUTCHINSON, D. W. RAHN, L. H. SIGAL, J. E. CRAFT, E. T. DeSANNA & S. E. MALAWISTA. 1983. Treatment of early manifestations of Lyme disease. Ann. Intern. Med. **99:** 22–26.
2. SVARTZ, N. 1946. Penicillin behandling vid dermatitis atrophicans Herxheimer. Nord. Med. **32:** 2783.
3. THYRESSON, N. 1949. The penicillin treatment of acrodermatitis chronica atrophicans (Herxheimer). Acta Derm. Venereol. (Stockholm) **29:** 572–621.
4. STEERE, A. C., J. GREEN, R. T. SCHOEN, E. TAYLOR, G. F. HUTCHINSON, D. W. RAHN & S. E. MALAWISTA. 1985. Successful parenteral penicillin therapy of established Lyme arthritis. N. Engl. J. Med. **312:** 869–874.
5. STEERE, A. C., A. R. PACHNER & S. E. MALAWISTA. 1983. Neurological abnormalities of Lyme disease: successful treatment with high-dose intravenous penicillin. Ann. Intern. Med. **99:** 767–772.
6. BARBOUR, A. G. 1984. Isolation and cultivation of Lyme disease spirochetes. Yale J. Biol. Med. **57:** 521–525.
7. JOHNSON, S. E., G. C. KLEIN, G. P. SCHMID & J. C. FEELEY. 1984. Susceptibility of the Lyme disease spirochete to seven antimicrobial agents. Yale J. Biol. Med. **57:** 99–103.
8. BERGER, B. W., M. H. KAPLAN, I. R. ROTHENBERG & A. G. BARBOUR. 1985. Isolation and characterization of the Lyme disease spirochete from the skin of patients with erythema chronicum migrans. J. Am. Acad. Dermatol. **13:** 444–449.
9. PREAC-MURSIC, V., B. WILSKE & G. SCHIERZ. 1986. European *Borrelia burgdorferi* isolated from humans and ticks: culture conditions and antibiotic susceptibility. Zbl. Bakt. Hyg. **263:** 112–118.
10. JOHNSON, R. C., C. KODNER & M. RUSSELL. 1987. *In vitro* and *in vivo* susceptibility of the Lyme disease spirochete, *Borrelia burgdorferi,* to four antimicrobial agents. Antimicrob. Agents Chemother. **31:** 164–167.
11. GARROD, L. P., H. P. LAMBERT & F. O'GRADY. 1987. Antibiotic Chemotherapy. Churchill Livingstone. New York.

12. NELL, E. 1954. Comparative sensitivity of treponemes of syphilis, yaws and bejel to penicillin *in vitro,* with observations on factors affecting its treponemicidal action. Am. J. Syph. Gonorrhea Vener. Dis. **38:** 92–105.

13. EAGLE, H. & A. D. MUSSELMAN. 1948. The rate of bactericidal action of penicillin *in vitro* as a function of its concentration, and its paradoxically reduced activity at high concentrations against certain organisms. J. Exp. Med. **86:** 99–131.

14. MORGAN, J. R., A. PAULL, M. O'SULLIVAN & B. D. WILLIAMS. 1985. The penetration of ceftriaxone into synovial fluid of the inflamed joint. J. Antimicrob. Chemother. **16:** 367–371.

15. SQUIRES, E. & R. CLEELAND. 1984. Microbiology and Pharmacokinetics of Parenteral Cephalosporins. Hoffmann-LaRoche. Nutley, NJ.

16. DATTWYLER, R. J., J. J. HALPERIN, H. PASS & B. J. LUFT. 1987. Ceftriaxone as effective therapy in refractory Lyme disease. J. Infect. Dis. **155:** 1322–1325.

17. DATTWYLER, R. J., J. J. HALPERIN, D. J. VOLKMAN & B. J. LUFT. 1988. Treatment of late Lyme disease. Lancet. In press.

Immunoperoxidase Staining of Spirochetes in Borrelial Skin Diseases

E. ABERER,[a] M. MAINITZ,[a] R. NEUMANN,[a]
AND G. STANEK[b]

[a]Department of Dermatology II
[b]Hygiene Institute
University of Vienna
A-1090 Vienna, Austria

Spirochetes have recently been visualized in skin biopsies of erythema chronicum migrans (ECM) by immunofluorescence.[1] The aim of our study was to look for spirochetes on histological sections in lesional skin of ECM, acrodermatitis chronica atrophicans (ACA), lymphadenosis cutis benigna (LCB), and 22 different dermatoses of unknown origin.

Formalin-fixed, paraffin-embedded skin sections of 87 biopsies were investigated by an avidin-biotin-immunoperoxidase method.[2]

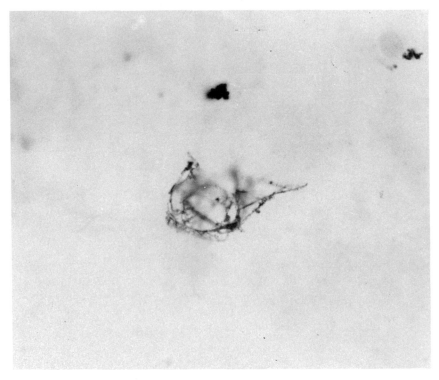

FIGURE 1. Granuloma annulare: historesin embedding, semithin section, with cluster of spirochetes. Magnification: 1000×.

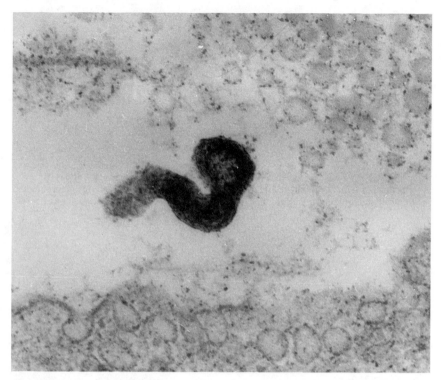

FIGURE 2. Electron micrograph of granuloma annulare, showing spirochete between collagen fibers. Magnification: 95,000×.

Additionally, formalin-fixed skin samples from one patient with granuloma annulare (GA) were embedded in Historesin® (LKB) and cut with an ultramicrotome.

Biopsies of two patients with GA were investigated ultrastructurally after embedding and routine staining by electron microscopy.

RESULTS

In one of three patients with ECM, thick heavily stained and thin single or conglomerated spirochetes could be seen histologically. Thin, single-lying, or more frequently, clusters of aggregated spirochetes situated in the dermal connective tissue were detected in two patients with ACA, one patient with LCB and three of five patients with granuloma annulare. In 4 of 13 patients with morphea and 6 of 13 patients with lichen sclerosus et atrophicans, thick "swollen" organisms could be found.

In one patient with GA identical microorganisms could be detected on semithin sections (FIG. 1). In the negative control sections similar structures could also be found, unstained.

By electron microscopy structures which appeared consistent with spirochetes could be detected intercellularly between the collagen fibers (FIG. 2).

DISCUSSION

In this study we demonstrated spirochetes in ECM, ACA, LCB, morphea, LSA, and GA on histological sections by an immunoperoxidase method. In GA spirochetes were also detected on semithin sections and ultrastructurally. As only culture procedures will definitely prove a spirochetal etiopathogenesis in the investigated dermatoses, further studies will be needed to elucidate the specificity of our findings.

REFERENCES

1. PARK, H. K., B. E. JONES & A. G. BARBOUR. 1986. Erythema chronicum migrans of Lyme disease: Diagnosis by monoclonal antibodies. J. Am. Acad. Dermatol. **15:** 406–410.
2. ABERER, E. & G. STANEK. 1987. Histological evidence for spirochetal origin of morphea and lichen sclerosus et atrophicans. Am. J. Dermatopathol. **9:** 374–379.

Isolation and Biological Activity of *Borrelia burgdorferi* Peptidoglycan[a]

GREGORY BECK AND GAIL S. HABICHT

Department of Pathology
SUNY at Stony Brook
Stony Brook, New York 11794

Peptidoglycan (PG) is an important component of bacterial cells. It is an essential cell wall polymer of most bacteria and has been isolated from many species of spirochetes. Spirochete PG is associated with the cytoplasmic membrane. PG consists of a glycan backbone with alternating β_{1-4}-linked residues of N-acetyl-D-glucosamine and muramic acid.[1] It is thought that PG is involved in maintaining cell rigidity and shape.[2] Therefore, it has been postulated that PG serves to maintain the coiled configuration of the spirochete.[2]

The biological activities of PG are diverse and complex. Its immunopotentiating activities have made it the subject of intense scrutiny. Some of the varied properties of PG include: induction of antibody formation, immunomodulation, complement activa-

TABLE 1. Induction of Fever by *B. burgdorferi* Peptidoglycan

Time (Minutes)	ΔT^a
0	0.0
30	0.5
60	1.3
90	1.4
120	0.9
160	1.9
240	0.7
330	0.3

[a]Measured in degrees centigrade. A rabbit pyrogen dose is defined as the quantity of PG that produces a peak rise above baseline of 0.6–0.9°C. A rise of <0.3°C was not considered significant.

tion, release of mediators, induction of inflammation, and increased macrophage phagocytosis.[1] Many of the symptoms of Lyme disease could be explained by the host response to spirochetal PG. These include fever, arthritis, erythema chronicum migrans, and malaise. Our interest in the host response in Lyme disease led us to study its PG. We therefore extracted and characterized the PG from *Borrelia burgdorferi*.

Spirochetal PG was isolated by solubilization of the cells with warm 1% SDS followed by digestion with proteases. The amino acid composition was consistent with that of PG isolated from other spirochetes and bacteria, with ornithine being the predominant amino acid.[3] We first investigated the ability of the PG to induce fever. Fifteen micrograms of PC was injected i.v. into New Zealand albino rabbits and the

[a]This work was supported by grant no. AR36028 from the National Institutes of Health.

365

TABLE 2. Mitogenic Activity of *B. burgdorferi* Peptidoglycan on Normal Human Peripheral Blood Mononuclear Cells

Dose (μg/ml)	dpm $\pm$ SE
0	1568 $\pm$ 141
1	1274 $\pm$ 63
7.5	1689 $\pm$ 219
15	1791 $\pm$ 268
30	1570 $\pm$ 157
125	1858 $\pm$ 155
250	1805 $\pm$ 180
500	1721 $\pm$ 18

rectal temperature was taken every 10 minutes. A biphasic fever was observed. The data are presented in TABLE 1. When 10 μg of PG were injected i.d. into normal human skin, a skin reaction characterized by erythema and swelling was observed. The reaction started a few minutes after injection, reached a peak by 36 hours, and then subsided. The lesions disappeared completely after a few days and no permanent damage was seen. The PG was found to stimulate murine macrophages to secrete interleukin-1 (IL-1). When 50 μg of PG were added to a confluent monolayer of P388D1 cells and the supernatant collected 24 hours later, it stimulated the cells in the thymocyte proliferation assay (Δdpm $\pm$ SE = 9550 $\pm$ 269; $p < .001$ as compared to P388D1 cells alone). When the PG was added to human peripheral blood mononuclear cells, no mitogenic activity was observed. TABLE 2 presents data from a representative experiment. Murine C3H/HeJ splenocytes were also unresponsive to the spirochetal PG (dpm $\pm$ SE = 4750 $\pm$ 237 without PG, as compared to 5375 $\pm$ 53 in the presence of 20 μg/ml PG).

The results of these studies are in agreement with those of other investigations of the biological activities of PG.[1,4] The role of PG in discussions of the pathogenesis of Lyme disease must now be taken into consideration. That *B. burgdorferi* PG and lipopolysaccharide (LPS) are both powerful immunomodulators and stimulators of IL-1 gives more credence to the importance of this cytokine in Lyme disease.[5] These new observations on the *in vitro* and *in vivo* activities associated with the cellular components of the *B. burgdorferi* spirochete provide further insight on how a small number of invading organisms can cause a multisystemic disease such as Lyme disease.

REFERENCES

1. HEYMER, B., P. H. SEIDL & K. H. SCHLEIFER. 1985. Immunochemistry and biological activity of peptidoglycan. *In* Immunology of the Bacterial Cell Envelope. D. E. S. Stewart-Tull & M. Davies, Eds.: 11–46. John Wiley & Sons. Chichester.
2. JOSEPH, R., S. C. HOLT & E. CANALE-PAROLA. 1973. J. Bacteriol. **115:** 426–434.
3. JOHNSON, R. C., F. W. HYDE & C. M. RUMPEL. 1984. Yale J. Biol. Med. **57:** 529–537.
4. UMEMOTO, T., T. OTA, H. SAGAWA, K. KATO, H. TAKADA, M. TSUJIMOTO, A. KAWASAKI, T. OGAWA, K. HARADA & S. KOTANI. 1981. Infect. Immun. **31:** 767–774.
5. BECK, G., G. S. HABICHT, J. L. BENACH, J. L. COLEMAN, R. M. LYSIK & R. F. O'BRIEN. 1987. A role for interleukin-1 in the pathogenesis of Lyme disease. Zbl. Bakt. Hyg. A **263:** 133–136.

Genetic Organization and Nucleotide Sequence of an Outer Surface Protein Gene of *Borrelia burgdorferi*

SVEN BERGSTRÖM

Department of Microbiology
University of Umeå
S-901 87 Umeå, Sweden

ALAN G. BARBOUR

Departments of Microbiology and Medicine
University of Texas Health Science Center
San Antonio, Texas 78284

Lyme borreliosis is a zoonosis caused by the tick-borne spirochete *Borrelia burgdorferi*.[1] After a tick bite the *B. burgdorferi* spirochete enters the vascular and lymphatic circulatory system and a systemic infection develops, which is characterized by a variety of syndromes including erythema chronicum migrans,[2] acrodermatitis chronica athrophicans,[3] lymphocytic meningoradiculitis,[2] and Lyme arthritis.[1] Chronic borreliosis is a consequence of either the host's inability to rid itself of the infecting agent or the development of an immunological reaction with autoimmune-like symptoms. The outer surface properties of the borrelia probably play a major role in the host-parasite interactions in borreliosis and are therefore important for the pathogenesis of this organism.

Immunochemical analysis of the type strain B31 of *B. burgdorferi* have revealed several antigens. Among these are two abundant proteins with molecular masses of 31,000 (31 kDa) and 34,000 (34 kDa), respectively. These two proteins, denoted OspA (31 kDa) and OspB (34 kDa), are located at the surface of the borrelia, embedded in its fluid membrane.[4,5]

The isolation and characterization of a recombinant plasmid, pTRH32, carrying a borrelia DNA insert coding for the OspA and OspB genes, has previously been described.[6] The *osp* genes were localized on 2-kb region of this borrelia DNA insert and it was found that these genes were transcribed together as a single transcriptional unit.[7]

Presented herein are a restriction map of pTRH44, a previously described plasmid[7] that carries *ospA* (FIG. 1), and a discussion of the nucleotide sequence of the *ospA* gene of *B. burgdorferi*. The *ospA* gene encodes a 273 amino-acid-long protein with a molecular weight of 29,334. Upstream from the translational starting point are two regions (P1 and P2) that mimic the consensus sequence for promoters found in *Escherichia coli*, with P1 being most like the consensus sequence. A possible start codon, present at position 151, is preceded by a strong Shine-Dalgarno sequence eight base pairs upstream from the ATG codon. The codon usage of the *ospA* gene does not differ significantly from the pattern found in *E. coli;* however, a preference for codons containing A and T was seen. This is not surprising, since borrelia DNA has a high AT content.

This is the first time a *B. burdorferi* gene, *ospA,* has been sequenced. The translated protein shows all the features exhibited by other outer membrane proteins,[8]

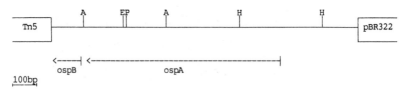

FIGURE 1. Physical map and gene organization of *osp* gene containing plasmid pTRH44. The rectangular areas represent Tn5 and pBR322 sequences, respectively. Restriction sites used in the subcloning into M13 phages mp18 and mp19 are indicated: *A, Aha* III; *E, Eco* RI; *P, Pst* I; *H, Hind* III.

i.e., a high content of charged amino acid residues (31%) and a hydropathic profile that does not show any long segments of hydrophobicity. This is not surprising since this protein is located in the outer membrane of *B. burgdorferi.*

REFERENCES

1. STEERE, A. C., R. L. GRODZICKI, A. N. KORNBLATT, J. E. CRAFT, A. G. BARBOUR, W. BURGDORFER, G. P. SCHMID, E. JOHNSON & S. E. MALAWISTA. 1983. N. Engl. J. Med. **308:** 733–740.
2. BENACH, J. L., E. M. BOSLER, J. P. HANRAHAN, J. L. COLEMAN, T. F. BAST, G. S. HABICHT, D. J. CAMERON, J. L. ZIEGLER, W. BURGDORFER, A. G. BARBOUR, R. EDELMAN & R. A. KASLOW. 1983. N. Engl. J. Med. **308:** 740–742.
3. ÅSBRINK, E., B. HEDERSTEDT & A. HOVMARK. 1984. Acta Derm. Venereol. **64:** 506–512.
4. BARBOUR, A. G., S. L. TESSIER & S. F. HAYES. 1984. Infect. Immun. **45:** 94–100.
5. BARBOUR, A. G., S. L. TESSIER & W. J. TODD. 1983. Infect. Immun. **41:** 795–804.
6. HOWE, T. R., L. W. MAYER & A. G. BARBOUR. 1985. Science **227:** 645–646.
7. HOWE, T. R., F. T. LAQUIER & A. G. BARBOUR. 1986. Infect. Immun. **54:** 207–212.
8. NIKAIDO, H. & M. VAARA. 1985. Microbiology Rev. **49:** 1–32.

An Unusual Isolate of *Borrelia burgdorferi* from a Tick in California

M. BISSETT, W. HILL, W. PROBERT, AND S. KURASHIGE

Microbial Diseases Laboratory
California Department of Health Services
Berkeley, California 94704

Two major surface proteins of *Borrelia burgdorferi* designated as OspA and OspB have been described,[1] and molecular analyses of these proteins have shown differences between North American and European isolates.[2] With few exceptions, both the North American and European strains bind OspA monoclonal antibody (mAb) H5332, but European isolates vary in their reaction with OspA mAb H3TS. Strains that do not react with OspA mAb (H5332 or H3TS) and that possess a major protein of 20-24–kDa apparent molecular weight have been reported from Europe, but not from North America.[2-4] One (DN 127) of 13 strains of *B. burgdorferi* isolated from adult *Ixodes pacificus* collected primarily from Northern California differed from any previously reported North American strain, but was similar to reported strains isolated in Europe. This report describes the molecular analyses of proteins of this strain and the reaction of a mAb prepared to a major protein of the strain.

The methods used, polyacrylamide gel electrophoresis (SDS-PAGE), Western blot (WB), and indirect immunofluorescence (IFA), have been described.[5] Monoclonal antibody for OspA (H5332 and H3TS), OspB (H6831 and H5TS), flagellin (H9724), and *B. hermsii* (H4825) were kindly supplied by Dr. A. Barbour. A mAb was prepared to the 25-kDa protein band of strain DN127 by excising the band from a Coomassie-blue-stained SDS-PAGE gel, electroeluting, and inoculating into Balb/c mice. Hybridomas were produced by fusion of spleen cells with P3x63–Ag8.653 myeloma cells. Supernatants of a cloned hybridoma (86 DN-1) did not react with strains of *Leptospira*, *Borrelia hermsii*, or *Treponema pallidum*. It was necessary to wash spirochetes in 0.5% formalinized phosphate-buffered saline before fixing to slides to obtain satisfactory IFA results with 86 DN-1 mAb.

The original DN-127 strain of *B. burgdorferi* showed only 10% of the spirochetes reacting with H5332. Limiting dilution cloning of this strain produced a clone (DN127 cl 9-2) that did not react with H5332 mAb in IFA tests, reacted very weakly or not at all in WB using H5332 mAb, was negative in WB and IFA with H3TS (OspA) and two OspB (H6831 and H5TS) mAb, and reacted with H9724 (flagellin) mAb but was negative in WB and IFA with *B. hermsii* (H4825) mAb. SDS-PAGE analysis showed no bands in the 31-kDa or 34-kDa region with the cloned strain, but a major protein in the 25-kDa region (FIG. 1A). 86 DN-1 mAb reacted strongly in WB to the 25-kDa protein and, interestingly, reacted with minor protein bands in the 20-24–kDa region of other California isolates (FIG. 1B). WB performed with patients' sera have shown that some patients have antibodies that are bound to a 25-kDa protein of the DN127 cl 9-2 strain.

Passage in BSK II affected the reaction of DN127 cl 9-2 with H5332 (FIG. 2). After eight weekly passages in BSK II, the DN127 cl 9-2 strain reacted as the original noncloned DN127 strain; *i.e.*, approximately 10% of the spirochetes reacted to mAb H5332 in IFA, a protein band of apparent 32 kDa molecular mass appeared in SDS-PAGE, and H5332 mAb was bound in WB. The presence of the 25-kDa major

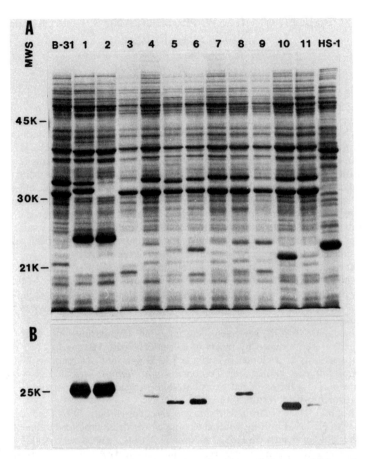

FIGURE 1. (A) Coomassie-blue-stained proteins of whole cell lysates of 11 strains of *B. burgdorferi* isolated from *Ixodes pacificus* and control strains B31 (type strain of *B. burgdorferi*) and HS1 (strain of *B. hermsii*) separated by SDS-PAGE (12.5% acrylamide concentration). Positions of molecular weight standards (MWS) are indicated to the left of the gel. (B) Western blot of protein bands transferred to nitrocellulose paper and reacted with monoclonal antibody 86 DN-1. Bound antibody was detected with horseradish-peroxidase-conjugated protein A. The position of the 25-kDa protein is indicated. Isolates: lane 1, DN127; lane 2, DN127 cl 9-2; lane 3, SON 188; lane 4, SON 2110; lane 5, SON 328; lane 6, SON 335; lane 7, HUM 115; lane 8, HUM 3336; lane 9, MEN 115; lane 10, MEN 2523; lane 11, LAKE 339.

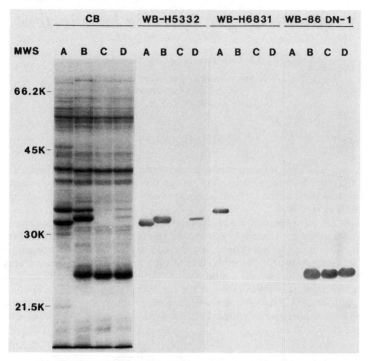

FIGURE 2. Coomassie-blue-stained (CB) proteins and Western blots (WB) of lysates of control strain B-31 (*A*), original DN127 isolate (*B*), low-passage cloned strain DN127 cl 9-2 (*C*), and cloned strain DN127 cl 9-2 after eight weekly passages in BSK II (*D*). Proteins of lysates were separated by SDS-PAGE and either stained with CB (first panel) or transferred to nitrocellulose paper for WB analysis. The blots were reacted with the following monoclonal antibodies: H5332 (OspA, second panel), H6831 (OspB, third panel), or 86 DN-1 (25-kDa protein, fourth panel). Bound antibody was detected by horseradish-peroxidase-conjugated protein A. Positions of the molecular weight standards (MWS) are indicated.

protein and its reaction with 86 DN-1 mAb in IFA or WB was not affected by passage.

Further studies with mAb 86 DN-1 will be helpful in demonstrating antigenic shifts within and between strains isolated from different geographic locations, and may have significance in the investigations to define the epidemiology and pathogenesis of Lyme disease.

REFERENCES

1. HOWE, T. R., L. W. MAYER & A. G. BARBOUR. 1985. Science **227:** 645–646.
2. BARBOUR, A. G., R. A. HEILAND & T. R. HOWE. 1985. J. Infect. Dis. **152:** 478–484.
3. STANEK, G., G. WEWALKA, V. GROH, R. NEUMANN & W. KRISTOFERITSCH. 1985. Lancet **1:** 401.
4. WILSKE, B., V. PREAC-MURSIC, G. SCHIERZ & K. V. BUSCH. 1986. Zbl. Bakt. Hyg. A **263:** 92–102.
5. BISSETT, M. & W. HILL. 1987. J. Clin. Microbiol. **25:** 2296–2301.

Lectin Binding to *Borrelia burgdorferi*[a]

JAMES L. COLEMAN AND JORGE L. BENACH

New York State Department of Health
SUNY at Stony Brook
Stony Brook, New York 11794

INTRODUCTION

The early antibody response to *Borrelia burgdorferi* is primarily directed against the endoflagella. Surface antigens are recognized as the disease progresses.[1,2] The possibility that some of the surface antigens may be carbohydrates of low immunogenicity led to these studies.

Lectins are substances with well-characterized affinities for specific carbohydrate groups. Concanavalin A (Con A) specifically reacts with α-linked mannose residues. *Dolichos biflorus* agglutinin (DBA) and soybean agglutinin (SBA) possess carbohydrate specificities toward *N*-acetylgalactosamine and galactose. Peanut agglutinin (PNA) and *Ricinus communis* agglutinin 120 (RCA 120) are specific for galactose. Wheat germ agglutinin (WGA) is specific for *N*-acetylglucosamine and *Ulex europaeus* agglutinin I (UEA I) is specific for fucose. In this study, affinity blotting with lectins against *B. burgdorferi* antigens was used to elucidate the presence or absence of spirochete carbohydrate.

MATERIALS AND METHODS

The Shelter Island, New York strain[3] of *B. burgdorferi* was used for all experiments and was grown in serum-free modified Kelly's medium.[4]

SDS-PAGE, transfer of electrophoretically separated proteins to nitrocellulose, and subsequent blotting was done according to previously described methods[1,5,6] with the following modification: Tris-buffered saline containing Tween 20 (20 mM Tris, 500 mM NaCl, 0.5% Tween 20) was used instead of bovine serum albumin (BSA) as a diluent and quenching agent for the blots. This was done in order to eliminate excessive background staining in the lectin experiments due to contaminating glycoproteins present in BSA.

Biotinylated lectin kit BK-1000 containing Con A, DBA, SBA, PNA, WGA, UEA I, and RCA 120 was obtained from Vector Laboratories, Burlingame, CA, and used at 10 μg/ml. All sugars in competition studies were used at 200 mM. Avidin conjugated to horseradish peroxidase was purchased from Hyclone Laboratories, Logan, UT.

The glycosidases α-mannosidase (40 U/ml), *N*-acetylgalactosaminidase (0.1 U/ml), α-galactosidase (10 U/ml), β-galactosidase (2 U/ml), fucosidase (0.42 U/ml) and *N*-acetylglucosaminidase (1.8 U/ml) were all purchased from the Sigma Chemical Co., St. Louis, MO. Enzyme treatments were done on whole *B. burgdorferi* at 37°C for a 24-hour period. Protease inhibitors EDTA (5 mM), phenylmethyl-sulfonyl

[a]This work was supported in part by United States Department of Health and Human Services grant no. AI–23167 from the National Institute of Allergy and Infectious Diseases of the National Institutes of Health.

fluoride (10 mM), and aprotinin (5 μg/ml) were included with glycosidases and controls during incubation.

RESULTS

In our experiments, all seven lectins were reactive, with numerous bands being resolved in all cases (FIG. 1). The total number of reactive sites was quite consistent

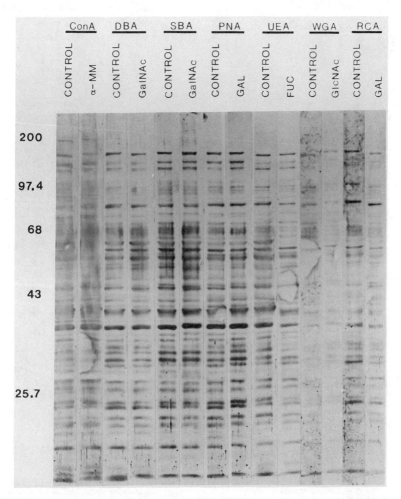

FIGURE 1. Blotting analysis of seven lectins (with inhibiting sugars) to *B. burgdorferi* whole cell lysates after SDS-PAGE and transfer to nitrocellulose. Analyzed were concanavalin A (*ConA*), *Dolichos biflorus* agglutinin (*DBA*), soybean agglutinin (*SBA*), peanut agglutinin (*PNA*), *Ulex europaeus* agglutinin I (*UEA*), wheat germ agglutinin (*WGA*), and *Ricinus communis* agglutinin 120 (*RCA*). The inhibiting sugars were α-methylmannoside (α-MM), N-acetylgalactosamine (*GalNAc*), galactose (*GAL*), fucose (*FUC*), and N-acetylglucosamine (*GLcNAc*).

from one lectin to another, ranging from a high of 51 for PNA to a low of 40 for RCA 120. Con A, DBA, UEA I, and WGA had 46, 42, 50, 48, and 42 sites, respectively. In addition, a vast majority of the sites were common to all of the lectins. In order to determine if the lectin binding was specific, competition experiments were done with the following cognate sugars: α-methylmannoside (for Con A), N-acetylgalactosamine (for DBA and SBA), galactose (for PNA and RCA 120), fucose (for UEA I), and N-acetylglucosamine (for WGA). Repeated experiments were unsuccessful in elimi-

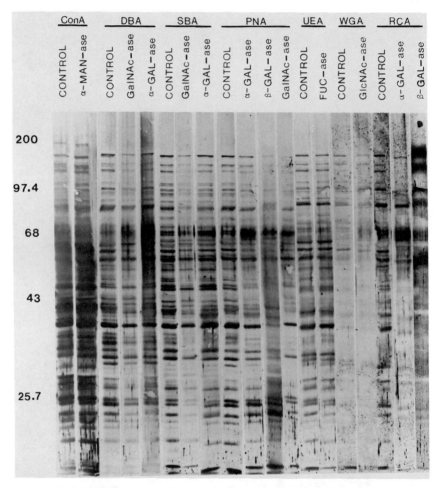

FIGURE 2. Blotting analysis of seven lectins to *B. burgdorferi* whole cell lysates after treatment with specific glycosidic enzymes followed by SDS-PAGE and transfer to nitrocellulose. Enzymes used were α-mannosidase (*α-MAN-ase*), N-acetylgalactosaminidase (*GalNAc-ase*), α-galactosidase (*α-GAL-ase*), β-galactosidase (*β-GAL-ase*), fucosidase (*FUC-ase*), N-acetylglucosaminidase (*GlcNAc-ase*). Lectins were concanavalin A (*Con A*), *Dolichos fiblorus* agglutinin (*DBA*), soybean agglutinin (*SBA*), peanut agglutinin (*PNA*), *Ulex europaeus* agglutinin I (*UEA*), wheat germ agglutinin (*WGA*) and *Ricinus communis* agglutinin 120 (*RCA*).

nating lectin reactivity. In addition, whole spirochetes were treated with specific glycosidic enzymes (FIG. 2). Con A reactivity was not affected by α-mannosidase. N-acetylgalactosaminidase eliminated or greatly reduced major bands with apparent M_rs of 31, 37, and 41 kDa for DBA. SBA showed reduction of reactive bands at 37, 41, and 45 kDa and PNA showed reduction of bands at 35, 37, and 41 kDa for N-acetylgalactosaminidase. Some changes in electrophoretic mobility of epitopes recognized by PNA and RCA 120 were caused by β-galactosidase. Other minor changes were also observed.

DISCUSSION

Specific lectin binding to a cell surface or to cell proteins immobilized on a solid matrix can be inhibited by coincubation with cognate sugars as well as treatment of the cells with specific glycosidases. Competition experiments with cognate sugars failed to eliminate lectin reactivity in affinity blots. Likewise, glycosidase treatment of spirochetes prior to SDS-PAGE and lectin blotting failed to eliminate a vast majority of the bands. This evidence suggests, with bands of 31, 35, 37, 41, and 45 kDa as possible exceptions, that lectin binding to *B. burgdorferi* is nonspecific and may be due to other mechanisms. Interaction with hydrophobic ligands, independent of the saccharide binding activity normally associated with these lectins, could be such a mechanism.

REFERENCES

1. COLEMAN, J. L. & J. L. BENACH. 1987. Isolation of antigenic components from the Lyme disease spirochete: Their role in early diagnosis. J. Infect. Dis. **155:** 756–765.
2. CRAFT, J. E., D. K. FISHER, G. T. SHIMATO & A. C. STEERE. 1986. Antigens of *Borrelia burgdorferi* recognized during Lyme disease: Appearance of a new immunoglobulin M response and expansion of the immunoglobulin G response late in the illness. J. Clin. Invest. **78:** 934–939.
3. BURGDORFER, W., A. G. BARBOUR, S. F. HAYES, J. L. BENACH, E. GRUNWALDT & J. P. DAVIS. 1983. Lyme disease—a tick-borne spirochetosis? Science **216:** 1317–1319.
4. BENACH, J. L., H. B. FLEIT, G. S. HABICHT, J. L. COLEMAN, E. M. BOSLER & B. P. LANE. 1984. Interactions of phagocytes with the Lyme disease spirochete: Role for the Fc receptor. J. Infect. Dis. **150:** 497–507.
5. LAEMMLI, U. K. & M. FAVRE. 1973. Maturation of the head of bacteriophage T4. I. DNA packaging events. J. Mol. Biol. **80:** 575–599.
6. TOWBIN, H., T. STAEHELIN & J. GORDON. 1979. Electrophoretic transfer of proteins from polyacrylamide gels to nitrocellulose sheets: Procedures and some applications. Proc. Natl. Acad. Sci. USA **76:** 4350–4354.

Identification of *Borrelia burgdorferi* Surface Components by Triton X-114 Phase Partitioning

T. M. CUNNINGHAM,[a] D. D. THOMAS,[a,c]
S. D. THOMPSON,[b]
J. N. MILLER,[a] AND M. A. LOVETT[a,b]

[a]*Departments of Microbiology and Immunology*
[b]*Department of Medicine*
University of California
Los Angeles, California 90024

Triton X-114 has been used to explore the protein composition of the *Borrelia burgdorferi* outer surface. The low cloud point of Triton X-114 (20°C) permits phase partitioning of detergent-solubilized proteins and recovery of proteins with hydrophobic character.[1] *B. burgdorferi* B31 was cultured in BSK II medium,[2] solubilized at 4°C in 50 mM Tris-50 mM EDTA, pH 7.6, containing 1% Triton X-114, and phase partitioned at room temperature. The phases were separated and the Triton phase was washed twice with Tris-EDTA. All fractions were acetone precipitated and resuspended in sample buffer containing SDS and 2-mercaptoethanol. Samples were boiled and subjected to SDS polyacrylamide gel electrophoresis in 12.5% gels. FIGURE 1 shows the Coomassie-blue-stained polypeptides after solubilization and phase partitioning of *B. burgdorferi* in Triton X-114. Most of the cellular proteins were not solubilized by TX-114, but solubilization of several proteins, including the OspA and OspB proteins,[3] was observed. Fourteen polypeptides, including six abundant species with apparent molecular weights of 66, 61, 39, 34, 31, and 23 kDa, partitioned into the detergent (hydrophobic) phase. These species were strongly reactive with rabbit anti-*B. burgdorferi* serum. Importantly, flagella (which reside in the periplasmic space) and penicillin binding proteins (also a periplasmic marker in many bacterial species) did not partition into the Triton X-114 phase, but remained associated with the insoluble cytoplasmic cylinders. In order to assess morphologically the effect of the detergent on the outer membrane, organisms were treated with Triton X-114 prior to whole mount or thin-section electron microscopy. The results are shown in FIGURE 2. Within 15 minutes of addition of Triton X-114 extraction solution, spirochetal diameters were reduced and extensive unwinding of periplasmic flagella was noted. Removal of surface material was attributed, at least in part, to a blebbing process. On thin sections, organisms treated with Triton X-114 appear to be devoid of outer membranes, whereas untreated control organisms have visible outer membranes and obviously contained periplasmic flagella.

Surface components, such as outer membrane proteins, may mediate the initial interaction between the host immune response and *B. burgdorferi*.[4] We were interested in exploiting new techniques for characterizing *B. burgdorferi* outer membrane components. Triton X-114 is a nondenaturing detergent that solubilizes proteins based

---

[c]Present address: Department of Microbiology and Immunology, Bowman Gray School of Medicine, Wake Forest University, 300 S. Hawthorne, Winston-Salem, North Carolina 27103.

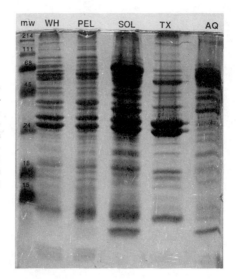

FIGURE 1. SDS-PAGE of phase-partitioned Triton X-114 solubilized *B. burgdorferi* surface proteins. Whole, untreated *B. burgdorferi* (lane 2) is compared with TX-114 insoluble (lane 3) and TX-114 soluble (lane 4) fractions. Hydrophobic phase partitioning of the soluble material (lane 4) yielded a hydrophobic detergent-soluble (lane 5) and a hydrophilic aqueous (lane 6) fraction.

on their hydrophobic transmembrane or anchor domains.[1] Our results indicate that Triton X-114 solubilizes a defined subset of hydrophobic proteins from *B. burgdorferi* and suggest that this detergent removes the outer membrane while leaving the insoluble cytoplasmic cylinders intact. Others have removed outer membrane material from this organism.[5,6] However, the nondenaturing effects of Triton X-114 are attractive when considering future functional studies of the spirochete-host interaction.

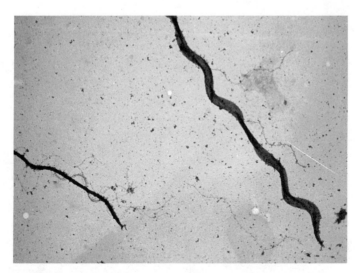

FIGURE 2. Electron microscopy of TX-114-treated *B. burgdorferi*. Diameters of organisms were diminished and periplasmic flagella were unwound after treatment.

REFERENCES

1. PRYDE, J. G. 1986. Trends Biol. Sci. **11:** 160–163.
2. BARBOUR, A. G. 1984. Yale J. Biol. Med. **57:** 521–525.
3. BARBOUR, A. G. 1984. Yale J. Biol. Med. **57:** 581–586.
4. CRAFT, J. E., D. K. FISCHER, G. T. SHIMAMOTO & A. C. STEERE. 1986. J. Clin. Invest. **78:** 934–939.
5. COLEMAN, J. L., J. L. BENACH, G. BECK & G. S. HABICHT. 1987. Zbl. Bakt. Hyg. A **263:** 123–126.
6. COLEMAN, J. L. & J. L. BENACH. 1987. J. Infect. Dis. **155:** 756–765.

A Model of the Spread of Lyme Disease in Natural Populations

Center for Coastal and Environmental Studies
Rutgers University
New Brunswick, New Jersey 08903

A discrete-time model was developed of the spread of Lyme disease spirochetes, *Borrelia burgdorferi*, in populations of northern deer ticks, *Ixodes dammini* (Acari: Ixodidae), and their vertebrate hosts. The model was based on a 2-year tick life cycle, with nymphs occurring earlier in the season than larvae (of a different generation).[1] Ticks acquire spirochetes primarily from their small-mammal hosts.[2-4] The prevalence of spirochetes among questing ticks (k_t') was calculated from spirochete prevalence in the previous stage (k_t) as follows: $k_t' = k_t + (\Sigma_h k_h i_h p_h) (1 - k_t)$, where k_t = proportion of ticks infected; k_h = proportion of host individuals infected (host species h); i_h = infectiousness of host species h (of uninfected ticks feeding on an infected host of

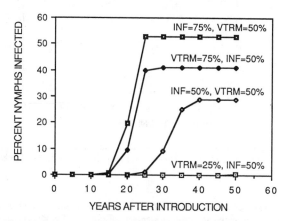

FIGURE 1. Predicted influence of infectiousness and degree of vertical transmission among hosts of immature ticks on prevalence of Lyme spirochetes in questing nymphal ticks: INF, percentage of uninfected ticks feeding on an infected host that become infected; VTRM, percentage of offspring of an infected host that are infected at birth.

species h, the proportion that become infected); and p_h = proportion of ticks that feed on host species h. Spirochete prevalence in hosts was modeled as: $k_h' = k_h + (1-(1-k_t)^n)(1-k_h)$, where n = average number of ticks per individual on host species h. The numbers of ticks per host were held constant during each run, and were based on data from Fire Island, NY collected by the author, C.P. Ewing, and A.F. O'Connell. Each run simulated the introduction of 10 infected nymphal ticks into a population of 10^6 uninfected nymphs, and followed the spread of spirochetes through tick and vertebrate populations for 50 years.

Four runs of the model (FIG. 1) showed spirochete prevalence staying quite low for several years, then increasing rapidly (in three cases) to a stable percentage of ticks infected. The greater the infectiousness of the vertebrate host to immature ticks, the faster the predicted increase and higher the ultimate prevalence of spirochetes in questing nymphs. Similarly, the greater the efficiency of vertical transmission among hosts, the faster the increase and higher the ultimate percentage of nymphs infected.

When vertical transmission among vertebrate hosts was efficient (*e.g.*, 50% of offspring of an infected mother infected at birth), turnover in host populations had little influence on predicted disease incidence. However, when vertical transmission was inefficient (*e.g.*, only 5% of offspring infected) turnover among vertebrate hosts had an important influence on spirochete prevalence. Turnover (= reproduction) of vertebrate hosts during the summer (between the nymphal and larval feeding peaks) had a far greater impact on spirochete prevalence than did early spring reproduction (FIG. 2). The presence of alternate hosts for immature ticks influenced the predicted

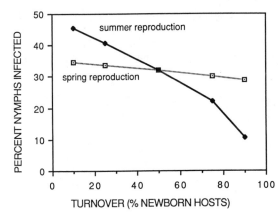

FIGURE 2. Predicted effect of host reproduction at various times of year on prevalence of Lyme spirochetes in questing nymphal ticks (50 years after introduction of infected ticks).

prevalence of Lyme disease when they differed from the primary host in infectiousness to ticks. The model suggests that infectiousness, efficiency of vertical transmission, and seasonal timing of reproduction of the predominant vertebrate hosts of immature ticks strongly influence the rate of increase and ultimate prevalence of Lyme disease in natural populations.

REFERENCES

1. SPIELMAN, A., M. L. WILSON, J. E. LEVINE & J. PIESMAN. 1985. Annu. Rev. Entomol. **30:** 439–460.
2. PIESMAN, J., J. G. DONAHUE, T. N. MATHER & A. SPIELMAN. 1986. J. Med. Entomol. **23:** 219.
3. BOSLER, E. M., J. C. COLEMAN, J. L. BENACH, D. A. MASSEY, J. P. HANRAHAN, W. BURGDORFER & A. G. BARBOUR. 1983. Science **220:** 321–323.
4. LEVINE, J. F., M. L. WILSON & A. SPIELMAN. 1985. Am. J. Trop. Med. Hyg. **34:** 355–360.

A Short Amino Acid Sequence Is Shared by Surface Antigens of *Borrelia duttonii,* *Borrelia hermsii,* and *Borrelia burgdorferi*

L. HAYES,[a,b] D. J. M. WRIGHT,[b] AND L. C. ARCHARD[a]

[a]*Department of Biochemistry*
[b]*Department of Medical Microbiology*
Charing Cross and Westminster Medical School
London W6 8RF, United Kingdom

The spirochetes *Borrelia duttonii* and *Borrelia hermsii* are agents of tick-borne relapsing fever; each of these borreliae is able to evade the host immune response by varying its major surface antigen (variant surface antigen; VSAg). As each successive antigenic type is cleared by the immune system, it is replaced by a different serotype. *Borrelia burgdorferi,* another tick-borne *Borrelia,* is the agent of Lyme disease. This condition is often chronic, suggesting that the host cannot effectively rid itself of the infecting organism.

Barstad *et al.*[1] have shown that several short amino acid sequences are shared in common between two VSAgs of *B. hermsii.* We have used a 20-base synthetic mixed oligonucleotide based on a seven amino acid sequence shared by these two VSAgs to probe DNA from *B. duttonii* and *B. burgdorferi* in an attempt to identify surface antigen genes in these two organisms. The shared amino acid sequence and corresponding oligonucleotide sequence are shown in FIGURE 1.

```
amino acid sequence:          Ser  Ala  Glu  Asn  Ala  Phe  Tyr


oligonucleotide sequence:  3' CN  CGN  CTY  TTR  CGN  AAR  ATR 5'
```

FIGURE 1. Oligonucleotide sequence derived from *Borrelia hermsii* VSAg amino acid sequence, where N = any nucleotide; Y = pyrimidine; R = purine; degeneracy = 1024. *B. hermsii* amino acid sequence data from Barstad *et al.*[1]

The mixed oligonucleotide was synthesized by the phosphotriester method, and end-labeled with ^{32}P using T4 polynucleotide kinase, to a specific activity of approximately 1×10^8 dpm/μg DNA.

Five hundred ng of each DNA species was dot blotted onto a nitrocellulose membrane, including the oligonucleotide and *E. coli* HB101 DNA as positive and negative controls, respectively. One μg of non-cleaved *B. duttonii* DNA was electrophoresed in one direction at 30 V for 90 hours through 0.6% agarose, then transferred to a nylon membrane by Southern blotting.

In each case the DNA was denatured in 0.5 M NaOH, 1.5 NaCl, neutralized in 0.5 M Tris Cl, pH 7.2, 1.5 M NaCl, and immobilized by baking. The filters were incubated with the oligonucleotide probe in 6×SSC, 5×Denhardt's solution, 0.1% SDS, 5 mM EDTA, 100 μg/ml denatured *E. coli* tRNA, for 16 hours at 45°C, then washed in 6×SSC, 0.1% SDS, 5 mM EDTA for 30 minutes at 45°C, and autoradiographed.

The VSAg-specific mixed oligonucleotide probe hybridized to both of the *Borrelia* spp. DNAs tested but not to *E. coli* HB101 DNA (FIG. 2A). We could not detect on the filter the presence of the oligonucleotide itself as it is too short to bind to the nitrocellulose under these conditions.

These results indicate that the seven amino acid peptide sequence common between at least two VSAgs of *B. hermsii* is also shared by *B. duttonii* and *B. burgdorferi*. This suggests that *B. burgdorferi* expresses surface antigens that are related to the VSAgs of the relapsing fever borreliae, and that this spirochete may itself undergo antigenic variation. This could explain the chronic nature of some manifestations of Lyme disease.

We have shown that the genetic complement of *B. duttonii* contains at least ten elements which are separable under certain conditions (FIG. 2B). Extrachromosomal DNA species have been described in *B. hermsii* and *B. burgdorferi*.[2] These two organisms also each possess a major chromosomal species, whereas in *B. duttonii* we

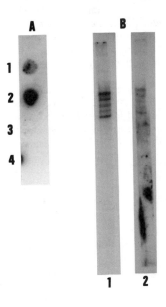

FIGURE 2. (A) Autoradiograph of dot blot of *Borrelia* spp. DNA hybridized to VSAg-specific mixed oligonucleotide probe. Lane 1, *B. burgdorferi* DNA; lane 2, *B. duttonii* DNA; lane 3, *E. coli* HB101 DNA; lane 4, oligonucleotide. (B) Autoradiographs of Southern blots of noncleaved *B. duttonii* DNA. Lane 1, probed with homologous total *B. duttonii* DNA, lane 2, probed with VSAg-specific oligonucleotide.

have found no genetic element that obviously corresponds to the chromosome. In *B. duttonii*, the VSA-specific oligonucleotide hybridizes to a family of seven genetic elements ranging in size from 24 to 150 kb (FIG. 2B). These seven DNA species virtually comigrate under conventional electrophoresis conditions, and they are present at high copy number with respect to two very high molecular weight species. We conclude that these are components of a segmented genome.

REFERENCES

1. BARSTAD, P. A., J. E. COLIGAN, M. G. RAUM & A. G. BARBOUR. 1985. Variable major proteins of *Borrelia hermsii:* Epitope mapping and partial sequence analysis of CNBr peptides. J. Exp. Med. **161:** 1302–1314.
2. PLASTERK, R. H., M. I. SIMON & A. G. BARBOUR. 1985. Transposition of structural genes to an expression sequence on a linear plasmid causes antigenic variation in the bacterium *Borrelia hermsii*. Nature **318:** 257–263.

Electron Microscope Characterization of Cloned and Uncloned Strains of *Borrelia burgdorferi*

STANLEY F. HAYES,[a] WILLY BURGDORFER,[a] AND
ALAN G. BARBOUR[b]

[a]*Laboratory of Pathobiology
Rocky Mountain Laboratories
Hamilton, Montana, 59840*

[b]*University of Texas Health Science Center
Department of Microbiology
San Antonio, Texas 78284*

Concern has been expressed[1] about the possibility of a mixed population (two morphologically different spirochetes) within strain B31, the original prototype of *Borrelia burgdorferi,* because this strain was found to possess either 7 or 11 endoflagella. The number of endoflagella and other factors, such as end shape,[2] have been used to differentiate spirochetes of the genus *Borrelia* from spirochetes of the genus *Treponema*. Therefore, we initiated an electron microscopy study to determine

TABLE 1. Random Endoflagella Counts on 10 Spirochetes of *B. burgdorferi* from B31 and IRS Strains

	B31 Clone x[a]	B31 Clone y[b]	B31[c]	IRS[c]	IRS[b]
	3	7	11	7	7
	9	9	7	7	9
	6	14	6	5	11
	7	11	7	8	7
	8	11	7	4	9
	9	9	4	7	13
	14	11	7	6	6
	7	7	6	7	9
	11	9	4	4	8
	7	7	7	7	11
AVERAGE[d]	8	10	7	6	9

[a]Late log phase.
[b]Early log phase.
[c]Old stationary culture.
[d]Averages rounded to nearest whole number.

whether the number of endoflagella and end shape are constant features or are subjects of phenotypic variation within Lyme disease spirochetes. Both cloned and uncloned cultures of isolates B31 and IRS, the latter derived from the European tick, *Ixodes ricinus,* were investigated. To establish the number of endoflagella possessed by each isolate, spirochetes from early through late log phase and also older cultures were

383

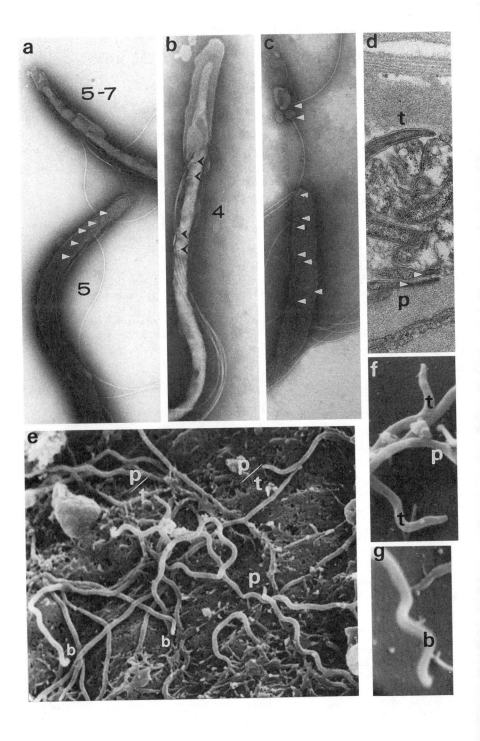

adsorbed to parlodion-coated, 300 mesh copper grids. They were then disrupted using DH_2O or 1% deoxycholate and negatively stained with pH 6.5–7.0 phosphotungstic acid. The results indicated a variability in both the number of endoflagella and the end shape, irrespective of cloning or not cloning. TABLE 1 reflects the varying numbers of endoflagella for both isolates. The highest endoflagella count (as many as 14) was recorded for young cultures in log phase. Variability was noted in all samples, however. Similar variability in endoflagella number has been noted by Ackermann *et al.* in studies of 19 uncloned *B. burgdorferi* isolates from *I. ricinus* ticks in West Germany.[3] FIGURE 1 shows spirochete profiles with variations in endoflagella number and end shapes. This figure also contains inserts of thin section and scanning electron micrographs for comparison. Spirochetes with pointed, truncated, and blunt ends are seen in the scanning micrograph, whereas spirochetes of the thin section profile exhibit only pointed or truncated configurations. These variations were always more apparent in negatively stained and scanning than in thin section preparations. Based upon our findings, we conclude that strains of *B. burgdorferi,* whether cloned or uncloned, exhibit variability in both the endoflagella number and end shape. Variation in endoflagella numbers may depend upon the physiologic state of the spirochete, while end-shape variations appear to be related to the negative staining technique.

REFERENCES

1. HOVIND-HOUGEN, K. 1984. Ultrastructure of spirochetes isolated from *Ixodes ricinus* and *Ixodes dammini*. Yale J. Biol. Med. **57:** 543–548.
2. HOVIND-HOUGEN, K. 1976. Determination by means of electron microscopy of morphologic criteria of value for clarification of some spirochetes, in particular, treponemes. Acta Pathol. Microbiol. Scand. Suppl. B **225:** 1–41.
3. ACKERMANN, R., J. KABATZKI, H. P. BOISTEN, A. C. STEERE, R. L. GRODZICKI, S. HARTUNG & U. RUNNE. 1984. *Ixodes ricinus* spirochete and European erythema chronicum migrans disease. Yale J. Biol. Med. **57:** 573–580.

FIGURE 1. (**a, b**) Negatively stained spirochetes with truncated or blunt ends possessing endoflagella numbers ranging from 4 to 9 (*arrows* denote insertion points). (**c**) Spirochetes treated with DOC, from an early log phase culture, with nine insertion points. (**d**) Thin section profile of the *I. ricinus* spirochete within hypodermal tissues adjacent to the basal lamina. (**e–g**) Scanning micrographs representing *B. burgdorferi* in *I. dammini* (**e**), associated with the midgut diverticular surface, and from BSK II cultural media (**f, g**). Abbreviations: *b*, blunt; *p*, pointed; *t*, truncated or tapered; *p/t*, pointed to truncated. (Scanning micrographs courtesy of M. D. Corwin, Rocky Mountain Laboratories, Hamilton, Montana.)

Western Blot Analysis of Serum and Cerebrospinal Fluid Antibodies to *Borrelia* Strains in Patients with *Borrelia* Meningitis

MATS KARLSSON, INGRID MÖLLEGÅRD,
BIRGIT SKÖLDENBERG, GÖRAN STIERNSTEDT,
EVA ÅSBRINK,[a] AND BENGT WRETLIND

Departments of Infectious Diseases and Clinical Bacteriology
Danderyd Hospital
S-18288 Danderyd, Sweden

[a]*Department of Dermatology*
Karolinska Institute at Södersjukhuset
Stockholm, Sweden

Since cultivation of *Borrelia* spirochetes from patients with *Borrelia* meningitis is seldom successful, the diagnosis depends on epidemiological, clinical, and serological data. Western blot technique might be used as a complement in serological diagnosis.[1,2] We used this technique to analyze the antibody response of patients with *Borrelia* meningitis to different strains of *Borrelia* spirochetes. Ten patients (three males and seven females), 21 to 81 years old, were studied. All patients had a positive ELISA test against *Borrelia*[3] in serum and/or in cerebrospinal fluid (CSF) and mononuclear pleocytosis in CSF. Between three and five pairs of serum and CSF samples from each patient were analyzed. The samples were drawn before antibiotic treatment between 3 weeks and 19 months after the onset of neurological symptoms, and between 2 weeks and 3.5 years (mean = 45 weeks) after treatment. Two strains of *Borrelia* isolated from Swedish *Ixodes ricinus* ticks, strain B31 isolated from *Ixodes dammini* in the United States, and three strains from Swedish patients with meningitis, acrodermatitis, and erythema migrans, respectively, were used. The strains were harvested after cultivation in modified Kelly's medium and sonicated. The cell lysates were subjected to SDS-PAGE (5–15% gradient of acrylamide), transferred to nitrocellulose,[4] and reacted with serum or CSF. IgG and IgM antibodies were detected with alkaline phosphatase conjugated swine and goat anti-human antibodies. The gels were stained with Coomassie blue.

The SDS-PAGE pattern of proteins of the six *Borrelia* strains did show considerable similarities, but differences were mainly seen in the 31–34 kDa region, where two major proteins with molecular mass of 32–33 kDa were seen. Four of the *Borrelia* strains (three human isolates) had major proteins of about 20 kDa.

All patients had IgG antibodies in both serum and CSF to at least one band in all strains studied. However, the strength and pattern of reactivity differed. The band patterns were generally similar in each patient against human and tick strains. All patients had IgG antibodies against one 41-kDa protein and against 1–4 proteins in the 56–60 kDa region at least in one serum specimen. Eight patients had antibodies to a 31–34 kDa protein, though some reactions were very weak. Four had antibodies to a 86 kDa protein, two to 82–83 kDa proteins, and six to 18–20 kDa proteins. TABLE 1 shows

TABLE 1. Serum IgG Antibodies to *Borrelia* Proteins in Patients with Meningitis[a]

Patient	Duration (Weeks) of Neurological Symptoms[b]	Molecular Mass of Proteins (kDa)
A	3	41
B	8	*59* 58 44 *41 32 23 18*
C	8	18
D	11	*83 59 57 56* 54 47 44 *41 39* 38 *32 18*
E	18	72 *58 57 42 41* 37
F	29	*72* 63 *57* 56 54 *47 42 41* 39 34 33 13
G	32	*85* 82 79 76 62 60 *58* 57 *56* 55 50 48 46 45 43 *41* 39 *38* 36 33 *31* 29 28 20 18
H	37	145 124 100 94 *86* 82 79 *74* 68 65 63 60 59 58 57 56 54 51 48 46 45 43 *41* 39 *38* 37 36 33 30 27 26 *19*
I	69	63 *58 57* 55 49 *48* 46 45 41 *39 38*
J	81	*82* 69 *56 55* 53 41 30 28 27 *18* 17 *16 15*

[a]*Borrelia* strain 20, isolated from CSF of a Swedish child with meningitis, was used as antigen. Serum dilution was 1 : 100. Major bands are shown in *italics*.
[b]Persistent headache included as symptom.

IgG antibodies to CSF strain 20 in the first serum sample from each patient. The IgM antibodies were mostly directed against the same antigens as the IgG antibodies. Patients with a longer history of neurological symptoms had a stronger immunization to additional proteins (≤ 20), and a weaker IgM reactivity. The antibody patterns in CSF did in most cases correspond to that found in serum but were stronger in CSF in some patients. In comparison with conventional ELISA based on whole-cell preparations, the Western blot was more sensitive in detecting early antibody production, especially in serum.

REFERENCES

1. BARBOUR, A. G., W. BURGDORFER, E. GRUNWALDT & A. C. STEERE. 1983. J. Clin. Invest. **72:** 504–515.
2. WILSKE, B., G. SCHIERZ, V. PREAC-MURSIC, K. VON BUSCH, R. KÜHBECK, H.-W. PFISTER & K. EINHÄUPL. 1986. J. Infect. Dis. **153:** 304–314.
3. STIERNSTEDT, G. T., M. GRANSTRÖM, B. HEDERSTEDT & B. SKÖLDENBERG. 1985. J. Clin. Microbiol. **21:** 819–825.
4. KYHSE-ANDERSEN, J. 1984. J. Biochem. Biophys. Methods **10:** 203–209.

The Role of Specific Antibody and Complement in Killing of *Borrelia burgdorferi* by Human Serum

SIMS K. KOCHI AND RUSSELL C. JOHNSON

University of Minnesota Medical School
Minneapolis, Minnesota 55455

Lyme disease is an arthropod-borne disease caused by the spirochete, *Borrelia burgdorferi*. The bacterium appears capable of evading the immune response of the host to persist in tissues. As a result, chronic arthritis and progressive neurological degeneration are frequent clinical manifestations. For this reason, research was conducted to investigate possible mechanisms employed by *B. burgdorferi* to evade host defenses.

In the case of a number of gram-negative bacterial infections, resistance to complement-mediated serum killing is an important factor in determining the ability of the infecting organism to establish infection. In this study, we evaluated the antibody and complement (C) requirements for serum killing of *B. burgdorferi* strain 297 by normal human serum (NHS).

Employing *in vitro* hemolytic assays, an evaluation of the ability of strain 297 to activate serum complement (C) was made. Activation of both the classical and alternative C pathways was observed, in the absence of detectable *Borrelia*-reactive antibodies, in both the fluid and solid phases. In 20% NHS, strain 297 consumed 100% of the available total hemolytic complement during a 60-min incubation at 37°C. In addition, consumption of 65%, 58%, and 100% of the available C components 3 (C3), 4 (C4), and 9 (C9), respectively, was observed. In serum pretreated with 10-mM ethyleneglycol-bis(B-aminoethylether)-N,N,N',N'-tetraacetic acid (EGTA), treated to block classical pathway activation, both C3 (34%) and C9 (70%) were consumed. C4 consumption was minimal. C component deposition studies using radioiodinated C3, C8, and C9 indicated that these components were being deposited on the bacterial cell surface.

In spite of C activation, no significant killing of strain 297 was observed in 1–30% NHS in an *in vitro* bactericidal assay. The addition, however, of high-titered human anti-*B. burgdorferi* IgG to NHS resulted in greater than 80% killing of strain 297 in 10% NHS. NHS immunochemically depleted of C1 was found to be bactericidal for strain 297 only in the presence of immune antibody.

The results of these experiments indicate that in spite of the activation of both C pathways, *B. burgdorferi* strain 297 is resistant to the nonspecific bactericidal activity of NHS. However, in the presence of immune antibody *B. burgdorferi* is killed through the activity of the classical C pathway. Deposition of C3, C8, and C9 further suggest that serum resistance of *B. burgdorferi* strain 297 to NHS is not due to an inability to activate or deposit complement.

B-Cell Response at Cellular Level in Cerebrospinal Fluid and Blood in Lyme Disease and Controls

HANS LINK, SHAHID BAIG, TOMAS OLSSON,
ANNE ZACHAU, AND GÖRAN STIERNSTEDT[a]

Karolinska Institute
Department of Neurology at Huddinge University Hospital
S-141 86 Huddinge, Sweden
and
[a]Department of Infectious Medicine
Danderyd Hospital
Stockholm, Sweden

Determinations of antibody (Ab) levels in body fluids—constituting the basis for confirming diagnosis of Lyme disease—have the following limitations: (1) Concentrations in CSF are dependent on functional status of blood-brain barrier, level of Ig or Ab in serum, and local production within the CSF-CNS. (2) Results are influenced by half-life and catabolism of Ab molecules, which vary among different classes and subclasses of Ig. (3) *In vivo* absorption of self-reactive Ab by circulating or tissue-bound autoantigens may interfere with their detection. (4) No information is obtained concerning precise anatomical location of Ab formation. It can be anticipated that determination of Ab secretion at cellular level circumvents most of these limitations.

We have adopted and modified a nitrocellulose immunospot assay[1] for enumeration of *Borrelia* Ab of IgG, IgA, and IgM isotypes among 10×10^3 lymphocytes isolated from CSF (CSF-L) and peripheral blood (PBL). In parallel, we have quantitated numbers of IgG-, IgA-, and IgM-producing cells per 10×10^3 CSF-L and PBL. FIGURE 1 gives a schematic presentation of the nitrocellulose immunospot assay.

Our material hitherto examined consists of paired CSF and peripheral blood (PB) from five patients with serologically verified *Borrelia*-induced CNS disease and from 14 patients with other inflammatory nervous system diseases.

TABLE 1 shows that all five patients with *Borrelia*-induced CNS disease had in their CSF cells secreting specific Ab of IgG, IgA, and IgM class, while no such cells were demonstrable in PB. Thus, the specific humoral immune response seems, in these patients, to be highly sequestrated to the CNS-CSF compartment.

The specificity of enumeration of *Borrelia* Ab secreting cells in CSF and PB was evaluated in 14 controls (TABLE 2). Five displayed in CSF, but never in PB, cells producing *Borrelia* Ab. Two of these patients had neurosyphilis and cells in CSF secreting *Borrelia* Ab of all three isotypes. The remaining three patients consisted of two with Guillain-Barré syndrome and one with Sjögren's syndrome. ELISA revealed marginal elevation of IgM antibodies against *Borrelia* in one of the patients with Guillain-Barré syndrome but otherwise normal values. Our data, although preliminary, indicate that the three latter patients may in fact have neurological diseases due to *Borrelia* infection despite normal serology. These patients will be admitted for penicillin treatment and followed regarding *Borrelia* immunospots. The positive results in the two patients with neurosyphilis most probably reflect the well-known cross-reactivity between antibodies against *Borrelia burgdorferi* and *Treponema pallidum*.

In conclusion, our data indicate that Lyme disease with CNS manifestations is accompanied regularly by the presence in CSF of cells secreting specific Ab of IgG, IgA, and IgM isotypes. No such immune response was demonstrable in the patients' PB. The presence of cells secreting *Borrelia* Ab observed in CSF from patients with certain neurological disorders and mostly negative *Borrelia* serology, as reflected by

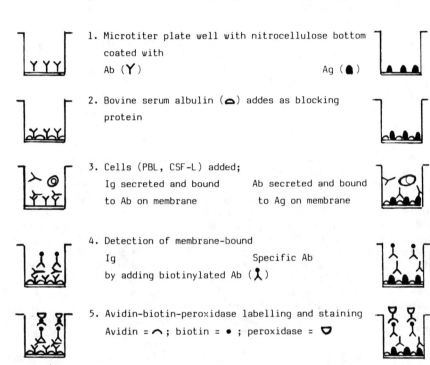

1. Microtiter plate well with nitrocellulose bottom coated with
   Ab (Y)   Ag (●)

2. Bovine serum albulin (◠) addes as blocking protein

3. Cells (PBL, CSF-L) added;
   Ig secreted and bound   Ab secreted and bound
   to Ab on membrane   to Ag on membrane

4. Detection of membrane-bound
   Ig   Specific Ab
   by adding biotinylated Ab (⅄)

5. Avidin-biotin-peroxidase labelling and staining
   Avidin = ◠; biotin = ● ; peroxidase = ▽

6. Counting of spots in dissection microscope
   1 Ig producing cell = 1 spot = 1 antibody-producing cell

FIGURE 1. Schematic presentation of nitrocellulose immunospot assay for enumeration of cells producing Ig (left) and specific antibodies (right) of different isotypes. Abbreviations: *Ab*, antibodies; *Ag*, antigen.

ELISA results, might indicate that enumeration of Ab-producing cells as carried out in this study is not only complementary in serologically well-defined *Borrelia* infections of the CNS, but might have diagnostic implications for patients with a neurological picture not incompatible with Lyme disease but for whom serology of CSF and serum remain negative. Another interesting observation based on this study is that the proportion of cells producing specific Ab usually amounted to 20–30% of the total

TABLE 1. Numbers of *Borrelia* Ig-Antibody–Producing Cells of G, A, and M Isotypes per 10×10^3 Lymphocytes in CSF and Peripheral Blood (PB) from Five Patients with CNS Disease Caused by *Borrelia* Spirochetes

Patient No.	Days after Onset of Neurological Symptoms	Clinical Characteristics	Mononuclear Cells ($\times 10^6/l$) in CSF	IgG		IgA		IgM	
				CSF	PB	CSF	PB	CSF	PB
1	33	erythema, lesions of cranial nerves VII and VIII, radiculopathy	112	2/28	0/6	2/26	0/12	3/7	0/3
	40	Pc,[a] progression of cranial nerve lesions	nd[b]	4/10	0/9	1/15	0/11	1/5	0/1
	50	Pc + steroids, improving	40	1/1	0/1	1/15	0/8	1/6	0/1
2	66	Radicular pains, meningitis, Pc	151	2/14	0/3	1/3	0/4	1/9	0/3
	72	Pc, improving	176	2/nd	0/2	1/15	0/8	2/8	0/5
	105	symptom free	10	2/3	0/2	0/0	0/5	0/2	0/3
3	32	erythema, radicular pains followed by meningitis	211	16/81	0/nd	6/6	0/7	2/6	0/4
	46	Pc, symptom free	111	3/12	0/4	3/11	0/6	2/8	0/1
	59	symptom free	21	6/10	0/3	11/4	0/4	3/5	0/0
	120	symptom free	20	10/12	0/2	0/0	0/5	0/2	0/3
4	90	paraplegia, ongoing tetracycline treatment, improving	91	43/15	0/4	27/10	0/1	7/nd	0/2
5	30	meningitis + radicular pains, Pc finished, recovered	136	3/128	0/8	6/7	0/12	7/80	0/3

[a]Pc = High-dose 10-day intravenous penicillin treatment.
[b]nd = not done.

TABLE 2. Numbers of Patients with Lyme Disease and Controls with Cells Secreting Antibodies of Different Isotypes against *Borrelia* Antigens per 10×10^3 Mononuclear Cells Isolated from CSF and Peripheral Blood (PB)

Diagnosis	Isotype	CSF	PB
Lyme disease with CNS symptoms	IgG	5	0
($n = 5$)	IgA	5	0
	IgM	5	0
Controls with other inflammatory	IgG	5	0
nervous system diseases	IgA	4	0
($n = 14$)	IgM	3	0

number of cells producing Ig of corresponding isotype. Since Ig-producing cells are rare in normal CSF, this means that only a minor part of the B-cell response compartmentalized to CSF in Lyme disease is specifically directed against the etiologic agent. This is in accordance with previous observations regarding systemic humoral immune response in systemic infections.

REFERENCES

1. MÖLLER, S. A. & C. A. K. BORREBAECK. 1985. J. Immunol. Methods **79:** 195.

Anti-Fab Antibodies in Lyme Disease

J. S. LOUIE,[a] J. E. PERSSELIN,[c] G. Y. SHI,[a] H. T. JOBE,[a]
M. R. LIEBLING,[a] A. C. STEERE,[b] AND R. H. STEVENS[c]

[a]Harbor-UCLA Medical Center
Torrance, California 90509

[b]Tufts Medical Center
Boston, Massachusetts 02111

[c]Department of Microbiology and Immunology
University of California at Los Angeles
Los Angeles, California 90024

Immunoglobins directed against the Fab portion of human IgG are a heterogeneous group of autoantibodies that occur in individuals with chronic illnesses, including malignancies, infections, and autoimmune disorders, and in some normal persons as well.[1-4] Lyme disease, a persistent infection with the spirochete *Borrelia burgdorferi*, presents as a clinical spectrum heralded by erythema chronicum migrans that progresses to heart, neurologic, and arthritic disease. Despite antibiotic therapy, the arthritis can become chronic, and result in destructive joint damage.[5] In rheumatoid arthritis (RA), a chronic autoimmune disease characterized by an erosive synovitis, serum anti-Fab antibodies (anti-FABA) are present in most patients and consist of polyclonal alkaline IgG_1 and clonally restricted acidic IgG_3 and IgG_4 populations.[6] In this study, we investigated whether similar anti-FABA occur in Lyme disease, especially in patients with arthritis, and whether the anti-FABA IgG subclasses and isoelectric focusing (IEF) spectrotypic expresson patterns were similar to those of RA.

IgG anti-FABA subclass distributions were determined in sera from Lyme patients with skin, neurologic, and arthritic disease and in RA, syphilis, pinta, and normal sera using ELISA assays. Briefly, 30 $\mu g/mL$ of Fab fragments of polyclonal human IgG were used to coat 96-well microtiter plates, blocked with 1% bovine serum albumin (BSA), incubated with serum samples, and then followed by mouse monoclonal anti-human IgG_1, IgG_2, IgG_3, or IgG_4 antibodies diluted with 1% BSA to 1 : 3200, 1 : 800, 1 : 3200, and 1 : 10,000 respectively. Binding of the monoclonals was detected by adding a 1 : 2400 dilution of an alkaline phosphatase conjugated goat anti-mouse antibody, followed by p-nitrophenyl phosphate substrate. All monoclonal antisera were mouse subclass IgG_1 and the same lot of conjugated goat anti-mouse was used for all subclass determinations. Optical densities (OD) were measured with a multichannel spectrophotometer and were converted to nanograms of mouse IgG bound based on a standard curve generated by coating wells with goat anti-mouse IgG and known quantities of mouse IgG.[7] The clonal heterogeneity of serum anti-FABA was determined by IEF spectrotypic analyses. Four μl serum samples were applied to sorbitol-agarose gels containing 6-M urea and 5% ampholines, pH 3.5–9.5 (BioRad, Richmond, CA). Gels were focused at constant power (6.25 W/110 mm gel) and incubated sequentially in sodium sulfate to precipitate the isolated proteins, dimethyl suberimidate to cross-link the proteins, and glycine to block any remaining reactive groups. Gels were overlaid with ^{125}I-Fab molecules diluted in 1% ovalbumin, washed, fixed with 10% trichlorecetic acid, stained with Coomassie blue, and autoradiographed on T-Mat G film (Kodak, Rochester, NY).[6]

ELISA assays demonstrated elevations of IgG$_1$ anti-FABA in the RA, Lyme, and pinta sera, when compared to those in normals. Interestingly, the elevated IgG$_1$ anti-FABA in Lyme sera were predominant in patients with arthritis (FIG. 1). IgG$_3$ anti-FABA were significantly higher in the RA and syphilis sera, and no significant differences of IgG$_2$ or IgG$_4$ were noted (data not shown).

IEF spectrotypic analyses revealed that 10 of the sera possessed alkaline anti-FABA spectrotypes (ST) with well-defined, individual bands, indicative of a clonally

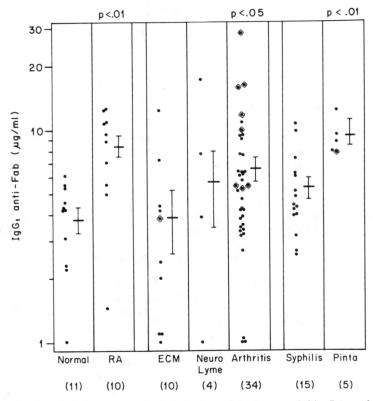

FIGURE 1. Serum IgG$_1$ anti-Fab (μg/ml) is elevated in Lyme arthritis, RA, and pinta (Wilcoxon rank sum). Mean and standard errors are recorded. Sera depicting restricted alkaline spectrotype patterns are enclosed in *squares*.

restricted antibody response. Furthermore, 8 of the 10 sera with these restricted alkaline bands were from patients with chronic Lyme arthritis, including 5 of the 6 highest IgG$_1$ anti-FABA levels in the Lyme arthritis group (FIG. 2). When these Lyme arthritis sera were subjected to affinity purification on staphylococcal protein A columns to recover IgG proteins, restricted alkaline anti-FABA ST patterns were detected that were identical to those in the whole sera (FIG. 3).

These data describe a subpopulation of clonally restricted alkaline anti-FABA unique to Lyme disease, and primarily confined to those individuals with chronic

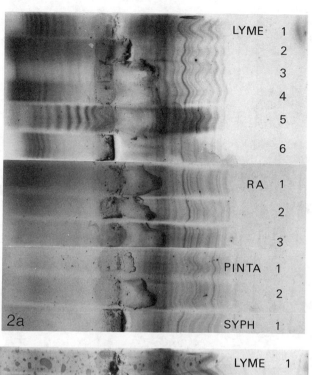

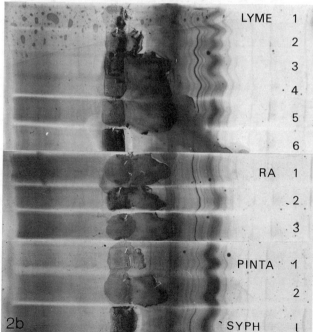

FIGURE 2. Spectrotypic analyses by IEF depict individual alkaline bands in Lyme sera (lanes 1–6) directed against ^{125}I-Fab in the radioautograph (**a**) when compared to the patterns of serum proteins stained by Coomassie blue. (**b**).

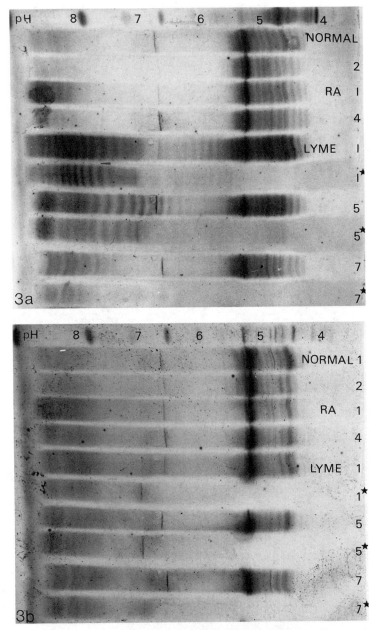

FIGURE 3. Spectrotypic analyses by IEF confirm the alkaline spectrotypes of anti-Fab in Lyme sera 1, 5, and 7, compared to normal and RA. The IgG fractions recovered from staphylococcus protein A (SPA) columns of Lyme sera 1*, 5* and 7* depicted the identical alkaline spectrotypes in the radioautograph (**a**) as compared to the protein stain (**b**). The deletion of the acidic spectrotypes suggests they were IgG3 anti-Fabs, since IgG3 is not taken up by SPA.

arthritis. Although there is a potential for the formation of immune complexes that could deposit into tissues or interact in other immune networks, the significance of these anti-FABA remains at present unclear. Studies are underway to determine whether they represent an antibody response to borrelia antigens that cross-react with epitopes present on human Fab molecules, or whether they reflect an anti-idiotypic response to chronic expression of antiborrelia antibodies. Such studies may lead to a better understanding of the host response to chronic infection and the involvement of autoimmune responses in the clinical expression of disease.

REFERENCES

1. DAVEY, M. P. & L. KORNGOLD. 1982. Association of anti-F(ab′)$_2$ antibodies (pepsin agglutinators) with immune complexes as determined by enzyme-linked immunosorbent assays. Int. Arch. Allergy Appl. Immunol. **67**: 278–283.
2. MORGAN, A. C., R. D. ROSSEN, K. J. McCORMICK, J. S. STEHLIN & B. C. GIOVANELLA. 1982. "Hidden" cytotoxic antibodies that react with allogenic cultured fetal and tumor cells contained in soluble immune complexes from normal human sera. Cancer Res. **42**: 881–887.
3. NASU, H., D. S. CHIA, D. W. KNUTSON & E. V. BARNETT. 1980. Naturally occurring human antibodies to the F(ab′)$_2$ portion of IgG. Clin. Exp. Immunol. **42**: 378–386.
4. PERSSELIN, J. E., J. S. LOUIE & R. H. STEVENS. 1984. Clonally restricted anti-IgG antibodies in rheumatoid arthritis. Arthritis Rheum. **27**: 1378–1386.
5. STEERE, A. C., J. GREEN, R. T. SCOHEN, *et al.* 1985. Successful parenteral penicillin therapy of established Lyme arthritis. N. Engl. J. Med. **312**: 869–874.
6. PERSSELIN, J. E. & R. H. STEVENS. 1985. Anti-Fab antibodies in humans. Predominance of minor immunoglobulin G subclasses in rheumatoid arthritis. J. Clin. Invest. **76**: 723–730.
7. PERSSELIN, J. E., B. KELD, L. FRIED & R. H. STEVENS. 1985. Subclasses of human IgG anti-Fab antibodies: Parameters for optimum detection. Int. Arch. Allergy Appl. Immunol. **78**:368–374.

Specificity of Human B-Cell Responses
of Immunodominant Antigens
of *Borrelia burgdorferi*

BENJAMIN J. LUFT,[a] RAYMOND J. DATTWYLER,[a]
JOHN J. HALPERIN,[b] PETER FALLDORF,[a]
AND DAVID J. VOLKMAN[a]

[a]*Department of Medicine*
[b]*Department of Neurology*
Health Science Center
SUNY at Stony Brook
Stony Brook, New York 11794

Serological testing for Lyme borreliosis has been hampered by the high level of cross-reacting antibody in the sera of patients with evidence of previous Lyme disease.[1] As a result, high levels of anti-*B. burgdorferi* antibody must be present in order for these titers to be considered significant. However, in cases of syphilis cross-reacting anti-*B. burgdorferi* antibodies may be present that further complicate the specificity of the test.[1,2] Although diagnostic tests for Lyme disease are being performed routinely, little is known about the specificity and persistence of antibodies to individual immunodominant antigens of *B. burgdorferi*. Using sera from patients with Lyme borreliosis characterized by arthritis, secondary and latent syphilis, or no evidence or history of previous infection, we compared the response to antigens of both *B. burgdorferi* and *T. pallidum*.

In order to characterize the antibody response of patients with late Lyme borreliosis, sera of seven patients were reacted with *B. burgdorferi* antigens separated by SDS-PAGE and electrophoretically transferred to nitrocellulose paper. Sera from patients with late Lyme borreliosis responded to well-defined antigens of 83, 66, 60, and 39–41 kDa. There was variable response to the antigens between 29 to 34 kDa (FIG. 1). In contrast, control subjects with no history of tick bite, skin rash, or arthritic or neurologic disease responded, although weakly, to the 41 kDa antigen (data not shown).

Sera from patients with secondary or latent syphilis also responded to *B. burgdorferi* antigens. Specifically, sera from these patients cross-reacted to the 66, 60, and 41 kDa antigens of *B. burgdorferi*. Notably, sera from these patients failed to respond to the 29–34 kDa antigens. Most remarkably, however, patients with syphilis also recognized an array of antigens between 41 and 66 kDa that sera from patients with Lyme borreliosis fail to recognize. This suggests that patients with severe *B. burgdorferi* infection recognize a restricted number of *B. burgdorferi* antigens. In contrast, sera from patients with Lyme borreliosis had extremely weak binding to the 44, 31, and 27 kDa treponemal antigens, whereas sera from patients with syphilis clearly recognized an array of *T. pallidum* antigens (data not shown). This further implies a restriction in the humoral response to *B. burgdorferi* antigens by patients with Lyme disease. Further studies are necessary to determine specific immunodominant epitopes of *B. burgdorferi* antigens that may aid in improving the sensitivity and specificity of the current serological tests.

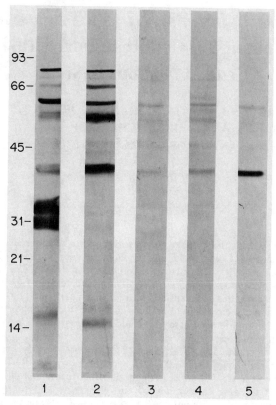

FIGURE 1. Immunoblotting analysis of *Borrelia burgdorferi* antigens by sera of patients with late Lyme borreliosis (Lanes 1 and 2), and secondary (lane 3) and latent (lanes 4, 5) syphilis. A sonicated preparation of the B31 strain of *B. burgdorferi* was solublized in running buffer containing 1% SDS and 2% 2-mercaptoethanol. Ten μg of protein was separated in 10% slab polyacrylamide gels in the presence of 0.1% SDS by the methods described by Laemmli[3] and electrophoretically transferred to nitrocellulose paper using the buffer system described by Towbin *et al.*[4] Antigens were detected by incubation of nitrocellulose paper with a 1 : 100 dilution of sera of patients before immunologic detection with alkaline phosphatase-conjugated goat anti-human IgG. The molecular weight standards are notated on the left-hand border of the figure.

REFERENCES

1. MAGNARELLI, L. A., D. S. ANDERSON & R. C. JOHNSON. 1987. Cross-reactivity in serological tests for Lyme disease and other spirochetal infections. J. Infect. Dis. **156**: 183–188.
2. HUNTER, E. F., H. RUSSELL, C. E. FARSLY, J. S. SAMPSON & S. D. LARSEN. 1986. Evaluation of sera from patients with Lyme disease in the fluorescent treponemal antibody absorption test for syphilis. Sex. Trans. Dis. **13**: 232.
3. LAEMMLI, U. K. 1979. Cleavage of structural proteins during the assembly of the head of bacteriophage T4. Nature (London). **227**: 680–685.
4. TOWBIN, H., T. STAEHELIN & J. GORDON. 1979. Electrophoretic transfer of proteins from acrylamide gels to nitrocellulose sheets: Procedure and some applications. Proc. Natl. Acad. Sci. USA **76**: 4350–4354.

Borrelia burgdorferi as a Trigger for Autoimmune T-Cell Reactions within the Central Nervous System

ROLAND MARTIN,[a] JOHANNES ORTLAUF,[a]
VERONIKA STICHT-GROH,[b]
AND HANS GEORG MERTENS[a]

[a]Department of Neurology
[b]Institute of Hygiene and Microbiology
University of Würzburg
8700 Würzburg, Federal Republic of Germany

Borrelia burgdorferi has been found to cause a number of different diseases of the central nervous system (CNS), including lymphomeningoradiculitis, radiculomyelitis, and even encephalomyelitis. Characteristic cerebrospinal fluid (CSF) findings consist of a lymphocytic pleocytosis, oligoclonal *Borrelia burgdorferi* (Bb) specific IgG bands, and high CSF: serum ratios of Bb antibody titers. When peripheral blood lymphocytes (PBL) and CSF mononuclear cells of patients suffering from lymphomeningoradiculitis were analyzed in proliferative assays, it could be demonstrated that they responded upon stimulation with Bb antigen.[1]

In the present study, 505 T-cell lines (TCLs) were directly expanded by the limiting dilution technique[2] using allogeneic, irradiated ($\times$5000R) feeder cells and interleukin-2 from the CSF of three patients suffering from chronic Lyme radiculomyelitis. The TCLs were later analyzed for phenotype and for antigen-specific proliferative responses using Bb antigen and a panel of CNS and peripheral nervous system (PNS) autoantigens in ^{3}H-thymidine incorporation assays.

When the CSF cells were seeded, about one out of 50 up to one out of 20 gave rise to a colony. The proliferative testing of CSF-derived TCLs gave the following results:

TABLE 1. Proliferative Responses of a Sample of Bb-specific TCLs Isolated from the CSF of Patients Suffering from Chronic Lyme Radiculomyelitis

	^{3}H-Thymidine Incorporation in the Presence of		
TCL No.	Bb Antigen	Medium	IL-2
E6/10B	119,810 $\pm$ 5,450	1,090 $\pm$ 280	13,020 $\pm$ 340
E9/30B	7,300 $\pm$ 870	660 $\pm$ 240	121,690 $\pm$ 7,180
D2/60	15,180 $\pm$ 5,500	1,120 $\pm$ 340	1,600 $\pm$ 120
H10/10B	15,630 $\pm$ 560	1,070 $\pm$ 90	1,920 $\pm$ 620
A9/3	9,930 $\pm$ 520	1,290 $\pm$ 150	2,200 $\pm$ 240

TCLs were tested in the presence of autologous antigen-presenting cells and results given in counts per minute (cpm).

[a]This work was supported by grant no. Sti 63/4–1 of the Deutsche Forschungsgemeinschaft.

400

TABLE 2. Proliferative Responses of a Representative Sample of MBP-specific TCLs Isolated from the CSF of Patients Suffering from Chronic Lyme Radiculomyelitis

	^{3}H-Thymidine Incorporation in the Presence of		
TCL No.	MBP	Medium	IL-2
B4/180	2,900 ± 550	180 ± 140	1,340 ± 50
H11/180B	1,930 ± 390	580 ± 50	500 ± 30
C2/180	14,870 ± 2,870	50 ± 40	21,510 ± 5,760
B9/90	13,430 ± 5,130	710 ± 210	6,010 ± 1,820
B3/180	870 ± 260	130 ± 70	4,410 ± 140

Cells were tested in the presence of autologous antigen-presenting cells and results expressed as cpm.

4.7–7.7% of tested TCLs responded to stimulation with Bb antigen, 2.2–5.3% to myelin basic protein (MBP), 5.9% to whole peripheral myelin (PM), 3.1% to galactocerebrosides (Gal), 0.4% to P2 protein, a basic myelin component of the peripheral nerve, and 0.4% to cardiolipin, which is found in mitochondrial membranes and bacterial cell walls. A minor fraction of TCLs was found to respond to both Bb antigen and MBP (0.7–1.8%), or to MBP and to PM (2.2%). A representative sample of Bb-specific and of MBP-specific TCLs is given in TABLES 1 and 2. Surface marker analysis revealed the majority of TCLs to be positive for CD3 (pan T cell), CD4 (helper-inducer subset), and HLA class II antigens and negative for CD8 (cytotoxic-suppressor subset). The antigen-specific proliferative responses were restricted by HLA class II molecules.

These data show that in patients suffering from chronic Lyme disease not only Bb-specific T cells, but also T cells reactive to CNS and PNS autoantigens can be isolated from the CSF. *Borrelia burgdorferi* is thus able to induce autoimmune T-cell reactions. Whether these autoreactive T cells cause demyelination in certain individuals rather than the *Borrelia* itself remains to be determined.

REFERENCES

1. PACHNER, A. R., A. C. STEERE, L. H. SIGAL & C. J. JOHNSON. 1985. Antigen-specific proliferation of CSF lymphocytes in Lyme disease. Neurology 35: 1642–1644.
2. MORETTA, A., G. PANTALEO, L. MORETTA, J. C. CEROTTINI & M. C. MINGARI. 1983. Direct demonstration of the clonogenic potential of every human peripheral blood T cell. J. Exp. Med. 157: 743–754.

Reducing Transmission of Lyme Disease Spirochetes in a Suburban Setting

THOMAS N. MATHER, JOSE M. C. RIBEIRO,
SEAN I. MOORE, AND ANDREW SPIELMAN

Department of Tropical Public Health
Harvard School of Public Health
Boston, Massachusetts 02115

Recently, a new method has been developed that distributes acaricide to white-footed mice (*Peromyscus leucopus*), the principal reservoir of the Lyme disease spirochete (LDS) *Borrelia burgdorferi,* in order to kill immature *Ixodes dammini* infesting these hosts.[1] This method relies on the nesting and foraging behavior of these mice. Standard cotton balls, impregnated with permethrin (7.4% w/w), are dispensed from weather-resistant tubes placed at 10-meter intervals in suitable mouse habitats. Mice collect the cotton as they forage for fibrous material to build their nests, thus incorporating the acaricide into their burrows.

This method, using such permethrin-treated cotton (PTC), was employed in a suburban community where ticks (*I. dammini*) are abundant and Lyme disease is endemic, in an attempt to reduce the risk of human exposure to LDS-infected ticks. The study area, located in Ipswich, Massachusetts, is bordered on its perimeter by salt marsh and is transected by a road. An 18-acre tract containing seven residences located on the south side of the road was selected for treatment with PTC. A total of 850 tubes, each packed with 4.5 grams of PTC, were distributed in grid fashion in all potential mouse habitats. The treated cotton was distributed in early May 1986, 15 August 1986, 10 May 1987, and 4 August 1987. Thus, PTC was distributed twice each summer during seasons corresponding to the feeding activity pattern of the immature stages of the tick.[2]

To evaluate the effectiveness of PTC in reducing tick infestations on *P. leucopus,* mice were live-trapped on the perimeter of yards located in the centers of the treated and nontreated sites. A total of 33 of 34 mice captured around five nontreated yards on 10 August 1986 were infested with an average of 20 larval and nymphal *I. dammini* each. In contrast, 39 of 40 mice captured on the same date around five yards in the treated site were found to be tick-free. The only tick-infested mouse captured in a treated yard had three larval ticks. Evaluations conducted prior to and following treatment during 1987 produced similar results. While ticks were found infesting 43 of 45 mice captured in nontreated yards, none of the 52 mice captured in treated yards were tick infested. Distribution of PTC appeared to be nearly completely effective in eliminating infestations of ticks on *P. leucopus.*

To determine whether such reduced tick infestations on the mouse reservoir indeed resulted in lowered transmission risk, we measured the relative abundance of host-seeking nymphal *I. dammini* in both treated and nontreated yards, as well as the LDS infection rate in samples of these ticks. Host-seeking nymphal *I. dammini* were collected on the perimeter of yards by dragging a 1-meter square flannel flag for a measured amount of time. Samples of nymphs collected in this manner were examined for LDS using a direct fluorescent antibody procedure.[3] Prior to treatment (in 1985) and following initial treatment (in 1986), the abundance of host-seeking nymphs varied from yard to yard but was statistically equivalent in yards throughout the study site. Furthermore, LDS infection rates in these nymphs were uniform. Host-seeking nymphs, collected in treated yards between 17 June and 28 July 1987, however, were nearly tenfold less abundant than were nymphs in nontreated yards (TABLE 1). In addition, the average LDS infection rate was 8.8% and 31% in nymphs from PTC-treated and nontreated yards, respectively. Using a transmission risk index (TRI), which considers both nymphal abundance and LDS infection rate, we determined that risk of human exposure to LDS-infected ticks was reduced by 97% following just one season of treatment with PTC.

TABLE 1. Relative Abundance of Host-Seeking Nymphal *Ixodes dammini*[a]

	No. of Samples	No. Man Hours Collecting	No. Host-seeking Nymphs Collected
PTC-treated Sites	8	7	49
Nontreated Sites	10	7	435

[a]Collections were made between 17 June and 28 July, 1987

In conclusion, it would appear that a tick control program using PTC applied just twice per season can dramatically reduce the risk of transmission of LDS in areas where human exposure to LDS-infected ticks is intense.

REFERENCES

1. MATHER, T. N., J. M. C. RIBEIRO & A. SPIELMAN. 1987. Lyme disease and babesiosis: Acaricide focused on potentially infected ticks. Am. J. Trop. Med. Hyg. **36:** 609–614.
2. WILSON, M. L. & A. SPIELMAN. 1985. Seasonal activity of immature *Ixodes dammini* (Acari: Ixodidae). J. Med. Entomol. **22:** 408–414.
3. STEERE, A. C., R. L. GRODZICKI, A. N. KORNBLATT, J. E. CRAFT, A. G. BARBOUR, W. BURGDORFER, G. P. SCHMID, E. JOHNSON & S. E. MALAWISTA. 1983. The spirochetal etiology of Lyme disease. N. Engl. J. Med. **308:** 733–742.

Colony Formation by Lyme Disease Spirochetes

U. G. MUNDERLOH,[a] T. J. KURTTI,[a] R. C. JOHNSON,[c]
AND G. G. AHLSTRAND[b]

[a]*Department of Entomology*
[b]*Department of Plant Pathology*
University of Minnesota
St. Paul, Minnesota 55108

[c]*Department of Microbiology*
University of Minnesota
Minneapolis, Minnesota 55455

Lyme spirochetes, *Borrelia burgdorferi*, were first isolated from *Ixodes dammini* ticks in Barbour-Stoenner-Kelley (BSK) medium.[1] Culture-adapted strains can be cloned in liquid medium[2] and grown as a "lawn" on solid BSK,[3] but isolated colonies do not arise. An agar-cloning procedure would facilitate the selection of variants, mutants, and

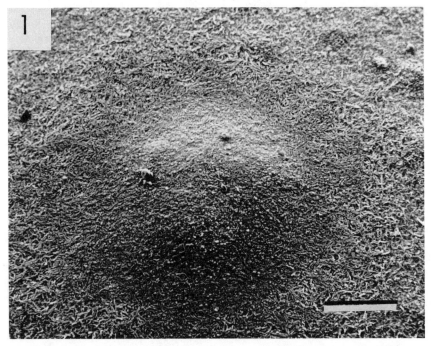

FIGURE 1. Scanning electron micrograph of *Borrelia burgdorferi* (strain 297) colony with raised center and surrounding flat spirochete layer. *Bar* represents 40 μm.

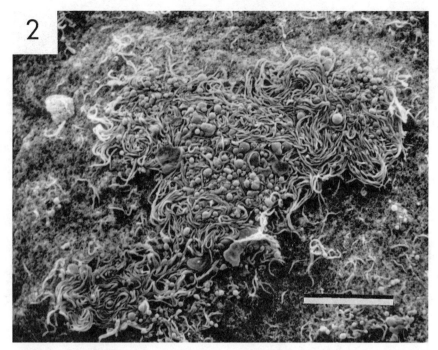

FIGURE 2. Scanning electron micrograph of a portion of a *Borrelia burgdorferi* (strain 297) colony, granular type, showing spirochetal aggregates. Note round bodies among spirochete bundles. *Bar* represents 15 μm.

recombinant clones. We describe here the electron microscopic appearance of *B. burgdorferi* colonies on agarose medium.

Strain 297 was grown in L-15B/S medium[4] to 2–3×10^7/ml in one week without forming clumps. BSK medium with twice the amount of gelatin and additional $NaHCO_3$ was solidified with 1.5% agarose[4] and poured into petri dishes. A high agarose concentration was critical, because at 1% the organisms did not form discrete colonies. Spirochete dilutions were spread onto the medium and incubated in candle jars at 34°C. After 2 to 4 weeks, the plates were examined with a dissecting microscope. In this system, the proportion of borreliae giving rise to colonies varied from 20% to 100%. The average colony diameter was 0.8 mm, ranging from 0.3 to 1.5 mm, with a maximum of 1.9 mm after 5 weeks. Spirochetes were clearly visible at the surface of the partially exposed colonies. Two morphologically distinct colony types developed within the surface layer: one shallow convex with smooth edges (FIG. 1), often with small satellite colonies nearby, the other granular and diffuse (FIG. 2). The former consisted of a flat layer of spirochetes, often with a raised center, while the latter comprised large numbers of small borrelial aggregates. Intermediate forms were also seen. Spherical bodies, possibly representing damaged or degenerate cells, were seen among bundles of spirochetes, especially in the center of the colonies.

The ability to grow *B. burgdorferi* as discrete colonies on solid medium opens new approaches to their genetic analysis and manipulation.

REFERENCES

1. BURGDORFER, W., A. G. BARBOUR, S. F. HAYES, J. L. BENACH, E. GRUNWALDT & J. P. DAVIS. 1982. Science **216:** 1317–1319.
2. BARBOUR A. G., W. BURGDORFER, S. F. HAYES, O. PETER & A. AESCHLIMANN. 1983. Curr. Microbiol. **8:** 123–126.
3. BARBOUR, A. G. 1984. Yale J. Biol. Med. **57:** 521–525.
4. KURTTI, T. J., U. G. MUNDERLOH, R. C. JOHNSON & G. G. AHLSTRAND. 1987. J. Clin. Microbiol. **25:** 2054–2058.

Presence and Effects of Lyme Disease in a Barrier Island Deer Population

ALLAN F. O'CONNELL, JR.,[a] MARK W. SAYRE,[b]
AND EDWARD M. BOSLER[c]

[a]National Park Service
Fire Island National Seashore
Patchogue, New York 11772

[b]Department of Forestry and Wildlife Management
University of Massachusetts
Amherst, Massachusetts 01003

[c]New York State Department of Health
Health Science Center
State University of New York at Stony Brook
Stony Brook, New York 11794

INTRODUCTION

As part of an investigation of the ecology of an unmanaged white-tailed deer (*Odocoileus virginianus*) population, the presence of *Borrelia burgdorferi* in ticks removed from deer and the serologic response of deer to the spirochete were examined. Further investigation was conducted to develop a standardized test for use in detecting *B. burgdorferi* antibodies in deer sera.

The study was conducted on Fire Island (lat. 40°41′ N, long. 73°00′ W), a 50-km barrier island parallel to the South Shore of Long Island, approximately 50 km east of New York City. Several levels of land use and management exist on the island, including federal, state and county parks, and private residential communities. Fire Island is a known endemic area for human Lyme disease.

METHODS

Ticks were collected from live and dead deer, triturated in phosphate-buffered saline (pH 7.4), and examined for spirochetes using dark-field microscopy.[1] Deer were either live-trapped using Clover traps or immobilized with a Capchur gun and darts® (Palmer Chemical and Equipment Co., Inc., Douglasville, GA) containing a mixture of xylazine hydrochloride (Rompun®; Haver Lockhart, Miles Laboratories, Inc., Shawnee, KS) and ketamine hydrochloride (Vetalar®; Parke-Davis, Division of Warner Lambert Co., Morris Plains, NJ). Yohimbine hydrochloride (Yohimbine®; Sigma F and D Division, Ltd., St. Louis, MO) was used as a drug antagonist. Twenty individuals were outfitted with radio collars (Telonics, Inc., Mesa, AZ) and all captured animals were marked with ear-tags for future identification. Blood samples were taken from the jugular vein for blood chemistry determination and *B. burgdorferi* serologies. Serum samples were collected to determine antibody levels and were frozen until processed. Deer capture was conducted over an 18-month period to collect serial blood samples, which were used to determine the presence and persistence of immunoglobulin levels.[2,3] Serum samples were examined for humoral IgG antibodies to *B. burgdorferi* using both an indirect fluorescent antibody (IFA) test and an enzyme-linked immunosorbent assay (ELISA). The ELISA procedure[4] was modified for deer serum by using alkaline-phosphatase anti-bovine IgG (heavy and light chain) immunoglobulin as the secondary antibody (Kirkegaard and Perry Laboratories, Gaithersburg, MD). The secondary IgG antibody used in the IFA tests was fluoroscein isothiocyanate conjugated goat derived anti-bovine (Kirkegaard and Perry Laboratories).

RESULTS

Three tick species, *Ixodes dammini, Amblyomma americanum,* and *Dermacentor varabilis* were collected from deer on Fire Island. Approximately 26% of total ticks collected and examined (*n* = 340) were infected with spirochetes. *I. dammini* and *A. americanum* both contained spirochetes. Nymphs from both species revealed at least a 50% infection rate, and only one larval *I. dammini* was infected. *I. dammini* was the predominant species found on Fire Island deer, representing 92% of all ticks collected. *I. dammini* were also distributed along the entire island and were recovered in all 20 areas from which deer were sampled. *A. americanum* were found in only seven areas, often separated by several kilometers. While infected *I. dammini* were recorded in both uninhabited park areas and residential communities, *A. americanum* were found to be infected with *B. burgdorferi* only within residential communities.

Although telemetry data revealed deer home ranges generally <5 km in length, movements were recorded in excess of 17 km traversing both park and community boundaries.

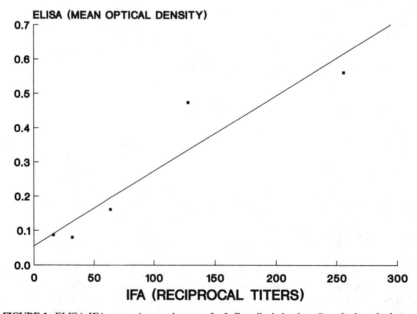

FIGURE 1. ELISA-IFA comparison on deer sera for IgG antibody levels to *Borrelia burgdorferi.*

TABLE 1. Antibody Levels for Serial Blood Samples Collected from White-tailed Deer on Fire Island, New York[a]

Deer No.	Antibody Level		
	Date 1	Date 2	Date 3
1	0.150 (12/04/85)	0.270 (3/17/86)	—
2	0.091 (2/26/86)	0.148 (4/30/86)	—
3	0.116 (2/28/86)	0.091 (3/28/86)	—
4	0.202 (3/27/86)	0.043 (12/01/86)	0.150 (12/17/86)
5	0.039 (3/28/86)	0.041 (4/02/86)	—
6	0.295 (12/01/86)	0.319 (12/05/86)	0.184 (12/18/86)

[a]Values listed represent optical density using an ELISA.

A comparison of serum IgG levels between ELISA and IFA tests showed a positive correlation ($r = .868$, $p < .01$) for both serological procedures (FIG. 1). Serial blood samples were collected from six deer; four deer demonstrated increased antibody levels over time as determined by two samples from each individual (TABLE 1). Two animals were sampled one additional time and had fluctuating titers. One of these two deer was sampled within a 3-week period, while the other was sampled over several months.

DISCUSSION

I. dammini and *A. americanum,* two vectors of Lyme disease, utilize the white-tailed deer as a host during all life stages.[1,5] Our results indicate that *A. americanum* populations are currently lower than *I. dammini* populations and are focal on the island. We speculate that these localized populations of *A. americanum* will be further distributed throughout the island by deer movements. Given the widespread distribution of *I. dammini* on Fire Island, the relatively small deer home ranges may serve to maintain local tick populations, once established. Movements of deer and associated ticks may also serve to spread *B. burgdorferi* in this insular environment.

The paired serum samples that exhibited rising antibody titers during the winter months suggest reexposure to spirochetes. One possible mechanism of reexposure could be via feeding adult ticks.

The ELISA developed in this study proved to be a successful procedure for the detection of serum IgG levels in response to *B. burgdorferi* in deer serum.

REFERENCES

1. BOSLER, E. M., B. G. ORMISTON, J. L. COLEMAN, J. P. HANRAHAN, & J. L. BENACH. 1984. Prevalence of the Lyme disease spirochete in populations of white-tailed deer and white-footed mice. Yale J. Biol. Med. **57:** 651–659.
2. WYAND, M. S. & S. W. NIELSEN. 1985. Lyme disease—a wildlife perspective. Trans. Northeast Sect. Wildlife Soc. **42:** 178–184.
3. MAGNARELLI, L. A., J. A. ANDERSON & W. A. CHAPPELL. 1984. Antibodies to spirochetes in white-tailed deer and prevalence of infected ticks from foci of Lyme disease in Connecticut. J. Wildl. Dis. **20:** 21–26.
4. COLEMAN, J. L. & J. L. BENACH. 1987. Isolation of antigenic components from the Lyme disease spirochete: Their role in early diagnosis. J. Infect. Dis. **155**(4): 756–765.
5. SCHULZE, T. L., G. S. BOWEN, E. M. BOSLER, M. K. LAKAT, W. E. PARKIN, R. ALTMAN, B. G. ORMISTON & J. K. SHISLER. 1984. *A. americanum:* A potential vector of Lyme disease in New Jersey. Science **224:** 601–603.

Assessment of *in Vitro* Growth of *Borrelia burgdorferi* by Tritiated Adenine Incorporation

CHARLES S. PAVIA AND SUSAN BITTKER

Departments of Medicine, Microbiology
and Immunology
New York Medical College
Valhalla, New York 10595

INTRODUCTION

The recent development of improved methods for culturing *B. burgdorferi*[1] has created new opportunities for studying the biology, biochemistry, immunology, and chemotherapy of these spirochetes. One factor limiting the rapidity with which these aspects can be explored is the time required to assess growth *in vitro* by long-term bulk cultures and by periodic microscopic examination of these cultures to determine spirochete levels and growth rates. We report here a radioisotopic method using tritiated adenine to assess spirochete growth, and describe some of the factors that influence the relationship between radioisotope incorporation and parasite numbers.

MATERIALS AND METHODS

The 297[2] and RF-1[3] strains of *B. burgdorferi* were grown continuously in stock cultures in complete BSK medium containing 100 μg/ml of nalidixic acid and 100 μg/ml of 5-fluorouracil.[1] Growth capability of spirochetes was assessed using a microculture system modified from a previously described assay.[4] Each well of flat-bottom microtiter plates contained 50 μl of different dilutions of *Borrelia* plus 100 μl of complete BSK medium. Control cultures contained 150 μl of complete BSK alone. Prior to incubation, all cultures were pulse-labeled by the addition of 50 μl of complete BSK medium containing 0.5 μCi of either ^{3}H-adenine, ^{3}H-hypoxanthine, ^{3}H-thymidine, or ^{3}H-uracil. All culture plates were placed in an air-tight chamber and incubated at 31–33°C. Twenty-four to 72 hours later, spirochetes were assayed for nucleic acid synthesis by first harvesting samples onto glass fiber filter paper, followed by extensive washing with distilled water using a semiautomated cell harvester (Bellco, Vineland, NJ). Samples were counted for radioactivity after each fiber filter disk was placed into a plastic scintillation vial containing a toluene-based scintillation fluid. Data are expressed as mean counts per minute (cpm) of ^{3}H-isotope incorporation and are taken from at least three replicate cultures. In other experiments, the antimicrobial agents penicillin G, cefotaxime sodium (Claforan), and gentamicin sulfate (Garamycin) were tested for antiborrelial activity using the microculture technique. These antibiotics were obtained as aqueous solutions and dilutions of these were made in complete BSK medium prior to their addition to selected wells of *Borrelia* microcultures and just before isotope labeling and incubation.

410

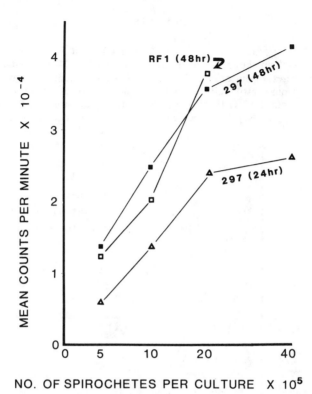

FIGURE 1. Relationship between spirochete numbers used to initiate cultures and ³H-adenine incorporation by *B. burgdorferi* (strains RF-1 and 297) after 24 and 48 hours. Cultures were established in separate wells of microtiter plates in a final volume of 0.2 ml of complete BSK medium containing 0.5 μCi ³H-adenine. Counts per minute for control cultures containing no spirochetes averaged 431. Data are taken from ten replicate experiments.

TABLE 1. Incorporation of Tritiated Nucleic Acid Precursors by *Borrelia burgdorferi* (Counts per Minute, in Thousands)

Culture Conditions[a]	24 h[b]	48 h	72 h
297 + ³H-adenine	26.3	37.9	41.4
297 + ³H-thymidine	0.97	0.91	1.8
297 + ³H-hypoxanthine	1.04	1.26	1.52
297 + ³H-uracil	0.6	0.53	0.67

[a]Each microculture contained 2×10^6 *Borrelia* plus the indicated isotope.
[b]Time in which cultures were harvested; data are from three replicate experiments.

RESULTS

With a starting concentration of *Borrelia* ranging from 5×10^5 to 4×10^6 per culture, the level of uptake of ^{3}H-adenine at the end of both a 24- and 48-hour pulse by growing spirochetes was linear (FIG. 1). An insignificant amount of isotope (431 cpm) was recovered from control cultures containing no spirochetes. In contrast, *Borrelia* exhibited poor uptake of ^{3}H-thymidine, hypoxanthine, and uracil at 24, 48, and 72 hours of culture (TABLE 1). When penicillin G, gentamicin, or cefotaxime were added

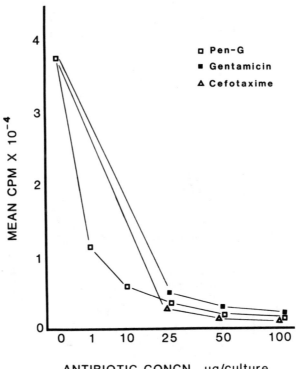

FIGURE 2. Comparative activity of penicillin G ($\square$), gentamicin ($\blacksquare$), and cefotaxime ($\triangle$) against *B. burgdorferi* (strain 297) *in vitro*. The cpm represent the uptake by spirochetes (2×10^6/culture) at each concentration of the drugs during a 48-hour culture period. Data are from five replicate experiments.

in various concentrations to cultures initiated with 2×10^6 *Borrelia*, ^{3}H-adenine incorporation was inhibited in a nearly linear fashion (FIG. 2). At antibiotic doses ranging from 25 to 100 μg per culture, the level of inhibition varied from 90% to 96%.

DISCUSSION

We chose ^{3}H-adenine as a tool to assess *Borrelia* growth *in vitro* because studies with another pathogenic spirochete, *Treponema pallidum*, showed that treponemes can utilize this purine well when synthesizing DNA and RNA.[5] The assay technique developed here showed that adenine was utilized with extremely high efficiency, whereas other nucleic acid precursors were incorporated poorly or not at all. It is probable that *B. burgdorferi*, like other bacteria,[6] possess transport mechanisms and enzymes that aid in the efficient uptake and incorporation of exogenous adenine, although specific assays for these activities in *B. burgdorferi* have not been performed.

Compared to traditional culture and microscopic methods used for measuring *Borrelia* growth, this assay system has several advantages. The rapid uptake of adenine allows the use of smaller culture volumes, increasing the possible number of samples per unit volume severalfold and, at the same time, reduces assay time considerably. These features permit the use of this technique for the detailed analysis of the optimal nutritional requirements and other environmental factors conducive to nucleic acid synthesis during short-term culture. In addition, it should be readily adaptable, as described here for evaluating antibiotic sensitivity, for studying the effects of various host-derived factors, such as immune serum or cells, on *Borrelia* growth.

SUMMARY

To evaluate rapidly *in vitro* the growth of two strains (297, RF-1) of *B. burgdorferi*, tritiated adenine was added to spirochete microcultures containing complete BSK medium, and radioisotope incorporation was measured. When culture parameters were carefully controlled, tritiated adenine incorporation was proportional to the number of spirochetes used to initiate culture. *Borrelia* exhibited a poor rate of isotope incorporation during short-term culture in the presence of tritiated hypoxanthine, thymidine, or uracil. For culture periods lasting from 24 to 72 hours, incorporation of tritiated adenine was inhibited by the antibiotics penicillin G, cefotaxime, and gentamicin. The minimum inhibitory concentration was determined for each of these antimicrobials, and these values ranged from 25 to 100 μg per culture. This rapid radiometric assay could be used to measure inhibition of *B. burgdorferi* growth by other antibiotics as well as to measure the antiborrelial activity of the various humoral and cellular components (such as antibodies and lymphocytes) derived from patients with Lyme disease or as a result of active immunization.

REFERENCES

1. BARBOUR, A. G. 1984. Yale J. Biol. Med. **57:** 521–525.
2. STEERE, A. C., R. L. GRODZICKI, A. N. KORNBLATT, J. E. CRAFT, A. G. BARBOUR, W. BURGDORFER, G. P. SCHMID, E. JOHNSON & S. E. MALAWISTA. 1983. N. Engl. J. Med. **308:** 733–740.
3. PAVIA, C. S., S. BITTKER & D. FISH. 1988. In preparation.
4. PAVIA, C. S., C. L. DIGGS & J. WILLIAMS. 1983. Am. J. Trop. Med. Hyg. **32:** 675–681.
5. NORRIS, S. J., J. N. MILLER & J. A. SYKES. 1980. Infect. Immun. **29:** 1040–1049.
6. BURTON, K. 1977. Biochem. J. **168:** 195–204.

Erythema Migrans Borreliosis: An HLA-associated Disease?

K. H. PFLÜGER,[a] C. D. REIMERS,[b,d] U. NEUBERT,[e]
C. MEISEL,[g] B. TRAPP,[a] J. LEITITIS,[c] B. VÖLKER,[e,h]
P. MÜNCHHOFF,[h] J. LITZENBERGER,[b]
H. HOLTHAUSEN[f] AND E. PONGRATZ[i]

[a]Department of Hematology
[b]Department of Neurology
[c]Department of Pediatrics
University of Marburg
Marburg, Federal Republic of Germany

[d]Friedrich Baur Institute
Department of Internal Medicine
[e]Department of Dermatology
[f]Department of Pediatrics
University of Munich
Munich, Federal Republic of Germany

[g]Private Dermatology Practice
Aüfsessplatz 21
Nuremberg, Federal Republic of Germany

[h]Occupational Health Service
Munich, Federal Republic of Germany

[i]Pediatric Hospital Josefinum
Augsburg, Federal Republic of Germany

Erythema migrans borreliosis is a complex multisystemic infectious disorder caused by the spirochetal species termed *Borrelia burgdorferi*. The clinical picture is characterized by affection of various organ systems such as skin, central and peripheral nervous system, heart, joints, and some other organs. Reports on HLA association to *Borrelia burgdorferi* infection (BBI) are still controversial. HLA-DR2 was found to be correlated to more severe and/or chronic courses of this infectious disorder.[1,2] However, this finding was not confirmed by others.[3] The purpose of this study was to investigate phenotype frequencies of HLA antigens in patients with different stages and manifestations of BBI. HLA antigen patterns of 52 A, B, C, and DR antigens have been determined in a group of 189 patients and were compared to the HLA antigen frequencies of 457 control persons. Both groups have been typed during the same time period by identical staff and antiserum sets. Statistical analysis was performed by Fisher's test for 2×2 contingency tables; p values obtained were corrected (p_{corr}) by multiplication with the total number of comparisons within a single gene locus. Related risk (RR) was calculated using the equation described by Haldane and Woolf. Patients' characteristics are summarized in TABLE 1. Inapparent infections present in a group of forest workers are characterized as stage 0 of the disease. The results of HLA antigens found to be different in patients and control persons are given in TABLE 2. HLA-Cw3 was found to be more frequent in patients suffering from BBI as compared to the control group (39.2% vs. 21.9%). This difference is statistically significant ($p_{corr} = 0.003$). RR was calculated to be 2.3 and etiologic fraction 0.22, respectively. In

TABLE 1. Patients and Diagnoses

Stage	Diagnosis	*n*
0	forest workers with asymptomatic infections	37
1	erythema migrans	53
	lymphadenosis benigna cutis	3
2	meningitis	7
	meningopolyneuritis	78
	myocarditis	2
3	encephalomyelitis	1
	acrodermatitis chronica atrophicans	27
		201[a]

[a]Seven patients showed two different manifestations.

addition, the antigen A2 was more frequent in the patients (56.7% vs. 42.7%, p_{corr} = 0.025, RR = 1.76). Thus the phenotype combination HLA-A2 and HLA-Cw3 was more frequent in the patients (25% vs. 11.8%, p = .00001). In contrast to antigens A2 and Cw3, DR3 was found to be significantly less frequent in patients (15.3% vs. 25.5%, p_{corr} = 0.045, RR = 0.5) as compared to the controls. DR2 was not differently distributed in controls and patients, but this antigen was more often found in stage 0 patients and exhibited decreasing frequency in more advanced stages. All other tested HLA antigens showed no significant differences between patients and controls. The frequency of HLA-DR2 decreased significantly from stage 0 to stage 3 of the disease (rank correlations coefficient of Spearman = -1.00, p = 0.05). An increased frequency of HLA-Cw3 and HLA-Cw4 in patients suffering from acute leukemia was reported and the authors discussed the possibility that these antigens may be markers for a low immune response to putative leukemia viruses.[4] In this sense, HLA-Cw3 may also dispose to BBI. HLA-DR2, being more frequently found in patients with lower stages of BBI, is thought to prevent more severe courses and complications of this infection. This finding compares favorably with the recent report of van Doorn[5] and differs from earlier reports,[1,2] which found an increased risk for complications in HLA-DR2 carriers.

TABLE 2. Woolf-Haldane Analysis of Frequencies of HLA Antigens Significantly Associated with *Borrelia burgdorferi* Infections

	Control group	Stage 0	Stage 1	Stage 2	Stage 3	Stages 1–3
A2 present	195/457	13/37	36/55	47/87	15/28	93/164
RR[a]	—	0.73	3.55	1.58	1.55	1.76
p_{corr}^{b}	—	ns[c]	0.008	ns	ns	0.025
CW3 present	100/457	14/37	19/53	33/86	13/28	62/162
RR	—	2.17	2.00	2.22	3.09	2.21
p_{corr}	—	ns	ns	0.013	0.04	0.0003
DR3 present	121/457	10/34	7/50	12/84	5/27	24/157
RR	—	1.16	0.45	0.46	0.63	0.50
p_{corr}	—	ns	ns	ns	ns	0.045
DR2 present	134/457	14/34	15/50	26/85	7/28	48/157
RR	—	1.69	1.03	1.06	0.80	1.03
p_{corr}	—	ns	ns	ns	ns	ns

[a]RR = relative risk.
[b]p_{corr} = p value after correction for multiple comparisons.
[c]ns = not significant.

REFERENCES

1. STEERE, A. C., A. GIBOFSKY, M. E. PATARROYO, R. J. WINCHESTER, J. A. HARDIN, S. E. MALAWISTA. 1979. Chronic Lyme arthritis. Ann. Intern. Med. **90**: 896–901.
2. STEERE, A. C., A. GIBOFSKY, J. A. HARDIN, R. J. WINCHESTER, S. E. MALAWISTA. 1979. Lyme arthritis: Immunologic and immunogenetic markers (abstract). Arthritis Rheum. **22**: 662–663.
3. KRISTOFERITSCH, W. & W. R. MAYR. 1984. HLA-DR in meningopolyneuritis of Garin-Bujadoux-Bannwarth: Contrast to Lyme disease? J. Neurol. **231**: 271–272.
4. D'AMARO, J., F. H. BACH, J. J. VAN ROOD, A. A. RIMM & M. M. BORTIN. 1984. HLA C associations with acute leukaemia. Lancet **ii**: 1176–1178.
5. VAN DOORN, P. A., A. BRAND, M. VERMEULEN & J. H. J. WOKKE. 1987. Antibodies against neural tissue and DR2 antigen in patients with Bannwarth's syndrome (abstract). Presented at the Lyme Borreliosis Update Europe Conference, Baden, June 2–4.

Vector Competence of Ticks in the Southeastern United States for *Borrelia burgdorferi*[a]

JOSEPH PIESMAN

Department of Epidemiology
School of Public Health
University of Alabama at Birmingham
Birmingham, Alabama 35294

Although human cases of Lyme disease have been reported from the southeastern United States,[1] the vector tick transmitting these infections has not been identified. The three principal person-biting tick species in the southeastern United States are *Amblyomma americanum*, *Dermacentor variabilis*, and *Ixodes scapularis*. The vector competence of these three tick species for *Borrelia burgdorferi* was tested.

All ticks were held at 21°C. *Ixodes* ticks were held at 97% relative humidity (RH), while *Amblyomma* and *Dermacentor* ticks were held at 85% RH. The strain of *A. americanum* used in these experiments originated from Gillespie Co., Texas, and was

TABLE 1. Ability of Larval *Amblyomma americanum* to Acquire *Borrelia burgdorferi* Infection[a]

Host No.	Species[b]	Days Postrepletion							Total
		0–1	1–2	2–3	7–8	9–10	19–20	≥40[c]	
1	Aa	0/15	—	—	—	0/15	0/15	0/82	0/127
	Id	1/6	—	—	—	4/6	5/6	4/5	14/23
2	Aa	0/10	—	—	—	0/10	0/10	0/48	0/78
	Id	2/6	—	—	—	4/6	4/6	6/9	16/27
3	Aa	0/6	—	—	—	0/6	0/6	0/18	0/36
	Id	2/6	—	—	—	6/6	6/6	10/10	24/28
4	Aa	0/33	0/27	0/20	0/15	—	—	0/20	0/115
	Id	7/33	12/27	11/20	9/15	—	—	15/20	54/115
Total	Aa	0/64	0/27	0/20	0/15	0/31	0/31	0/168	0/356 (0%)
	Id	12/51	12/27	11/20	9/15	14/18	15/18	35/44	108/193 (56%)

[a]Measured as no. infected/no. examined.
[b]Aa, *Amblyomma americanum;* Id, *Ixodes dammini.*
[c]Postmolting to nymphs (40–69 days postrepletion).

kindly supplied by Dr. J. George (United States Department of Agriculture). The *I. scapularis* and *D. variabilis* ticks were from Alabama, and the *I. dammini* ticks were from a colony originating on Great Island, Massachusetts. The strain of *B. burgdorferi* used in these experiments (JD1) was isolated and maintained as previously described.[2] Hamsters were infected with spirochetes by serving as hosts to infected nymphal *I.*

[a]This work was supported in part by National Institutes of Health Grant no. AI22847.

417

dammini as previously described.[2] At 3–4 weeks postnymphal exposure, test larvae were allowed to feed on these hamsters. Larval ticks were subsequently examined for spirochetes by dark-field and direct fluorescent antibody methods previously described.[3]

A total of four simultaneous feedings of larval *A. americanum* and *I. dammini* were conducted (TABLE 1). The majority (56%) of *I. dammini* proved to be infected, while 0 out of 356 *A. americanum* were infected. In a single trial, larval *D. variabilis* contained spirochetes when examined within 3 days of repletion (7/37 = 19%); but, only 1 of 12 larvae examined at 10 days postrepletion, and 0 of 20 examined postmolting to nymphs, contained spirochetes (TABLE 2).

Unlike *Amblyomma* and *Dermacentor,* larval *I. scapularis* were efficient in acquiring and maintaining *B. burgdorferi*. In three trials, 25 out of 30 (83%) *I. scapularis* fed as larvae on hamsters were infected when examined as resultant nymphs. In transmission trials with these resultant nymphal *I. scapularis,* 4 out of 4 hamsters exposed to 1, 2, 7, or 14 infected nymphs acquired spirochetal infection.

TABLE 2. Ability of Larval *Dermacentor variabilis* to Acquire *Borrelia burgdorferi* Infection[a]

Species[b]	Days Postrepletion					Total
	0–1	1–2	2–3	9–10	≥38[c]	
Dv	3/15	2/10	2/12	1/12	0/20	8/69 (12%)
Id	7/15	9/10	6/7	6/7	7/7	35/46 (76%)

[a]Measured as no. infected/no. examined.
[b]Dv, *Dermacentor variabilis;* Id, *Ixodes dammini*.
[c]Postmolting to nymphs (38–42 days postrepletion).

The high vector competence of *I. dammini,*[2] *I. scapularis,*[4] *I. ricinus,*[5] and *I. pacificus*[6] for *B. burgdorferi* has been reported previously. In contrast, ticks in other genera (i.e., *Amblyomma, Dermacentor*) appear to acquire and maintain Lyme disease spirochetes inefficiently. There may be unique physiological characteristics of ticks in the genus *Ixodes* that enable them to serve as vectors of *B. burgdorferi*.

REFERENCES

1. Morbid. Mortal. Wkly. Rep. 1985. **34:** 376–378, 383–384.
2. PIESMAN, J., T. N. MATHER, R. J. SINSKY & A. SPIELMAN. 1987. J. Clin. Microbiol. **25:** 557–558.
3. PIESMAN, J., T. N. MATHER, J. G. DONAHUE, J. LEVINE, J. D. CAMPBELL, S. J. KARAKASHIAN & A. SPIELMAN. 1986. Acta Trop. **43:** 263–270.
4. BURGDORFER, W. & K. L. GAGE. 1986. Zbl. Bakt. Hyg. A **263:** 15–20.
5. BURGDORFER, W., A. G. BARBOUR, S. F. HAYES, O. PETER & A. AESCHLIMANN. 1983. Acta Trop. **40:** 79–83.
6. BURGDORFER, W., R. S. LANE, A. G. BARBOUR, R. A. GRESBRINK & J. R. ANDERSON. 1985. Am. J. Trop. Med. Hyg. **34:** 925–930.

Efficacy of Nucleic Acid Hybridization Probes for the Detection and Identification of *Borrelia burgdorferi*

TOM G. SCHWAN

Rocky Mountain Laboratories
National Institute of Allergy and Infectious Diseases
Hamilton, Montana 59840

ALAN G. BARBOUR

University of Texas Health Science Center
San Antonio, Texas 78284

Historically, spirochetes of the genus *Borrelia* have been identified by their arthropod host and geographical place of origin.[1] More recently, guanine-plus-cytosine composition of total genomic DNA has been used to examine species and their taxonomic relationship within the genus.[2] Currently, *Borrelia burgdorferi* is most often identified by reactivity to monoclonal antibodies specific for epitopes associated with outer surface proteins unique to this spirochete.[3]

In the last 15 years, the use of specific sequences of DNA as probes for the sensitive and specific recognition of homologous sequences in numerous cell types has become a powerful tool for molecular biologists, including those interested in infectious diseases.[4] Because of several potential problems in identifying *Borrelia burgdorferi* (and other *Borrelia* species) using serological tests, we examined the potential use of two sequences of DNA as hybridization probes for the specific identification of the Lyme disease spirochete.

Starting with the cloned plasmid-encoded gene for the outer surface protein A of *B. burgdorferi*,[5] we subcloned two fragments and used them as DNA hybridization probes for both purified plasmid DNA and whole spirochetes of three strains of *B. burgdorferi*, as well as *B. hermsii, B. parkeri, B. turicatae, B. coriaceae, B. crocidurae,* and *B. anserina*. Plasmid DNA was purified as described previously,[6] except that cesium chloride density gradient centrifugation was not done. DNA concentration and purity were determined by UV absorbance at 260 nm and 280 nm. DNA sequences used as probes were nick-translated using a commercial kit and labeled with ^{32}P-dCTP following instructions of the manufacturer (BRL, Gaithersburg, MD). Hybridizations were done on GeneScreen *Plus* following the instructions of the manufacturer (NEN, Boston), and membranes were exposed to Kodak X-OMAT film at −70°C with an intensifying screen and developed with a Kodak X-OMAT M20 processor. Spirochetes were cultured in BSK-II medium[7] and counted by dark-field microscopy using Stoenner's method.[8]

Probe 3G (0.445-kilobase *Pst* I–*Hind* III fragment, FIG. 1) and probe 16H (0.32-kilobase *Hind* III–*Hind* III fragment) both hybridized strongly with plasmid DNA and whole spirochetes of two North American strains of *B. burgdorferi* (B31 and HB19), but only weakly with a strain from Germany identified as *B. burgdorferi* by reactivity with mAb H5332. Both probes also hybridized weakly with *B. hermsii* but not with the other species tested. Probe 3G, being approximately 125 bases larger, was slightly more sensitive than probe 16H, and was able to detect down to 500 picograms

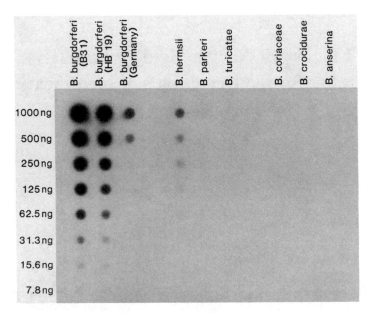

FIGURE 1. Hybridization of probe 3G with serial dilutions of purified plasmid DNA of three strains of *Borrelia burgdorferi* and six other *Borrelia* species. GeneScreen *Plus* was presoaked in 0.5 M Tris, pH 7.55, for 30 minutes and then placed in a 96-well blot manifold (BioRad) and tightened under vacuum. Serial dilutions of DNA in 0.125 N NaOH, 0.125×SSC (1× SSC = 0.15 M sodium chloride, 0.015 M sodium citrate) were loaded in wells and pulled onto the membrane with vacuum. The membrane was air dried (37°C), denatured with 0.5 N NaOH (twice, 2 minutes each), neutralized with 1 M Tris (twice, 2 minutes each), and air dried. The membrane was prehybridized with 50% formamide, 6×SSC, 5× Denhardt's solution, 0.5% SDS, 0.1% sodium pyrophosphate, and denatured salmon sperm DNA for 24 hours at 42°C, followed by probe hybridization for 16 hours at the same temperature. The membrane was washed twice 5 minutes each in 2×SSC at room temperature, twice 15 minutes each in 2×SSC, 1% SDS at 65°C, and twice 15 minutes each in 0.1×SSC at 65°C.

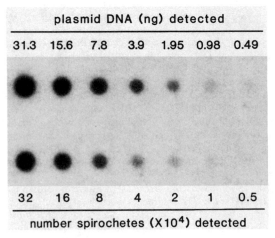

FIGURE 2. Limits of sensitivity of probe 3G hybridized with purified plasmid DNA and whole spirochetes of *Borrelia burgdorferi* (B31).

of DNA and 10,000 spirochetes (FIG. 2). Both probes failed to detect spirochetes in midgut tissues of infected *Ixodes dammini*. With reduced exposure times of hybridization membranes to film, cross-reactivity with *B. hermsii* can be eliminated, giving these probes the required specificity to identify North American isolates of *B. burgdorferi* after the number of spirochetes have been amplified in culture.

REFERENCES

1. DAVIS, G. E. 1948. Ann. Rev. Microbiol. **2:** 305–334.
2. HYDE, F. W. & R. C. JOHNSON. 1984. J. Clin. Microbiol. **20:** 151–154.
3. BARBOUR, A. G., R. A. HEILAND & T. R. HOWE. 1985. J. Infect. Dis. **152:** 478–484.
4. LERMAN, L. S., Ed. 1986. DNA Probes: Applications in Genetic and Infectious Disease and Cancer. Cold Spring Harbor Laboratory. New York.
5. HOWE, T. R., F. W. LAQUIER & A. G. BARBOUR. 1986. Infect. Immun. **54:** 207–212.
6. BARBOUR, A. G. & C. F. GARON. 1987. Science **237:** 409–411.
7. BARBOUR, A. G. 1984. Yale J. Biol. Med. **57:** 521–525.
8. STOENNER, H. G. 1974. Appl. Microbiol. **28:** 540–543.

IgM in the Sera of Patients with Lyme Neurologic Disease Bind to Cross-reacting Neuronal and *Borrelia burgdorferi* Antigens

L. H. SIGAL AND A. H. TATUM

Departments of Medicine and Pathology
VAMC/SUNY-Health Science Center
Syracuse, New York 13210

We tested sera of patients with ECM, arthritis, and neurologic manifestations of Lyme disease (LD) for their ability to bind to human nerve in indirect immunofluorescence (IIF). Neurologic patients had IgM anti-*B. burgdorferi* antibodies that cross-react with human axons. Thus, the specific humoral response to *B. burgdorferi* may produce antibodies capable of binding to host tissues. These auto-antibodies may play a role in the immunopathogenesis of the neurologic lesions of LD.

MATERIALS AND METHODS

A sonicate of *B. burgdorferi* was prepared (BAg) as previously described.[1] Normal spinal cord was homogenized and extracted in 3% Triton X in saline (NAg). Sera (seven from patients with ECM, six with chronic arthritis, and seven with neurologic damage) were randomly chosen from a bank of LD sera. Normals and patients with diabetic neuropathy and Guillain-Barré syndrome (previously found to have serum IgM anti-axonal antibodies) and osteoarthritis and rheumatoid-factor-positive rheumatoid arthritis were also studied. Monoclonal antibodies to *B. burgdorferi* OspA, OspB, and flagellin were obtained.[2,3] IIF was done on sections of normal human nerve. After incubation with sera, the sections were overlaid with fluorosceinated anti-human IgM, rinsed, and viewed. Sera positive at a 1 : 5 dilution were serially diluted twofold until they reacted <1+. Sera four times more concentrated than this were then incubated with the BAg or NAg, centrifuged, and the clarified sera tested.

RESULTS

LD neurologic disease sera had IgM that bound to human axons (TABLE 1). LD arthritis patients had less reactivity and those with ECM usually had none. Only one ECM patient had binding; she was studied 7 days after onset of ECM with uncomplicated disease, but had *in vivo* and *in vitro* evidence of extreme B-cell hyperactivity.[4] Sera from normals and patients with non-LD arthritis did not bind. The IgM anti-axonal activity in diabetic neuropathy and Guillain-Barré syndrome was not affected by absorption with BAg, but was eliminated by absorption with NAg.

LD anti-axonal binding was also eliminated by NAg absorption. However, unlike the other groups the LD sera's anti-axonal binding was eliminated by absorption with BAg.

Monoclonal antibodies to OspA and OspB did not bind to human nerve sections. The antiflagellin antibody bound to axons, in a pattern identical with that of the LD sera.

DISCUSSION

The presence of anti-axonal antibodies in neurologic patients as early as the first week of LD suggests that the anti-axonal reactivity is not due to an immune response to axonal antigens liberated from previously damaged nerves. The cross-reactivity is unlikely to be coincidental; none was demonstrated in the non-LD neuropathies. The reactivity of the antiflagellin antibody with human axons suggests that flagellin is an antigen responsible for the cross-reactivity.

Anti-axonal binding may represent the potential to develop neurologic damage. Other, perhaps cellular, mechanisms may be required; BAg-reactive cells have been

TABLE 1. Indirect Immunofluorescence, Using Sera from Patients with Lyme Disease and Controls Diluted in PBS[a]

	0	1 : 5	1 : 10	1 : 20	1 : 40
Lyme disease					
Neurologic disease ($n = 7$)					
Cranial nerve palsies		1	0	1	2
Meningoencephalitis			1	2	
Arthritis ($n = 6$)	3	2	1		
ECM ($n = 7$)	6			1	
Controls					
Normal sera ($n = 8$)	8				
Rheumatoid arthritis ($n = 4$)	4				
Osteoarthritis ($n = 4$)	4				
Diabetic neuropathy ($n = 2$)				1	1
Guillain-Barré syndrome ($n = 2$)				1	1

[a]Results indicate the highest dilution at which the serum gave definite 1+ anti-axonal reactivity.

found in the cerebrospinal fluid of patients with LD meningo-encephalitis.[5] It is also possible that a subclinical neuropathy was present in the case of ECM and LD arthritis with anti-axonal activity.

Antibodies made as part of the specific immune response to *B. burgdorferi* also bind to human axons and are found preferentially in the serum of patients with LD neurologic disease. One cross-reacting borrelial antigen may be flagellin. This study suggests that LD neurologic disease may be due to the production of cross-reacting auto-antibodies, produced by molecular mimicry.

REFERENCES

1. SIGAL, L. H., A. C. STEERE, D. H. FREEMAN & J. M. DWYER. 1986. Proliferative responses of mononuclear cells in Lyme disease: Reactivity to *Borrelia burgdorferi* antigens is greater and the response to mitogens is less in joint fluid than in blood. Arthritis Rheum. **29**: 761–769.

2. BARBOUR, A. G., S. F. HAYES, R. A. HEILAND, *et al.* 1986. A *Borrelia*-specific monoclonal
    antibody to a flagellar epitope. Infect. Immun. **52**: 549–554.
3. BARBOUR, A. G., S. L. TESSIER & S. F. HAYES. 1984. Variation in a major surface protein of
    Lyme disease spirochetes. Infect. Immun. **45**: 94–100.
4. SIGAL, L. H., A. C. STEERE & J. M. DWYER. 1988. *In vivo* and *in vitro* B cell hyperactivity in
    Lyme disease. J. Rheumatol. **15**: 648–654.
5. PACHNER, A. R., A. C. STEERE, L. H. SIGAL & C. J. JOHNSON. 1985. Antigen-specific
    proliferation of CSF lymphocytes in Lyme disease. Neurology **35**: 1642–1644.

Interaction between *Borrelia burgdorferi* and Polymorphonuclear Leukocytes

Phagocytosis and the Induction of the Respiratory Burst

ANDREW SZCZEPANSKI AND HOWARD B. FLEIT

Department of Pathology
SUNY at Stony Brook
Stony Brook, New York 11794

INTRODUCTION

The ability of polymorphonuclear leukocytes (PMN) to engulf and kill bacteria is of major importance in host defense against bacterial infection. An important microbicidal mechanism of phagocytic cells is the formation of toxic oxygen metabolites following the stimulation of the respiratory burst. The phagocytosis of *Borrelia burgdorferi* by phagocytic cells has been described.[1,2] The ability of the spirochetes to induce the respiratory burst in PMN was also examined using a chemiluminescence assay.[2] Both of these studies described the phagocytosis of spirochetes in the presence and absence of immune serum, however little is known about the mechanism of uptake of these spirochetes in the absence of serum opsonins. In the present studies the early events in the phagocytosis of unopsonized *Borrelia burgdorferi* were examined ultrastructurally. In addition, the induction of the respiratory burst in PMN by opsonized and unopsonized spirochetes was compared using the nitroblue tetrazolium (NBT) reduction assay.[3]

METHODS

For ultrastructural studies of phagocytosis the spirochetes and PMN were centrifuged into a pellet at 4°C and warmed to 37°C. Spirochete to PMN ratios of 50 : 1 and 100 : 1 were used. Phagocytosis was terminated by fixing the pellets with 3% glutaraldehyde in 0.2M sodium cacodylate buffer. Fixed specimens were then osmicated, dehydrated in a graded series of ethanol solutions, and embedded in epon. Thin sections were prepared, stained with uranyl acetate and lead citrate, and observed in a transmission electron microscope. Some specimens were prepared using 0.1% ruthenium red during fixation in glutaraldehyde and osmication in order to stain for cell surface carbohydrate.[4] NBT reduction to formazan was examined on cytospin preparations of PMN-spirochete suspensions. PMN used in this study were isolated from normal healthy donors by Ficoll-Hypaque centrifugation followed by dextran sedimentation and osmotic lysis to remove red blood cells. Prior to use, both spirochetes and PMN were washed and resuspended in RPMI-1640. NBT (Sigma Chem. Co.) was prepared the day of use as a 0.2% stock solution in Hanks balanced salt solution.

RESULTS AND DISCUSSION

The phagocytosis of unopsonized *Borrelia burgdorferi* by polymorphonuclear leukocytes was observed as early as 1 minute following warming to 37°C of spirochete-PMN pellets. Ruthenium red, a stain that identifies cell surface carbohydrates for ultrastructural analysis, demonstrated the direct contact between spirochete outer

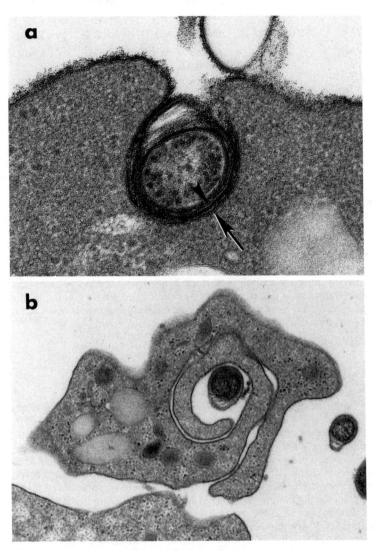

FIGURE 1. Phagocytosis of unopsonized *Borrelia burgdorferi*. (a) A ruthenium red stained pellet demonstrates the close apposition of spirochete outer membrane (*arrowhead*) to the neutrophil plasma membrane (*arrow*); (magnification: 116,000 ×). (b) In certain instances pseudopod coils were observed around unopsonized spirochetes; (magnification: 38,400 ×).

TABLE 1. NBT Reduction by Polymorphonuclear Leukocytes

Stimulus	Percent Cells Reducing NBT[a]
Experiment 1: Dose Response to Spirochetes	
Control[b]	1.3
10 ng/ml PMA	94.3
100 ng/ml PMA	95.5
5×10^5 spirochetes	7.5
5×10^6 spirochetes	51.0
5×10^7 spirochetes	99.0
Experiment 2: Effect of Opsonization on NBT Reduction	
Control[b]	1.0
1 ng/ml PMA	18.4
10 ng/ml PMA	68.1
100 ng/ml PMA	91.3
5×10^5 IS[c] opsonized spirochetes	8.8
5×10^6 IS[c] opsonized spirochetes	24.0
5×10^5 NHS[d] opsonized spirochetes	8.3
5×10^6 NHS[d] opsonized spirochetes	20.0
5×10^5 unopsonized spirochetes	4.7
5×10^6 unopsonized spirochetes	18.0

Each sample contained 5×10^5 PMN in a total volume of 0.2 ml containing 0.1% nitroblue tetrazolium (NBT). Cells were incubated with spirochetes or phorbol myristate acetate (PMA), as a positive control, for 30 minutes at 37°C on an orbital shaker.

[a]Percentage of cells containing blue-black formazan deposits as determined by see title page.

membrane and neutrophil plasma membrane (FIG. 1a). During the phagocytosis of spirochetes the coiling of pseudopods around unopsonized spirochetes was observed (FIG. 1b). The pseudopod coils were similar in appearance to the process of coiling phagocytosis described for unopsonized *Legionella pneumophila*.[5] The ability of *Borrelia burgdorferi* to induce the respiratory burst in PMN was examined by the NBT reduction assay (TABLE 1). The percent of PMN containing reduced NBT increased as a function of spirochete number. Ninety-nine percent of the PMN contained reduced NBT at a spirochete-to-PMN ratio of 100 : 1. Opsonization of the spirochetes with immune serum produced a slight increase in the percentage of NBT-positive PMN using spirochete to PMN ratios of 1 : 1 and 10 : 1, but the effect of opsonization on NBT reduction was much less dramatic than that of spirochete concentration. These studies demonstrate that (1) the phagocytosis of unopsonized *Borrelia burgdorferi* by PMN is initiated by direct contact of the spirochete outer membrane with the plasma membrane of the PMN; (2) some *B. burgdorferi* are internalized by PMN by coiling phagocytosis as observed previously with unopsonized *L. pneumophila;* (3) the induction of the respiratory burst in PMN was dependent on the number of unopsonized spirochetes.

ACKNOWLEDGMENTS

These studies were supported by the Sinsheimer Foundation.

REFERENCES

1. BENACH, J. L., H. B. FLEIT, G. S. HABICHT, J. L. COLEMAN, E. M. BOSLER & B. P. LANE. 1984. Interactions of phagocytes with the Lyme disease spirochete: Role of the Fc receptor. J. Infect. Dis. **150:** 497–507.
2. PETERSON, P. K., C. C. CLAWSON, D. A. LEE, D. J. GARLICH, P. G. QUIE & R. C. JOHNSON. 1984. Human phagocyte interaction with the Lyme disease spirochete. Infect. Immun. **46**(2): 608–611.
3. BAEHNER, R. L. & D. A. NATHAN. 1968. Quantitative nitroblue tetrazolium test in chronic granulomatous disease. N. Engl. J. Med. **278:** 971–976.
4. CHAMBERS, V. C. 1973. The use of ruthernium red in an electron microscope study of cytophagocytosis. J. Cell Biol. **57:** 874–878.
5. HORWITZ, M. A. 1984. Phagocytosis of the Legionnaire's disease bacterium *(Legionella pneumophila)* occurs by a novel mechanism: Engulfment with a pseudopod coil. Cell **36:** 27–33.

Incompetence of Deer as Reservoirs of *Borrelia burgdorferi*

SAM R. TELFORD III, THOMAS N. MATHER,
SEAN I. MOORE, MARK L. WILSON, AND ANDREW
SPIELMAN

Department of Tropical Public Health
Harvard School of Public Health
Boston, Massachusetts 02115

An effective reservoir must be physiologically and ecologically competent to deliver a given pathogen. Many mammalian species have been considered to be reservoirs of the Lyme disease spirochete, *Borrelia burgdorferi*, yet, with one exception, none have been rigorously tested for both criteria. The white-footed mouse, *Peromyscus leucopus*, effectively transmits *B. burgdorferi* to the vector tick, *Ixodes dammini*.[1] Furthermore, a major fraction of immature *I. dammini* are fed by this mouse,[2] and it is by far the most abundant host.

White-tailed deer (*Odocoileus virginianus*) feed all stages of *I. dammini*. It is therefore not surprising that deer are infected by *B. burgdorferi* in enzootic areas.[3] Whether larval *I. dammini* are infected by feeding upon deer has not been demonstrated, nor has the contribution of deer relative to that of the white-footed mouse in feeding larval ticks been quantified. To implicate deer as major reservoirs[4] is unjustified.

Accordingly, we shot 19 deer from two intensely enzootic sites, Hog and Naushon Islands in coastal Massachusetts, during September 1986, to evaluate the reservoir competence of deer for the Lyme disease spirochete. Nymphal activity is maximal in June and July.[5] Therefore, deer in these localities were assumed to have been heavily exposed to infection, since 10–25% of questing nymphs are infected with *B. burgdorferi*. To be effective as a reservoir, deer must be infective during August and September, during the peak of larval tick activity.

An average of 342 ($\pm$115 SE) larval *I. dammini* infested each deer. We collected engorged larvae from 14 deer, and allowed them to molt to nymphs, 185 of which were examined for *B. burgdorferi* by a direct fluorescent antibody procedure. Two nymphs, derived from separate deer, were infected. This rate of infection (1.1%) is low when compared with that of nymphs derived from *P. leucopus* (46.9%), and is consistent with estimates of the prevalence of transovarially infected ticks in these sites.[6]

Deer are abundant, vagile, and long-lived. They serve as host to all stages of *I. dammini,* and are probably the only rivals to *P. leucopus* in terms of their contribution towards feeding immature ticks. Ecologically, they could be important reservoirs of a tick-transmitted pathogen. They are, however, physiologically incompetent in transmitting *B. burgdorferi* to larval *I. dammini.*

REFERENCES

1. DONAHUE, J. G., J. PIESMAN & A. SPIELMAN. 1987. Am. J. Trop. Med. Hyg. **36:** 92–96.
2. PIESMAN, J. & A. SPIELMAN. 1979. Ann. Entomol. Soc. Am. **72:** 829–832.

3. MAGNARELLI, L. A., J. F. ANDERSON & W. A. CHAPPELL. 1984. J. Wildl. Dis. **20:** 21–26.
4. BOSLER, E., B. G. ORMOSTON, J. L. COLEMAN, J. P. HANRAHAN & J. L. BENACH. 1984. Yale J. Biol. Med. **57:** 651–659.
5. WILSON, M. L. & A. SPIELMAN. 1985. J. Med. Entomol. **22:** 408–414.
6. PIESMAN, J., J. G. DONAHUE & A. SPIELMAN. 1986. J. Med. Entomol. **23:** 219.

Immunoregulatory Abnormalities in
Borrelia burgdorferi Infection

J. A. THOMAS, R. LIPSCHITZ, M. G. GOLIGHTLY,
AND R. J. DATTWYLER

Department of Pathology
University Hospital
SUNY at Stony Brook
Stony Brook, NY 11794

Previously we have found that peripheral blood mononuclear cells (PBMC) from patients with Lyme borreliosis (LB) have strong proliferative responses to *Borrelia burgdorferi* (Bb), but a decreased response to the mitogen concanavalin A (ConA).[1,2] A similar disparity between antigen-mitogen responsiveness has been described in synovial fluid mononuclear cells (SFMC) from patients with rheumatoid arthritis (RA) and juvenile rheumatoid arthritis (JRA).[3-5] These arthritides have many clinical and pathological features in common with the inflammatory arthritis of LB that may be linked to a common immunoregulatory abnormality. A subpopulation of CD4[+] cells that expresses the antigen 2H4 is responsible for the induction of suppression. This subpopulation has a strong proliferative response to ConA but proliferates poorly to soluble antigens.[6] In contrast, the CD4[+]4B4[+] population, which is responsible for B-cell help, is known to have a strong proliferative response to soluble antigens but a relatively poor response to ConA.[7] In this study we have phenotypically characterized PBMC and SFMC from patients with LB and other inflammatory arthritides using two-color immunofluorescence and flow cytometry to determine the involvement of these and other immunoregulatory cells in the pathophysiology of these diseases.

Sixteen synovial fluid samples were obtained for analysis: 5 LB, 5 RA, 1 JRA, 1 polychondritis, and 4 traumatic. The traumatic SFs yielded an insufficient number of mononuclear cells for analysis. In addition, 32 PB were studied: 13 LB, 5 RA, 1 JRA, and 13 normal controls. TABLE 1 shows the results of phenotypic characterization of T-cell subpopulations from the PB and SFMCs. In both LB and non-LB SF the percentage of CD3[+] cells did not differ, but the CD4[+]:CD8[+] ratio was significantly different ($p < .005$). This ratio was markedly higher in the SF from LB patients. Activated T cells were demonstrated by the presence of HLA-DR. Although the relative percentages of activated T cells within each subpopulation were similar in both SF groups, the absolute number of activated CD8[+] cells was higher in the non-LB SF, while the absolute number of activated CD4[+] cells was higher in the Lyme SF. A significant number of activated CD8[+] cells ($p < .025$) was detected in LB PB but not in the RA or control PB. In the PB of patients with LB there was a significant reduction ($p < .025$) in the percentage of the suppressor-inducer (SI) subpopulation (CD4[+]2H4[+]) when compared to either RA patients or normal controls. This immunoregulatory imbalance was much more pronounced in all SFs studied, as evidenced by the virtual absence of the SI subpopulation and the predominance of helper-inducer (HI) subpopulation. TABLE 2 displays the results of additional phenotypic analysis of SFMCs. There was a significant increase in the percentage of NKH-1[+] cells in the LB SF, whereas no differences were noted in the expression of other NK cell antigens (CD16[+], Leu-7[+]). In addition, the percentages of Leu-M3[+], CDw13[+], and CDw14[+] cells were similar.

431

TABLE 1. T Cell Subpopulations in PB and SFMC: A Comparison of LB and Other Inflammatory Athritides

	PBMC			SFMC	
Phenotype	Control	LB	RA	LB	Non-lyme[a]
CD3$^+$CD4^{+e}	44.4 ± 2.4	43.0 ± 2.9	41.4 ± 4.5	43.7 ± 4.6^c	27.7 ± 3.6
CD3$^+$CD8^{+e}	17.9 ± 1.7	15.5 ± 2.3	9.2 ± 1.9^b	14.4 ± 1.3^c	30.4 ± 4.4
CD4$^+$HLA-DR^{+d}	0.3 ± 0.3	1.2 ± 0.8	1.7 ± 1.0	26.0 ± 8.3	27.0 ± 5.1
CD8$^+$HLA-DR^{+g}	3.5 ± 1.3	13.8 ± 4.9^b	0.2 ± 0.1	56.6 ± 9.9	51.0 ± 12.4
CD4$^+$2H4^{+d}	44.5 ± 3.8	30.7 ± 3.6^b	49.8 ± 3.0	4.9 ± 3.0	4.5 ± 2.5
CD4$^+$4B4^{+d}	48.0 ± 3.7	56.9 ± 9.9^c	42.4 ± 3.9	88.7 ± 4.7	93.3 ± 4.4
CD2^{+e}	73.8 ± 5.3	84.4 ± 1.3^b	79.8 ± 3.8	79.6 ± 3.8	74.0 ± 7.3
CD4$^+$/CD8^{+f}	2.9 ± 0.4	3.7 ± 0.7	4.9 ± 1.3	3.2 ± 0.5^c	1.1 ± 0.3
CD4$^+$2H4$^+$/ CD4$^+$4B4^{+f}	1.2 ± 0.2	2.4 ± 0.4^{b,c}	0.9 ± 0.1	18.1 ± 2.1	20.7 ± 2.3

PBMC, peripheral blood mononuclear cells; SFMC, synovial fluid mononuclear cells; LB, Lyme borreliosis; RA, rheumatoid arthritis.
[a]Non-LB includes RA, JRA, and polychondritis.
[b]Statistically significant ($p < .05$) when compared to control group.
[c]Statistically significant ($p < .05$) when test groups are compared.
[d]Numbers are expressed as a percentage of CD4$^+$ cells.
[e]Numbers are expressed as a percentage of lymphocytes.
[f]Numbers are expressed as a ratio.
[g]Numbers are expressed as a percentage of CD8$^+$ cells.

The imbalance between CD4$^+$2H4$^+$ (SI) and CD4$^+$4B4$^+$ (HI) regulatory T cells demonstrated offers an explanation for the disparity in antigen-mitogen responsiveness of SFMC. This immunoregulatory imbalance provides a model for a sustained inflammatory response due to the loss of suppressor-inducer activity in joints of patients with inflammatory arthritis. Since it has been demonstrated that the induction of suppression by the CD4$^+$2H4$^+$ population is antigen-specific,[8] it is possible that the local production of antigen-specific antibodies in SF becomes uncontrolled after initial stimulation. This could lead to the deposition of immune complexes that may result in a chronic inflammatory response. In conclusion, these findings indicate a significant role of the cellular immune response in the pathogenesis of LB and other inflammatory arthritides.

TABLE 2. Additional Phenotypical Characterization of SFMC

Phenotype	LB	Non-LB
CD20$^+$ (B1)	5.2 ± 2.5	4.1 ± 1.0
CDW13$^+$ (MY7)	32.6 ± 8.8	25.3 ± 6.6
CDW14$^+$ (MY4)	27.3 ± 4.9	22.0 ± 4.0
Leu M3$^+$	22.2 ± 3.7	15.5 ± 5.5
Leu 7$^+$	9.3 ± 2.7	9.4 ± 3.3
CD16$^+$(Leu-11)	14.5 ± 3.9	12.1 ± 2.8
NKH-1$^+$	25.6 ± 3.9^a	8.5 ± 3.7

All numbers are expressed as a percentage of mononuclear cells; LB, Lyme borreliosis; non-LB represents SF from RA, JRA, and polychondritis.
[a]Statistically significant ($p < .005$) when compared to other test groups.

REFERENCES

1. DATTWYLER, R. J., J. A. THOMAS, J. L. BENACH & M. G. GOLIGHTLY. 1986. Cellular immune response in Lyme disease: The response to mitogens, live *Borrelia burgdorferi*, NK cell function, and lymphocyte subsets. Zbl. Bakt. Hyg. A **263:** 151–159.
2. DATTWYLER, R. J., J. A. THOMAS, J. L. BENACH, *et al.* 1985. Serum immunoregulatory factors in Lyme disease. Clin. Res. **33**(2): 399A.
3. ABRAHAMSEN, T. G., S. S. FROLAND & J. B. NATVIG. 1978. *In vitro* mitogen stimulation of synovial fluid lymphocytes from rheumatoid arthritis and juvenile rheumatoid arthritis patients: Dissociation between the response to antigens and polyclonal mitogens. Scand. J. Immunol. **7:** 81–90.
4. PETERSEN, J., V. ANDERSEN, G. BENDIXEN, *et al.* 1982. Functional characteristics of synovial fluid and blood mononuclear cells in rheumatoid arthritis and traumatic synovitis. Scand. J. Rheumatol. **11:** 75–80.
5. PETERSEN, J., V. ANDERSEN, T. INGEMANN-HANSEN, *et al.* 1983. Synovial fluid and blood monocyte influence on lymphocyte proliferation in rheumatoid arthritis and traumatic synovitis. Scand. J. Rheumatol. **12:** 299–304.
6. MORIMOTO, C., N. L. LETVIN, J. A. DISTASO, *et al.* 1985. The isolation and characterization of the human suppressor inducer T cell subset. J. Immunol. **134**(3): 1508–1515.
7. MORIMOTO, C., N. L. LETVIN, A. W. BOYD, *et al.* 1985. The isolation and characterization of the human helper inducer T cell subset. J. Immunol. **134**(6): 3762–3769.
8. MORIMOTO, C., N. L. LETVIN, J. A. DISTASO, *et al.* 1986. The cellular basis for the induction of antigen-specific T8 suppressor cells. Eur. J. Immunol. **16:** 198–204.

Detection of Antibodies to Salivary Gland Components of *Ixodes dammini*[a]

CHRISTINE M. WHEELER, JAMES L. COLEMAN,
EDWARD M. BOSLER, AND JORGE L. BENACH

New York State Department of Health
SUNY at Stony Brook
Stony Brook, New York 11794

INTRODUCTION

Acquired resistance to antigens derived from the feeding activities of ticks can result in lower engorgement weights and even death of the tick while still attached.[1,2] Evidence for antibody and cellular immune responses to tick antigens are known to occur.[3] In this study, we present evidence for *Ixodes dammini* salivary gland antigen-specific antibody responses in two species of mammals and lack of evidence for the presence of spirochetes in salivary gland preparations of *I. dammini* females.

METHODS

Ixodes dammini were collected in eastern Long Island and placed in plastic capsules bound to New Zealand white rabbits. The weights of engorged females and the sizes of tick lesions were recorded. Salivary glands of unengorged female *I. dammini* were homogenized in PBS and the total protein content of the soluble fraction was determined. Five μg of salivary gland protein was subjected to SDS-PAGE (12.5% acrylamide) and transferred to nitrocellulose. Western blots were done with serum from rabbits and dogs previously exposed to multiple *I. dammini* feedings.

RESULTS

There was a significant decrease in the engorgement weight of *I. dammini* as a result of repeated tick feedings on rabbits (first feeding, $\bar{x} \pm SD = 166$ mg $\pm$ 89; second feeding, 139 mg $\pm$ 76; third feeding, 34 mg $\pm$ 23; Student's *t* test, $p \leq .05$). The diameter of the tick lesions was also reduced after subsequent feedings (first feeding, 4 mm $\pm$ 0.5; third feeding, 3 mm $\pm$ 0.05). Only 64% of the females survived the engorgement period on the rabbit during the second and third feedings. Both rabbits and dogs produce antibodies to salivary gland antigens of *I. dammini* (FIG. 1). The rabbits produced antibodies to a salivary gland antigen with a M_r of 12 kDa and the dogs produced antibodies to a salivary gland protein with a M_r of 18 kDa as well as to other salivary gland antigens with approximate M_rs of 53 kDa and 120 kDa. In

[a]This work was funded by grant no. AI-23167 from the National Institutes of Health to Jorge L. Benach.

434

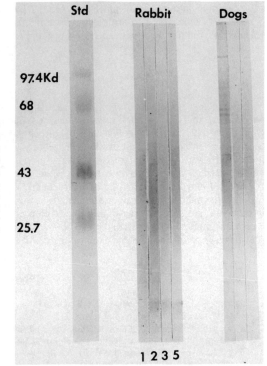

FIGURE 1. Western blots of salivary gland antigen using serum from rabbits and dogs exposed to female *I. dammini* followed by horseradish-peroxidase-conjugated anti-rabbit and anti-dog Ig with 4-chloro-1-naphthol as substrate. Molecular weight markers are the first lane on the left. The numbers under the rabbit strips refer to the number of tick feedings.

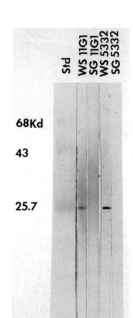

FIGURE 2. Western blots of salivary gland and whole spirochete antigen treated with monoclonal 11G1 and H-5332 followed by horseradish-peroxidase-conjugated anti-mouse IgM and IgG, respectively, with 4-chloro-1-naphthol as substrate. Molecular weight markers are the first lane on the left. Abbreviations: *WS*, whole spirochete; *SG*, salivary gland.

addition, murine monoclonal antibodies H5332 (courtesy of Dr. Alan Barbour) and NYS-11G1, which bind to antigenic determinants of the OspA antigen of *Borrelia burgdorferi*, did not react with the salivary gland preparation (FIG. 2).

DISCUSSION

It is unclear whether *I. dammini* transmits the Lyme disease spirochete, *Borrelia burgdorferi*, to its host via the saliva or regurgitation of midgut contents. The salivary gland should be the most likely source of spirochetal antigen, since large quantities of saliva are released to the host during tick feedings. However, our findings suggest that if the spirochete is present in the salivary gland extract, it is present in such low numbers that it can not be detected by Western blot analysis. Monoclonal antibody NYS-11G1 can detect up to 10 pg of spirochetal OspA in Western blots.

Rabbits and dogs produce antibodies to salivary gland antigens, indicating that as in other animal species,[4] these animals develop antibody responses to tick antigens. These antibodies may contribute to the low engorgement weights of ticks fed on previously exposed animals and even to tick death.

REFERENCES

1. BROWN, S. J. 1982. Antibody- and cell-mediated immune resistance by guinea pigs to adult *Amblyomma americanum* ticks. Am. J. Trop. Med. Hyg. **31**(6): 1285–1290.
2. BROWN, S. J. & P. W. ASKENASE. 1983. Immune rejection of ectoparasites (ticks) by T cell and IgG antibody recruitment of basophils and eosinophils. Fed. Proc. **42**: 1744–1749.
3. BENACH, J. L., G. S. HABICHT, B. L. GOCINSKI & J. L. COLEMAN. 1984. Phagocytic cell responses to *in vivo* and *in vitro* exposure to the Lyme disease spirochete. Yale J. Biol. Med. **57**: 599–605.
4. WIKEL, S. K., J. E. GRAHAM & J. R. ALLEN. 1978. Acquired resistance to ticks. Immunology **34**: 257–263.

Microgeographic Distribution of Deer and of *Ixodes dammini*

Options for Reducing the Risk of Lyme Disease[a]

MARK L. WILSON,[b,e] THOMAS S. LITWIN,[c] AND
THOMAS A. GAVIN[d]

[b]*Department of Tropical Public Health*
Harvard School of Public Health
Boston, Massachusetts 02115

[c]*Seatuck Research Program*
Cornell Laboratory of Ornithology
P.O. Box 31
Islip, New York 11751

[d]*Department of Natural Resources*
Cornell University
Ithaca, New York 14853

The distribution and abundance of *Ixodes dammini* is influenced by availability of suitable hosts, movement of infested vertebrates, and possibly climate or geography.[1] Among the hosts for adult ticks, white-tailed deer (*Odocoileus virginianus*) are most heavily parasitized. Studies have shown that the abundance of this host was correlated with that of the tick,[2] and virtual eradication of deer decreased tick density.[3] Various medium-sized mammals, however, are also infested by this tick.[1] We examined the relative importance of other mammals as hosts for adult ticks, and the small-scale spatial distribution over which deer and tick densities might be correlated. Our study was conducted at the 80 ha Seatuck National Wildlife Refuge (lat. 40°43' N, long. 73°13' W) in Islip, NY (FIG. 1). Many mammal species were abundant, including numerous deer; *I. dammini* were frequently encountered and cases of Lyme disease had been diagnosed there. To estimate tick and host abundances, we periodically captured, examined and released deer, racoons, opossums, and domestic animals during September through December, when adult ticks are most active.[1] As a measure of feeding success, female ticks were weighed. During this time we also used radiotelemetry to determine systematically the relative frequency with which deer were found in 0.25-ha quadrants of the refuge. The abundance of immature ticks was then estimated during the following summer, when these stadia are most active,[4] by examining white-footed mice (*Peromyscus leucopus*) captured on the quadrants. Relative densities of hosts were determined by enumeration, trapping success, or capture-recapture estimates.

Deer harbored the most female ticks per individual and, although their density was

[a]This work was supported by the New York State Department of Environmental Conservation's Gift to Wildlife Program, Cornell University (Hatch Project 147442), the United States Fish and Wildlife Service, the National Institute of Alergy and Infectious Diseases (no. AI 19693), and the Seatuck Research Program.
[e]Present address: Institut Pasteur, B.P.: 220, Dakar, Senegal.

437

less than that of racoons, they hosted 94.6% of the feeding tick population. Racoons, cats, and opossums provided blood-meals to 3.6%, 1.6%, and 0.2% of female ticks, respectively. The engorgement success of ticks feeding on cats and racoons, however, was better than that on deer. Frequency of deer sightings per quadrant was positively correlated with mean number of larval ($p < .001$) and nymphal ($p < .012$) *I. dammini* per mouse (TABLE 1).

Although deer are not reservoirs for *Borrelia burgdorferi*,[5] this one species is a crucial determinant of the density and spatial distribution of the vector tick. Other hosts harbor few adult ticks, and therefore, most reproduction of *I. dammini* results from blood-meals taken from deer. The spatial distribution of tick-infested deer during fall corresponded to that of larval and nymphal ticks the following summer. Replete adult *I. dammini* presumably drop from deer most frequently at sites that they use most extensively. Eggs are laid there, larvae emerge, and then quest for hosts. Thus, over the scale of tens of meters, deer density and activity appear to determine the local abundance of immature ticks. *I. dammini*-borne disease depends largely upon human-

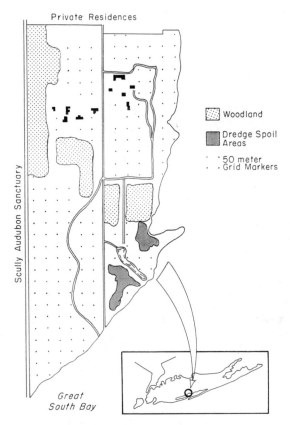

FIGURE 1. Map of the Seatuck National Wildlife Refuge, Islip, NY, showing the 0.25-ha quadrants that served as the spatial unit of analysis. *Stippled areas* indicate those woodland quadrants on which relative densities of deer, white-footed mice, and immature *I. dammini* were estimated.

TABLE 1. Correlations among Relative Densities of Deer, White-footed Mice, and *Ixodes dammini* Larvae and Nymphs on 43 Quarter-Hectare Woodland Quadrants at the Seatuck National Wildlife Refuge, Islip, NY

Host or Tick	n	Relative Density[a] Mean ± SD	Correlation[b] with:			
			Deer	Mice	Larvae	Nymphs
Deer	102	2.4 ± 3.0	—	ns	<0.001	<0.012
Mice	208	4.9 ± 2.3		—	ns	ns
Larvae	8975	43.2 ± 42.9			—	<0.001
Nymphs	163	0.8 ± 1.3				—

Density estimates of radio-collared deer were made during September through December 1985, when most adult tick feeding occurs, and observations of ticks on mice were made the following August through September (1986), when immature ticks are most abundant.

[a]Number of deer or mice per quadrant, and mean number of $\log_{10}$-transformed larval and nymphal *I. dammini* per mouse per quadrant.

[b]*p* Value is probability of greater linear correlation coefficient (r^2).

tick contact and disease prevention should focus on this interface. Our results suggest that the risk of Lyme disease may be decreased by reducing contact between humans and sites used intensively by deer.

ACKNOWLEDGMENT

We thank Mary C. Capkanis, Anne M. Ducey, David C. MacLean, and David Peterson for field assistance.

REFERENCES

1. SPIELMAN, A., M. L. WILSON, J. F. LEVINE & J. PIESMAN. 1985. Ecology of *Ixodes dammini*-borne human babesiosis and Lyme disease. Annu. Rev. Entomol. **30:** 439–60.
2. WILSON, M. L., G. H. ADLER & A. SPIELMAN. 1985. Correlation between deer abundance and that of the tick, *Ixodes dammini* (Acari : Ixodidae). Ann. Entomol. Soc. Am. **78:** 172–176.
3. WILSON, M. L., J. PIESMAN, S. R. TELFORD III & A. SPIELMAN. 1987. Reduced abundance of vector ticks following elimination of deer. J. Med. Entomol. In press.
4. WILSON, M. L. & A. SPIELMAN. 1985. Seasonal activity of immature *Ixodes dammini* (Acari : Ixodidae). J. Med. Entomol. **22**(4): 408–414.
5. TELFORD, S. R., III, T. M. MATHER, S. I. MOORE, M. L. WILSON & A. SPIELMAN. 1987. Incompetence of deer as reservoirs of *Borrelia burgdorferi*. Am. J. Trop. Med. Hyg. In press.

Observations of Two High-Risk Populations from the Swiss Plateau, a Region Heavily Infested with *Ixodes ricinus*/*Borrelia burgdorferi* Complex[a]

A. AESCHLIMANN,[b] L. GERN,[b] E. ZHIOUA,[b]
E. FROSSARD,[c] A. WALTER,[c] H. FAHRER,[d]
M.-J. SAUVAIN,[d] S. VAN DEN LINDEN,[d]
AND N. GERBER[d]

[a]*Zoological Institute*
University of Neuchâtel
Neuchâtel, Switzerland

[b]*District Hospital of Aarberg*
Aarberg, Switzerland

[c]*Department of Rheumatology*
University of Bern
Bern, Switzerland

INTRODUCTION

In western Europe, Lyme borreliosis develops after tick bites of *Ixodes ricinus* infected with *Borrelia burgdorferi*. In Switzerland, no population of this tick species devoid of infection has been detected to date.[1]

Two groups of people considered high-risk populations because of their frequent contact with the woods were studied: (1) sportsmen (such as orienteerers), who spend a lot of their time running in the forest, which increases their risk of coming in contact with *I. ricinus* and thus *B. burgdorferi* infections, and (2) a population without clinical signs of Lyme borreliosis, but living in a rural area (Aarberg) in the Swiss Plateau where biotopes favorable to *I. ricinus* are numerous.

METHODS

The sportsmen were asked to donate blood in the spring of 1986 (sample I) and to answer a questionnaire about their training habits, history of tick bites, and Lyme symptomatology. This procedure was repeated in the fall of the same year (sample II) and will be done twice again during 1987. Of the original 964 subjects, 565 have been retested so far (samples I and II). The tests used were indirect immunofluorescence test (IF)[2] for sample I and enzyme-linked immunosorbent assay (ELISA)[3] for samples I and II.

The other studied population consisted of 491 persons entering the hospital of

[a]This work was supported by the Swiss National Research Foundation.

Aarberg. None of these patients presented with any signs of Lyme borreliosis. Each individual had to fill out a questionnaire concerning professional and leisure activities in the woods and history of tick bites. The sera were tested by ELISA.

RESULTS

Nearly 80% of the orienteerers have a history of tick bites. Among the participants, 19.8% presented positive IgG titers ($\geq 1/128$; sample I, IF). Analyzing the reported symptoms, we found that 28% of the 107 persons with clearly high IgG titer had mentioned skin, joint, or nervous involvement, whereas 18.4% of the subjects with low titers presented the same manifestations ($p < 0.05$). Twenty-one orienteerers had very high IgG titers (1/1024). Only one had a history of probable arthritis, the remainder

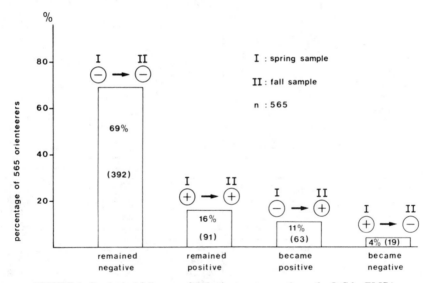

FIGURE 1. Serological follow-up of 565 orienteerers over 6 months, IgG by ELISA.

reported no symptoms. During the first year, the majority of the titers remained stable. A shift from negative to positive was seen in 11.1% (FIG. 1). Two of the persons who presented with a seroconversion had developed symptoms: one an ECM, one a facial palsy; their titers rose from negative up to 1/1024 (IgG).

Of the 491 sera of patients of Aarberg without clinical symptoms of Lyme borreliosis, 26.6% presented positive titers (IgG). We tried to find a correlation between age and value of antibody titers, in view of the relatively high mean age of the studied population (56.5 years). No correlation could be found between these two parameters. It has not been possible to explain the high percentage of positive individuals by a higher exposure to such risks as professional and leisure contacts with woods or history of tick bites referring to the questionnaire (FIG. 2). On the other hand, the results have demonstrated that the percentage of men with positive antibody titers was higher than the percentage of positive women ($\chi^2 = 11.7447, p = 0.001$).

DISCUSSION

In the orienteerers study, the most astonishing finding is the relative lack of symptoms in the group with the highest titers, hinting that nonapparent infections with the spirochete seem to be important. During the half year, the majority of the titers remained stable; 11.1% shifted from negative to positive. This was probably due to recent contact with infected ticks but was accompanied in only two cases by disease manifestations.

The population of Aarberg that did not present symptoms of Lyme disease presented a high percentage of positive individuals, which was surprising. We can

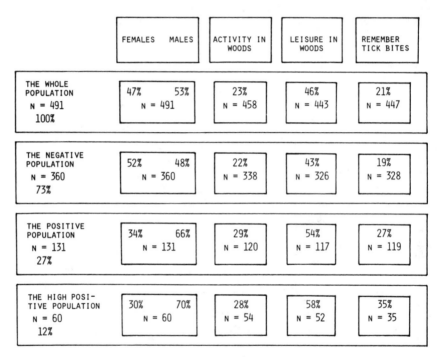

FIGURE 2. Percentages of rural population exposed to different risks.

explain this only by the rural behavior of the people of the studied region, which in itself is a risk factor. The persons, mainly living in small villages, have close contact with nature and ticks, even though tick bites are not often remembered. Such contacts are probably more frequent for men than for women.

What is important to point out in these studies is the high prevalence of nonapparent *B. burgdorferi* infections in the sportsmen, who belong to a population directly exposed to infected tick bites and are fully aware of this risk (80% remembered tick bites), as well as in the rural population of Aarberg, which does not have the same awareness of the encountered risks (21% remembered tick bites) but which is also directly exposed to tick bites because of its rural life style.

REFERENCES

1. AESCHLIMANN, A., E. CHAMOT, F. GIGON, J.-P. JEANNERET, D. KESSELER & C. WALTHER. 1987. *B. burgdorferi* in Switzerland. Zbl. Bakt. Hyg. A **263:** 450–458.
2. CHAMOT, E. Contribution à l'étude de l'Erythema migrans Krankheit en Suisse. Thesis. University of Neuchâtel. Neuchâtel.
3. RUSSELL, H., J.-S. SAMPSON, G. P. SCHMID, H. W. WILKINSON & B. PLIKAYTIS. 1984. Enzyme-linked immunosorbent assay and indirect immunofluorescence assay for Lyme disease. J. Infect. Dis. **149:** 465–470.

Borrelia burgdorferi Survival
in Human Blood Samples

GUY BARANTON AND ISABELLE SAINT-GIRONS

Leptospirosis Laboratory
Institut Pasteur
75724 Cedex 15, Paris, France

INTRODUCTION

Lyme borreliosis may be considered as a blood-borne infection because it is generally transmitted by tick bites.[1] Dissemination in the organism of its etiological agent, *Borrelia burgdorferi,* may occur at various stages of evolution,[2] sometimes at a late stage. The manner of dissemination remains uncertain, but the large spectrum of infected organs (*e.g.,* mainly the presence of *B. burgdorferi* in the endocardium,[3] as well as possible materno-fetal transmission,[4] suggest that blood plays a major role. However, blood isolations of *B. burgdorferi* are quite rare.[5]

Having observed that a strain could remain alive several months in BSK II medium kept at +4°C and that the strains we isolated from cerebrospinal fluid of patients[6] had survived despite several days' transportation, we attempted to determine whether a killing effect of the blood is obvious and therefore whether *B. burgdorferi* transmission by transfusion is in practice impossible.

MATERIAL AND METHODS

Twenty-five blood samples from 10 normal donors were collected on citrate phosphate dextrose preservative (CPD) as is usual in blood banks. As soon as the flasks were filled they were inoculated with *B. burgdorferi* and cooled at +4°C. The B31 *B. burgdorferi* strain was grown 7 days in BSK II medium, washed twice, and suspended at 10^8/ml in PBS, pH 7.6. 250μl of the suspension was added to each flask (10^6 *B. burgdorferi* per ml in final suspension). The rubber-tapped flasks maintained at +4°C were checked weekly by sampling an aliquot from each one. Forty μl from this aliquot were inoculated in 2 ml of BSK II medium and examined within 10 days incubation at +30°C for spirochetes under dark-field illumination.

RESULTS

All the cultures remained positive from the first day until the twenty-fifth day, which was the end of the experiment for nine flasks. The tenth was tested again until the sixtieth day and was still positive.

DISCUSSION

The temperature (+4°C) might inhibit phagocytosis and decrease *B. burgdorferi* sensitivity to low pH (pH of flasks was between 6.5 and 7.1), because incubation of such an inoculated blood flask at 30°C leads to a quick disappearance of *B. burgdorferi*.

CONCLUSION

B. burgdorferi may survive in fresh whole blood samples kept at +4°C in blood banks and therefore could be transmitted by transfusion. The possibility of such an event should be evaluated among recipients.

REFERENCES

1. BURGDORFER, W., A. G. BARBOUR, *et al.* 1982. Science **216:** 1317–1319.
2. STEERE, A. C., N. H. BARTENHAGEN, *et al.* 1986. Zbl. Bakt. Hyg. A **263:** 201–205.
3. DURAY, H. P. & A. C. STEERE. 1986. Zbl. Bakt. Hyg. A **263:** 169–178.
4. SCHLESINGER, P. A., H. P. DURAY, *et al.* 1983. Ann. Intern. Med. **103(1):** 67–68.
5. BENACH, J. L., E. M. BOSLER, *et al.* 1983. N. Engl. J. Med. **308:** 740–742.
6. ALLAL, J. P., P. THOMAS, J. MAZZONELLI & G. BARANTON. 1986. Med. Mal. Infect. **16(6):** 445–446.

Lyme Disease in Rhode Island

J. BRONDUM, M. A. RITTMANN, B. A. DeBUONO, AND
L. LaFAZIA

Rhode Island Department of Health
Providence, Rhode Island 02908

Lyme disease (LD) became officially reportable in Rhode Island in 1982, when 14 cases were reported to the Rhode Island Department of Health (RIDH). Since then, the number of annual LD cases in Rhode Islanders has risen in each successive year, to 55 in 1986; as of July 31, 21 cases had been reported in 1987, making a total of 182 case reports since 1982. The corresponding number of physicians reporting LD rose from two in 1982 to 37 in 1986, suggesting that the increased reporting was far more a function of better disease recognition than one of increased incidence. While onset of illness was reported in every month of the year, 114 (63%) onsets occurred in June through August. One hundred thirteen (62%) cases were reported from Washington County, the southernmost county in the state, and 46 (41%) of these were from one municipality (Block Island).

Median age of LD patients was 36 years (range 1–90 years); 86 (47%) cases were in females, none of whom were pregnant at the time of their illness. Of the 167 cases whose race was known, 158 (95%) were white, three (2%) black, three Hispanic, two (1%) Asian, and one (1%) Native American.

Erythema chronicum migrans (ECM) was seen in 115 (63%). The most commonly named symptom of systemic illness was myalgia (42%), followed by fever (37%) and headache (34%). Arthritis was diagnosed in 84 (46%) cases, neurological involvement in 26 (14%), and cardiac involvement in eight (4%). Sixty-eight (37%) reported a tick bite within 1 month of onset of their illness, and 100 (55%) felt that they had acquired LD in Rhode Island.

Patients with ECM were significantly more likely to report headache than those without ECM (OR = 2.6; 95% confidence interval: 1.2–5.8), and to have reported a tick bite within 1 month of the onset of illness (OR = 0.3; 95% CI: 1.4–6.7). They were less likely to report arthritis (OR = 0.3; 95% CI: 0.1–0.6). Serum was drawn from 133 (73%) cases a median of 14 days after onset in those with ECM and 28.5 days after onset in those without.[a] In all other ways the two groups were similar. Overall, only 25% of LD cases had received antimicrobial therapy at the time of the report to RIDH.

Characterization of the epidemiology of LD in RI is still evolving. Future intervention by the RIDH must focus on informing the public about high-risk areas and months of the year for acquiring LD in the state and increasing physician awareness of the disease, including placing greater emphasis on providing antibiotic therapy early in the course of the disease.

---

[a] The RIDH Serology Laboratory performs an indirect immunofluorescence assay (IFA) as a diagnostic aid. All IFA reagents are prepared and standardized within the laboratory except for the anti-human immunoglobulin conjugate (Cappell Laboratories). An IFA result of 1:64 with a polyvalent conjugate (IgM, IgG, IgA) is considered significant in patients with chronic Lyme disease manifestations. If clinical disease is absent but there is a titer of 1:64, it is recommended that the patient be retested in 1 month.

Evaluation of Rapid Enzyme Immunoassay for Canine Lyme Disease Antibody Detection

JEFFREY BRYANT,[a] ARTHUR YI,[a] DAVID SAVUKINAS,[b]
STUART HODDER,[b] AND ROBERT GILFILLAN[b]

[a] Cambridge BioScience Corporation
365 Plantation
Worcester, Massachusetts 01605
[b] Tufts University School of Veterinary Medicine
Boston, Massachusetts 02130

INTRODUCTION

A rapid enzyme immunoassay (EIA) for the detection and measurement of antibody to *Borrelia burgdorferi* has been developed. The assay has been used to evaluate dog serums that were tested for presence of antibodies to Lyme disease on immunofluorescence assay (IFA) and on Western blot. Requiring just two hours to complete, the EIA utilizes partially purified spirochetal antigen coated to polystyrene

TABLE 1

	Western Blot		IFA	
	+	−	+	−
EIA				
+	22	2	22	2
−	0	31	7	24
Sensitivity	100%		76%	
Specificity	94%		92%	
Total Agreement	97%		84%	

A score of 3 or greater is considered positive on the Western blot. This score, due to a lack of sample characterization, cannot be used as a standard of Lyme disease in the patient. OD of greater than .30 is considered a positive on the EIA assay. A titer of 1:32 or greater is considered a positive on the IFA assay.

microwells. Using as little as 1 μl of serum, the test is run using a peroxidase-labeled goat anti-dog (heavy- and light-chain specific) antibody, and a urea peroxide/ tetramethylbenzidine (TMB) substrate/chromogen system.

RESULTS

The results of these experiments are summarized in TABLE 1.

CONCLUSIONS

1. The sensitivity of the EIA, when compared with the results of the Western blot, was 100%. The specificity of the EIA, when compared with the results of the Western blot, was 94%. This indicates that, with the exception of two samples out of 55 samples tested, there is agreement between the amount of antibody detected by means of EIA and by means of Western blot.
2. The Western blots also indicate that bands at 31 kDa, 66 kDa and approximately 90 kDa are major sites for specific binding of canine antibody. It must be emphasized that, due to the lack of characterization of the samples, we can not at this time be sure how the Western blots correlate to actual disease in the patients, and thus how the EIA results correlate to actual disease in the patients. We believe, however, that with access to well-characterized samples we would be able to further optimize the assay. Potentially, the specificity of the EIA could be further increased, using the Western blot as a standard.
3. The turnaround time for EIA results is less than 2 hours, with minimum hands-on time.
4. The EIA procedure is very simple, and is easy to perform in a reproducible manner.

Lyme Borreliosis in Children

A Prospective Clinical-Epidemiological Study

HANS-JÜRGEN CHRISTEN,[a] FOLKER HANEFELD,[a]
NICOL BARTLAU,[a] KLAUS WASSMANN,[b] AND
REINER THOMSSEN[b]

[a]Department of Pediatrics
[b]Department of Medical Microbiology
University of Göttingen
3400 Göttingen, Federal Republic of Germany

Lyme borreliosis is now frequently observed in children.[1-3] Because of their behavior, it should be expected even more frequently than in adults. Up to now, however, very little knowledge has existed about the clinical course of Lyme borreliosis in childhood and possible differences between adults and children. In order to investigate the clinical spectrum of Lyme borreliosis in childhood, a prospective hospital-based multicenter study was started in August 1986 that included seven pediatric departments serving a geographically well-defined region in the Northeast of Germany with a population of 2 million people. Special emphasis was placed on the relative frequency of Lyme borreliosis among acute neurologic disorders in children. Diagnosis of Lyme borreliosis was based on the detection of specific IgM antibodies in serum and—in all neurologic cases—in CSF, using an IgM capture assay. Nonspecific cross-reactions, especially against *Treponema pallidum* and Epstein-Barr virus, were excluded in all positive cases. In order to evaluate the sensitivity and specificity of the test, all patients, including the initially negative ones, were followed up with repeated controls of antibody titer for a period of 6 months (after 2 and 6 weeks as well as after 4 and 6 months). In cases with neurologic disorders, identified as Lyme borreliosis, a second CSF examination was done after 4 to 6 months. The relative frequency of Lyme borreliosis among the cases investigated over the first 10 months of the study, *i.e.*, 33 out of 87 cases, is given in TABLE 1. The age of the positive cases ranged from 2 to 15 years. Two-thirds of them were boys. The most common neurologic feature was a peripheral N. VII palsy (14 out of 20 cases). In contrast to idiopathic Bell's palsy, all these IgM positive cases showed a pleocytosis in CSF irrespective of whether clinical symptoms of meningitis were present (TABLE 2). In aseptic meningitis (8 out of 39 cases), cell count and protein content of CSF allow no differentiation according to the etiology. Among the other neurologic disorders, there was one case with a characteristic Guillain-Barré syndrome (CSF findings: 10 cells, protein 1.2 g/l; decreased nerve conduction velocities) in whom Lyme borreliosis could be verified. This disorder has rarely been reported among neurologic presentations of Lyme borreliosis.[4] In cases with gonarthritis, Lyme borreliosis could be verified in two out of nine children by detection of IgM antibodies in joint effusion. All children who were initially seronegative for IgM antibodies remained so during the follow-up of 6 months. This gives support for the high sensitivity of the methods used. Another problem concerns the discrepancy of antibody results in serum and CSF. One case was observed in whom a significantly elevated antibody titer was missing in serum but present in CSF at the onset of the disease. The possibility of initially false-negative results has to be kept in mind if only serum titers are studied. Concerning the clinical outcome, all children improved quickly and without any residual symptoms following antibiotic therapy. All children with neurologic symptoms or arthritis received high-dose penicillin given

TABLE 1. Clinical Spectrum of Lyme Borreliosis in Childhood and Its Relative Frequency among the Illnesses Investigated (Results Refer to the First 10 Months of the Prospective Study)

	Unknown Etiology (*n*)	Lyme Borreliosis (*n*)	Tick Bite (*n*)	Erythema Migrans (*n*)
Neurological disorders	47	28	14	8
Peripheral facial palsy	6	14		
Aseptic meningitis	31	8		
Guillain-Barré syndrome	1	2		
Acute ataxia	2	1		
Meningoencephalitis	1	1		
Severe headache	2	2		
Multiple sclerosis	1	—		
Pseudotumor cerebri	1	—		
Acute hemiplegia	1	—		
Multiple cranial nerve disorder	1	—		
"Postinfectious arthritis"	7	2	1	—
Erythema migrans	—	3	3	3
TOTAL	54	33	18	11

intravenously over 10 days. The cases with erythema migrans only were treated orally with erythromycin. None of the children has shown a relapse up to now. Nevertheless, five out of seven children with neurologic symptoms, in whom a reexamination of CSF was done after 6 months, revealed a persistent slightly elevated IgM titer, whereas cell count and protein concentration were normal. The implication of these findings in respect to the efficiency of antibiotic therapy remains unclear.

CONCLUSION

The spectrum of Lyme borreliosis in children differs from adults. Although there is a clear preponderance of peripheral facial palsy, the leading neurologic feature of

TABLE 2. CSF Findings in Peripheral N. VII Palsy and Meningitis

	n	Bilateral	Stiff Neck	CSF Findings	
				Cell Count ($\times 10^6$/l) $\bar{x}$ (Range)	Protein (g/l) $\bar{x}$ (Range)
N. VII palsy					
Lyme borreliosis	14	3	3	155 (13–463)	0.88 (0.20–2.51)
Unknown etiology	6	—	—	7 (2–14)	0.33 (0.21–0.49)
Meningitis					
Lyme borreliosis	8		8	183 (16–430)	0.69 (0.27–1.36)
Unknown etiology	31		31	165 (17–1067)	0.42 (0.13–1.18)

Lyme borreliosis in adults,[5-6] the Bannwarth's syndrome, was not observed among children in the present study. Because of characteristic CSF findings, CSF examination including serological testing for *B. burgdorferi* should be performed in any unexplained neurologic disorder of acute onset.

REFERENCES

1. WILLIAMS, C. L., A. S. CURRAN, A. C. LEE & V. O. SOUSA. 1986. Am. J. Public Health **76:** 62–65.
2. JOERBECK, H. J. A., P. M. GUSTAFSSON, H. C. F. LIND & G. T. STIERNSTEDT. 1987. Acta Paediatr. Scand. **76:** 228–233.
3. CHRISTEN, H.-J. & F. HANEFELD. 1986. Zbl. Bakt. Hyg. A **263:** 337–342.
4. STERMAN, A. B., S. NELSON & P. BARCLAY. 1982. Neurology **32:** 1302–1305.
5. PACHNER, A. R. & A. C. STEERE. 1985. Neurology **35:** 47–53.
6. PFISTER, H. W., K. M. EINHÄUPL, B. WILSKE & V. PREAC-MURSIC. 1986. Zbl. Bakt. Hyg. A **263:** 343–347.

Clinical Manifestations of Tick-Borne Erythema in the USSR

EUGENIJ P. DEKONENKO

Department of Neuroinfectious Diseases
Institute of Poliomyelitis and Viral Encephalitides
of the AMS USSR
Moscow oblast, 142782, USSR

Tick-borne erythema migrans was first mentioned in the USSR as long ago as the 1920s. During the forties and fifties, due to investigations connected with tick-borne encephalitis (TBE), these erythemas were more frequently diagnosed.[1] According to some investigators, erythema makes up from 3% to 15% of the suspected cases of TBE.[2] For many years these diseases were confused with or thought to be a part of tick-borne encephalitis. It is now well known that erythema is the best clinical marker for Lyme disease.[3] The independent existence of Lyme borreliosis (LB) and its wide distribution in the forest zone of the USSR has been confirmed.[1,4]

During a more than 10-year period 90 patients with erythema appearing after tick bites were investigated. The onset of the erythema was between May and October. The disease developed into areas endemic for TBE, where *Ixodes persulcatus* and *Ixodes ricinus* predominated. The median age was 44 years (range 2–70 years). Out of 90 patients, 50 were men. There were patients from several geographic regions of the USSR. Two types of erythema were noted: annular and homogeneous. The median time from tick bite to onset of erythema was 10 days (range 1 to 53 days). We observed that erythema could disappear without treatment between 10 and 20 days or remained for months.

In an acute phase of the disease general symptoms were found in 74 (82%) of the 90 patients (TABLE 1). Patients were studied at different periods of erythema and there were different complaints and symptoms depending on the stage of the disease. There were three general stages of the disease. The first stage included common infectious symptoms accompanied by skin lesion (duration up to 1 month); at the second stage

TABLE 1. General Signs and Symptoms of Tick-borne Erythema

Signs and Symptoms	Number of Patients	%
Elevated temperature (37–40°C)	74	82
Malaise and fatigue	67	74
Headache	52	58
Pain in an area of an erythema	27	30
Myalgias	24	27
Arthralgias	22	24
Regional lymphadenopathy	15	17
Dizziness	10	11
Nausea and vomiting	9	10
Sore throat	8	9
Sleep disturbances	8	9
TOTAL	90	100

TABLE 2. Neurologic Abnormalities following Tick-borne Erythema

Type of Disturbance	Number of Patients (Total = 58)	%
Radicular symptoms	37	64
Cranial nerve abnormalities (except facial nerve)	31	53
Disturbances of reflexes	19	33
Aseptic meningitis	14	24
Facial paralysis	8	14
Cerebellar abnormalities	5	9
Paralysis of upper extremities	4	7
Muscle atrophy of shoulder girdle	3	5

neurologic manifestations occurred (duration 2 weeks to 4 months) and the third stage appeared as arthritis (duration from 3 to 4 weeks up to 2 years).

Neurologic disturbances were found in 58 patients (64%). The most common neurologic involvements were disturbances of peripheral nervous system such as radiculitis, brachial plexitis, mononeuritis, etc. Thirty-seven of the 58 patients (64%) had peripheral nervous system involvement (TABLE 2). Cranial nerves were affected slightly (III, IV, VI, V, XII) in 31 patients (58%). Facial palsy was observed in eight patients (14%). In most of these (seven) unilateral involvement was found. Fourteen of the 58 patients had aseptic meningitis (24%). It should be noted that aseptic meningitis alone was observed only in three patients. The other eleven patients had signs of meningitis with superimposed radiculopathy, facial palsy, paresis of extremeties, etc. The cerebrospinal fluid (CSF) contained on the average 100 cells/mm^3 (predominantly lymphocytes, with a range of 5.5–378). Four patients had paresis of the upper extremities. Two of them had monoparesis and two had flaccid paraparesis of the extremities accompanied by paresis of the neck.

Sera and CSF from some patients were tested by indirect immunofluorescence[4] and enzyme-linked immunosorbent assay.[5] Titers to *B. burgdorferi* were discovered in most of them.

REFERENCES

1. DEKONENKO, E. P., YU. K. SMIRNOV & K. G. UMANSKY. 1985. Z. Nevr. Psychiatr. **4:** 539–545 (in Russian).
2. SHAPOVAL, A. N. 1980. Tick-borne encephalomyelitis (in Russian). Moscow.
3. STEERE, A. C., N. H. BARTENHAGEN, J. E. CRAFT, J. GORDON, M. D. HUTCHINSON, J. H. NEWMAN, D. W. RAHN, L. H. SIGAL, P. N. SPIELER, K. S. STENN & S. E. MALAWISTA. 1983. Ann. Intern. Med. **99:** 76–82.
4. KORENBERG, E. I., V. N. KRUCHECHNIKOV, E. P. DEKONENKO, S. V. SHCHERBAKOV & YU. V. ANANYINA. 1986. ZhMEI **6:** 111–113 (in Russian).
5. DEKONENKO, E. P. & A. C. STEERE. Submitted.

Lyme Disease Presenting as Seronegative Rheumatoid Arthritis

ANDREA DLESK, DAVID F. BJARNASON, PAUL
MITCHELL, AND PAT McCARTY

Marshfield Clinic
Marshfield, Wisconsin 54449

The arthritis of Lyme disease (LD) usually is a transient, intermittent, monoarticular or oligoarticular process most commonly affecting large joints, particularly knees.[1-3] It generally occurs about 6 weeks after infection. Joints affected, in decreasing order of frequency, are knees, shoulders, elbows, temporomandibular joints, ankles, wrists, hips, and rarely, small joints of the hands and feet. Arthritis occurs in about 50% to 60% of LD patients. It generally lasts days to weeks and spontaneously resolves. Up to 10% of patients with LD develop chronic Lyme arthritis (LA).[4]

TABLE 1. American Rheumatism Association Criteria for the Diagnosis of RA[a]

1. Morning stiffness
2. Pain on motion or tenderness in at least one joint
3. Swelling of one joint, representing soft tissue or fluid
4. Swelling of at least one other joint (soft tissue or fluid) with an interval free of symptoms no longer than 3 months
5. Symmetrical joint swelling (simultaneous involvement of the same joint, right and left)
6. Subcutaneous nodules over bony prominences, extensor surfaces or near joints
7. Typical roentgenographic changes, which must include demineralization in periarticular bone as an index of inflammation; degenerative changes do not exclude diagnosis of RA
8. Positive test for rheumatoid factor in serum
9. Synovial fluid; a poor mucin clot formation on adding synovial fluid to dilute acetic acid
10. Synovial histopathology consistent with RA
    a. Marked villous hypertrophy
    b. Proliferation of synovial cells
    c. Lymphocyte/plasma cell infiltration in subsynovium
    d. Fibrin deposition within or upon microvilli
11. Characteristic histopathology of rheumatoid nodules biopsied from any site

[a]Seven criteria are required for diagnosis of classic RA, five for definite RA, and three for probable RA. To meet criteria 1 to 5, symptoms or signs must be present for at least 6 weeks.

LA is generally not thought of as a symmetric inflammatory polyarthritis affecting primarily small joints of the hands and feet. At our institution in Central Wisconsin, an area endemic for LD, we speculated that some patients with LD might present in this fashion. The following study was designed to determine if the arthritis of LD could be mistaken for seronegative rheumatoid arthritis (SNRA).

Lyme titers (LT) by immunofluorescence assay (IFA) were obtained on patients with diagnoses of SNRA. LT was considered significantly positive if 1 : 256. All patients fulfilled American Rheumatism Association criteria for definite RA (TABLE

1). All were negative for rheumatoid factor by latex fixation. Antinuclear antibodies were absent on Hep-2 sustrate. Age, sex, initial hemoglobin, erythrocyte sedimentation rate (ESR) Westegren, time from onset of symptoms to initial clinical presentation, length of follow-up, and response to therapy were recorded for LT positive (LT$^+$) and LT negative (LT$^-$) groups.

Between October 1984 and August 1987, 102 patients were studied. There were 42 males and 60 females averaging 52.9 years of age. Twenty-seven had a positive Lyme titer $\geq 1 : 256$ by IFA. Eleven males and 16 females were in this group, compared to 31 males and 44 females in the LT$^-$ group. The mean age in the LT$^+$ group was 43.2 years and in the LT$^-$ group 56.4 years. Differences in sex and age were not statistically significant. No differences were found in mean Hgb between the two groups (13.5 g/dl LT$^+$ vs. 13.4 g/dl LT$^-$) or in ESR at the time of presentation (25 mm/h and LT$^+$ vs. 23 mm/h LT$^-$).

Of the 27 LT$^+$ patients, 10 had LT of 1 : 256 and 13 had titers of 1 : 512. In addition, there were two individuals each with LT of 1 : 2048 and 1 : 4096. All 27 patients received antibiotic therapy and 18 (67%) responded to antibiotic therapy with resolution of joint symptoms. Of the LT$^-$ patients, 22 (29%) were free of joint symptoms or signs at their last visit. Fifty-three (71%) had persistently active synovitis. Statistically, significantly fewer LT$^+$ patients were symptomatic at follow-up ($p <$ 0.001). Mean length of follow-up in the LT$^+$ group was 7.4 months; in the LT$^-$ group, 16 months.

Because of the favorable response to antibiotic therapy with either resolution or abrogation of joint symptoms among the LT$^+$ group of SNRA patients, we conclude that LD should be checked for among patients presenting with SNRA in endemic areas.

REFERENCES

1. STEERE, A. C. *et al.* 1977. Lyme arthritis: An epidemic of oligoarticular arthritis in children and adults in three Connecticut communities. Arthritis Rheum. **20:** 7–17.
2. STEERE, A. C. *et al.* 1979. Lyme arthritis: Correlation of serum and cryoglobulin IgM with activity, and serum IgG with remission. Arthritis Rheum. **22:** 471–483.
3. KELLEY, W. N. *et al.* 1986. Textbook of Rheumatology. Saunders. Philadelphia.
4. STEERE, A. C. *et al.* 1979. Chronic Lyme arthritis: Clinical and immunogenetic differentiation from rheumatoid arthritis. Ann. Intern. Med. **90:** 896–901.

A Survey of Tick Bites Acquired in a Lyme Disease Endemic Area in Southern New York State

R. C. FALCO AND D. FISH

Westchester County Health Department
White Plains, New York 10601
and
New York Medical College
Valhalla, New York 10595

Westchester County, located in southern New York State, is a Lyme disease endemic area.[1] Unsolicited tick specimens that had bitten humans in the county during 1985 were identified and background information was obtained.

A total of 126 ticks were examined: 96 (76.2%) *Ixodes dammini*, 26 (20.6%) *Dermacentor variabilis*, 2 (1.6%) *Amblyomma americanum*, and 2 (1.6%) unidentifiable. *I. dammini* was found biting humans in all months of the year but February and December. The seasonal distribution of nymphal bites was greatest between May 16 and June 30, when 74.4% of the bites occurred. Adult *I. dammini* bites were more evenly distributed throughout the year, with 53.5% occurring between October 1 and November 30, and 44.2% occurring between March 1 and June 15. Only one larval *I. dammini* was submitted (in September).

Ages of *I. dammini* bite victims ranged from 0.5 years to 84 years, with a mean age of 24.5 years (SD = ± 4.72). Age classes for victims were skewed, with 39.0% of all victims in the 0–9 year age class. A significant positive correlation (Spearman rank test, $r_s = 0.90$, $p < 0.02$, $n = 8$) was found between the age classes of tick bite victims and Lyme disease cases reported from Westchester County in a previous study.[1]

The site of attachment for biting *I. dammini* was determined for 84 ticks (TABLE 1). More nymphal bites (37.2%) occurred on the lower extremities than on any other body area. Adult ticks were most commonly found on the head (22.0%). Forty-eight (68.6%) of 70 respondents reported tick bites acquired in their own yard. These data support our previous findings that many cases of Lyme disease in Westchester County are acquired in the immediate vicinity of the patients' homes.[2] Other sites included schools, parks, and work places (TABLE 2).

TABLE 1. Attachment Sites of *I. dammini*, Westchester Co., NY, 1985

Body Area	No. (%) of Nymphs	No. (%) of Females
Head	4 (9.3)	9 (22.0)
Neck	5 (11.6)	3 (7.3)
Shoulder/back	3 (7.0)	8 (19.5)
Upper extremities	6 (14.0)	7 (17.1)
Chest	2 (4.7)	0 (0.0)
Abdomen/groin	6 (14.0)	7 (17.1)
Lower extremities	16 (37.2)	6 (14.6)
Buttocks	1 (2.3)	1 (2.4)
TOTAL	43 (100.1)	41 (100.0)

TABLE 2. Locations of *I. dammini* Human Bite Acquisition, Westchester Co., NY, 1985

Location	No. (%) of Bites
Yard	48 (68.6)
School/camp	8 (11.4)
Park/recreation	6 (8.6)
Employment	3 (4.3)
Other	3 (4.3)
Hunting	2 (2.9)
TOTAL	70 (100.1)

Follow-up information from 71 *I. dammini* bite victims indicated that 49 (69.0%) consulted a physician regarding the bite, which resulted in 29 (40.8%) of the victims receiving antibiotic therapy. Two of the victims who were not treated prophylactically developed erythema migrans at the site of tick attachment and were diagnosed as having Lyme disease. Based upon the 381 cases of Lyme disease reported in Westchester County during 1985, we estimate that approximately 14,000 people were bitten by *I. dammini* during that year.

REFERENCES

1. WILLIAMS, C. L., A. S. CURRAN, A. C. LEE & V. O. SOUSA. 1986. Lyme disease: Epidemiologic characteristics of an outbreak in Westchester County, N. Y. Am. J. Public Health. **76:** 62–65.
2. FALCO, R. C. & D. FISH. 1988. Prevalence of *Ixodes dammini* near the homes of Lyme disease patients in Westchester County, N. Y. Am. J. Epidemiol. **127:** 826–830.

Detection of Lyme Disease in Dogs by Indirect Immunofluorescent Antibody Assays

ROBERT GILFILLAN,[a,b] DEBORAH KANE,[b]
MARY E. O'BRIEN,[b] DOMINIQUE ROUVET,[c]
AND JAMES DASBACH[c]

[a]Department of Pathology
[b]Tufts Veterinary Diagnostic Laboratories
Tufts University School of Veterinary Medicine
Boston, Massachusetts 02130

[c]MSPCA
Nantucket Animal Hospital
Nantucket, Massachusetts 02534

The incidence of Lyme disease in man, dogs, and horses has increased over the past several years in New England as the spread of this tick-borne infection continues to be detected in larger and larger geographic areas throughout the country. The range of susceptibility to this spirochete, *Borrelia burgdorferi*, in both wild and domestic animals has continued to expand also as the recognition and the means to identify this affliction have become available. Although still incomplete, systematic studies on vector ecology will likely indicate still more potential for higher levels of infection. Funding for basic and applied research on both human and animal disease and for tick surveillance programs remains inadequate.

Following the characterization of the disease in man by Steere *et al.*[1] and identification of the etiologic agent by Burgdorfer *et al.*[2] Lissman *et al.*[3] described Lyme disease in a dog suffering from a disabling arthritis. In 1984, our laboratory initiated efforts to search for and to identify antibody to Lyme disease spirochetes in the horse[4] by conventional IFA techniques, employing acetone-fixed spirochetes propagated in modified Kelly's medium. At this time, we also initiated and standardized an IFA antibody assay in the dog, employing reference sera obtained from Dr. Paul Urband.[5] Dr. Willy Burgdorfer, Rocky Mountain Laboratories, Hamilton, Montana provided assistance in the standardization of the assay by examining the specificity and sensitivity of our antigen and reference sera with those prepared and used in his laboratory.[2]

From 1984 through 1986, 1073 symptomatic dogs and 274 horses have been tested. Infection rates, including current and past infections in the dog, progressed from 63% to 72%. Antibody titers ranging from 64 to 4086 were scored positive, employing polyvalent FITC conjugate. Serum specimens from 231 dogs were tested at the same time by conventional indirect immunofluorescent antibody (IFA) for Rocky Mountain spotted fever (RMFS), an enzootic disease localized primarily in the eastern part of Massachusetts. Twenty-seven dogs demonstrated high levels of antibody (≥ 64) to both *B. burgdorferi* and RMSF, suggesting coinfections. In a separate study, 36 dogs from Missouri with clinical serologic evidence of *Ehrlichia canis* infections were tested for antibody to Lyme disease spirochetes. Ten of these dogs demonstrated antibody levels of 1 : 32 or greater, suggesting past infection with this spirochete.

In 1986, collaborative efforts were undertaken by investigators from Cambridge Biosciences, Inc. (Worcester, MA) to develop a more sensitive ELISA assay for Lyme disease antibody employing partially purified antigens extracted from spirochetes. Western blot analysis using labeled canine serum showed good correlation between ELISA and IFA assays as described by Bryant *et al.* (this volume).

Carefully conducted, well-defined prospective clinical and model studies on the immune response are needed with both dogs and horses to document IgM and IgG changes over the course of the disease in order to more accurately interpret serologic assays and to differentiate among primary infection, reactivated infection, or reinfection, particularly in animals residing in areas perennially infested with tick vectors. Such studies have been undertaken.

REFERENCES

1. STEERE, A. C., S. E. MALAWISTA, J. A. HARDIN, *et al.* 1977. Erythema chronicum migrans and Lyme arthritis. Ann. Intern. Med. **86:** 685–698.
2. BURGDORFER, W., A. G. BARBOUR, S. F. HAYES, *et al.* 1982. Science **216:** 1317–1319.
3. LISSMAN, B. A., E. M. BOSLER, H. CAMAY, *et al.* 1984. Spirochete-associated arthritis (Lyme disease) in a dog. J. Am. Vet. Med. Assoc. **185:** 219–220.
4. MARCUS, L., M. PATTERSON, R. GILFILLAN & P. URBAND. 1985. Antibodies to *Borrelia burgdorferi* in New England horses: Serologic survey. Am. J. Vet. Res. **46:** 2570–2572.
5. KORNBLATT, A. N., P. H. URBAND & A. C. STEERE. 1985. Arthritis caused by *Borrelia burgdorferi* in dogs. J. Am. Vet. Med. Assoc. **186:** 964–969.
6. BRYANT, J., A. YI, D. SAVUKINAS, S. HODDER & R. GILFILLAN. 1988. Evaluation of rapid enzyme immunoassay for canine Lyme disease antibody detection. This volume.

Serologic Reactivity to *Borrelia burgdorferi* in Rheumatoid Arthritis Patients

PAUL E. LAVOIE

Pacific Presbyterian Medical Center
San Francisco, California 94115

WILLY BURGDORFER

Rocky Mountain Laboratory
Hamilton, Montana 59840

INTRODUCTION AND PURPOSE

Lyme borreliosis is a common infectious multisystem disorder in endemic regions where the *Ixodes* tick vector has a high incidence of *Borrelia burgdorferi* infection.[1] The borreliosis shares many symptoms and signs with other established diseases, thereby raising the possibility of diagnostic confusion especially in regions of low tick vector infection incidence.[2] To investigate this we studied a series of patients presenting to a metropolitan rheumatology practice in northern California, a region of low endemic infection.

MATERIALS AND METHODS

Two hundred and four sera were collected from 174 patients over approximately 1 year. The patient mix was representative of the practice. The Lyme borreliosis sera were studied separately earlier. The sera were enumerated serially and processed without name or diagnosis. Where more than one sera was collected from a patient, the highest positive dilution was later assigned to that patient.

The control population consisted of patients without evidence for a primary inflammatory disorder. Included here were those with hypertension, gout, pseudogout, osteoarthritis, coronary artery disease, temporomandibular joint (TMJ) syndrome, asthma, obesity, as well as true normals.

The sera were examined for antibodies against methanol-fixed B31 organisms by standard indirect immunofluorescence antibody (IFA) techniques.[3] The fluoresceinated goat anti-human globulin serum (BBL Microbiology Systems, Benton Dickinson & Co., Cockeysville, MD) was used in a 1 : 200 dilution of 1% BSA in PBS. All sera except for the previously studied Lyme borreliosis sera were assayed by doubling dilutions to a titer limit of 1 : 256.

Criterion for positive reaction was fluorescence of spirochetes greater than the background staining of rat erythrocytes on the smear.

RESULTS

Based on the control population, the threshold for seropositivity by this IFA method was calculated (control mean plus 2 SD) to be at titer $\geq$ 1 : 80. Those patients achieving a titer of $\geq$ 1 : 128 were deemed seropositive.

The miscellaneous inflammatory patients were assigned to a single category when it was determined that none of these other inflammatory disease groups achieved statistical significance. These were: angioimmunoblastic lymphadenopathy with dysproteinemia (AILD, $n = 1$); ankylosing spondylitis ($n = 4$); CREST (calcinosis, Raynaud's phenomenon, esophageal dysmotility, sclerodactyly, telangiectasias) syndrome ($n = 1$); dermatomyositis ($n = 1$); eosinophilic fasciitis ($n = 1$); nonspecific inflammation, *e.g.,* unexplained high erythrocyte sedimentation rate, polyclonal

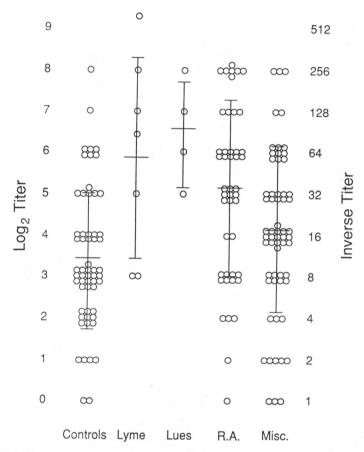

FIGURE 1. Compiled results. Each *circle* represents a single patient. Mean values and standard deviations are shown for each group.

gammopathy ($n = 7$); polymyalgia rheumatica ($n = 8$); progressive systemic sclerosis ($n = 2$); psoriasis ($n = 6$); psoriatic arthritis ($n = 15$); Reiter's ($n = 7$); systemic lupus erythematous ($n = 7$).

Five in the miscellaneous category had positive titers: They had the following diseases: AILD ($n = 1$), nongonoccal urethritis ($n = 1$), psoriasis ($n = 1$), psoriatic arthritis ($n = 1$), and Reiter's syndrome ($n = 1$).

The Lyme borreliosis, late latent lues, and rheumatoid arthritis groups achieved statistical significance by the chi-square method at $p < 0.01$.

The percentage of significant titers were: controls, 2/58 (3%); Lyme borreliosis, 3/7 (43%); late latent lues, 2/4 (50%); rheumatoid arthritis, 11/45 (24%); miscellaneous inflammatory, 5/60 (8%).

The percentage of significant titers within the rheumatoid arthritis group were as follows. For the American Rheumatism Association rheumatoid arthritis classes, none

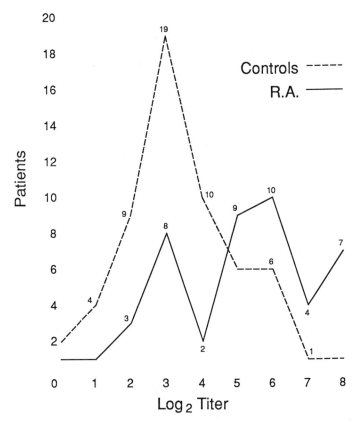

FIGURE 2. Graphical comparison of borrelial serum response of rheumatoid arthritis patients versus controls.

had significant borrelia seropositivity in the probable class. Three of sixteen (19%) were positive in the definite class. Eight of twenty-six (31%) in the classical class were positive.

When the presence of IgM rheumatoid factor (R.F.) and positive borrelia antibodies in rheumatoid arthritis patients were compared, 8 of 28 (29%) R.F.-positive patients were found to be also borrelia seropositive, while three of seventeen (18%) of

R.F.-negative patients had borrelia seropositivity. The classical and R.F.-positive subsets achieved significance at $p < 0.01$.

The results of this study are compiled in FIGURE 1. The graphical comparison of the rheumatoid arthritis versus the control sera is displayed in FIGURE 2.

DISCUSSION

Cross-reactivity between late latent lues serum and *B. burgdorferi* was predictable, based on the work of Barbour *et al.*[4] The serologic correlation between rheumatoid arthritis and *B. burgdorferi* does not establish causality but it does raise serious considerations.

Rheumatoid arthritis and Lyme borreliosis share some important findings: (i) the erosive articular injury is difficult to separate on clinical, radiologic, and pathologic examinations[5]; (ii) multisystem involvement is seen at times in rheumatoid arthritis as it is commonly recognized in Lyme borreliosis[6]; (iii) the juvenile onset patterns are often indistinguishable clinically; (iv) the recent finding of HLA-DR4 in patients with erosive Lyme arthritis offers a genetic similarity between the diseases.[7]

The potential for rheumatoid factor contributing to serologic inaccuracies is recognized.[8,9] It was not within the scope of this work to attempt correction for this possible difficulty, because the effort was designed simply as a population study. Since rheumatoid factors are found within many chronic disorders including Lyme borreliosis, it would have required removal of these globulins from all sera.[10] Future investigation of this type may be indicated.

CONCLUSIONS

Seroreactivity to *Borrelia burgdorferi* is inadequate in separating Lyme borreliosis from rheumatoid arthritis. Some patients with Lyme borreliosis may present as rheumatoid arthritis.

REFERENCES

1. MATUSCHKA, F. R. & A. SPIELMAN. 1986. The emergence of Lyme disease in a changing environment in North America and Central Europe. Exp. Appl. Acarol. **2:** 337–353.
2. STEERE, A. C., N. H. BARTENHAGEN, J. E. CRAFT, G. J. HUTCHINSON, J. H. NEWMAN, D. W. RAHN, L. H. SIGAL, P. N. SPIELER, K. S. STENN & S. E. MALAWISTA. 1983. The early clinical manifestations of Lyme disease. Ann. Intern. Med. **99:** 76–82.
3. BARBOUR, A. G., S. J. TESSIER & H. G. STOENNER. 1982. Variable major proteins of *Borrelia hermsii*. J. Exp. Med. **156:** 1312–1324.
4. BARBOUR, A. G., W. BURGDORFER, E. GRUNWALDT & A. C. STEERE. 1983. Antibodies of patients with Lyme disease to components of the *Ixodes dammini* spirochete. J. Clin. Invest. **72:** 504–515.
5. STEERE, A. C., A. GIBOFSKY, M. E. PATARROYA, R. J. WINCHESTER, J. A. HARDING & S. E. MALAWISTA. 1979. Chronic Lyme arthritis. Ann. Intern. Med. **90:** 896–901.
6. DECKER, J. L. & P. H. POLTZ. 1985. Extra-articular rheumatoid disease. *In* Arthritis and Allied Conditions, 10th edit. D. J. McCarty, Ed.: 620–642. Lea & Febiger. Philadelphia, PA.
7. STEERE, A. C. & R. J. WINCHESTER. Personal communications.

8. SHIRODARIA, P. V., K. B. FRASER & F. STANFORD. 1973. Secondary fluorescent staining of virus antigens by rheumatoid factor and fluorescein-conjugated anti-IgM. Ann. Rheum. Dis. **32:** 53–57.

9. SALONEN, E. M., A. VAHEVI, J. SUNI & O. WAGER. 1980. Rheumatoid factor in acute viral infections. J. Infect. Dis. **142(2):** 250–255.

10. KUJALI, G. A., A. C. STEERE & J. S. DAVIS IV. 1987. IgM rheumatoid factor in Lyme disease. J. Rheum. **14(4):** 772–776.

Lyme Disease in the United Kingdom

An ELISA Study of Dog Sera with Antigen Comparison between the American B31 Strain and a British IWG Strain

YAN-MING LIU,[a] CLIVE E. BENNETT,[a] JOHN E. WHITE,[b]
AND SHEENA A. WAITKINS[c]

[a]Department of Biology
University of Southampton
Southampton SO9 3TU, United Kingdom

[b]Royal South Hants Hospital
Southampton SO9 4PE, United Kingdom

[c]Leptospira Reference Unit
Hereford County Hospital
Hereford HR1 2ER, United Kingdom

Recently, Lyme disease was found in England[1,2] and one strain of spirochete (IWG strain) was isolated by one of us (SAW) from a hard tick taken from a dog in Hereford, U.K. The spirochete of *Borrelia burgdorferi* had been isolated from dogs in the USA.[3] The objective of this study was to determine if dogs have been infected by the spirochete in the U.K. and to discover any relationship between the B31 strain from the USA and the IWG strain.

MATERIALS AND METHODS

Blood

One hundred and fifty-six dog samples were taken from England and Wales, U.K. Four positive and five negative control sera were obtained from the Connecticut Agricultural Experiment Station, Connecticut, and I.C.I. Macclesfield, U.K.

ELISA Method

Microtiter plate wells were coated with 100-μl sonicated antigen-coupling buffer (3.2 μg antigen protein per ml) at 37°C overnight. Dilutions of sera made in 1% BSA/PBS (100 μl/well) were inoculated and incubated for 1.5 hours. After washing, 100 μl of peroxidase-conjugated anti-dog IgG (1 : 2000) was added and incubated for 1 hour. Substrate was O-phenylenediamine di-HCl. Cut-off OD values were 2.4 SD above the mean optical density values of 1.512 dilutions of sera from five negative samples. Thirty-two samples were used in a comparative study of B31 and IWG strains. To confirm the sensitivity and specificity of the ELISA method, four sera from the USA and four from the U.K. were reacted with antigen of B31 stain in an ^{125}I-labeled protein A Western blotting assay.[4]

TABLE 1. Titers of Antibody Responses to *Borrelia burgdorferi* B31 Strain, Determined by ELISA[a]

| Group[b] | Negative | | | | Positive | | | | Total Number |
	<1:64	1:64	1:128	1:256	1:512	1:1024	1:2048	1:4096	
1		1	1	2			2	2	8
2	1								1
3	7	43	46	16	2		1		115
4	2	9	15	11	2	1	1		41
TOTAL NUMBER	10	53	62	29	4	1	4	2	165

[a]All sera had titers below 1 : 64 when they were reacted in antigen-free wells.
[b]Groups: 1, control samples from the USA ($n = 8$); 2, control sample of a disease-free dog from I.C.I. Macclesfield, U.K.; 3, sera from Hampshire, U.K. ($n = 115$); 4, sera from Hereford, U.K. ($n = 41$).

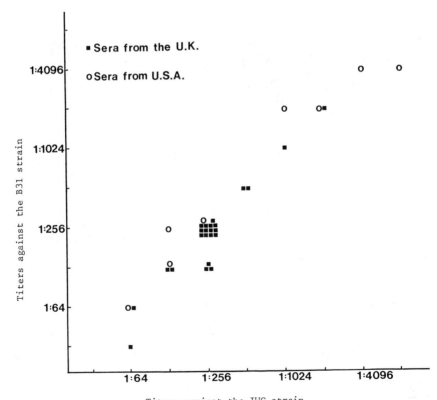

FIGURE 1. Antigen comparison between the B31 strain of *Borrelia burgdorferi* and the IWG strain from the U.K.

RESULTS AND DISCUSSION

ELISA results of antibody responses to *Borrelia burgdorferi* B31 strain are shown in TABLE 1. Of 156 dog sera tested the following had positive titers 1 : 512 or above: 3 of 115 from Hampshire and 4 of 41 from Hereford. This shows that endemic areas of Lyme disease exist in the U.K.

The antigen comparison test results are shown in FIGURE 1. Both antigens of strain B31 and strain IWG had similar reaction patterns with the 32 sera tested. Only a few samples (three of the sera from the USA and four of the sera from the U.K.) gave a little deviation. This result suggests that these two strains could be the same species, *Borrelia burgdorferi*.

In the Western blot assay both positive sera from the USA and the U.K. gave the same polyband reaction pattern to the antigen of B31 strain and the negative sera gave a single-band or no-band pattern. These results confirmed the specificity of the ELISA results. But some of the negative control sera (with ELISA titers of 1 : 256 or 1 : 128) from the USA also gave a similar polyband reaction pattern when the blots were overdeveloped. It is suggested that there are specific antibodies in some of the control sera from the USA, which could have reduced the positive rate in our ELISA test. We estimate that at least one-fifth of our dog sera had specific antibodies to *Borrelia burgdorferi*.

REFERENCES

1. MUHLEMANN, M. F. 1984. Br. J. Dermatol. **111**(3): 335–339.
2. WILLIAMS, D., *et al.* 1986. Br. Med. J. **292**(6535): 1560–1561.
3. BURGESS, E. C. 1986. Lab. Anim. Sci. **36**(3): 288–290.
4. BARBOUR, A. G. 1984. Yale J. Biol. Med. **57**: 581–586.

Concurrent Neocortical Borreliosis and Alzheimer's Disease

Demonstration of a Spirochetal Cyst Form

ALAN B. MacDONALD

Southampton Hospital
Southampton, New York 11968

A 71-year-old man died in Arizona 3 years after the onset of progressive dementia. A diagnosis of probable Alzheimer's disease was based on clinical criteria. The brain was removed at autopsy, frozen (unfixed), and transported to the Department of Pathology, University of California, San Diego, School of Medicine where it was stored at −70°C for further study. The author received the frozen brain and utilized methods previously described[1] for *in vitro* culture, cytologic, immunohistochemical, and silver impregnation studies. Argyrophilic plaques and neurofibrillary tangles were found in the frontal lobe and hippocampal formation in sufficient number to establish the neuropathologic diagnosis of Alzheimer's disease (FIG. 1A). Spirochetes were visualized in imprint preparations of freshly thawed frontal lobe cortex with monoclonal antibody H5332, which specifically binds to the outer surface membrane of *Borrelia burgdorferi* (FIG. 2). *Borrelia* spirochetes were recovered from cultures of freshly thawed cerebral cortex and hippocampus in Barbour-Stoenner-Kelly medium. An unexpected observation was the identification of cystic forms of the *Borrelia* spirochete in dark-field preparations of cultured hippocampus, and in imprints of hippocampus using the monoclonal antibody H9724, which binds to class-specific axial filament proteins of *Borrelia* spirochetes. Oil immersion examination of sections from the hippocampus impregnated with silver disclosed a rare cystic structure (FIG. 1B). Previous workers have identified spirochetal cyst forms in cultures of nonpathogenic treponemal spirochetes and have suggested that spirochetes have a complex life cycle.[2-5] Dark-field examination of aged cultures of the B31 reference strain of *Borrelia burgdorferi* disclosed cystic structures similar to the cysts found in the autopsy brain culture.

The following hypothesis is offered based on these observations. Borrelia spirochetes have a complex life cycle which includes corkscrew-shaped forms, uncoiled filamentous forms, L-forms lacking a cell wall, cystic and ameboid forms, and granular forms. These forms may exist as either extracellular or intracellular pathogens. The cystic form of *Borrelia* may explain the Pick body, which is found in Pick's disease, and the granular form of *Borrelia* may explain granulovacuolar degeneration of nerve cells in the hippocampal formation in Alzheimer's disease. A cystic form of the *Borrelia* spirochete would explain the ability of the microbe to persist in the host during a prolonged period of asymptomatic clinical latency, which spans the period between primary infection and the expression of tertiary manifestations of neuroborreliosis.

REFERENCES

1. MacDONALD, A. B. & J. M. MIRANDA. 1987. Concurrent neocortical borreliosis and Alzheimer's disease. Hum. Pathol. **18:** 759–761.

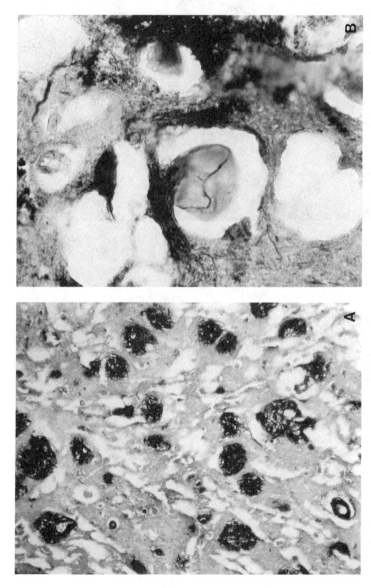

FIGURE 1. Autopsy hippocampus, ammoniacal silver stain. (A) Argyrophilic plaques; magnification: 100×. (B) Cyst form near plaque; magnification: 500×.

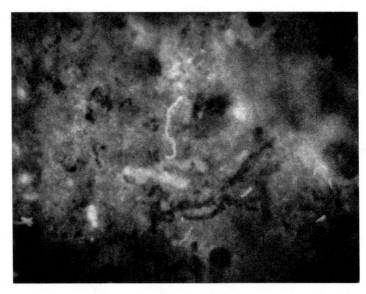

FIGURE 2. *Borrelia* spirochete in imprint of unfixed frontal lobe of brain, revealed using murine monoclonal antibody H5332 for outer surface membrane of *Borrelia burgdorferi*. Magnification: 1000×.

2. REIN, M. F. 1976. Biopharmacology of syphilotherapy. J. Am. Vener. Dis. Assoc. **3**(2): 109–127.
3. OVCINNIKOV, N. M. & V. V. DELEKTORSKIJ. 1971. Current concepts of the morphology and biology of *Treponema pallidum* based on electron microscopy. Br. J. Vener. Dis. **47**: 315–328.
4. COUTTS, W. E. & W. R. COUTTS. 1953. *Treponema pallidum* buds, granules, and cysts as found in human syphilitic chancres and seen in fixed unstained smears under darkground illumination. Am. J. Syph. Gonorrhea Vener. Dis. **37**: 29–35.
5. DELAMMATER, E. D., M. HAANES & R. H. WIGGALL. 1951. Studies on the life cycle of spirochetes V. The life cycle of the Nichols nonpathogenic *Treponema pallidum* in culture. Am. J. Syph. Gonorrhea Vener. Dis. **35**: 164–179.

Determination of Class and Specificity of Antibodies to *Borrelia burgdorferi* in Lyme Disease

JAMES J. MARX, JR., CYNTHIA MOTSZKO,
PAUL MITCHELL, AND ANDREA DLESK

*Marshfield Medical Research Foundation and the Marshfield Clinic
Marshfield, Wisconsin 54449*

The serologic response to *B. burgdorferi* is a major criterion used for the diagnosis of Lyme disease. The methods used for antibody determination are far from standardized.

The serologic reactivity of 2618 sera submitted for Lyme disease testing from patients was determined using an immunofluorescent assay (IFA) and an enzyme immunoassay (EIA). Commercial preparations of antihuman immunoglobulin ($\gamma + \mu + \alpha$) were routinely used in both assays. Serologic reactivity was defined as an

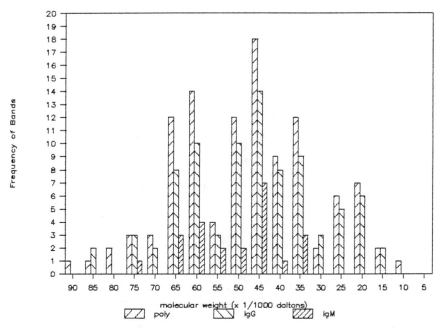

FIGURE 1. Frequency of response to antigenic components of *Borrelia burgdorferi*. Molecular weight distribution of antigenic fragments was determined by separation on SDS-PAGE (12% gel) and developed using alkaline-phosphatase-labeled antihuman polyvalent (H + L chain specific), IgG (γ-chain specific), or IgM (μ-chain specific) antisera. Frequency is a cumulative frequency of the reactivity of 23 sera from patients with Lyme disease.

IFA ≥256. EIA reactivity was defined as >2 SD above the mean of 100 nondiseased individuals residing in central and northern Wisconsin, an area endemic for Lyme disease. The results of the EIA are reported as a ratio of the OD compared to a high-titered reference serum. The same isolate of *B. burgdorferi* was used for both assays. The soluble extracts for the EIA were prepared according to the method described by Russell *et al.*[1] There was a strong correlation ($r = 0.684$, $p < 0.000$) for the regression of the results of these methods. The immunoglobulin class was determined in each of these sera. All of the sera that were positive by EIA also had demonstrable antibody of the IgG and/or IgM classes. There were, however, a significant number of sera ($n = 133$) that had markedly elevated IgM titers without elevations in the routine IFA or EIA. These elevations were not associated with any apparent common denominator.

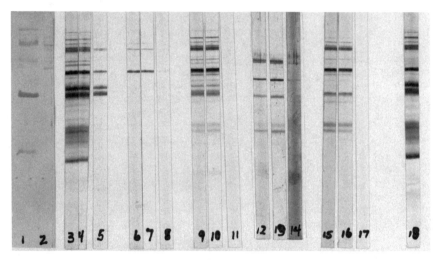

FIGURE 2. Various patterns of reactivity on immunoblots from SDS-PAGE stained with five lyme disease sera. Lane 1, low molecular weight standard; lane 2, *Borrelia burgdorferi* extract; lane 3-5, patient SA; lane 6-8, patient Ab; lane 9-11, patient St; lane 12-14, patient Vo; lane 15-17, patient Do; lane 18, rabbit antisera to *B. burgdorferi* extract. Blots were stained sequentially for polyvalent antibodies, IgG antibodies and IgM antibodies in each patient's serum. The rabbit antibody was stained for polyvalent antibody.

The diversity of the antibody response was determined using Western blot techniques with a polyvalent antiserum, IgG specific, or IgM specific antiserum. The results are summarized in FIGURE 1. The bands with the highest frequency of occurrence in 23 sera from patients appear to be in the range of 60–65 kDa, 45 kDa, and 35 kDa. This is also true when class-specific antisera are used. FIGURE 2 summarizes the type of patterns seen in patients' samples. These results are consistent with the reports of Craft *et al.*[2] and Coleman *et al.*[3] on the major components of the organism.

Western blots using a hyperimmune rabbit sera demonstrated that antigenic extracts were consistent from batch to batch. Further, elevations of IgM titers in the absence of a polyvalent titer (IFA or EIA) were not reacting specifically to the extract of *B. burgdorferi* as suggested by the lack of demonstrable bands on Western blots.

REFERENCES

1. RUSSELL, H., J. S. SAMPSON, G. P. SCHMID, H. W. WILKINSON & B. PLIKAYTIS. 1984. Enzyme-linked immunosorbent assay and indirect immunofluorescence assay for Lyme disease. J. Infect. Dis. **149:** 465–470.
2. CRAFT, J. E., D. K. FISCHER, G. T. SHIMAMOTO & A. C. STEERE. 1986. Antigens of *Borrelia burgdorferi* recognized during Lyme disease. J. Clin. Invest. **78:** 934–939.
3. COLEMAN, J. L. & J. L. BENACH. 1987. Isolation of antigenic components from the Lyme disease spirochete: Their role in early diagnosis. J. Infect. Dis. **155:** 756–765.

A Comparison of Test Procedures for the Detection of Antibody to *Borrelia burgdorferi*

L. E. MERTZ, G. H. WOBIG, J. DUFFY,
AND J. A. KATZMANN

*Mayo Clinic/Foundation
Rochester, Minnesota 55905*

Three procedures were established for the detection of antibody to *Borrelia burgdorferi*. An indirect immunofluorescence assay (IFA) used intact organisms as the substrate; the upper limit of normal was the serum dilution at which 95% of normals were negative (2 SD limit = 1 : 256). An ELISA assay used the filtrate from sonicated organisms; the upper limit of normal was the assay result at which 99% of normals were negative (3 SD limit = 250 antibody response units). An adsorbed ELISA (ELISA-ABS) was identical to the above assay except that serum samples were preincubated with a *Treponema phagedenis* (Reiter) adsorbent. We tested Lyme, infectious disease, and autoimmune sera (TABLE 1).

All three assays were sensitive in detecting neurologic and arthritic Lyme disease; the increase in sensitivity with the ELISA was due to detection of erythema migrans (EM) Lyme sera. The adsorption step preferentially reduced reactivity of normal compared to Lyme sera and allowed a further small increase in sensitivity for EM sera. The decrease in false positives in the autoimmune group was due to loss of reactivity of rheumatoid factor positive sera in the ELISA. The decrease in false positives in the infectious disease group was due to a decrease of reactivity of leptospirosis, pinta, yaws, and FTA-ABS positive sera. Six of the 12 false positives in the ELISA-ABS assay, however, were from yaws patients. The Lyme ELISA-ABS was the most sensitive and specific assay tested and was introduced into routine use.

During the 6 months of October 1986 to March 1987, we tested 453 patient samples in the ELISA-ABS. Of these 453, 427 (94%) were negative (<250 ABR) and 26 (6%) were positive. The medical histories of patients with positive test results were

TABLE 1. Performance of Three Lyme Assays with Defined Sample Populations

Disease (No. of Sera)	Number Positive		
	IFA	ELISA	ELISA-ABS
Lyme[a] (29)	19	23	25
Autoimmune[b] (112)	5	2	2
Infectious[c] (106)	23	16	12
Sensitivity	66%	79%	86%
% False positive	13%	8%	6%

[a]Erythema migrans (10), neurologic (9), and arthritic (10).
[b]Positive ANA (64), positive anti-DNA (16), positive RF (15), and monoclonal gammopathy/cryoglobulin (17).
[c]Yaws (10), pinta (5), leptospirosis (6), syphilis (40), hepatitis B (15), mononucleosis (15), and streptococcus (15).

TABLE 2. Diagnosis of Patients with Positive Lyme ELISA-ABS Test

	ELISA-ABS (ABR units)	
	250–999	>1000
No. of patients with positive ELISA	19	7
No. of patients (%) diagnosed as definite/probable Lyme disease	7 (37%)	5 (71%)

reviewed, and patients with definite and probable Lyme disease were identified (TABLE 2). These 453 results contained 14 false positives. Five of seven patients with an ELISA-ABS result of >1000 ABR had Lyme disease diagnosed; their test results ranged from 3480 to 8260 ABR. Diagnoses of the two other patients with ELISA-ABS results >1000 ABR included lymphocytic meningitis with possible Lyme disease and radiculitis/disk disease.

These data show that in our clinical practice a positive Lyme serology has a positive predictive value of approximately 50% (12/26); a positive result >1000 ABR has a positive predictive value of approximately 70% (5/7, *i.e.* results >1000 ABR have a 70% chance of being from a Lyme patient). Lyme disease serology is useful in confirming clinical suspicion, and our results emphasize the need to interpret serologic data in the context of epidemiologic and clinical features.

Borrelia burgdorferi Infections in Bavarian Forest Workers

A Follow-up Study[a]

UWE NEUBERT,[b] PETER MÜNCHHOFF,[d]
BERNHARD VÖLKER,[b,d] CARL D. REIMERS,[c]
AND KARL H. PFLÜGER[e]

[b] *Department of Dermatology*
[c] *Friedrich Baur Institute*
University of Munich
Munich, Federal Republic of Germany

[d] *Occupational Health Service Munich*
Munich, Federal Republic of Germany

[e] *Department of Hematology/Oncology*
University of Marburg
Marburg, Federal Republic of Germany

Erythema migrans borreliosis, the European equivalent of Lyme borreliosis, is endemic in Bavaria, situated in the Southeast of West Germany. It seems of particular interest to what extent a population group especially prone to tick bites by its occupation shows clinical and serological hints to an infection with *Borrelia burgdorferi* (Bb). In 1983 we examined 211 forest workers from different regions of Upper Bavaria clinically and tested their sera with regard to antibodies (Ab) against Bb by means of an indirect immunofluorescence assay.[1] Two and a half years (y) later 53 of initially 71 seropositive forest workers could be reexamined. The clinical course was determined utilizing a standard questionnaire and further clinical data applied by family doctors. Serum Ab titers were reevaluated; additionally syphilis serology was performed, and rheumatoid factors, antinuclear antibodies, and HLA phenotypes determined. Of the collective initially examined ($n = 211$; age 17–68, median 49 y), 71 (33.6%) proved to be seropositive (reciprocal IgM and/or IgG titers ≥ 10). The percentage of seropositivity increased with rising age (median age of 71 seropositives 56 y, of 140 seronegatives 46.5).[2] IgG Ab were found in 84.5%, IgM Ab in 53%, IgG and IgM Ab in 38% of the 71 sera. Slight differences between seronegative and seropositive forest workers turned out in tick bite history (never bitten by tick 25% of the seronegatives, 10% of the seropositives; $p = 0.01$, Fisher's exact test), elevated erythrocyte sedimentation rates (7% in seronegatives vs. 16% in seropositives), in heart symptoms such as arrythmia, tachycardia, dycardia as well as in verified cardiac disease (9% in seronegatives vs. 14% in seropositives), manifest joint involvement (22% vs. 23.6%), nervous system disorders (6% vs. 7%) and in history of erythema migrans (0.7% vs. 2.8%). No actual cutaneous manifestations of erythema migrans borreliosis were observed in the initial collective.

[a]This investigation was in part supported by a grant (no. Ne 329/1-1) from Deutsche Forschungsgemeinschaft.

476

Three years later (1986, t_3) 53 of the 71 forest workers found seropositive and meanwhile untreated could be reexamined clinically and serologically (FIG. 1). In 12 (23%) elevated Ab titers were no longer found. IgG Ab were shown in 36 (initially 47), 34 (94%) already being IgG-antibody positive in 1983 (t_0). Thirteen (initially 29) forest workers exhibited IgM Ab, nine (69%) being already positive at t_0. IgG and IgM

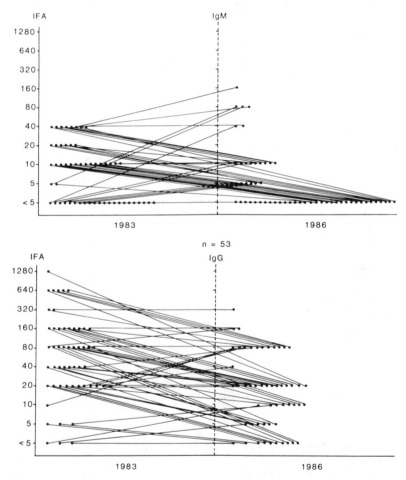

FIGURE 1. Course of reciprocal IgM and IgG serum antibody titers against *B. burgdorferi* in 53 Bavarian forest workers from 1983 to 1986. Indirect immunofluorescence assay.[1]

Ab were found in 10 (initially 23) forest workers, six (60%) being already positive at t_0. Thirty-three forest workers (70%) showed a significant ($\geq$fourfold) decrease in IgG Ab titers, 23 (79%) in IgM Ab titers. Sixteen IgG and 25 IgM titers did not significantly alter. Six of eight forest workers having developed a fourfold rise in IgG and/or IgM-Ab titers had a history, symptoms or signs compatible with Bb infection of skin, joints or nervous system. For instance, a 60-year-old man with steeply increasing serum Ab titers from 1983 to 1986 and 1987 (reciprocal Ab titers: IgG 10, 80, 1280; IgM 40, 10, 160) exhibited a discrete histologically confirmed acrodermatitis chronica atrophicans of the left leg with associated neuropathy accompanied by impaired capacity of reaction and concentration.

As TABLE 1 shows, differences were found concerning the incidence of symptoms affecting skin, joints, heart, and nervous system between 33 forest workers showing significant decrease of serum IgG Ab titers and 20 forest workers with increased or not significantly altered IgG titers. Moreover, 41% of 17 forest workers whose IgG and/or IgM titers rose ≥twofold had shown an elevated erythrocyte sedimentation rate, and 24% a verified cardiac disease at t_0. In 1986, 35% of the same group reported cardiac symptoms and 76% suffered from joint disorders. Rheumatoid factors were detected in

TABLE 1. History of Skin Lesions and Symptoms and Signs Affecting Joints, Heart, and Nervous System in Bavarian Forest Workers (Follow-up Collective 1986, $n = 53$)

	IgG Ab Titer Decreased ≥ Fourfold (%)	IgG Ab Titer Risen or Not Significantly Altered (%)
Skin lesions		
Specific[a]	9	30
Small transient	52	45
Never	39	25
Symptoms and signs affecting:		
Joints[b]	51.5	75
Heart[c]	18	35
Nervous system[d]	33	45

Incidence of lesions and symptoms in one group ($n = 33$) showing significant (≥fourfold) decrease of serum IgG antibody titers and another group ($n = 20$) exhibiting risen or not significantly altered IgG antibody titers against *B. burgdorferi*.

[a]Erythema migrans, lymphadenosis cutis benigna, acrodermatitis chronica atrophicans.
[b]Most frequent: Recurrent asymmetrical obligoarthralgias.
[c]Most frequent: Absolute tachyarrhythmia, AV block.
[d]Most frequent: Paresthesias, hypesthesias, radicular pain.

12 (23%) sera of the follow-up group. HLA phenotypes CW3 and DR2 were each found in 19 (35%) out of 54 seropositive forest workers reexamined (see K.H. Pflüger et al.,[3] this volume). Altogether, regardless of the serological course, 14 forest workers (26%) showed a definite history or findings compatible with manifest erythema migrans borreliosis. Thirty-seven (70%) had no hints of manifest infection; in two cases unequivocal information was not obtained.

In conclusion, the significant decrease of Ab titers and the lack of evidence for manifest erythema migrans borreliosis in about two-thirds of our forest workers found initially seropositive and left untreated lead to the assumption that infections by Bb usually may take an inapparent and possibly self-healing course. On the other hand, a heightened incidence of various symptoms in seropositive forest workers, and especially in those showing rising antibody titers, recommend an early and adequate antibiotic treatment of all seropositive persons.

REFERENCES

1. NEUBERT, U., H. E. KRAMPITZ & H. ENGL. 1986. Microbiological findings in erythema (chronicum) migrans and related disorders. Zbl. Bakt. Hyg. A **263:** 237–252.
2. MÜNCHHOFF, P., B. WILSKE, V. PREAC-MURSIC & G. SCHIERZ. 1986. Antibodies against *Borrelia burgdorferi* in Bavarian forest workers. Zbl. Bakt. Hyg. A **263:** 412–419.
3. PFLÜGER, K. H., C. P. REIMERS, U. NEUBERT, C. MEISEL, B. TRAPP, J. LEITITIS, B. VÖLKER, P. MÜNCHHOFF, J. LITZENBERGER, H. HOLTHAUSEN & E. PONGRATZ. 1988. Erythema migrans borreliosis: An HLA-associated disease? This volume.

Sclerotic Skin Lesions as Manifestations of *Ixodes*-borne Borreliosis[a]

INGEGERD OLSSON,[b] ANDERS HOVMARK,[b]
EVA ÅSBRINK,[b] AND EVA BREHMER-ANDERSSON[c]

[b]Department of Dermatology
[c]Department of Pathology
Södersjukhuset, 10064 Stockholm, Sweden

Localized scleroderma and lichen sclerosus et atrophicus (LSA) are both sclerotic cutaneous disorders of unknown etiology. It is as yet not settled whether they represent different manifestations of a single disease process or are separate but related disorders. It has long been known that scleroderma-like skin lesions can occur concomitantly with acrodermatitis chronica atrophicans (ACA). In some of these patients sclerotic lesions dominate and inflammatory ACA lesions can be slight and therefore may be overlooked. These patients will sometimes be diagnosed as suffering from scleroderma or LSA.[1] Studies have recently been performed concerning the frequency of serological evidence of borreliosis among patients with localized scleroderma but the conclusions reached are inconsistent.[2–4]

MATERIAL AND METHODS

The occurrence of sclerotic skin lesions among patients seen at our department with a diagnosis of ACA or Borrelia lymphocytoma has been recorded since 1982.

Sera from patients with a diagnosis of scleroderma or LSA, but without clinical

TABLE 1. Frequency of Positive Borrelial Antibody Titers, Measured by an ELISA, in Sera of Patients with a Diagnosis of Scleroderma or Lichen Sclerosus et Atrophicus (LSA)[a]

	No.	Disease Duration Median (Range)	Positive Titers in IgG and/or IgM[b]
Localized scleroderma	15	2 years (3 months–12 years)	2
Generalized scleroderma	4	11 months (2 months–14 years)	0
LSA, including extragenital involvement	14	3.5 years (3 months–10 years)	3
LSA with anogenital involvement alone	36	1.5 years (1 month–10 years)	5

[a]A positive titer is defined as a titer above the 95th percentile of healthy individuals.
[b]Six patients were positive in IgG alone and three patients in IgM alone.

[a]This work was supported by a grant from the Swedish Medical Research Council (no. 7935).

480

TABLE 2. Titers of IgG Antibodies against *Borrelia*

	≤410	>410–1000	>1000–3000	>3000
Sc	17	2	—	—
LSA	45	5	—	—
EM	72	10	6	—
BL	5	6	6	2
ACA	—	10	21	56
HI	176	9	—	—

Titers were measured by an ELISA in sera of 19 patients with localized or generalized scleroderma (Sc), 50 patients with lichen sclerosus et atrophicus (LSA), 88 patients with uncomplicated erythema migrans (EM), 19 patients with Borrelia lymphocytoma (BL), and 87 patients with acrodermatitis chronica atrophicans (ACA) and 185 healthy individuals (HI).

signs of ACA or Borrelia lymphocytoma, have been examined from 1984 for the presence of antibodies to Borrelia. In most cases, diagnoses of scleroderma or LSA were histopathologically confirmed. The presence of IgG and IgM antibodies was established with an ELISA, as has elsewhere been described.[5]

RESULTS

Among 87 patients with ACA, seven had clinically and histopathologically scleroderma- or LSA-like skin lesions. One patient with a Borrelia lymphocytoma on areola mammae simultaneously developed a LSA lesion on one arm. The effect of antibiotic treatment on the sclerotic lesions in these patients varied from a complete cure to a slight improvement.

Serological examination was performed on a total of 19 patients with scleroderma and 50 patients with LSA. The results are shown in TABLE 1. The IgG titers are correlated to those of healthy individuals and patients with diagnosed borreliosis in TABLE 2. It is noteworthy that the titers in the patients with sclerotic skin lesions did not in any cases exceed the highest titers found in the healthy individuals. The same was true for the IgM titers. Thus, the by-definition positive titers were insufficient for a definite serological diagnosis of borreliosis. Ten of the 69 patients with a diagnosis of scleroderma or LSA received antibiotics, but without any obvious effect on the skin lesions when followed up 3–24 months after the treatment.

CONCLUSION

Sclerotic skin lesions, clinically and histopathologically similar to or indistinguishable from scleroderma or LSA, can occur in association with borreliosis. However, in the majority of patients with scleroderma or LSA we did not find serological evidence of borrelial etiology.

REFERENCES

1. ÅSBRINK, E., E. BREHMER-ANDERSSON & A. HOVMARK. 1986. Am. J. Dermatopathol. **8:** 209–219.

2. RUFLI, T., S. LEHNER, A. AESCHLIMANN, E. CHAMOT, F. GIGON & J.-P. JEANNERET. 1986. Hautarzt **37:** 597–602.
3. HANSEN, K., J. SERUP & S. HOYBYE. 1987. Lancet **i:** 682.
4. ABERER, E., G. STANEK, M. ERTL & R. NEUMAN. 1987. Acta Derm. Venereol. (Stockholm) **67:** 225–231.
5. ÅSBRINK, E., A. HOVMARK & B. HEDERSTEDT. 1985. Acta Derm. Venereol. (Stockholm) **65:** 509–514.

An Indirect Quantitative Fluorescence Immunoassay for the Detection of Lyme Disease Serum Antibody

DANIEL R. PENNELL,[a] PHILIP J. WAND,[a]
AND RONALD F. SCHELL[a,b]

[a]Wisconsin State Laboratory of Hygiene
[b]Department of Medical Microbiology
University of Wisconsin
Madison, Wisconsin 53706

Determination of serum antibody levels to *Borrelia burgdorferi* is often helpful in the diagnosis of Lyme disease. Established procedures include the indirect fluorescent antibody (IFA) test[2–5] and enzyme-linked immunosorbent assay (ELISA).[1–3,5] In this study an indirect quantitative fluorescence immunoassay (FIAX) was evaluated. A total of 247 sera were tested by FIAX and the conventional IFA test, including 46 normal individuals from a nonendemic area (Maryland), 147 patients meeting case definition (presence of erythema migrans, EM), and 54 patients with other spirochetal or autoimmune diseases. In addition, 50 sera from individuals residing in an endemic area (Northern Wisconsin) and 72 patients with neurologic disease were tested by FIAX alone.

TABLE 1. FIAX Serum Reactivity by Geographic Area and Disease

Sera	No. Tested	No. Positive (%)	Mean ΔFSU[a]
Nonendemic area	46	0 (0.0)	7.9
Lyme endemic area	50	9 (18.1)	10.0
Lyme case	147	120 (81.6)	25.3
Rheumatoid factor	12	2 (16.7)	12.1
Antinuclear antibody	12	5 (41.7)	13.3
Syphilis	18	17 (94.4)	39.5
Leptospirosis	9	3 (33.3)	14.2
Relapsing fever borreliosis	3	1 (33.3)	23.7
Multiple sclerosis	24	5 (20.8)	11.2
Amyotrophic lateral sclerosis	48	10 (20.8)	11.4

[a]Mean of all sera test. ΔFSU = fluorescence signal units after subtraction of nonspecific reactivity. ΔFSU $\leq$ 14.9 interpreted as negative.

FIAX correlated well with IFA (Pearson correlation coefficient = 0.72). A FIAX precision analysis yielded interassay coefficients of variation (CV) of 15.3%, 12.1%, and 12.5% (seven replicates) and intra-assay CV of 14.9%, 2.9%, and 4.7% (six replicates) for low-, medium-, and high-reacting sera, respectively. When a FIAX activity level was established such that all normal, nonendemic sera were interpreted as negative (TABLE 1), 120 case sera were positive (TABLE 2, sensitivity = 81.6%). FIAX sensitivity improved to 85.6% when results for sera collected during the first 2 weeks after onset of disease were omitted. A low proportion of positive to negative results for sera collected early after onset of Lyme disease has been previously observed for IFA and ELISA.[3]

Reactivity to FIAX antigen was seen in 2 of 12 sera positive for rheumatoid factor, 5 of 12 sera positive for antinuclear antibody, 17 of 18 sera positive for syphilis, 3 of 9 sera positive for leptospirosis, and 1 of 3 sera positive for relapsing fever borreliosis (TABLE 1). Such cross-reactivity has been observed with IFA and ELISA tests for Lyme disease.[3] Reactivity was also seen in 5 of 24 patients with multiple sclerosis (MS), and 10 of 48 patients with amyotrophic lateral sclerosis (ALS).

Mean FIAX reactivity was greater for sera obtained from individuals residing in an area endemic for Lyme disease in comparison to individuals from a nonendemic area (TABLE 1), demonstrating the presence of greater antibody background in this population. This mean reactivity was, however, less than that seen in MS and ALS patients.

Serological analysis remains the most appropriate approach for the clinical laboratory in offering diagnostic assistance in potential cases of Lyme disease. FIAX is a convenient and dependable means of evaluating sera for this purpose. Additional

TABLE 2. FIAX Results for Lyme Case Defined Sera

| | Weeks After Disease Onset | | |
	≤2	>2	Total
No. positive	25	95	120
No. negative	11	16	27
Sensitivity (%)	69.4	85.6	81.6

efforts should concentrate on evaluating serological capacities for the identification of non-EM cases and reducing cross-reactivity.

REFERENCES

1. CRAFT, J. E., R. L. GRODZICKI & A. C. STEERE. 1984. Antibody response in Lyme disease: Evaluation of diagnostic tests. J. Infect. Dis. 149: 789–795.
2. MAGNARELLI, L. A., J. M. MEEGAN, J. F. ANDERSON & W. A. CHAPPELL. 1984. Comparison of an indirect fluorescent-antibody test with an enzyme-linked immunosorbent assay for serological studies of Lyme disease. J. Clin. Microbiol. 20: 181–184.
3. RUSSELL, H., J. S. SAMPSON, G. P. SCHMID, H. W. WILKINSON & B. PLIKAYTIS. 1984. Enzyme-linked immunosorbent assay and indirect immunofluorescence assay for Lyme disease. J. Infect. Dis. 149: 465–470.
4. STEERE, A. C., R. L. GRODZICKI, A. N. KORNBLATT, J. E. CRAFT, A. G. BARBOUR, W. BURGDORFER, G. P. SCHMID, E. JOHNSON & S. E. MALAWISTA. 1983. The spirochetal etiology of Lyme disease. N. Engl. J. Med. 308: 733–740.
5. STIERNSTEDT, G. T., M. GRANSTROM, B. HEDERSTEDT & B. SKOLDENBERG. 1985. Diagnosis of spirochetal meningitis by enzyme-linked immunosorbent assay and indirect immunofluorescence assay in serum and cerebrospinal fluid. J. Clin. Microbiol. 21: 819–825.

Corticosteroids for Radicular Pain in Bannwarth's Syndrome

A Double-blind, Randomized, Placebo-controlled Trial

H. W. PFISTER, K. M. EINHÄUPL, P. FRANZ,
AND C. GARNER

Neurological Department
University of Munich, Klinikum Grosshadern
D-8000 Munich, Federal Republic of Germany

Severe radicular pain that usually does not respond to analgesics and nonsteroidal antiphlogistics is the clinical hallmark of Bannwarth's syndrome (BS). Some case reports and our own experience demonstrated the prompt and sufficient improvement of pain after corticosteroid therapy. In order to assess the efficacy of corticosteroids in the treatment of radicular pain in acute BS, we performed a double-blind, randomized, placebo-controlled trial.

PATIENTS AND METHODS

We randomly assigned 21 patients with BS who complained of intense radicular pain to 7-day treatment with either methylprednisolone (60 mg orally per day) or

TABLE 1. Clinical Data of 21 Patients with Bannwarth's Syndrome

	Penicillin and Corticosteroid ($n = 11$)	Penicillin and Placebo ($n = 10$)
Age (years)	56.7 ± 15.9[a]	50.2 ± 10.2
Sex	4 M, 7 F	3 M, 7 F
Arthropod bite	10	9
Erythema migrans[b]	3	7
Neurologic abnormalities		
Radicular pain	11	10
Headache	2	1
Stiff neck	1	2
Facial palsy	3	2
Pareses of extremities	5[c]	3[d]
Cerebrospinal fluid		
Lymphocytic pleocytosis		
(cells/μl)	267 ± 320	142 ± 95
Total protein (mg/dl)	79 ± 34	72 ± 37
Duration onset of pain to		
onset of therapy (days)	26.3 ± 19.7	12.0 ± 6.5

[a]Data expressed as mean ± standard deviation.

[b]In one patient of the corticosteroid group and in two patients of the placebo group erythema migrans was still present when neurological symptoms and signs developed.

[c]Weakness left arm (1); incomplete cauda syndrome (1); weakness right foot extensor (1); weakness left leg (2).

[d]Paraparesis both arms (1); quadriceps and iliopsoas paresis left (1); quadriceps paresis right (1).

485

placebo. In addition, all patients were treated with antibiotics, 19 patients with penicillin parenterally over 10 days and 2 patients, allergic to penicillin, with doxycycline orally over 4 weeks. Patients who had been pretreated with corticosteroids were excluded from the study. Clinical data of all patients are shown in TABLE 1. The diagnosis of BS was confirmed by elevated IgG or IgM antibody titers against *Borrelia burgdorferi* as measured by indirect immunofluorescence in 18 patients ($\geq 1 : 64$). Neurological examination was performed daily for 7 days. The daily dose of analgesics was recorded during the 7-day period. Intensity of pain was assessed by magnitude

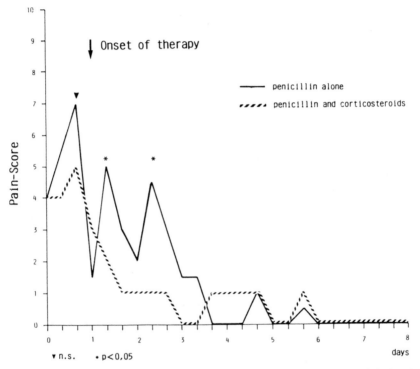

FIGURE 1. Radicular pain in Bannwarth's syndrome (magnitude estimation: 0–10) during the 7-day treatment period with penicillin and corticosteroids ($n = 11$) as compared to penicillin and placebo ($n = 10$). The curves represent medians of corresponding pain scores in all patients of the corticosteroid and placebo group, respectively. In the first two days of treatment, especially at night, improvement of radicular pain is faster when corticosteroids are added to penicillin therapy.

estimation three times a day over the whole treatment period using a score from 0 to 10. The principal statistical method was the Wilcoxon rank-sum test. Clinical reexamination was performed 3 to 18 months after therapy.

RESULTS

Group differences in sex, age, and neurological symptoms were not evident. The mean duration from onset of radicular pain to onset of therapy was different in both groups (TABLE 1). The total amount of analgesics taken was similar in both groups. The effect of penicillin treatment on radicular pain begins 24 to 48 hours after the onset of therapy and pain disappeared completely in nearly all patients after the fourth to fifth day. During the first 2 days of treatment, especially at night, improvement of radicular pain seemed to be faster when corticosteroids were added to penicillin therapy (FIG. 1) At the end of the trial period radicular pain had almost completely resolved in both groups. We observed two patients in each group whose neurological symptoms (facial palsies or pareses of extremities) deteriorated during the treatment period. During the follow-up period 3 to 18 months after therapy no relapse of symptoms was observed. At clinical reexamination no patient presented with functional motor deficits.

DISCUSSION

Clinical observations of BS therapy in the preantibiotic era suggested that radicular pain promptly resolves by corticosteroid therapy.[1,2] Surprisingly, our results show that penicillin alone diminishes radicular pain within a few days. Because of the scatter of the pain scores before the onset of therapy and the relatively small number of patients in this study, only a trend of the efficacy of corticosteroids could be demonstrated. As radicular pain improves very quickly by therapy with penicillin alone, additional corticosteroids should be taken into consideration only in selected cases in which intense radicular pain does not respond to analgesics and nonsteroidal antiphlogistics.

The observation of clinical worsening in a few patients of both groups indicates that either penicillin might not be the antibiotic of choice or the neurological symptoms are due to secondary, probably immunological, mechanisms following initial borrelial infection; in addition clinical deterioration might be explained in part by Herxheimer reaction.

REFERENCES

1. SCHALTENBRAND, G. 1966. Durch Arthropoden übertragene Infektionen der Haut und des Nervensystems. Münch. Med. Wochenschr. **108:** 1557–1562.
2. PFISTER, H. W., K. M. EINHÄUPL, C. GARNER & R. HABERL. 1985. Corticosteroids versus penicillin in the treatment of meningoradiculitis of Bannwarth (Bannwarth's syndrome). J. Neurol. **232** (Suppl.): 293.

Suspected Borreliosis in Cattle

JOHN E. POST,[a] ERIC E. SHAW,[a]
AND SCOTT D. WRIGHT[b]

[a]University of Connecticut
Storrs, Connecticut 06268

[b]University of Florida
Gainesville, Florida 32610

Serological and microbiological studies have shown that many species of mammals in *Ixodes* tick infested areas are infected with *Borrelia burgdorferi*.[1] However, clinical disease associated with these infections has been only reported in humans, horses,[2,3] and dogs.[4] We briefly reported two suspected cases in cows in 1986[5] and now report clinical and experimental studies involving 13 mature lactating cows having suspected clinical borreliosis.

Clinical signs, similar in all, included erythema, warmth, swelling and hypersensitivity to touch of the skin of the ventral udder and lower rear legs. There was mild lameness and pastern and fetlock joints were swollen. Milk production was diminished probably because pain interfered with milk "letdown." Although mastitis was suspected, laboratory tests for common pathogens and inflammatory cells were negative. Body temperatures and hemograms were normal. Cows treated intravenously with 3 gm of oxytetracycline once or twice daily for 3 to 5 days recovered in this time period, but recovery in untreated animals took 2 to 3 weeks.

IFA tests for serum antibodies to *Borrelia burgdorferi* were positive in 4 of 6 cows tested. Titers ranged from 1 : 64 to 1 : 128. Similar IFA tests for five common *Leptospira* serotypes that infect cattle were negative. Spirochetes with Borrelia morphology were observed in the urine of two cows by dark-field microscopy. Attempts to culture organisms from blood, urine, and milk of three cows were not successful.

A mature cat fed 4 ml of milk from an affected cow seroconverted from a negative IFA *B. burgdorferi* antibody titer to a positive titer of 1 : 64. Similarly, five negative *Peromyscus leucopus* mice all developed titers of 1 : 8 to 1 : 32 when inoculated subcutaneously with 0.1 ml of the same milk. Five additional mice, each inoculated the same way, with 0.1 ml of urine from the affected cow developed IFA titers ranging from 1 : 32 to 1 : 64. None of the experimental animals developed clinical signs.

The observations described suggest that cows develop clinical borreliosis with an ECM lesion like humans, and the limited experimental animal exposure studies indicate that infectious spirochetes may be transmitted in urine and milk.

REFERENCES

1. MAGNARELLI, L. A., J. F. ANDERSON, A. F. KAUFMANN, L. L. LIEBERMAN & G. D. WHITNEY. 1985. J. Med. Entomol. **21:** 52.
2. BURGESS, E. C., D. GILLETTE & J. P. PICKETT. 1986. J. Am. Vet. Med. Assoc. **189:** 1340–1342.
3. POST, J. E., E. E. SHAW & F. PALKA. 1986. Proc. 32nd Conv. Am. Assoc. Equine Practitioners. pp. 415–421.
4. LISSMAN, B. A., E. M. BORLER, H. CAMAY, B. G. ORMISON & J. L. BENACH. 1984. J. Am. Vet. Med. Assoc. **184:** 219.
5. SHAW, E. E., J. E. POST & F. C. PALKA. 1986. Am. Assoc. Vet. Lab. Diag. 29th Ann. Proc. pp. 231–242.

The Prevalence of Antibody to *Borrelia burgdorferi* among Patients with Undiagnosed Central Nervous System Disease in California

JULIE A. RAWLINGS

Texas Department of Health
Bureau of Laboratories
Austin, Texas 78756-3194

ROBERT S. LANE

University of California
Berkeley, California 94720

Borrelia burgdorferi is capable of causing central nervous system (CNS) abnormalities throughout the course of Lyme disease.[1-3] With this in mind, we began a retrospective serosurvey for the detection of antibodies to *B. burgdorferi* in California patients with undiagnosed CNS disease. Acute and convalescent sera were collected between 1968 and 1976 from three geographic regions: 53 specimen pairs from the northwestern coastal counties (FIG. 1), 54 pairs from the southwestern coastal counties, and 127 pairs from counties in the Central Valley.

Altogether, 234 patients were tested using the indirect fluorescent antibody (IFA) procedure.[4] Of these, 52 patients (22%) had positive antibody titers: 13 showed fourfold rises in titer between the acute and convalescent phase and 39 showed either twofold rises to ≥1 : 256 or static titers of 1 : 256 or greater. By geographic areas, 14 patients (26%) from the north coastal counties had positive titers, seven (13%) from the southern region were seropositive, and 31 (24%) from the Central Valley had positive titers. The lowest percentage of positives (5%) was detected in sera collected in 1968; the highest percentage (53%) was detected in sera collected in 1975 (FIG. 2).

A brief list of symptoms was received for 20 of the positive patients. The most common complaints included fever (*n* = 15), headache (*n* = 11), and nausea or vomiting (*n* = 6). Physicians suspected viral encephalitis or meningitis for 15 patients and Rocky Mountain spotted fever for four patients. There was documentation of tick exposure for four patients and a ground squirrel bite for one. One patient became ill after camping at Sequoia National Park, another after receiving an "insect bite" while exploring a cave in Texas.

Lyme disease is presently the most prevalent tick-borne illness in California (personal communication, R. A. Murray). However, it is likely that some patients in this study suffered from a cross-reacting tick-borne relapsing fever infection, as *Borrelia hermsii*, *Borrelia parkeri*, and *Borrelia turicatae* and their associated vectors are endemic to California. Tick-borne relapsing fever spirochetes are capable of causing chronic CNS manifestations similar to those associated with *B. burgdorferi*.[5,6] Perhaps the cases identified in our survey can be attributed to any of several *Borrelia* species. If this is so, collectively they may be responsible for a chronic borreliosis syndrome.

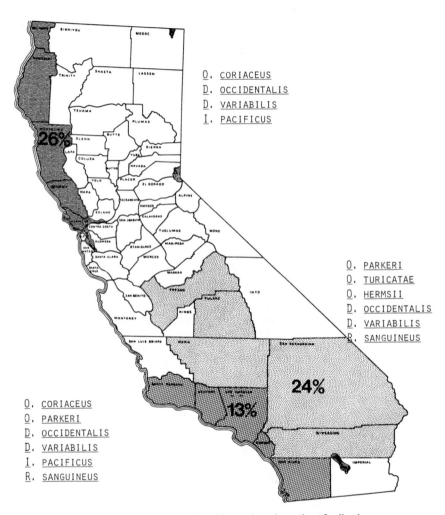

FIGURE 1. Percentage of positive patients by region of collection.

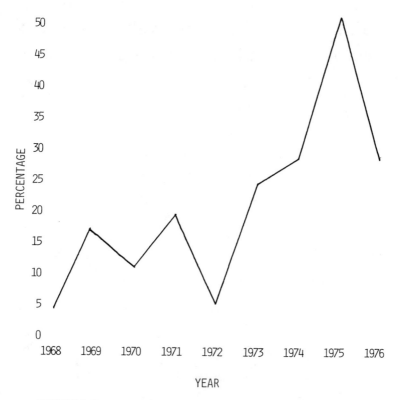

FIGURE 2. Percentage of positive patients by year of specimen collection.

REFERENCES

1. PACHNER, A. R. & A. C. STEERE. 1985. Neurology **35:** 47–53.
2. PACHNER, A. R. & A. C. STEERE. 1986. Zbl. Bakt. Hyg. A **263:** 301–306.
3. REIK, L. A., A. C. STEERE, N. H. BRATENHAGEN, R. E. SHOPE & S. E. MALAWISTA. 1979. Medicine **58:** 281–294.
4. RUSSELL, H., J. S. SAMPSON, G. P. SCHMID, H. W. WILKINSON & B. PLIKAYTIS. 1984. J. Infect. Dis. **149:** 465–470.
5. SCOTT, R. B. 1944. Lancet **2:** 436–439.
6. SOUTHERN, P. M. & J. P. SANFORD. 1969. Medicine **48:** 129–149.

Differentiation of Progressive Borrelia Encephalomyelitis from Multiple Sclerosis

B. REHSE-KÜPPER,[a] R. ACKERMANN,[b] J. KABATZKI,[b]
AND S. HARTUNG[b]

[a]Universitäts-Nervenklinik Köln
Joseph-Stelzmann-Strasse 9
5000 Köln 41, Federal Republic of Germany

[b]Medizinisch-Diagnostisches Laboratorium
Hohenzollernring 14
5000 Köln 41, Federal Republic of Germany

INTRODUCTION

Though patients with progressive borrelia encephalomyelitis (PBE) can show higher pleocytosis, impaired blood/CSF barrier, and sometimes more severe mental disorders, multiple central nervous symptomatology, CSF alterations, and chronic remittant course often are similar to multiple sclerosis (MS).[1,2] PBE can be treated specifically and immunosuppression can be harmful. It is therefore important to differentiate PBE from MS. We investigated unclassified MS patients with "definite" diagnosis from 20 neurologic departments in the Federal Republic of Germany for serum antibodies against *Ixodes ricinus* borrelia (strain S_2N_{34}) by ELISA.[3] In order to assess an involvement of the nervous system we looked for intrathecally synthesized

TABLE 1. Serum and CSF Ab against *Ixodes ricinus* Borrelia in MS Patients, $n = 633$, Average Age 47 (19–78), 230 Male, 403 Female

Serum Ab 200 U[a]/Total	Ab per 1 μg IgG	
	CSF Ab = Serum Ab/CSF Ab > Serum Ab	
90/633 (14%)	59/3 (5%)	

[a]0–95 units (U) = negative; 100–195 U = borderline; 200 U = positive.

borrelia Ab of seropositive patients. For this purpose specific borrelia Ab activities per unit weight of IgG in CSF and serum were compared by ELISA. Higher Ab titers per μg IgG in CSF than in serum indicate the presence of additional Ab from local synthesis and herewith activity of the pathogen in the nervous system (TABLE 1–3).[4]

FOLLOW-UP EXAMINATIONS

Patient 1. After 3½ years nuerologic deficiencies had slowly progressed. CSF findings were identical with the former ones. The result of a recent i.v. penicillin treatment is still unknown.

TABLE 2. MS Patients with Locally Synthesized CSF AB against *Ixodes ricinus* Borrelia: Clinical Picture

Patient	Age	Sex	Duration of Disease	Clinical Syndrome	CSF
1	48	M	10 y	Tetraspastic cerebellar syndrome	IIGG[a] OCB[b]
2	31	F	6 mo.	Opticusneuritis, sensibility disorders	IIGG OCB
3	30	M	10 d	Nonsystemic sensibility disorders, strengthened tendon reflexes	OCB

[a]Intrathecally produced IgG
[b]Oligoclonal IgG bands

Patient 2. After three months without antibiotic treatment the patient showed a visus deficit on the left; nonsystemic sensitivity disorders, signs of demyelination in NMR, and oligoclonal IgG bands in the CSF, but no more intrathecally produced borrelia Ab.

Patient 3. After 1½ years, half a year after a 10-day oral treatment with 200 mg doxycyclin per day, the patient still complained about slight sensitivity disorders. In the CSF he showed oligoclonal IgG bands but no more intrathecally produced borrelia Ab.

CONCLUSIONS

1. The 14% infection rate of *Ixodes ricinus* borrelia of our MS patients is similar to the rate found among healthy adults in Germany (11–30%).[5] Our result does not support the hypothesis of a frequent etiologic role of this pathogen in MS.
2. Most (95%) of the 62 investigated seropositive MS patients did not show intrathecally produced borrelia Ab. This means that their nervous system was not affected by the borrelia infection. Only three patients showed intrathecally produced antibodies.
3. In two of these three cases later on autochthonal CSF borrelia Ab with and without antibiotic therapy disappeared but signs of MS persisted. Obviously latent borrelia infection of the NS can be combined with MS. Autochthonal CSF AB against other pathogens like measles, rubella, VZV, mumps, HSV, vaccinia, etc. are well known in MS.[4]
4. In order to differentiate PBE as a rare event from MS, demonstration of

TABLE 3. Serologic Results

Patient	Serum Ab	Ab per 1 μg IgG	
		CSF	Serum
1	250 U	8	4
2	250 U	8	4
3	220 U	8	4

[a]Reciprocal titer.

    intrathecally synthesized CSF Ab to *Ixodes ricinus* borrelia *and* complete normalization of the CSF after specific therapy is necessary.

5. Regardless of manifest involvement of the nervous system, MS patients seropositive to *Ixodes ricinus* borrelia should be treated specifically with respect to the risk of a latent borrelia infection, especially when the patient undergoes immunosuppressive therapy.

REFERENCES

1. ACKERMANN, R., E. GOLLMER & B. REHSE-KÜPPER. 1985. Progressive Borrelian-Enzephalomyelitis. Dtsch. Med. Wochenschr. **110:** 1039–1042.
2. PACHNER, A., A. STEERE & Y. HAVEN. 1986. Neurologic involvement in the third stage of Lyme disease: CNS manifestations can mimic multiple sclerosis and psychiatric illness. Neurology **36** (Suppl. 1): 286.
3. REHSE-KÜPPER, B. & R. ACKERMANN. 1987. Demonstration of locally synthesized borrelia antibodies in cerebrospinal fluid. Zbl. Bakt. Hyg. A **263:** 407–411.
4. FELGENHAUER, K., H.-J. SCHÄDLICH, M. NEKIC & R. ACKERMANN. 1985. Cerebrospinal fluid virus antibodies. A diagnostic indicator for multiple sclerosis? J. Neurol. Sci. **71:** 291–299.
5. SCHMIDT, R., J. KABATZKI, S. HARTUNG & R. ACKERMANN. 1986. Erythema chronicum migrans in the Federal Republic of Germany. Zbl. Bakt. Hyg. A **263:** 435–441.

Unusual Neurological Manifestations of Second-Stage Lyme Borreliosis

E. SCHMUTZHARD,[a] P. POHL,[a] G. STOCKHAMMER,[a]
B. KLEEDORFER,[a] AND G. STANEK[b]

[a]Department of Neurology
University Hospital Innsbruck
Innsbruck, Austria

[b]Hygiene Institute
University of Vienna
Vienna, Austria

INTRODUCTION

Pachner and Steere have outlined the classical triad of neurological signs and symptoms of the second-stage Lyme borreliosis.[1] Lately the discussion has concentrated on the chronic or relapsing demyelinating form of this disease as part of its third stage.[2,3] Nevertheless, we would like to report unusual neurological manifestations which we could observe during the course of second-stage Lyme borreliosis.

CAUDITIS

Two female patients (67 and 75 years old) presented with painful lesion of cauda equina. CSF findings and serological examinations of blood and CSF established the diagnosis of cauditis caused by *Borrelia burgdorferi*. High-dosage penicillin led to complete recovery within 3 and 5 weeks, respectively.

FOCAL NODULAR MYOSITIS

A 52-year-old female was admitted because of bilateral facial paresis, painful atrophy of both biceps and triceps muscles, and severe local tenderness of these muscles.

Raised creatininkinase (CK), electromyography, and muscle biopsy lead to the diagnosis of meningopolyneuritis Bannwarth with focal nodular myositis. Serologic examination confirmed the etiologic role of *B. burgdorferi*. Adequate penicillin therapy led to dramatic improvement of local tenderness, normalization of CK, and most importantly, to the disappearance of inflammatory signs in control biopsy 8 weeks after antibiotic treatment.

CEREBRAL VASCULITIS ASSOCIATED WITH MENINGITIS

A 44-year-old female was seen because of left-sided sudden hemiparesis. CAT scan (2 days later) showed a right parietal hypodense area suggestive of recent arteria cerebri media infarction, magnetic resonance imaging confirming the diagnosis of infarction. In lumbar puncture a pleocytosis of 130 lymphocytes/mm^3 and intrathecal IgG, IgM, and IgA production was found. Serologic examination yielded a high titer of *Borrelia burgdorferi* antibodies in blood and CSF. Unfortunately, angiography of intracranial arteries was performed only 10 days after the onset of illness. It did not show any abnormalities. Adequate-high dosage penicillin therapy cleared the CSF, the serological titers returned to normal within 4 months; the left-sided hemiparesis, however, improved only partially.

CONCLUSION

Thus, in view of previous[4-6] and, particularly, these case reports, we suggest that the spectrum of signs and symptoms of second-stage Lyme borreliosis be extended to include cauditis, focal nodular myositis, and vasculitis, leading to cerebral infarction, as rare conditions.

REFERENCES

1. PACHNER, A. R. & A. C. STEERE. 1985. The triad of neurologic manifestations of Lyme disease: Meningitis, cranial neuritis and radiculoneuritis. Neurology **35:** 47–53.
2. ACKERMANN, R., E. GOLLMER & B. REHSE-KÜPPER. 1985. Progressive Borrelien-Encephalomyelitis. Dtsch. Med. Wochenschr. **110:** 1039–1042.
3. PACHNER, A. R. & A. C. STEERE. 1986. CNS manifestations of third stage Lyme disease. Zbl. Bakt. Hyg. A **263:** 301–306.
4. SCHMUTZHARD, E., J. WILLEIT & F. GERSTENBRAND. 1986. Meningopolyneuritis Bannwarth with focal nodular myositis: A new aspect in Lyme borreliosis. Klin. Wochenschr. **64:** 1204–1208.
5. MIDGARD, R. & H. HOFSTAD. 1987. Unusual manifestations of nervous system *Borrelia burgdorferi* infection. Arch. Neurol. **44:** 781–783.
6. CAMPONOVO, F. & C. MEIER. 1986. Neuropathy of vasculitic origin in a case of Garin-Bujadoux-Bannwarth syndrome with positive borrelia antibody response. J. Neurol. **233:** 69–72.

Antibody Titer Determinations against *Borrelia burgdorferi* in Blood Donors and in Two Different Groups of Patients

V. STICHT-GROH,[a] R. MARTIN,[b]
AND I. SCHMIDT-WOLF[a]

[a]*Institute of Hygiene and Microbiology*
[b]*Department of Neurology*
University of Würzburg
8700 Würzburg, Federal Republic of Germany

The purpose of the study was to determine the percentage of significant titers against *Borrelia burgdorferi* in blood donors ($n = 1033$) and in two different groups of patients. The first group ($n = 212$) originated from the Department of Neurology and all had a working diagnosis of Lyme meningoradiculitis. The second group of patients was randomly selected ($n = 419$) and came from the Department of Medicine and Surgery.

TABLE 1. Antibody Titer Determinations against *Borrelia burgdorferi* by IFA According to Origin of Sera ($n = 1664$)

	IFA Titers			
	1 : <64	1 : 64	1 : >64	Total Number
Blood donors				
Number	921	56	56	1033
% Lines	89.15%	5.42%	5.42%	
% Columns	63.43%	48.28%	58.33%	(62.08%)
Patients with suspected Lyme meningoradiculitis				
Number	170	23	19	212
% Lines	80.19%	10.85%	8.96%	
% Columns	11.70%	19.83%	19.79%	(12.74%)
Other patients				
Number	361	37	21	419
% Lines	86.16%	8.83%	5.01%	
% Columns	24.86%	31.90%	21.87%	(25.18%)
Total number	1452	116	96	1664
	(87.26%)	(6.97%)	(5.77%)	

We tested 1664 sera in toto both in IFA (indirect immunofluorescence assay, polyvalent conjugate, Dakopatts, F 200)[1] and in IgG ELISA (enzyme-linked immunosorbent assay, Dakopatts, P 214).[2] IgG-ELISA titer was considered significant if it yielded a net absorbance greater than the total derived by adding three standard deviations (SD) to the mean ($\geq \bar{x} \pm 3$ SD) of the absorbance for a group of eight negative controls.[2,3] Borderline results were calculated by adding two SD to the mean of the absorbance for a group of eight negative controls ($\geq \bar{x} \pm 2$ SD). All syphilitic sera were excluded.

IFA antibody determinations against *B. burgdorferi* showed that 5.42% of sera from blood donors, 8.96% of sera from patients with suspected Lyme meningoradiculitis, and 5.01% of sera from patients with a diagnosis other than borreliosis had significant titers (TABLE 1). IgG-ELISA showed relevant titers in 10.84% of sera from blood donors, 16.98% of sera from patients with suspected Lyme meningoradiculitis, and 9.31% of sera from patients with a diagnosis other than borreliosis (TABLE 2). A discrepancy in the significant titers between IgG-ELISA and IFA was found to be 2.22% in blood donors, 2.36% in the first group, and 4.05% in the second group of patients.

TABLE 2. Antibody Titer Determinations against *Borrelia burgdorferi* by ELISA (IgG) According to Origin of Sera ($n = 1664$)

	ELISA (IgG)			
	1 : <100	1 : 100	1 : >100	Total
Blood donors				
Number	829	92	112	1033
% Lines	80.25%	8.91%	10.84%	
% Columns	64.16%	49.73%	59.89%	(62.08%)
Patients with suspected Lyme meningoradiculitis				
Number	144	32	36	212
% Lines	67.92%	15.09%	16.98%	
% Columns	11.15%	17.30%	19.25%	(12.74%)
Other patients				
Number	319	61	39	419
% Lines	76.13%	14.56%	9.31%	
% Columns	24.69%	32.97%	20.86%	(25.18%)
Total number	1292	185	187	1664
	(77.64%)	(11.12%)	(11.24%)	

In all three groups no specific age and sex distributions could be detected. In the blood donor groups no specific blood group or Rh type prevalance could be found.

It is interesting to note that the first group of patients with a suspected Lyme meningoradiculitis had significant titers in IgG-ELISA in 16.98%, while in the blood donor group significant titers were found in 10.84%. It could not be excluded however, that among the second group of patients and blood donors some actually did not suffer from Lyme disease. A chi-square test was carried out to compare the different groups of sera. It was found that for the above reason the test was unsuitable to evaluate the results.

In conclusion, due to the high percentage of significant titers found in the blood donor group by IgG-ELISA and IFA, it is necessary that the diagnosis of Lyme borreliosis only be made in conjunction with the clinical findings and not on the basis of a high titer alone.

REFERENCES

1. STEERE, A. C., R. L. GRODZICKI, A. N. KORNBLATT, *et al.* 1983. The spirochetal etiology of Lyme disease. N. Engl. J. Med. **308:** 733–740.
2. CRAFT, J. E., R. L. GRODZICKI & A. C. STEERE. 1984. Antibody response in Lyme disease: Evaluation of diagnostic tests. J. Infect. Dis. **149:** 289–295.

Prevalence of *Borrelia burgdorferi* Antibodies in Dogs in Northern California

Risk Factors and Zoonotic Implications[a]

JOAN TEITLER,[b] JOHN MADIGAN,[c] ELFRIEDE DeROCK,[c]
NIELS PEDERSEN,[c] TIM CARPENTER,[b]
AND CHARLES FRANTI[b]

[b]*Department of Epidemiology and Preventive Veterinary Medicine*
[c]*Department of Medicine*
School of Veterinary Medicine, University of California
Davis, California 95616

Due to their relationship as companion animals, dogs have been suggested as sentinels for zoonotic disease outbreaks to evaluate risk factors shared with humans.[1,2] Therefore, to clarify Lyme disease (LD) host, environment, and agent/vector interactions in Northern California, we estimated the prevalence of *B. burgdorferi* (Bb) antibodies in dogs and correlated these titers with risk factors shared with humans.

Dogs were tested in Mendocino and Humboldt Counties, two California counties reporting a high incidence of human LD. The Pacific Ocean dominates the weather patterns in both counties, causing cool coastal temperatures that contrast with warm inland temperatures. Of 345 dogs tested, 91 (26%) had serum antibodies at dilutions 1:64 or greater, identified by indirect immunofluorescent antibodies as described by Wilkinson.[3] Titers ranged from nonreactive to greater than 1 : 4096. Information was obtained from owners via questionnaires concerning eighteen putative risk factors including environmental indexing, host signalment and clinical signs, and insect control measures. These risks factors were evaluated for association with Bb titers in dogs using chi-square tests and logistic regression (TABLES 1 and 2). Our data indicate a negative association between canine Bb titers (7–8% seroreactive) and cool coastal temperatures (<70°F mean July temperature). Studies with *Ixodes Pacificus*, the proposed California vector, similar to those conducted on *B. duttoni* previously, may be productive in determining if a minimum temperature threshold is necessary for spirochetal development within the tick or arthropod vector.[4] The focal distribution of canine Bb titers in southern Humboldt County (48% seroreactive) provided a common link with the epidemiology of LD on the east coast. In areas of New England, forest encroachment on relinquished farmland appears to favor dissemination of LD by creating areas for proliferation of ticks, mice and deer close to human/dog homes. In southern Humboldt County homes are also constructed in areas of new growth deciduous—conifer forests previously harvested for redwoods. Exposure to Bb was also associated with moderate to warm summer climates. Additional associations were whether or not the dogs frequently were permitted to roam unconfined, if the dogs had contact with wildlife, and with the type of insect control used on the dog by the owner. FIGURE 1 depicts the association between temperature, environment, Bb antibody titers in dogs, and distribution of human cases. Future studies to determine important

[a]This work was funded by a grant from the Companion Animal Fund, School of Veterinary Medicine University of California, Davis, California 95616

TABLE 1. Categorical Variables Associated with Antibodies to *Borrelia burgdorferi* in Dogs in Southern and Northern Humboldt and Mendocino Counties, California, 1986

Variable	Chi-Square
Environmental	
Average yearly rainfall	$p = .01$
Mean July temp.	$p = .006$
County	$p = .0000$
Residential vegetation	n/a
Agent/vector	
Insect control	$p = .06$
Ticks found on dog	$p = .008$
Time of day tested	n/a
Month tested	n/a
Host	
Unidentified lameness in dog	$p = .05$
Referring complaint	$p = .04$
Animal contacts	$p = .03$
Confined	$p = .002$
Weight	n/a
Travel history	n/a
Hair length	n/a
Breed	n/a
Sex/age	n/a

n/a = Variable not associated with canine *B. burgdorferi* titer.
$p > .05$.

TABLE 2. Estimated Model For Risk Factors: Model = Insect Control + County + Interaction with Degree of Confinement

Variable	Coefficient
intercept	−2.03
no insect control	−0.29
South Humboldt	2.80
S. Humboldt × not confined	1.63
bath	−1.00
not confined	0.92
Mendocino	1.05
Mendocino × not confined	0.39

Intercept-reference category for each variable + constant (e.g., "flea collar" is reference for insect control, "yes confined" is reference for confined, N. Humboldt is reference for county, "N. Humboldt × confined" is reference for county × confined interaction.) "Bath" = bath and multiple types of insect control used on dog by owner (e.g., dusting, sprays, hand removal, etc.).

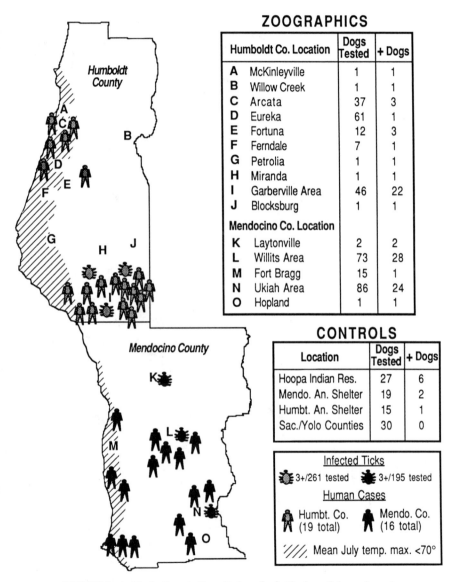

ZOOGRAPHICS

Humboldt Co. Location	Dogs Tested	+ Dogs
A McKinleyville	1	1
B Willow Creek	1	1
C Arcata	37	3
D Eureka	61	1
E Fortuna	12	3
F Ferndale	7	1
G Petrolia	1	1
H Miranda	1	1
I Garberville Area	46	22
J Blocksburg	1	1
Mendocino Co. Location		
K Laytonville	2	2
L Willits Area	73	28
M Fort Bragg	15	1
N Ukiah Area	86	24
O Hopland	1	1

CONTROLS

Location	Dogs Tested	+ Dogs
Hoopa Indian Res.	27	6
Mendo. An. Shelter	19	2
Humbt. An. Shelter	15	1
Sac./Yolo Counties	30	0

Infected Ticks
3+/261 tested   3+/195 tested
Human Cases
Humbt. Co. (19 total)   Mendo. Co. (16 total)
Mean July temp. max. <70°

FIGURE 1. Antibody titers to *Borrelia burgdorferi* in dogs, ticks, and people.

reservoirs/vectors and risk factors should be directed to high-risk regions rather than areas with naturally inhibitive climates.

When working with disease complexes such as Lyme disease, veterinarians, physicians, and other public health workers need to consider an interactive environment in assigning disease causality and designing strategies to prevent exposure of susceptible populations.

REFERENCES

1. SCHULZE, T. L., E. M. BOSLER, J. K. SHISLER, I. C. WARE, *et al.* 1986. Zbl. Bakt. Hyg. A **263:** 427–434.
2. GLICKMAN, L. & L. DOMANSKI. 1986. Alternatives to Laboratory Animals **13:** 267–285.
3. WILKINSON, H. W. 1984. Yale J. Biol. Med. **57:** 567–572.
4. FENG, L. C. & H. L. CHUNG. 1938. Chin. Med. J. Suppl. **2:** 555–562.

Lyme Disease during Pregnancy

A Cord Blood Serosurvey

CHRISTINE L. WILLIAMS,[a] JORGE L. BENACH,[b]
ANITA S. CURRAN,[c] PAUL SPIERLING,[d] AND
FRANK MEDICI[e]

[a]Department of Pediatrics
New York Medical College
Valhalla, New York 10595

[b]New York State Department of Health
Stony Brook, New York 11794

[c]Westchester County Health Department
White Plains, New York 10601

[d]Department of Obstetrics and Gynecology
Northern Westchester Hospital
Mt. Kisco, New York 10549

[e]Department of Pediatrics
Nyack Hospital
Nyack, New York 10960

Because both the spirochetal agents of relapsing fever and syphilis can be passed transplacentally, much concern has been expressed recently with respect to the potential adverse effects of Lyme disease during pregnancy. Untreated syphilis may be transmitted to the fetus during pregnancy and may result in fetal loss, stillbirth, and congenital infection. Human transplacental transmission of spirochetes of the genus *Borrelia* has also been reported to result in fetal infection and sometimes death. In addition, a *Borrelia*-like spirochete has been isolated from ticks implicated in outbreaks of epizootic bovine abortion in the western United States, a disease responsible for loss of up to 60% of calves in some herds.

In 1985, the Centers for Disease Control published a report of 19 cases of Lyme disease during pregnancy, five of which were associated with adverse fetal outcomes (prematurity, cortical blindness and developmental delay, intrauterine fetal death, syndactyly, rash). Since all of the outcomes differed, no conclusions could be drawn about the association of maternal Lyme disease with the adverse outcome.

Transplacental transmission of *B. burgdorferi* has now been reported by several investigators. In two cases of untreated first trimester maternal Lyme disease, both newborns at autopsy were found to have malformations of the heart (one baby was stillborn; one expired at 39 hours of life).

During late 1984 we proposed a serological comparison of two cohorts of babies, one born in a hospital located in a Lyme disease endemic area and the other born in a nonendemic area. This 6-month 1985 pilot study is the subject of this report. During the study period cord sera were obtained on all infants born in the participating hospitals. Consenting mothers were asked to fill out a detailed questionnaire, and neonatal status was assessed by review of hospital discharge summaries. Cord blood sera were analyzed for antibody to *B. burgdorferi* by both IFA and ELISA, and results were sent to the infant's pediatrician along with a request for a follow-up at 6 months of age (TABLE 1).

A total of 463 infants were enrolled, 282 from the endemic area and 181 from the control. Of these infants, 421 cord blood sera were obtained (91%), 255 from the endemic cohort and 166 from the control. Overall, 30 newborns (7.1%) were born with some detectable antibody to *B. burgdorferi*, 26 (10.2%) in the endemic cohort and 4 (2.4%) in the nonendemic cohort. (All of the sera with detectable antibody were negative for IgM-specific antibody). Six newborns had significant antibody levels (IFA 1 : 64 or above, or ELISA >.200). Five of these six infants were from the endemic area, and in two cases Lyme disease had been documented during pregnancy.

A total of 45 (9.7%) ICDA-codable malformations were reported, 25 (8.9%) among the 282 endemic infants and 20 (11.0%) among the 181 controls. Major

TABLE 1. Antibody to *B. burgdorferi* by Presence or Absence of Any Codable Malformation and by Hospital of Birth (Lyme Endemic vs. Nonendemic[a]

	Lyme Endemic Cohort Malformations		Nonendemic Cohort Malformations		
	Present	Absent	Present	Absent	
B. burgdorferi Antibody Present					
no.	1	25	0	4	30
row %	3.3	83.3	0	13.3	100%
col. %	4.5	10.7	0	2.7	
B. burgdorferi Antibody Absent					
no.	21	208	16	146	391
row %	5.4	53.2	4.1	37.3	100%
col. %	95.5	90.3	100	97.3	
Total					
no.	22	233	16	150	421
col. %	100%	100%	100%	100%	

[a]$n = 421$ infants with cord blood sera available.

malformations included 10 (3.5%) among the endemic infants and 8 (4.4%) for the controls. There was no association between the presence of antibody to *B. burgdorferi* and occurrence of a congenital malformation. Infants with detectable Lyme disease antibody were somewhat more likely to be of lower birthweight (150 grams less than seronegative babies) and small for gestational age compared with seronegative infants (6.9% vs. 2.8%), and to have had some degree of neonatal jaundice (43.3% vs. 24.8%), although these differences were not statistically significant. Conversely, occurrence of rash or heart murmur during the neonatal period did not differ among babies with and without detectable Lyme antibody.

In summary, no association between congenital malformations and the presence of detectable antibody to *B. burgdorferi* in cord blood could be established in the present pilot study. There was a tendency for babies with detectable antibody to be of lower birthweight, small for gestational age, and to have had some degree of neonatal jaundice, however these trends were not statistically significant. A larger study of 4000 infants is currently in progress which will examine these issues further.

REFERENCES

1. HARTER, C. A. & K. BENIRSCHKE. 1976. Fetal syphilis in the first trimester. Am. J. Obstet. Gynecol. **123:** 705–711.
2. FUCHS, P. C. & A. A. OYAMA. 1969. Neonatal relapsing fever due to transplacental transmission of *Borrelia*. J. Am. Med. Assoc. **208:** 690–692.
3. LANE, R. S., W. BURGDORFER, S. F. HAYES & A. G. BARBOUR. 1985. Isolation of a spirochete from the soft tick *Ornithodoros coriaceus,* a possible agent of epizootic bovine abortion. Science **230:** 85–87.
4. MARKOWITZ, L. E., A. C. STEERE, J. L. BENACH, J. D. SLADE & C. V. BROOME. 1986. Lyme disease during pregnancy. J. Am. Med. Assoc. **255:** 3394–3396.
5. SCHLESINGER, P. A., P. H. DURAV, B. A. BURKE, A. C. STEERE & M. T. STILLMAN. 1985. Maternal fetal transmission of the Lyme disease spirochete. Ann. Intern. Med. **103:** 67–68.
6. MACDONALD, A. 1986. Human fetal borreliosis, toxemia of pregnancy, and fetal death. Zbl. Bakt. Hyg. A **263:** 189–200.
7. WILLIAMS, C. L., A. C. CURRAN, A. C. LEE & V. O. SOUSA. 1986. Lyme disease: Epidemiological characteristics in an outbreak in Westchester County, N.Y. Am. J. Public Health **76:** 62–65.

Postviral Fatigue and Borrelial Antibodies

D. J. M. WRIGHT,[a] D. F. MULHEMANN,[a]

D. G. WILLIAMS[b] AND P. O. BEHAN[c]

[a]Departments of Medical Microbiology and Dermatology
Charing Cross Hospital
London W6 8RF, United Kingdom

[b]Division of Clinical Immunology
Kennedy Institute, London W6 7DW, United Kingdom

[c]Department of Neurology
University of Glasgow
Glasgow GF51 4TF, United Kingdom

INTRODUCTION

Postviral fatigue, otherwise known as myalgic encephalomyelitis (ME), has become increasingly recognized.[1-4] The anecdotal improvement of such patients on antibiotics renders viral cause unlikely and has led us to investigate a bacterial cause for ME. Malaise and fatigue are often a persistent symptom in Lyme disease. In our series of 201 patients with Lyme disease, the diagnosis was based on positive serological tests.[5,6] Twelve had severe malaise and fatigue and in two persistence of these phenomena for over 8 months was the sole finding. Sera from patients with ME were therefore examined for borrelia antibodies.

PATIENTS

Sixty patients were studied in whom the diagnosis of myalgic encephalomyelitis had been made according to the criteria adopted by Behan.[7] The disease had persisted in these patients for at least 2 years. The fatigue had been so severe that they were unable to continue employment. Their immunological and biochemical tests were normal. However, muscle biopsies from these patients had shown areas of focal muscle necrosis and a conspicuously increased jitter on their electromyograms. All patients had originated from different parts of the United Kingdom. There was no consistent history of tick bite or contact with deer or other wildlife.

METHODS

All sera were screened by indirect immunofluorescence for IgG and IgM antibodies and the positive tests confirmed by ELISA. Indirect immunofluorescence was carried out as previously described[8] using the American B31 strain as antigen. A titer of 256 was taken as being positive for serum with 2⁺ and 3⁺ fluorescence regarded as positive. The positive sera were screened with VDRL, TPHA, and autoimmune

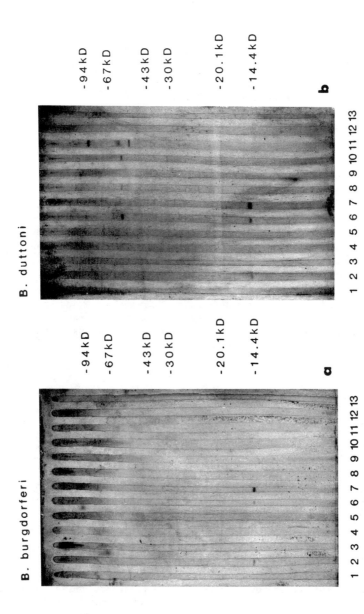

FIGURE 1. Immunoblots using (a) *B. burgdorferi* or (b) *B. duttonii* antigens. Lanes: 1–4, Sera from patients with multiple sclerosis with positive immunofluorescent *B. burgdorferi* antigen[1]; 5–10, sera from patients with ME; 11, serum from patients with multiple sclerosis but negative immunofluorescent tests using *B. burgdorferi* antigen; 12–13, casein.

serological tests. ELISA was carried out as described in the method of Magnarelli[9] with a sonicate of B31 antigen. Positive results were calculated by the following formula:

$$U/ml = \text{absorbance of } \frac{\dfrac{(\text{specimen}) - (\text{control})}{(\text{control})}}{\dfrac{(\text{standard}) - (\text{controls of standard})}{(\text{control})}} \times U/ml$$

All sera were tested in duplicate at a dilution of 1 : 160. The positive standard was arbitrarily taken as 270 units in sera, giving an immunofluorescence test positive at 1 : 256. All sera positive in the immunofluorescence and ELISA tests were then submitted for immunoblotting. The technique of immunoblotting was by electrophoretic transfer from 5–15% linear gradient polyacrylamide slab gel, stained with antihuman IgG horseradish peroxidase followed by diamino-benizidine. The antigens were derived by sonication of *Borrelia burgdorferi* B31 and *Borrelia duttonii* (Wellcome mouse) strains.

RESULTS

The sixty sera tested from patients with ME gave six positives. Three titers in the immunofluorescent test were 256, two 512 and one 2048. All had ELISA units greater than 580. In two of the sera, in which the immunofluorescence titer with anti-IgG conjugate was 256, the titer of IgM antibodies was 16, in the remaining four the IgM titer was less than 8. The patients with a positive test were indistinguishable on clinical or laboratory findings from those with negative tests. The immunoblots showed that in ME a common antibody bound to polypeptide (15 kDa) in the *B. duttonii* and *B. burgdorferi* tracks. However, with *B. duttonii* as antigen, antibody-bound polypeptides (55 kDa and 94 kda) were found (see FIGURE 1). Using sera from Lyme disease antibodies to polypeptides 15 kDa, 40 kDa, and 49 kDa were found using the *B. burgdorferi* derived antigen (tracks not shown). It therefore appears that antibodies to the 15 kDa polypeptides occur in both Lyme and ME, but antibodies to the 55-kDa and 94-kDa polypeptides were absent in Lyme disease.

CONCLUSIONS

Lack of specificity of the immunofluorescent and ELISA tests for Lyme disease is demonstrated. Only 6 of 60 ME sera gave positive tests in the above immunofluorescent and ELISA tests. None of the ME sera with positive immunofluorescent tests with IgG conjugate showed appreciable quantities of IgM antibodies, despite the suggestion that IgM is nonspecifically raised in ME. Immunoblots show that antibodies to the 15-kDa polypeptide occur in conditions other than Lyme. New antibodies were detected in a selected group of ME patients. Sera from patients with multiple sclerosis and positive Lyme serology used as a control failed to demonstrate these antibodies (see FIGURE 1). This new approach may lead to a diagnostic test for a proportion of patients with ME.

REFERENCES

1. BEHAN, P. O., W. M. H. BEHAN & E. J. BELL. 1985. J. Infect. **10:** 211–222.
2. WOOKEY, C. 1986. Post-viral fatigue syndrome and how to cope with it. *In* Myalgic Encephalomyelitis. Groom Helm. Beckenham, Kent. pp. 36–48.
3. THOMAS, P. K. 1987. Lancet **i:** 218–219.
4. MATTHEWS, W. B. 1986. Oxford Textbook of Medicine I. D. S. Wetherill, J. G. G. Ledingham & D. A. Warrell, Eds. Oxford University Press. Oxford.
5. STEINSTEDT, G. T. *et al.* 1986. Zbl. Bakt. Hyg. A **263:** 289–296.
6. STEERE, A. C. *et al.* 1986. Zbl. Bakt. Hyg. A **263:** 201–205.
7. BEHAN, P. O. J. R. Soc. Med. In press.
8. MUHLEMANN, M. F. & D. J. M. WRIGHT. 1987. Lancet **i:** 260–262.
9. MAGNARELLI, L. A., J. M. MEEGAN, J. F. ANDERSON & W. A. CHAPPELL. 1984. J. Clin. Microbiol. **20:** 181–184.
10. WILLIAMS, D. G., M. R. STOCKS, P. J. CHARLES & R. N. MAINI. 1986. J. Immunol. Methods **91:** 65–73.
11. MUHLEMANN, M. F., D. J. M. WRIGHT, *et al.* Zbl. Bakt. Hyg. A. In press.

Index of Contributors

511